ENDOMETRIOSIS
Current Management
and
Future Trends

ENDOMETRIOSIS
Current Management and Future Trends

Albany College of Pharmacy and Health Sciences
Vermont Campus

Juan A García-Velasco
MD PhD
Medical Director
IVI Madrid, Spain
Associate Professor
Rey Juan Carlos University
Madrid, Spain

Botros RMB Rizk
MD MA FACOG FACS HCLD FRCOG FRCS (C)
Professor and Head
Division of Reproductive Endocrinology and Infertility
Medical and Scientific Director
USA IVF Program
University of South Alabama College of Medicine
Alabama, USA

JAYPEE BROTHERS MEDICAL PUBLISHERS (P) LTD

St Louis (USA) • Panama City (Panama) • New Delhi • Ahmedabad • Bengaluru
Chennai • Hyderabad • Kochi • Kolkata • Lucknow • Mumbai • Nagpur

Published by

Jitendar P Vij

Jaypee Brothers Medical Publishers (P) Ltd

Corporate Office

4838/24 Ansari Road, Daryaganj, **New Delhi** 110 002, India, Phone: +91-11-43574357, Fax: +91-11-43574314

Registered Office

B-3 EMCA House, 23/23B Ansari Road, Daryaganj, **New Delhi** 110 002, India
Phones: +91-11-23272143, +91-11-23272703, +91-11-23282021,
+91-11-23245672, Rel: +91-11-32558559 Fax: +91-11-23276490, +91-11-23245683
e-mail: jaypee@jaypeebrothers.com, Website: www.jaypeebrothers.com

Branches

❑ 2/B, Akruti Society, Jodhpur Gam Road Satellite
   Ahmedabad 380 015   Phones: +91-79-26926233,   Rel: +91-79-32988717
   Fax: +91-79-26927094   e-mail: ahmedabad@jaypeebrothers.com

❑ 202 Batavia Chambers, 8 Kumara Krupa Road, Kumara Park East
   Bengaluru 560 001   Phones: +91-80-22285971, +91-80-22382956
   +91-80-22372664,   Rel: +91-80-32714073
   Fax: +91-80-22281761   e-mail: bangalore@jaypeebrothers.com

❑ 282 IIIrd Floor, Khaleel Shirazi Estate, Fountain Plaza, Pantheon Road
   Chennai 600 008   Phones: +91-44-28193265, +91-44-28194897
   Rel: +91-44-32972089 Fax: +91-44-28193231   e-mail: chennai@jaypeebrothers.com

❑ 4-2-1067/1-3, 1st Floor, Balaji Building, Ramkote Cross Road
   Hyderabad 500 095   Phones: +91-40-66610020
   +91-40-24758498,   Rel:+91-40-32940929
   Fax:+91-40-24758499,   e-mail: hyderabad@jaypeebrothers.com

❑ No. 41/3098, B & B1, Kuruvi Building, St. Vincent Road
   Kochi 682 018, Kerala   Phones: +91-484-4036109, +91-484-2395739
   +91-484-2395740   e-mail: kochi@jaypeebrothers.com

❑ 1-A Indian Mirror Street, Wellington Square
   Kolkata 700 013   Phones: +91-33-22651926, +91-33-22276404
   +91-33-22276415, Fax: +91-33-22656075,   e-mail: kolkata@jaypeebrothers.com

❑ Lekhraj Market III, B-2, Sector-4, Faizabad Road, Indira Nagar
   Lucknow 226 016   Phones: +91-522-3040553, +91-522-3040554
   e-mail: lucknow@jaypeebrothers.com

❑ 106 Amit Industrial Estate, 61 Dr SS Rao Road, Near MGM Hospital, Parel
   Mumbai 400012   Phones: +91-22-24124863, +91-22-24104532,
   Rel: +91-22-32926896 Fax: +91-22-24160828,   e-mail: mumbai@jaypeebrothers.com

❑ "KAMALPUSHPA" 38, Reshimbag, Opp. Mohota Science College, Umred Road
   Nagpur 440 009 (MS)   Phone: Rel: +91-712-3245220
   Fax: +91-712-2704275   e-mail: nagpur@jaypeebrothers.com

North America Office
1745, Pheasant Run Drive, Maryland Heights (Missouri), MO 63043, USA, Ph: 001-636-6279734
e-mail: jaypee@jaypeebrothers.com, anjulav@jaypeebrothers.com

Central America Office
Jaypee-Highlights Medical Publishers Inc. City of Knowledge, Bld. 237, Clayton, Panama City, Panama   Ph: 507-317-0160

Endometriosis: Current Management and Future Trends

© 2010, Jaypee Brothers Medical Publishers

This book has been published in good faith that the material provided by contributors is original. Every effort is made to ensure accuracy of material, but the publisher, printer and editors will not be held responsible for any inadvertent error(s). In case of any dispute, all legal matters to be settled under Delhi jurisdiction only.

First Edition: **2010**

ISBN   978-81-8448-808-1

Typeset at   JPBMP typesetting unit
Printed at   Ajanta Offset & Packagings Ltd., New Delhi

To

Carmela, Maria and Jaime,
my strongest supporters and
my greatest motivation
—Juan A García-Velasco

My very dear wife and life partner
Mary for her love, support
and sacrifice
—Botros RMB Rizk

Contributors

A Schally
Veterans Affairs Medical Center and
South Florida VA Foundation for
Research and Education, Miami, and
Department of Pathology and Division
of Hematology and Oncology
Department of Medicine, the Miller
School of Medicne, University of Miami
Miami, Florida, USA

Alka Prakash
University Department of
Obstetrics and Gynaecology
University of Cambridge
United Kingdom

Anabel Salazar
IVI Madrid
Rey Juan Carlos University
Madrid, Spain

Andre van As
Repros Therapeutics Inc
The Woodlands, Texas, USA

Andrea G Edlow
Department of Obstetrics and
Reproductive Biology, Brigham and
Women's Hospital; Harvard Medical
School, Boston, Massachusetts, USA

Andrew Prentice
University Department of
Obstetrics and Gynaecology
University of Cambridge
United Kingdom

Anjali Chandra
Center for Reproductive Medicine,
Glickman Urological and Kidney
Institute and Obstetrics-Gynecology
and Women's Health Institute;
Cleveland Clinic, Cleveland, USA

Anna Sokalska
Department of Obstetrics
Gynecology and Gynecological
Oncology, Karol Marcinkoswski
University of Medical Sciences
Poland

Antoni J Duleba
Department of Obstetrics and
Gynecology, University of California
Davis, Sacramento, California, USA

Antonio Pellicer
Fundación IVI
Instituto Universitario IVI
Valencia University, Valencia, Spain

Antoine Watrelot
Centre de recherché et d´Etude de la
Stérilité, Lyon, France

Ashok Agarwal
Professor of Surgery and Director
Center for Reproductive Medicine
Infertility, and Sexual Function
Glickman Urological and Kidney
Institute and Department of Obstetrics
and Gynecology, The Cleveland Clinic
Foundation, Cleveland, USA

Attila Bokor
Leuven Unoversity Center
Dept of Obstetrics and Gynecology
UZ Gastthuisberg, 3000
Leuven, Belgium

Botros RMB Rizk
Professor and Head
Division of Reproductive Endocrinology
and Infertility, Medical and Scientific
Director, USA IVF Program
University of South Alabama
College of Medicine, Alabama, USA

Bruno Borghese
Université Paris Descartes
Service de Gynécologie Obstétrique II et
Médecine de la Reproduction
Unité de Chirurgie Gynecologique CHU
Cochin-Saint Vincent de Paul Paris,
France

Carlos Simón
Fundación IVI
Instituto Universitario
IVI Valencia University
Valencia, Spain

Caroline E Gargett
Centr for Women's Health Research
Monash Institute of Medical Research
and Monash University
Department of Obstetrics and
Gynaecology, Monash Medical Center
Clayton, Victoria, Australia

Carolyn JP Jones
Maternal and Fetal Research Centre
School of Clinical and Laboratory
Science, Univeristy of Manchester
UK

Chakib M Ayoub
MBA, Associate Professor
Department of Anesthesiology
American University of Beirut
Beirut, Lebanon
Clinical Assistant Professor
Department of Anesthesiology
Yale University School of Medicine
New Haven, CT USA

Charles Chapron
Service de Gynécologie Obstétrique
II et Médecine de la Reproduction
Unité de Chirurgie Gynécologique
CHU Cochin-Saint Vincent de Paul
Paris, France

Charles Countant
Service de Gynécologie-Obstétrique
Hôpital Tenon, Assistance Publique des
Hôpitaux de Paris, Université Pierre et
Marie Curie, Paris, France

Christopher B Rizk
Rice University
Houston, Texas
USA

David Redwine
St. Charles Medical Center
Bend, Oregon
USA

David Smart
Enovapharma
London, United Kingdom

Deborah Eapen
Center for Reproductive Medicine
Glickman Urological and Kidney
Institute and Obstetrics-Gynecology
and Women's Health Institute
Cleveland Clinic, Cleveland, USA

Dominique de Ziegler
Université Paris Descartes, Service de
Gynécologie Obstétrique II et Médecine
de la Reproduction, Unité de Chirurgie
Gynecologique, CHU Cochin-Saint
Vincent de Paul, Paris, France

Donald P Brawn
Institute for the Study and
Treatment of Endometriosis
Chicago, IL, USA

Edgardo Somigliana
Fondazione Hospédale Maggiore
Policlinio, Mangiagalli e Regina Elena
Milan, Italy

Edurne Novella-Maestre
Valencia University
Valencia, Spain

Emile Daraï
Service de Gynécologie-Obstétrique,
Hôpital Tenon, Assistance Publique des
Hôpitaux de Paris, Université Pierre et
Marie Curie, Paris, France

Engel, JB
Universitätsfrauenklinik Würzburg,
Würzburg, Germany

Eric S Surrey
Colorado Center for Reproductive
Medicine Lone Tree, CO, USA

Felice Petraglia
Obstetrics and Gynecology
Department of Pediatrics
Obstetrics and Reproductive Medicine
University of Siena, Siena, Italy

Francisco Domínguez
Fundación IVI
Instituto Universitario
IVI Valencia University
Valencia, Spain

Friedrich Wieser
Department of
Gynecology and Obstetrics
Emory University School of Medicine
Atlanta, Georgia, USA

Gareth C Weston
Center for Women's Health Research
Department of Obstetrics and
Gynaecology and
Monash Institute of Medical Research
Monash University Melbourne, Australia

Gil Dubernard
Service de Gynécologie-Obstétrique,
Hôpital Tenon, Assistance Publique des
Hôpitaux de Paris, Université Pierre et
Marie Curie, Paris, France

Ioannis Vasilopulos
Université Paris Descartes Hôpital
Cochin, Reprod Endocr and Infertility,
Dept of Ob Gyn II, Paris, France

Irving M Spitz
Institute of Hormone Reseach and Ben
Gurion University of the Neveg
Jerusalem, Israel

Isabelle Streuli
Department of Obstetrics and
Gynecology, Hôpital de Morges
Switzerland

Jaques Donnez
Department of Gynecology
Université Catholique de Louvain
Cliniques Universitaires
St Luc, Brussels, Belgium

Jean-Christophe Lousse
Department of Gynecology
Université Catholique de Louvain
Brussels, Belgium

Jean Squifflet
Department of Gynecology
Université Catholique de Louvain
Brussels, Belgium

José Schneider
Department of Obstetrics and
Gynaecology, Rey Juan Carlos
University, Madrid, Spain

Juan A García-Velasco
Medical Director, IVI Madrid, Spain
Associate Professor, Rey Juan Carlos
University, Madrid, Spain

Juan Balasch
Professor and Chairman, Institute Clinic
of Gynecology, Obstetrics and
Neonatology. Hospital Clinic
Institut d´Investigacions Biomèdiques
August Pi I Sunyer (IDIBAPS), Facultad
of Medicine-University of Barcelona
Barcelona, Spain

Karamouti M
Department of Obstetrics and
Gynecology, University of Crete
Greece

Lone Hummelshoj
Endometriosis.org
London, England

Luciano G Nardo
Department of Reproductive Medicine
St Mary's Hospital, Manchester, UK
Maternal and Fetal Health Research
Centre, School of Clinical and
Laboratory Science, University of
Manchester, UK

Makrigiannakis A
Department of Obstetrics and
Gynecology, University of Crete
Greece

Marc Bazot
Service de Radiologie, Hôpital Tenon,
Assistance Publique des Hôpitaux de
Paris, Université Pierre et Marie Curie
Paris, France

Marc Princivalle
Enovapharma
London, United Kingdom

Marc R Laufer
Chief of Gynecology, Department of
Surgery, Children's Hospital; Division
of Reproductive Endocrinology
Department of Obstetrics
Gynecology and Reproductive Biology
Brigham and Women's Hospital
Harvard Medical School, Boston
Massachusetts, USA

Marcos Ballester
Service de Gynécologie-Obstétrique,
Hôpital Tenon, Assistance Publique des
Hôpitaux de Paris, Université Pierre et
Marie Curie, Paris, France

Marie-Madeleine Dolmans
Department of Gynecology
Université Catholique de Louvain
Brussels, Belgium

Marina Bellavia
Unité de medicine de la Reproduction,
CHUV, Lausanne, Switzerland

Mary Lou Ballweg
President/Executive Director
Endometriosis Association (International)
USA

Michelle Nisolle
Gynecology-Obstetrics Department
CHR de la Citadelle
University of Liège, Belgium

Mohamed Aboulghar
Professor of Obstetrics and Gynecology
Faculty of Medicine, Cairo University
Egypt

Mohamed FM Mitwally
Reproductive Endocrinology and
Infertility Specialist TCART (Toronto
Center for Advanced Reproductive and
Technology), University of Toronto
Toronto, Ontario, Canada

P Cobos
Human Reproduction Unit
Department of Obstetrics and
Gynecology, Cruces Hospital
País Vasco University
Baracaldo, Vizcaya, Spain

P Nervo
Gynecology-Obstetrics Department
CHR de la Citadelle
University of Liège, Belgium

Paola Vigano
AO Sant'Anna, Como and Center for
Research in Obstetrics and Gynecology
(CROG), Milan, Italy

Peter AW Rogers
Center for Women's Health Research
Department of Obstetrics and
Gynaecology and
Monash Institute of Medical Research
Monash University Melbourne,
Australia

Pascale Jadoul
Department of Gynecology
Université Catholique de Louvain
Brussels, Belgium

Rana Skaf
FACOG Active Staff
Greenwood OBGYN Associates
Greenwood, MS USA

Richard P Dickey
Clinical Professor and Division Head
Louisiana State University and
Medical Director, Fertility Institute of
New Orleans, New Orleans
Louisiana, USA

Roberto Matorras
Human Reproduction Unit
Department of Obstetrics and
Gynecology, Cruces Hospital
País Vasco University, Baracaldo
Vizcaya, Spain, IVI-Bilbao, Spain

Robert F Casper
Reproductive Endocrinology and
Infertility Specialist TCART (Toronto
Center for Advanced Reproductive and
Technology), University of Toronto
Toronto, Ontario, Canada

Robert N Taylor
Department of Gynecology and
Obstetrics, Emory University School of
Medicine, Atlanta, Georgia, USA

Roman Rouzier
Service de Gynécologie-Obstétrique,
Hôpital Tenon, Assistance Publique des
Hôpitaux de Paris, Université Pierre et
Marie Curie, Paris, France

Ronald D Wiehle
Repros Therapeutics Inc
The Woodlands, Texas, USA

Sajal Gupta
Center for Reproductive Medicine
Glickman Urological and Kidney
Institute and Obstetrics-Gynecology
and Women's Health Institute;
Cleveland Clinic, Cleveland, USA

Stefano Luisi
Obstetrics and Gynecology
Department of Pediatrics
Obstetrics and Reproductive Medicine
University of Siena
Siena, Italy

Shubbangi Kesavan
Center for Reproductive Medicine,
Glickman Urological and Kidney
Institute and Obstetrics-Gynecology
and Women's Health Institute;
Cleveland Clinic
Cleveland, USA

Sun-Wei Guo
Renji Hospital and Institute of
Obstetric and Gynecologic Research
Shanghai Jiao Tong University
School of Medicine
Shanghai 200001, China

Thomas M D'Hooghe
Leuven Unoversity Center
Dept Obstetrics and Gynecology
UZ Gastthuisberg, 3000
Leuven, Belgium

Tony G Zreik
MBA, Associate Professor
Assistant Dean for Clinical Affairs
Dept OB/GYN, Lebanese American
University School of Medicine
Beirut, Lebanon
Clinical Assistant Professor
Dept of Obstetrics, Gynecology and
Reproductive Sciences, Yale
University School of Medicine
New Haven, CT USA

W Paul Dmowski
Institute for the Study and
Treatment of Endometriosis
Chicago IL, USA

Preface

Writing a book in the 21st century may seem outdated, when information flows quickly through the web, papers are read prior to being published as e-papers, abstracts are easily accessed through Internet and PDF files of books or journals sent by e-mail. Blogs and web pages may also offer a tremendous amount of information to the basic scientist of the clinician. However, still a book has many advantages over the other type of information, which undoubtedly is extremely useful now and in the future. But a book binds together judicious information from world-known experts, with not only longstanding deep knowledge of the disease—each one of them on different, specific areas—but also with a capacity to critically analyze the recent developments of this very enigmatic and frustrating disease, endometriosis.

In this book, we have tried to compile the most up-to-date knowledge on endometriosis, from sociological and epidemiological point of view to future treatments, covering the theories on the pathogenesis, current and future diagnostic methods, therapeutic alternatives, and side fields such as fertility preservation, cancer possibilities, and quality of life in these patients.

All together, this book offers you, the readers, a detailed and complete explanation of the disease in 2009 and hopefully, will help you not only understand but also provide a better management of this disease to your patients.

Front cover pictures are a courtesy of Dr Novella-Maestre and Dr Martinez-Salazar.

Juan A García-Velasco
Botros RMB Rizk

Contents

Section 1
Epidemiology

Section 2
Pathogenesis of the Disease

Section 3
Diagnostic Dilemmas

Section 4
Clinical Relevance and Treatment Options

Section 5
Surgical Treatment

Section 6
Classical Medical Treatments

Section 7
New Medical Treatments

Section 8
Future Trends

Introduction

"Even if peritoneal endometriosis arises from the implantation of endometrial and tubal tissue on the surface of the peritoneum, as I believe it does, this does not prove that all instances of endometrium-like tissue involving the peritoneum arise from this source."

—John A Sampson, 1927

In almost every textbook endometriosis is characterized as *"enigmatic"*. Every woman, at every menstrual period shows some degree of retrograde menstruation. Menstrual debris reaches the peritoneal cavity every month. So, why do not all women develop endometriosis? After all, the viable regurgitated endometrial fragments constitute "self tissue" and they should not lead to activation of the peritoneal immune system. Still, that is exactly what happens. Peritoneal macrophages are activated, the menstrual fragments are digested, and the peritoneal cavity is cleaned month after month. Only if the menstrual reflux is too voluminous, or if the peritoneal defense system is too weak, does endometrium implant into the peritoneal lining and develop into endometriosis. Or, does it? In 1994, while reviewing the literature on occult endometriosis for Human Reproduction, I used the title *"Endometriosis does not exist, all women have endometriosis"* to stress that, apart from the many visible lesions, on purely theoretical grounds many more (as yet) invisible lesions can be expected to exist, waiting to develop into visible endometriosis.[1] So it depends on the definition you use and the meticulousness with which you scrutinize the peritoneal cavity whether endometriosis occurs frequently, always, or not at all.

Retrograde Menstrual Shedding of Viable Endometrial Tissue Fragments

What indeed is endometriosis? Is it always what we call a disease? Although the disease endometriosis can simply be defined as the presence of endometrial tissue, containing both glands and stroma, at locations outside the uterine cavity, emerging evidence indicates that to be pathologic, such tissue should not merely be there, it must persist and progress.[2] The simple existence of subperitoneal implants of endometrial tissue does not imply a pathologic condition as such. This suggests that attachment to, and subsequent invasion of the peritoneal lining by the refluxed endometrial tissue fragment is only phase I in the development of the disease. Phase II consists of the ensuing growth and proliferation of the seeded endometrium, interacting with the surrounding tissue of the peritoneal lining. If retrograde menstruation is a universal phenomenon in women,[3, 4] why do not all women develop endometriosis?[1] The puzzle of the sequence of events leading to the development of ectopic endometrial implants and eventually, in some women, to endometriosis, is gradually becoming unravelled. This book presents the state of the art of our knowledge of endometriosis. We have come a far way from the days of Karl Freiherr Von Rokitansky, who is often credited as the first one, in 1860, to describe the disease,[5] although Daniel Shroen, in 1690, already had mentioned typical "ulcers" on the surface of the bladder, intestines and broad ligament that gave rise to adhesions between the visceral organs.[6] The *magnum opus*, however, was written by John Sampson who presented in 1927, in his beautifully illustrated, 47 pages long paper *"Peritoneal endometriosis due to the menstrual dissemination of endometrial tissue into the peritoneal cavity"*[7] his regurgitation-implantation theory of endometriosis development, still the most widely accepted theory of the development of endometriosis today: Viable endometrial tissue fragments reflux during menstruation through the fallopian tubes into the abdominal cavity, where the first line of defence, the cellular and humoral peritoneal immune system is on the alert. A local, peritoneal inflammatory response occurs, the immune system is upregulated, and as a result individual tissue fragments are broken down into single cells to render them amenable to phagocytosis and subsequent digestion by the hyperactivated peritoneal macrophages. If occasionally one or more intact tissue fragments escape this peritoneal garbage collection and disposal system (e.g. by their sheer numbers, or by innate defects of the peritoneal defence system), apposition, attachment and invasion of the peritoneal lining – although so far never having been observed *in vivo*[8] – must follow to allow for the development of (subperitoneally located) endometriotic lesions. The fragments then may grow until a critical tissue volume of about one cubic millimetre. Up to this size, oxygen and nutrients may reach the newly established implant by diffusion. Further growth and proliferation, however, require the development of a new vascular supply tree by angiogenesis.[9, 10] Only after it will have become connected to the host vascular system will the explant be able to grow beyond one cubic millimetre and become visible to the naked (laparoscoped) eye. Hence, in order for us to better understand the difference between the *disorder* 'endometrial explant' and the *disease* 'endometriosis', this critical tissue level of one cubic millimetre is pivotal. It is the maximum volume of tissue that is able to survive on diffusion alone, and it is at the same time the minimum volume of tissue identifiable at laparoscopy. In dealing with clinical endometriosis we will therefore have to realize that apart from the few visible lesions in early endometriosis, dozens, or may be even hundreds, of still-invisible submicroscopic lesions do exist that are not yet discernible to the naked eye. In fact, surgical pathology of blind biopsies of visually normal peritoneum in endometriosis patients has shown 14% occult endometriotic lesions.[11-13] The corresponding figure for blind biopsies of normal peritoneum in non-endometriosis patients is 6%.[12, 13] By extrapolation, if in every patient these authors would have taken 16 biopsies instead of a single one, all women with normal looking peritoneum would have shown evidence of endometriosis.

Where are we now?

This is where we are in 2009. The number of publications on endometriosis has rapidly risen, from 119 per year in 1968 to 131 in 1978, 334 in 1988, 408 in 1998, and to 715 in 2008. All have contributed to our increased understanding of the disease. We now know that viable endometrium reaches the peritoneal cavity during menses. We know that it activates the peritoneal immune system and that it elicits an inflammatory response. The next thing we know is that occult, microscopic endometrial implants have been found submesothelially in visually normal peritoneum, even in women without identifiable endometriosis. The phase in between these two stages of development, however, is still a black box: sophisticated *in vitro* experiments suggest that endometrial fragments rather than single cells have the capacity to remodel the mesothelium and bypass the peritoneal lining. This is how clinical endometriosis may start. But this represents only one of the many theories of endometriosis development. Some lesions may not depend on menstrual regurgitation and implantation of shed endometrium at all. They rather may result from coelomic metaplasia, from dedifferentiation of mesothelium, or from the late outgrowth of persisting embryonic rests. (Epi)genetic background and environmental factors play a role. In this book, internationally recognized experts in the field present their views on the development of endometriosis, on its pathophysiology, etiology and symptomatology, and on the most appropriate methods of (biomarker) screening, clinical diagnosis and treatment.

Johannes LH Evers
President, World Endometriosis Society
Professor, Department of Obstetrics and Gynaecology
Center for Reproductive Medicine and Biology
GROW, School for Oncology and Developmental Biology
Maastricht University Medical Center
P.O. Box 5800
6202AZ Maastricht
The Netherlands

References

1. Evers JL. Endometriosis does not exist; all women have endometriosis. Hum Reprod 1994;9:2206-09.
2. Holt VL, Weiss NS. Recommendations for the design of epidemiologic studies of endometriosis. Epidemiology 2000;11:654-59.
3. Liu DT, Hitchcock A. Endometriosis: its association with retrograde menstruation, dysmenorrhoea and tubal pathology. Br J Obstet Gynaecol 1986;93:859-62.
4. Eskenazi B, Warner ML. Epidemiology of endometriosis. Obstet Gynecol Clin North Am 1997;24:235-58.
5. Von Rokitansky K, Über uterusdrüsenneubildung. Z Gesellsch Ärtzte (Wien)1860; 16;577.
6. Shroen DC. Disputatio inauguralis medica de ulceribus uteri. Krebs publishers, Jena 1690, pp 6-17.
7. Sampson JA. Peritoneal endometriosis due to the menstrual dissemination of endometrial tissues into the peritoneal cavity. Am J Obstet Gynecol 1927;14:422.
8. Redwine D, Is "microscopic" peritoneal endometriosis invisible? Fertil Steril 1988; 50:665.
9. McLaren J. Vascular endothelial growth factor and endometriotic angiogenesis. Hum Reprod Update 2000;**6**:45–55.
10. Maas JW, Groothuis PG, Dunselman GA, De Goeij AF, Struijker Boudier HA, Evers JL. Development of endometriosis-like lesions after transplantation of human endometrial fragments onto the chick embryo chorioallantoic membrane. Hum Reprod 2001;16:627-31.
11. Murphy AA, Guzick DS, Rock JA. Microscopic peritoneal endometriosis. Fertil Steril. 1989;51:1072-74.
12. Nisolle M, Paindaveine B, Bourdon A, Berliere M, Casanas-Roux F, Donnez J. Histologic study of peritoneal endometriosis in infertile women. Fertil Steril. 1990;53:984-88.
13. Balasch J, Creus M, Fabregues F, Carmona F, Ordi J, Martinez-Roman S, Vanrell JA. Visible and non-visible endometriosis at laparoscopy in fertile and infertile women and in patients with chronic pelvic pain: a prospective study. Hum Reprod. 1996;11:387-91.

Section 1

Epidemiology

Lone Hummelshoj

Chapter
1

Endometriosis— How Big is the Problem?

Introduction

A 'problem' is defined as "any thing, matter, person, etc., that is difficult to deal with" and "a puzzle, question, etc., set for solution".[1] Endometriosis is certainly difficult to deal with, and a solution to this particular puzzle has yet to be found, so this disease definitely qualifies as "a problem".

But, how big is the problem of endometriosis? And, is there a solution?

Endometriosis affects an estimated 10% of women in the reproductive age group, rising to 30-50% in women with infertility and/or pain.[2] This equates to approximately 100 million women across the world, *during the prime of their lives*, whose physical, mental and social well-being are impacted by the disease, potentially affecting their ability to finish an education and maintain a career, with effect on their relationships, social activities, and fertility. There is no known cure.

From a medical perspective endometriosis is defined as the presence of endometrial-like tissue outside the uterus, which induces a chronic, inflammatory reaction, predominantly in women of reproductive age, from all ethnic and social groups.[3]

From a woman's perspective, however, endometriosis is a disease of many illnesses which is surrounded by taboos, myths, delayed diagnosis, hit-and-miss treatments, and a lack of awareness, overlaid on a wide variety of symptoms that embody a stubborn, frustrating and, for some, chronic condition. These women are given a life sentence and are trapped by endometriosis **(Figure 1-1)**.

"In its worst stages, this disease affects the well-being of the female patient totally and adversely, her whole spirit is broken, and yet she lives in fear of still more symptoms such as further pain …". These are the words of Louis Brotherson MD, written in 1776,[4] and these words

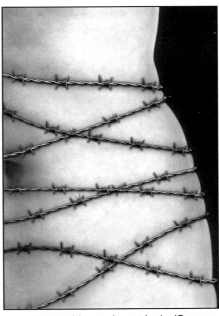

FIGURE 1-1: Trapped by endometriosis (Source: © 2008 World Endometriosis Research Foundation)

so accurately describe what many women with endometriosis face today—233 years later.

Unfortunately little has changed in the last 200 years. This is the problem!

This problem of endometriosis is further intensified when we remind ourselves that this disease is not only a significant problem for the woman, and her family, who has to deal with its impacts on a day-to-day basis.

The problem extends to the physician, who may struggle to aid this woman in getting her symptoms under control and restore her quality of life and, for some, fertility due to a lack of efficacious treatments; many of which have significant side-effects, which further compromise these women's lives.

In addition, from a societal perspective, endometriosis compounds into a much wider issue, where the cost of illness is estimated at more than US $ 22 billion a year in the USA alone. These costs are considerably higher than those related to Crohn's disease or to migraine – illnesses much better understood and socially acknowledged.[5]

Thus, the problem that is endometriosis cannot continue to be ignored – from any perspective.

Problem of Endometriosis

Endometriosis: A Disease of Many Illnesses

Endometriosis can affect women in many different ways. For some it is pain. For some it is infertility. For some it is a myriad of associated symptoms, including fatigue, fibromyalgia, irritable bowel syndrome, compromised sexuality, chronic pelvic pain, allergies, interstitial cystitis, and a low resistance to fevers. However, symptoms may not always reflect disease extent,[6,7] and establishing the diagnosis of endometriosis on the basis of symptoms alone can be difficult because the presentation is so variable and there is considerable co-morbidity.[3,7]

Consequently these factors contribute to a diagnostic delay ranging from 4-12 years in various health care settings between symptom onset, presenting with symptoms, and a definitive diagnosis, where endometriosis-related infertility is typically diagnosed sooner than endometriosis-related pain, and with a variance in whether the woman was seen within the context of a public or a private practice.[8-11]

Diagnostic Delay

The question of whether the diagnostic delay in endometriosis matters has arisen in recent years, and Ballard et al claim that it does.[11] They conducted semi-structured interviews where women recorded their experience of being diagnosed with endometriosis. Overall, very early experiences of pain were rarely disclosed to friends or family, partly due to embarrassment but also because these women did not want to appear weak or unable to cope with what they thought were normal—though very painful periods. Consequently the women lacked any comparative evidence from other women to indicate that their symptoms warranted medical intervention, and instead often withdrew from social activities, spending time in bed, and, at times, taking potentially harmful levels of analgesia.

This "normalization" of symptoms, where pain is seen to be "part of being a woman, mean that women tended to consider their experiences as normal, even when periods were recognised as problematic and disruptive to their lives. They considered themselves "unlucky" rather than ill. And, if the mother had had similar symptoms this tended to further delay these women seeking medical help.

At a medical level there will by definition always be somewhat of a diagnostic delay for the pure reason that a definitive diagnosis requires a laparoscopy – an invasive procedure. Nonetheless, Ballard showed that the delay in referral from primary to secondary care varied from 1 month to 22 years, with most women reporting multiple visits to their primary physician before referral to a specialist. Women were often "dismissed" by their primary physician, who also "normalized" their painful periods.[11]

It is clear, however, that the diagnostic delay goes both ways, and to a large extent is due to a breakdown in communication between the patient and physician. Without mutual physician-patient rapport and trust, and time to ask questions and "tease out" answers, establishing the diagnosis can be difficult because the symptoms of endometriosis may be one of those things we don't allow ourselves talk about.

Taboos

There are a lot of things that we as human beings choose not to talk about. Most often, it is because it embarrasses us. We would have to cross personal barriers to address certain issues – and endometriosis can be one of them.

Abdominal pain and/or bloating, irregular or excessive menstrual bleeding, pain during sexual intercourse, abdominal pain, nausea, diarrhea, back pain, and urinary retention are not topics that are addressed over Sunday lunch with friends and family, nor—often through embarrassment—with a physician, and thus remain unsaid and unacknowledged.

Furthermore, in terms of obtaining a diagnosis of endometriosis, these exact symptoms listed above taken together, or in combination with other physical symptoms, describe a mental disorder called "somatization disorder" according to the American Psychiatric Association.[12]

Whereas it is essential to assess the psychological status of any patient, it can be very detrimental to a woman, whose complaint of pain is valid, to be too easily dismissed as a "psychological case" because an organic cause of her symptoms have not been identified due to a persistent overall lack of awareness of the (combination of) major symptoms that indicate that she may suffer from endometriosis.

Hit and Miss Treatments

The problem of how to deal with endometriosis, however, does not stop at recognition and diagnosis. Managing the disease is a huge problem! Having obtained that—potentially elusive—diagnosis, the next challenge is finding a treatment that works. With no cure, symptomatic patients are typically treated by analgesics, hormones, surgery, assisted reproduction, complementary therapies, or a combination of these with the goal of:

1. Treating the symptoms.
2. Preventing recurrence.
3. Eliminating the endometriotic lesions.

Two and three may be interchangeable depending on definitions. Definitions, however, mean less to women with endometriosis; they want number one: they want to be symptom free!

Cure is, of course, the ultimate goal, but symptom management is more often the reality in endometriosis. Since evidence supporting the use of most medical therapies for endometriosis may not be as robust as we might wish to believe, and since the success rate of surgery is surgeon dependent,[13] treatment failures within this field are subsequently common.

Following a diagnosis, many women are therefore subjected to a roller-coaster of "hit and miss" treatments, with or without acceptable side effects, and/or repeat surgeries, with a subsequent impact on their quality of life.

Prevention and cure remains elusive. The problem of endometriosis has not yet been resolved.

Semi-solutions: Specialist Care, Communication, and Setting Expectations

In the meantime, however, we must be practical. We do not have solutions, but we must apply the knowledge we have today – combined with a bit of common sense: in addition to surgery and medical treatments, which may or may not work for a given population, effective disease management requires a multi-disciplinary treatment approach carried out within a specialized setting, where realistic expectations are well communicated and practitioners are prepared to "think outside the box".[3,7]

Women with endometriosis may also need to learn coping mechanisms and consider adopting lifestyle changes in order to create a life with a disease, which for many is long term and chronic. This is not ideal—yet may be reality for the time being, if they do not have access to specialist care.

Reminding ourselves that the problem of how to deal with endometriosis does not stop at recognition and diagnosis alone: disbelief may be an early emotion that is felt by the woman, closely followed by a fear of the unknown, just as Brotherson described in 1776.[4]

• Will the pain ever end?
• Will she ever be able to have children?
• What will happen if she does not get treatment?
• Will it get worse?
• Will the disease recur?
• Will the disease lead to a hysterectomy?
• Will endometriosis lead to cancer?
• Will she pass it to her daughter?

She may fear further tests and treatments, and experience anxiety when having to face unfamiliar medical tests or invasive procedures. This woman is entering a whole new world where she has to navigate the patient-doctor relationship, the bureaucracies of hospitals and insurance companies – whilst still having to attempt to keep her day-to-day life together on a personal and professional level and deal with the disruption this chronic illness brings in its wake. Denial, anxiety, and/or helplessness are all emotions that now need to be tackled in parallel with coping with pain and/or infertility.

Gomel, in his 2007 opinion paper, summarized this perfectly: patients arrive frustrated with themselves, their partners, and the health care system, having lost trust in physicians as a result of having consulted many without any satisfactory outcome. The initial consultation with many such patients who have become difficult to communicate with may also be frustrating for the physician. It is important therefore to assign appropriate time for the initial consultation of patients with chronic pelvic pain and to adopt an attentive and interested approach.[7]

Early, specialist care, through careful attention and communication therefore, may take women with endometriosis off the roller coaster of taboos, hit and miss treatments, and mis-communication and ensure they get early, timely, specialized care.

Thus, any practitioner must never hesitate to seek advice, where appropriate, from more experienced colleagues or refer the woman to a center with the necessary expertise to offer all available treatments in a multi-disciplinary context, including advanced laparoscopic surgery.[3,7]

This referral becomes crucial as soon as surgery is necessary since it is well accepted that the first surgery is the most important one. Thus, choosing a skilled endometriosis surgeon is extremely important. Inadequate and/or incomplete surgery, where for example the removal of endometriosis is not carried out during the same procedure as the diagnosis, will make subsequent surgery much more difficult and will ultimately impair outcome for the woman – and make the job for the next surgeon even more challenging!

Specialist Care/Centers of Excellence

"Centers of excellence" has been a much coined phrase in recent years. However, providing expertise in just one of the treatment disciplines required for the effective management of endometriosis does not constitute a "center of excellence". It takes an integrated approach involving a multi-disciplinary team that is centered on the woman and the "endometriosis specialist" (the decision making team!) to ensure the continuity of care which is so very important for those with persistent illnesses. This team may consist of:

- Gynecologists who not only understand reproductive medicine but also chronic pelvic pain;
- A surgical team led by a gynecologist specialized/accredited[13] in endometriosis surgery, including bowel surgeons and urologists;
- Pain specialists;
- Nurses;
- Physiotherapists;
- Counsellors;
- Psychologists/psychiatrists;
- Nutritionists/dieticians;
- Patient support organizations;
- Non-traditional practitioners;
- ...and probably many more (don't rule anyone out!)

All of these practitioners, with their different sets of skills, may play an important role in providing a holistic solution to an individual woman's needs. Assessment of therapeutic effectiveness may not exclusively rely on clinical data, but should incorporate patient based outcome measures and a willingness to explore combination therapies. If all these cogs in this treatment and management wheel are well-linked, the likelihood of positive long-term results become greater.[14]

Communicating and Setting Realistic Expectations

Treating a multi-dimensional disease such as endometriosis is a challenge for any physician and the cornerstone of any practice, multi-disciplinary or not, is to communicate information and set realistic expectations. "Let's see what happens" is potentially the most damaging phrase to patient confidence,[15] whereas through listening to the patient, communicating in a positive language, and involving the woman in decisions about her treatment, her fears may be alleviated, expectations may be more realistic, and outcomes may consequently improve.[3, 7]

Information is the cornerstone for any patient to understand what is happening in her body and to enable her to make informed decisions about her health care. Only the woman herself can decide how she values the benefits and risks associated with any given treatment, at any given time, and therefore it is crucial that she partakes in the decision making process not only in terms of investigations but also in the choice of the treatment of available options.[3,7] A well-informed patient is much more able to deal with any potential side-effects that may occur. As mentioned above, the resentment and frustration, which many with chronic diseases develop over time, more often than not, result in a disconnect between clinical management and the patient's expectations— expectations, which may have left the woman unprepared for the possibility of recurrence after treatment. It is important to not lose sight of this.

For example, if a patient has been promised a 100% "cure", and yet she finds herself only 80% symptom free following treatment, the outcome in the patient's view was not successful. However, if it has been communicated to her, that any given treatment may only give her 75% or even 50% relief, and indeed it does, then expectations have been met, even if that treatment has not provided a long-term curable effect. Therefore, setting realistic expectations is vital, although this can be difficult when dealing with someone who just wants pain relief – or a child – and wants it now!

It is only fair to the woman to let her know what her chances are.

Semi-solutions: Coping and Living with a Chronic Disease, and Tackling its Taboos

Having a diagnosis, and thus a name for her symptoms, provides a woman with a language in which to discuss her condition, and also sanctions access to social support and legitimizes absences from social and work obligations.[11]

Nonetheless, several hundred years after endometriosis was first described in the literature[16] we are no further in terms of satisfactory treatments. For women with endometriosis it thus becomes paramount to come to terms with living with a potentially chronic disease: to face the life sentence of pain and/or infertility they may have been given. But, this in itself brings limitations that are a challenge for anyone to cope with. As one woman with endometriosis expressed: "When you are healthy you have many dreams – when you are ill you have just one…".

In terms of coping a woman may be asked to indicate on a VAS scale of 1-10 how she *feels* (i.e. how severe is the pain?), but when it comes to coping, it may be more important to consider how she *functions*. Questions that may need to be asked include:
- Am I better on this particular/current treatment or not? If not, what needs to change?
- Do I need to make lifestyle changes in order to cope? If so, which ones?
- What is my total pain burden overall? How does that affect my ability to function?
- If my ability to function is affected, do I need to adjust work and social engagements? How do I do so?

Her answers to these questions may assist her in "tailoring" her own response to her disease and to determine, which adjustments she needs to make in order to exist with endometriosis as part of her life. Because she is not given a choice as to whether she wants to have endometriosis or not, this is not necessarily an easy task to accept or to carry out. But for women with endometriosis it is necessary to accept this process and to ultimately find a solution, which enables her to accept that endometriosis may have limited some of her choices in life, and that her life has to be led with these limitations.

It does, however, bring us back to the topic of taboos. Because living a life of limitations exposes us to society and its perceptions of what is "normal" and what is not – and, what we choose/dare to talk about.

Recognizing What We Don't Talk About

The two illnesses primarily associated with endometriosis are pain and/or infertility. But for many they are exactly the topics we are not comfortable talking about with our friends, colleagues, or even family.

Pain

Pain is a major public health issue throughout the world. In fact, the relief of pain and suffering has been the challenge of medicine from time immemorial; and despite the tremendous progress over the centuries, it remains a challenge.[7]

"Pain is a more terrible lord of mankind than even death itself" said Schweitzer.[17] Many women with endometriosis will agree with this. Unfortunately pain is not well understood or accepted in society unless it is in connection with a physically visible injury: we feel sympathetic towards a person who has broken her arm; we will enquire about the healing process, when the cast comes off, and how the physiotherapy is progressing. After some six to eight weeks, the woman can report that her arm is back to normal, and everyone heaves a sigh of relief. A person gets sick, she gets treatment, and she gets better.

Except this is not always the case with endometriosis. Furthermore, because most people are not aware of chronic pain, persistent disease processes, or "invisible" illnesses, women with endometriosis will to a large extent have to "cope" with their pain alone.

With their pain alone— and deal with her challenges on her own because endometriosis is hard for others to understand.

Explaining the disease, with its difficult-to-pronounce name takes a degree of candor about her body, which not every woman possesses. It requires at least some discussion of female anatomy and menstrual cycles, which can be uncomfortable topics for both the 'explainer' and the 'listener'.

Infertility

For endometriosis-related infertility it is similar: children are not necessarily a given. Failure to deliver that much desired child – or grandchild – can bring about a complete loss of respect from the family, resulting in feelings of personal failure and disgrace. Even in today's multi-cultural societies it can be difficult to be constantly mindful of the culturally personal aspects involved when fertility becomes an issue.

Like pain, infertility is not a topic easily discussed at social gatherings, and thus can become a personal and private grief – a grief that is intangible because the couple's sense of loss is invisible. There is no funeral, no body, no flowers, and no messages of comfort; the pain and losses are invisible and subsequently difficult for others to understand. The couple may chose to not talk about their feelings to family and friends, and start avoiding situations that remind them of their infertility, including socializing with couples who have children.[18]

This combination of grief and the eternal hope of "maybe next month" should be borne in mind and acknowledged by those dealing with couples with endometriosis-related sub-fertility – even if such issues are not yet discussed socially and to a large extent remain a taboo in today's society.

Endometriosis—The Way Forward

This is where we are in 2009:
- Millions of women are coping with endometriosis as it ravages their lives.
- Society does not acknowledge or deal with a common benign female disease despite its impact on society itself.
- Endometriosis remains a challenge for those who live with it.
- Endometriosis remains a challenge for those who seek to treat it.

When a disease affects an estimated 100 million women during the prime of their lives, the goal must be a future in which no woman's life is at risk of being compromised by endometriosis. Indeed a future in which these women's daughters should not fear what 10% of this generations' women have had to endure.

To achieve this we need to agree to a vision of a future in which millions of women are not prevented from fulfilling their dreams of completing their education, maintaining a career and having children because of a disease which could be prevented if only adequate funding for research was available.

To achieve this, four steps must be accomplished:
- There is increased awareness of endometriosis, its symptoms, effects and treatment options.
- All health professionals understand what endometriosis is, its symptoms, effects and treatment options.
- All women have ready access to timely diagnosis, appropriate treatment, care and support.
- Endometriosis becomes a high priority, with appropriate funding for research.

This cannot happen without all stakeholders collaborating: i.e. women with endometriosis, clinicians, scientists/researchers, governments, and industry must come together.

Conclusion

The problem of endometriosis is substantial and very real: we are dealing with a multi-dimensional disease, which affects an estimated 100 million of women across the globe. For some of these women endometriosis becomes a life sentence of living in pain or with infertility. Their lives, and those of their families, are severely compromised. That's a big problem.

The problem that needs solving is that collectively we need to find a way of taking care of women with endometriosis to safeguard our future. In other words:

without significant investment into causal research it becomes impossible to safeguard that future. Developing treatments that actually work will for women with endometriosis mean preservation of their fertility, improved quality of life, and reduced socio-economic costs – and a life without pain.

Today, effective disease management requires a multi-disciplinary treatment approach carried out within a specialized setting, where realistic expectations are well communicated. For now, women with endometriosis may also have to learn coping skills and consider lifestyle changes in order to create a life with a disease, which for many is long term and chronic.

However, it is said that to every problem there is a solution. For endometriosis this solution remains elusive; but, through global collaboration, prioritisation and coordination of research, and an open and inquisitive mind, we may just get there!

In conclusion: to solve the problem of endometriosis we need to apply and coordinate all of our faculties. The Danish philosopher, Piet Hein, summarized this perfectly:
"Our so-called limitations, I believe,
apply to faculties we don't apply.
We don't discover what we can't achieve
until we make an effort not to try"[19]

I encourage everyone to:
- Not limit themselves.
- Apply all of their faculties.
- Discover what they might just achieve.
- Make an effort to try—please!

With such commitment we can challenge the problem that is endometriosis and find a solution to improve the lives of those affected by the disease. With such commitment we can release these women – and future generations of women – from a life sentence of pain.

Until this happens, however, endometriosis will remain an unnecessary problem for too many millions of women worldwide.

References

1. The Collins concise dictionary of the English language, 2nd edition. Glasgow, Williams Collins Sons & Co, 1988.
2. Rogers PA, D'Hooghe TM, Fazleabas A, Gargett C, Giudice L, Montgomery GW, et al. Priorities for endometriosis research: recommendations from an international consensus workshop. Reprod Sci 2009;16:335-46.
3. Kennedy S, Bergqvist A, Chapron C, D'Hooghe T, Dunselman G, Greb R, et al. ESHRE Special Interest Group for Endometriosis and Endometrium Guideline Development Group. ESHRE guideline on the diagnosis

and treatment of endometriosis. Human Reprod 2005; 20(10):2698-2704.

4. Brotherson L. Dissertio medica inauguralis de utere inflammatione ejusdem. Edinburgh, Balfour and Smellie, 1776:16-22.

5. Simoens S, Hummelshoj L, D'Hooghe T. Endometriosis: cost estimates and methodological perspective. Hum Reprod Update 2007;13:395-404.

6. Vercellini P, Fedele L, Aimi G, Pietropaolo G, Consooni D, Crosignani PG. Association between endometriosis stage, lesion type, patient characteristics and severity of pelvic pain symptoms: a multivariate analysis of over 1000 patients. Human Reprod 2007;22(1):266-71.

7. Gomel V. Chronic pelvic pain: a challenge. JMIG 2007; 14:521-26.

8. Dmowski WP, Lesniewicz R, Rana N, Pepping P, Noursalehi M. Changing trends in the diagnosis of endometriosis: a comparative study of women with pelvic endometriosis presenting with chronic pelvic pain or infertility. Fertil Steril 1997;67(2):238-43.

9. Husby GK, Haugen RS and Moen MH. Diagnostic delay in women with pain and endometriosis. Acta Obstet Gynecol Scand 2003;82:649-53.

10. Arruda MS, Petta CA, Abrao MS and Benetti-Pinto CL. Time elapsed from onset of symptoms to diagnosis of endometriosis in a cohort study of Brazilian women. Hum Reprod 2003;18:4-9.

11. Ballard K, Lowton K, Wright J. What's the delay? A qualitative study of women's experiences of reaching a diagnosis of endometriosis. Fertil Steril 2006;86(5):1296-301.

12. American Psychiatric Association: Diagnosis and Statistical Manual of Mental Disorders. Washington DC, American Psychiatric Press, 1994:446-50.

13. Koninckx PR. Videoregistration of surgery should be used as a quality control. JMIG 2008; 15(2):248-53.

14. D'Hooghe T, Hummelshoj L. Multi-disciplinary centers/ networks of excellence for endometriosis management and research: a proposal. Human Reprod 2006;21(11): 2743-48.

15. Ogden J, Fuks K, Gardner M, Johnson S, McLean M, Martin P, Shah R. Doctors expressions of uncertainty and patient confidence. Patient Educ Couns 2002;48(2):171-6.

16. Knapp V. How old is endometriosis? Late 17th and 18th century description of the disease. Fertil Steril 1999;72(1):10-14.

17. Schweitzer A. On the edge of the primeval forest. New York, MacMillan, 1931.

18. Hummelshoj L, Bush D. Emotional aspects of endometriosis-related infertility. In: Allahbadia G, Merchant R, De Wilde RL, Verhoeven HC, eds. Gynecological Endoscopy and Infertility. India, Jaypee Brothers, 2005:400-03.

19. Piet Hein. Collected Grooks II. Copenhagen, Borgens Forlag A/S, 1973, ISBN 87-418-1090-92.

Roberto Matorras, P Cobos

Chapter 2

Epidemiology of Endometriosis

Introduction

The epidemiological approach to endometriosis is controversial since there are a number of methodological problems that preclude a correct analysis. The first problem concerns the diagnosis, namely that endometriosis can be asymptomatic and therefore its diagnosis requires performing an operative intervention (laparoscopy or laparotomy). Additionally, the diagnosis of endometriosis is not always histology based, and conversely, in a number of cases, normally appearing peritoneum reveals endometriotic lesions.

Limiting the case definition of endometriosis to women with a laparoscopic diagnosis may introduce a selection bias. For instance, it is possible that patients with greater access to medical care or with more advanced or aggressive endometriosis may be more likely to undergo investigative laparoscopy.[1] Furthermore, women with endometriosis whose symptoms are improved by first-line medical treatments may never need an invasive, albeit confirmatory, diagnosis.[1] It has been suggested that the diagnosis of endometriosis should require the presence of symptoms, but in the diagnostic work-up of an infertile couple there is much controversy as to whether the presence of minimal (or even mild) endometriosis in the absence of anatomical distortion, means that the infertility should be considered as being caused by the endometriosis or as an infertility of unknown cause.

The populations studied also differ widely: ranging from infertile women to women with pelvic pain, women undergoing tubal sterilization, women undergoing laparoscopies because of different reasons and women unexposed to spermatozoa.

A detection bias may also exist, as the thoroughness of examination differs between cases identified during an evaluation for infertility or pelvic symptoms and controls that were declared to be free of endometriosis during a tubal sterilization or other surgical procedure not initiated by symptoms.[1-3]

It is therefore no wonder that reports concerning the epidemiology of endometriosis show a wide variation in prevalence rates and report numerous discrepancies.

Endometriosis in Animal Models

Retrograde menstruation is known to occur only in women and in non-human primates, and in a few exceptional species, such as the elephant shrew and the bat.[4] The most widely studied animal model for endometriosis research is the baboon. The prevalence of spontaneous endometriosis in the baboons in captivity is close to 20%, with most of cases involving minimal disease.[5] The frequency of endometriosis has been found to increase with prolonging the time of captivity. It seems to indicate that most baboons develop some degree of endometriosis if they are maintained for long enough in captivity with regular menstrual cycles and without intervening pregnancy.[4]

Prevalence of Endometriosis

Prevalence Based on Population Data

Classically it has been claimed that about 10% of women in the reproductive age have endometriosis,[6] although such affirmation lacks of a solid background. Endometriosis is the third leading cause of gynecologic hospitalization in the United States.[7] In an interview survey, 50% of women who reported endometriosis had required bed rest for at least one day because of endometriosis at some time during the past year, with average number of days of bed rest being 17.8.[8]

A population-based study during the 1970s using medical records suggested an incidence of surgically or pathologically confirmed disease of 1.6 per 1000 white females aged 15-49.[9] Similarly, in a study based on hospital discharges, endometriosis was found as first listed diagnosis in 1.3 per 1000 discharges in women aged 16 to 44.[10] In Norway, the frequency of endometriosis was investigated by means of a questionnaire which was sent to all female inhabitants from a geographic area born between 1950 and 1952. The prevalence of endometriosis was 2.0% and the annual incidence was less than 0.3%.[11] The woman's life-time risk for endometriosis was calculated to be 2.2%.[11]

Prevalence of Endometriosis in Selected Populations

Prevalence in Women Undergoing Laparoscopy because of Infertility (Table 2-1)

In the 52 different reports we analyzed, the range for endometriosis prevalence within infertile populations ranges from 2.1% to 77.1% (**Table 2-1**). If the 22,904 cases are analyzed together, 26.13% prevalence would result. A single prevalence estimate for the entire fertile or infertile group may be too simplistic at best.[12]

Many of these differences are likely to be due to the different access to laparoscopy (indications, previous work-up, general availability of infertility treatments). The prevalence rates have been shown to increase with the year of publication and to decrease with sample size.[12]

Prevalence in Women Undergoing Laparoscopy because of Pelvic Pain (Table 2-2)

Among women admitted to a hospital because of pelvic pain, endometriosis prevalence ranges from 2.15 to 83.6%. If the 6815 cases from these 33 reports are analyzed together, 17.74% (1209 /6815) prevalence would result.

In a recent analysis it has been shown that the frequency of reporting endometriosis in women with pelvic pain was not influenced by the year of publication.[13]

Prevalence in Women Undergoing Laparoscopy because of Tubal Sterilization (Table 2-3)

Among women who seek tubal sterilization, the reported prevalence of endometriosis ranges from 1.4% to 50%. If the 9,811 cases from the 16 reports were analyzed together, 5.68% (558/9,811) prevalence would result, with extreme values ranging from 1.4% to 50%.

Table 2-1: Prevalence of endometriosis in infertile women (adapted from Eskenazi and Warner, 1997 and Guo and Wang, 2006)

Estimated prevalence of endometriosis in infertile women undergoing laparoscopy: review of the literature

First author	Year	Population	%
Fear	1968	27	3.7
Peterson	1970	204	33.3
Duignan	1972	675	7.7
Pent	1972	22	4.5
Liston	1972	197	5.6
Blunt	1972	41	21.95
Kleppinger	1974	27	25.9
Cohen	1976	1,380	23.2
Goldenberg	1976	112	25.9
Hasson	1976	66	22.7
Drake	1980	38	48
Strathy	1982	100	21
Cameron	1982	300	20
Musich	1982	182	34.6
Strathy	1982	100	21
Nordenskjold	1983	433	16
Stillman	1984	377	38.7
Moeloek	1984	199	49.7
Berger	1986	50	40
Cramer	1986	576	38.7
Cramer	1986	233	16.3
Cramer	1986	370	10
Cramer	1986	211	19.9
Cramer	1986	212	26.9
Cramer	1986	278	14
Sarram	1986	200	15.5
Chang	1987	2,053	2.1
Federici	1988	2,055	7.9
Dunphy	1989	731	22.3
Filer	1989	498	20.3
Singh	1989	91	16.5
Mahmood	1989	490	20.6
Cornillie	1990	105	77.1
Koninckx	1991	416	68
Rawson	1991	5	60
Mahmood	1991	654	21
Fedele	1992	545	38.5
Arumugam	1992	202	51
Waller	1993	174	20.7
Forman	1993	104	38.5
Beral	1994	1,750	11.08
Grupo Italiano	1994	660	29.5
El-Yahia	1994	130	27.7
Ajossa	1994	59	30.5
Matorras	1995	602	28.9
Woodworth	1995	165	39.4
Balasch	1996	52	50
Corson	2000	100	43
Matorras	2001	750	34.5
Hemmings	2004	2,777	55
Calhaz-Jorge	2004	1079	47.08
Nakawama	2007	47	44.68

Total prevalence: 26.13 % (5985/22,904)

Table 2-2: Prevalence of endometriosis in pelvic pain (adapted from Eskenazi and Warner, 1997 and Guo and Wang, 2006)

Estimated prevalence of endometriosis in patients undergoing laparoscopy due to pelvic pain: review of the literature

First author	Year	Population	%
Fear	1968	23	21.73
Blunt	1972	41	21.95
Liston	1972	134	4.47
Duignan	1972	180	7.22
Pent	1972	38	18.42
Lundberg	1973	91	14.28
Frangenheim	1974	302	27.48
Talbot	1974	85	21.17
Kleppinger	1974	28	7.14
Hasson	1976	120	12
Renaer	1981	108	20.37
Kresch	1984	100	32
Rosenthal	1984	60	16.66
Levitan	1985	186	2.15
Rapkin	1986	100	7.20
Bahary	1987	130	5.38
Vercellini	1989	126	32.53
Cornillie	1990	60	81.66
Longstreth	1990	76	19.73
Mahmood	1991	156	15
Rawson	1991	14	42.85
Peters	1991	49	8.16
Konincks	1991	170	70.58
Ajossa	1994	40	45
Grupo Italiano	1994	409	45.23
Taskin	1996	96	83.6
Balasch	1996	18	44.44
Ling	1999	95	82.10
Hemmings	2004	358	46
Rawson	1991	8	50
Sangi	1995	3,384	3.7
Balasch	1996	30	43.3

Total prevalence: 17.74% (1209/6815)

Endometriosis and Autoimmune Diseases

It has been reported that the frequency of autoimmune diseases among members of the Endometriosis Association who responded to a mailed questionnaire was much higher than expected according to Census data.[14] When medical records of patients with endometriosis were revised, however, similar frequencies of systemic lupus erythematous (SLE) and of Sjögren syndrome were found compared with women without endometriosis. Similarly, when the medical records of patients with SLE and Sjögren syndrome were revised, a similar frequency of endometriosis was found compared to in women without these autoimmune diseases.[15] These differences are probably due to a selection bias (patients with recurrent endometriosis are prone to be members of patients' association and to respond to the interview, especially if suffering from a severe concomitant disease).

Table 2-3: Prevalence of endometriosis in women undergoing sterilization (adapted from Eskenazi and Warner, 1997 and Guo and Wang, 2006)

Estimated prevalence of endometriosis in women undergoing sterilization: review of the literature

First author	Year	Population	%
Hasson	1976	296	1.4
Drake	1980	43	4.7
Strathy	1982	200	2
Kirshon	1989	566	7.4
Drake	1980	43	5
Kresch	1984	50	16
Liu	1986	75	43
Moen	1987	108	18
Wheeler	1989	3,060	1.6
Trimbos	1990	200	2.5
Moen	1991	107	22.4
Mahmood	1991	598	6
Rawson	1991	8	50
Sangi	1995	3,384	3.7
Balasch	1996	30	43.3
Hemmings	2004	1043	18

Total prevalence: 5.68% (558/9,811)

Endometriosis after the Menopause

Although endometriosis is diagnosed almost exclusively during the reproductive life, cases before menarche or after menopause are not exceptional.[16, 17] Thus, in a survey of 601 pathologically confirmed endometriosis cases, 9% were found to be in women older than 50 (2,9% in women older than 55).[17]

Prevalence in Unselected Populations (Table 2-4)

From a practical point of view it is important to elucidate the relationship between endometriosis findings and women's symptoms. It is well known that a number of women with endometriosis have no symptoms and, conversely, no pathological abnormalities at all are found in a number of cases of infertility or pelvic pain. Although

Table 2-4: Prevalence of endometriosis at different stages in women unexposed to spermatozoa and infertile women with normal partner's sperm (From Matorras et al, 2001)

	Women unexposed to spermatozoa (n =150) (%)	Infertile women with normal partner's sperm (n = 750) (%)
Stage I	26	19.3
Stage II	3.3	5.7
Stage III	1.3	3.1
Stage IV	1.3	8.4
Endometriosis (total)	32	34

it is tempting to establish a causal relationship between the symptoms and endometriosis findings, this is not necessarily true, especially in minimal-mild endometriosis. It would therefore be of interest to determine the prevalence of endometriosis in asymptomatic women, but subjected to the same diagnostic protocol as "symptomatic" women. Such a study had not been conducted until recently, mainly because of the ethical constraints (performing a laparoscopy on a "healthy" woman) and operational limitations. It is widely felt that the knowledge about the epidemiology of endometriosis is hampered by the impossibility of diagnosing this disease in the general population.

We have reported a very high prevalence of endometriosis in a population mimicking the normal population without children.[18] We studied 150 women who were unable to conceive because they had not been previously exposed to spermatozoa (the majority because of having an azoospermic partner), who underwent artificial insemination with sperm donor (AID). The control group consisted of 750 women from infertile couples in which the male had a normal sperm. All of them were subjected to diagnostic laparoscopy as a part of our systematic work-up at that time for the systematic study of the infertile couple as well as before undergoing artificial insemination donor (AID). The prevalence of endometriosis was similar (32% and 34.5%) in women not exposed to spermatozoa and in the controls. Rates of stage I were also similar in both

groups (26% and 19.3%). However there was a significant trend toward higher stages of endometriosis in infertile women (stage II 3.3% vs 5.7%; stage III 1.3% vs 3.1% and stage IV 1.3% vs 6.4%). Thus, stage I endometriosis was not more common in infertile women than in unselected women, whereas stages II-IV were more frequent in infertile women. We concluded that whereas a relationship between stage I endometriosis and infertility seemed unlikely, the relationship between stages II to IV and infertility seemed possible.

Other prevalences reported in different population settings are shown in **Table 2-5.**

Is Endometriosis always a Disease?

Some authors make a distinction between two different entities: endometriosis-disease and the physiologic endometriosis or "non-disease endometriosis".[19] The "non-disease endometriosis" would appear in the majority of women at some stage during their reproductive life.

It has been suggested that the definition of endometriosis should include not only the histological criteria (functional endometrial glands outside the uterine cavity) but also the presence of symptoms. Thus, only women with histologically confirmed endometriosis and symptoms should be considered as having endometriosis. This approach also raises important methodological problems however,

Table 2-5: Prevalence of endometriosis in population settings				
Estimated prevalence of endometriosis in populational settings: Review of the literature				
First author	*Year*	*Population number*	*Setting*	*%*
Houston	1987	31,703	White females of reproductive age (15-49 years) in Rochester, Minnesota, during 1970-1979	1.22
Mahmood	1991	134	Pre-menopausal women, undergoing abdominal hysterectomy for dysfunctional uterine bleeding in UK	25
Vessey	1993	17,032	Women attending family planning clinics, with follow up for up to 23 years, in England and Scotland	1.83
Moen	1997	4,034	Norwegian women aged 40 to 42. Cross-sectional study, in connection with a cardiovascular screening program	2
Matorras	2001	150	Spanish women unable to conceive because they had not been exposed to spermatozoa, undergoing artificial insemination donor	32.0
Hemmings	2004	2,777	Ten clinical institutions in the Montreal area. Women who underwent surgery between January 1998 and July 2002	32.04
Missmer	2004	116.678	USA women, Nurses' Health Study II with 10 years of follow-up	1.47
Missmer	2006	379,422	USA women, Nurses' Health Study II with 10 years of follow-up	0.29
Mirkin	2007	4×10^6	USA women, database of insurance company, 1999-2003	0.7
Flores	2008	1,193	Puerto Rican women. Questionnaires	4

especially concerning the relationship with infertility. It is well known that endometriosis is common in infertile women, but it is difficult to ascertain whether in cases with minimal endometriosis and no additional infertility factors the infertility is caused by endometriosis or the case should be considered as an infertility of unknown cause.

Although microscopic confirmation of endometriosis is desirable, such a criterion may be dependent upon the surgeon's intention and ability to excise lesions as well as the pathologist's interpretation of the histological findings.[20] On the other hand, this diagnostic method does not consider a large number of cases were lesions are very small and difficult to be excised to give a confirmatory diagnosis of endometriosis. Finally, the generalization of histology based studies to real-world diagnosis of endometriosis is highly questionable.[20]

Some authors have suggested that endometriosis should be defined not only by the presence of ectopic endometrium but also by evidence that the lesions are active cellularly or even have affected normal physiology.[1] Examples of cellular activity or physiologic effect might include evidence that the lesions are deep (> 5 mm), manifest as ovarian endometriomas, or are associated with pelvic adhesions not attributable to other causes.[1]

Other authors have suggested that since minimal and mild endometriosis are asymptomatic in a large number of cases, epidemiological studies should be directed only to advanced endometriosis, which are usually symptomatic.

A description of the endometriosis stage is mandatory for a better understanding of epidemiological reports on endometriosis. Thus, although a high frequency of endometriosis can be reported in "normal" populations, the majority of cases correspond to stages I and II.[18] Hemmings et al have reported that in their series the disease was stages III and IV in 30.7% of patients undergoing hysterectomy, and 23% undergoing laparoscopy, but only in 3.7% of cases of tubal ligation/ reanastomosis.[20]

Risk Factors (Table 2-6)

The aforementioned considerations concerning the limitations of epidemiological studies on the prevalence of endometriosis are also valid regarding the investigation of risk factors. It is therefore no surprise that a number of discrepancies exist between the different reports in this area.

Parameters that are most consistently reported as risk factors for endometriosis are those related with menstrual

Table 2-6: Risk factors in endometriosis (Adapted from Missmer et al, 2003)	
Summary of risk factors for endometriosis	
Risk factor	*Direction and consistency of effect*
Menstrual and reproductive factors	
Earlier age of menarche	↑ ↑, consistent
Shorter menstrual cycle length	↑ ↑, consistent
Heavier menstrual volume	↑, limited study
Irregular cycle duration	—, inconsistent
Tampon use	—, inconsistent
Oral contraceptive use	—, inconsistent
Greater parity	↓ ↓, consistent
Lactation	↓, limited study
Body habitus	
Greater height	↑, inconsistent
Greater weight	↓, inconsistent
Greater body mass index	↓, consistent
Greater waist-to-hip-ratio	↓, limited study
Red hair	↑, inconsistent
White race	—, inconsistent
Afroamerican women	↓, consistent
Lifestyle and environmental factors	
Regular exercise	↓, limited study
Cigarrette smoking	↓, inconsistent
Alcohol use	↑, limited study
Caffeine intake	↑, limited study
PCB, dioxine exposure	↑, consistent in primates but inconsistent in women
Immune disorder comorbidity	
Diagnosis with an autoimmune disorder	↑, inconsistent
Arrows indicate the approximate magnitude of the relation: ↑, slight to moderate increase in risk; ↑↑, moderate to large increase in risk; ↓, slight to moderate decrease in risk; ↓↓, moderate to large decrease in risk; —, no association.	

and reproductive factors. Risk of endometriosis seems to be greater in the presence of factors associated with an increased exposure to menstruation, such as early menarche, shorter menstrual cycle length, longer duration of flow, greater menstrual volume or flow, and reduced parity.[1,3,6] It has also been reported that a reduced lifetime of lactation is an endometriosis risk factor.

A genetic predisposition to endometriosis has been supported by the high concordance of the disease among identical twins. A familial predisposition with no clear Mendelian inheritance, but rather with multifactorial polygenic traits, has been investigated in severe endometriosis. Anyway, this topic will be extensively covered in another chapter in this book.

Weak inverse associations between endometriosis and weight and body mass index have been found.[2, 21] It has been speculated that this could be related to an increased rate of anovulatory cycles, irregular menstrual cycles or abnormalities in the androgen metabolism.

Lifestyle factors, such as smoking, exercise, and consumption of alcohol and caffeine, have also been related to an altered risk of endometriosis. Smoking has been found to be inversely related with endometriosis,[3, 21] but others have found no association.[22] It has also been reported that such an inverse relationship is present only in infertile women.[16] Exercising more than four hours per week has been reported to decrease the risk of endometriosis.[2, 23] The hypothesized mechanism is the reduction in estrogen levels.

Environmental Factors

Exposure to polychlorinated biphenyl (PCB) and dioxins has been associated with endometriosis in rhesus monkeys,[24] but studies in humans are controversial. On the other hand, smoking, which seems to be associated to a reduction in the risk of endometriosis, is a source of dioxins.

Increasing Frequency of Endometriosis

It seems that there is an increasing frequency of reporting endometriosis, although it is not clear whether this corresponds to a true increase in the occurrence of endometriosis ("endometriosis epidemic") or to improved diagnosis and awareness: greater availability of laparoscopy, improvement in the laparoscopy systems and technique, diagnosis of both classical forms and atypical forms, better patient selection due to progress in ultrasonography, etc.

For some authors, however, the increase in dioxins and some of the aforementioned changes in lifestyles and reproductive patterns could be responsible for a genuine increase in the incidence of endometriosis.

In two recent meta-analysis it was reported that among infertile women and in previously fertile women there was an increased prevalence with the year of publication.[12] but not in cases of pelvic pain.[13] More precise prevalence estimates, likely to be age-dependent, await carefully designed and executed studies that will also record covariates such as age at surgery and referral patterns.[12]

References

1. Missmer S, Cramer D. The epidemiology of endometriosis. Obstet Gynecol Clin N Am 2003; 30:1-19.
2. Signorello LB, Harlow BL, Cramer DW, Speigelman D, Hill JA Epidemiologic determinants of endometriosis: a hospital-based case-control study. Ann Epidemiol 1997;7:267-74.
3. Matorras R, Rodiguez F, Pijoan JL,, Ramón O, Gutierrez de Terán G, Rodríguez-Escudero FJ. Epidemiology of endometriosis in infertile women. Fertil Steril 1995;63:34-8.
4. D'Hooghe TM, Debrock S. Endometriosis, retrograde menstruation and peritoneal inflammation in women and in baboons. Hum Reprod Update 2002; 8: 84-88.
5. D'Hooghe TM, Bambra CS, Cornillie FJ, Isahakia M, Koninckx PR. Prevalence and laparoscopic appearance of spontaneous endometriosis in the baboon. Biol Reprod 1991; 45: 411-16.
6. Eskenazi B, Warner ML. Epidemiology of endometriosis. Obstet Gynecol Clin North Am 1997; 24:235-58.
7. Velebil P, Wingo PA, Xia Z, Wilcox LS, Peterson HB. Rate of hospitalization for gynecologic disorders among reproductive- age women in the United States. Obstet Gynecol 1995; 86: 764-69.
8. Kjerulff KH, Erickson BA, Langenberg PW. Chronic gynecological conditions reported by US women: findings from the National Health Interview Survey, 1984 to 1992. Am J Public Health 1996; 86: 195-99.
9. Houston DE, Noller KL, Melton LJ 3rd, Selwyn BJ. Incidence of pelvic endometriosis in Rochester, Minnesota, 1970-1979. Am J Epidemiol 1987;125:959-69.
10. National Center for Health Statistics. Ambulatory and inpatient procedures in the United States, 1994. Vital Health Stat 1997;132:1-113.
11. Moen MH, Schei B. Epidemiology of endometriosis in a Norwegian county. Acta Obstet Gynecol Scand 1997;76: 559-62.
12. Guo SW, Wang Y. Sources in heterogeneities in estimating the prevalence of endometriosis in infertile and previously fertile women. Fertil Steril 2006; 85: 1584-95.
13. Guo SW, Wang Y. The prevalence of endometriosis in women with chronic pelvic pain. Gynecol Obstet Invest. 2006;62:121-30.
14. Sinaii N, Cleary SD, Ballweg ML, Nieman LK, Stratton P. High rates of autoimmune and endocrine disorders, fibromyalgia chronic fatigue syndrome and atopic diseases among women with endometriosis: a survey analysis. Hum Reprod 2002;17:2715-24.
15. Matorras R, Ocerin I, Unamuno M, Nieto A, Peiró E, Burgos J, Expósito A. Prevalence of endometriosis in women with systemic lupus erythematosus and Sjogren's syndrome. Lupus. 2007;16:736-40.
16. Missmer SA, Hankinson SE, Spiegelman D, Barbieri RL, Marshall LM, Hunter DJ. Incidence of laparoscopically confirmed endometriosis by demographic, antropometric, and lifestyle factors. Am J Epidemiol 2004: 160: 784-96.
17. Elorriaga MA, Rodríguez F, Matorras R, Prieto B, Pijoan JL, Rodriguez-Escudero FJ. Postmenopausal endometriosis: a not exceptional condition. Obst Ginecol Españ 2000;9: 45-48.
18. Matorras R, Rodríguez F, Pijoan JL, Etxanojauregui A, Neyro JL, Elorriaga MA et al. Women who are not exposed to spermatozoa and infertile women have similar rates of stage I endometriosis. Fertil Steril 2001;76: 923-28.

19. Koninckx PR. Is mild endometriosis a condition occurring intermittently in all women? Hum Reprod 1994;9:2202-05.

20. Hemmings R, Rivard M, Olive DL, Poliquin-Fleury J, Gagné D, Hugo P, Gosselin D. Evaluation of risk factors associated with endometriosis.Fertil Steril 2004: 81:1513-21.

21. Cramer DW, Wilson E, Stillman RJ, Berger MJ, Belisle S, Schiff I, Albrecht B, Gibson M, Stadel BV, Schoenbaum SC. The relation of endometriosis to menstrual characteristics, smoking, and exercise. J Am Med Assoc 1986; 255: 1904-08.

22. Sangi-Haghpeykar H, Poindexter AN. Epidemiology of endometriosis among parous women. Obstet Gynecol 1995;85:983-92.

23. Bérubé S, Marcoux S, Maheux R. Characteristics related to the prevalence of minimal or mild endometriosis in infertile women. Epidemiology 1998;9:504-10.

24. Rier SE, Martin DC, Bowman RE, Dmowski WP, Becker JL. Endometriosis in rhesus monkeys (Macaca mulatta) following chronic exposure to 2,3,7,8-tetrachlorodibenzo-p-dioxin. Fundam Appl Toxicol 1993; 21: 433-41.

Pathogenesis of the Disease

Paola Vigano

Chapter 3

Implantation or Metaplasia: What Type of Disease?

Introduction

For more than 70 years, various theories have been promulgated to explain the pathogenesis of endometriosis. These theories included the induction theory, the celomic metaplasia theory, the embryonic rests theory.[1] Although some of these theories have not been completely abandoned, at present, retrograde menstruation is considered the _primum movens_ responsible for the development of the disease, at least in its form of peritoneal implants.[2] Therefore, there is a general consensus concerning the genesis of peritoneal lesions that would be attributed to the survival, adhesion, proliferation, invasion and vascularization of endometrial tissue regurgitated through the fallopian tubes during menstruation, an idea referred to as "implantation theory".[3] Conversely, the pathogenesis of ovarian endometriosis and of specific forms of deep endometriosis is still controversial.[4] Thus, presently, one of the main source of debate is whether or not the different forms of the disease have a unique common etiology or, conversely, represent three separate entities with different pathogeneses.

Implantation Theory

The mechanism of histogenesis referred to as implantation theory or Sampson's theory suggests that endometriotic lesions would result from reflux of viable endometrial tissue through the fallopian tubes and implant on peritoneal surface or pelvic organs.[5] Substantial evidence exist to support this hypothesis **(Table 3-1)**: (1) viable endometrial cells have been demonstrated in the menstrual effluent and peritoneal fluid; (2) endometrium can be implanted experimentally and grown within the peritoneal cavity; (3) all women have some degree of retrograde menstruation; (4) there is an association between

Table 3-1: Evidence supporting implantation theory
• Viable cells obtained from menstrual effluent and peritoneal fluid
• Endometrial cells can grow in peritoneal cavity
• Retrograde menstruation almost universal phenomenon
• Association of endometriosis with obstruction to the menstrual flow
• Transtubal, lymphatic, hematologic or iatrogenic deposition

obstructed menstrual outflow and endometriosis.[5] Transtubal dissemination appears to be the most common route of dissemination by far, although several other routes of dissemination of transplanted endometrial cells have been observed, including lymphatic and vascular channels and iatrogenic deposition.[5] According to the strong supporters of this theory, the pathogenesis of all forms of endometriosis, and not only of peritoneal lesions, has to be based on the implantation of endometrial fragments regurgitated in peritoneal cavity with retrograde menses.

"Metaplasia Theory" and the Different Entities of the Disease

According to some authors, peritoneal endometriosis, endometriosis of the ovary and endometriosis of rectovaginal septum must be considered as three separate entities with different pathogeneses[6] **(Table 3-2)**. Three different models have been proposed to explain the pathogenesis of typical ovarian endometriosis. It is very intriguing to observe that from 1919, each of these theories has been repetitively reproposed by different investigators who supported them with different and novel arguments. This unfortunately gives an idea of both the complexity of the disease and the limited progress made in terms of finding its exact cause.[4]

Table 3-2: Evidence supporting metaplasia theory

- Peritoneal disease: metaplastic potential of pelvic mesothelium
- Ovarian endometriosis
  - invagination of the cortex
  - metaplasia of coelomic epithelium
- Rectovaginal nodules
  - metaplasia of müllerian rests into endometriotic glands
  - secondary infiltration of peritoneal endometriosis of Douglas pouch

---

The formation of typical *chocolate cysts* might be due to:

- Inversion and progressive invagination of the ovarian cortex after the accumulation of menstrual debris derived from bleeding of superficial endometriotic implants, which are located on the ovarian surface and adherent to the peritoneum;
- The secondary involvement of functional ovarian cysts by endometrial implants located on the ovarian surface;
- Metaplasia of the coelomic epithelium covering the ovary.

The first demonstration in favor of the first hypothesis was by Hughedson who, by serial sections of ovaries containing an endometrioma, reported that the first momentum in the formation of 90% of typical chocolate cysts would be represented by the implantation of regurgitated endometrial tissue on the ovarian surface and subsequent adhesion to the pelvic peritoneum.[4] Most endometriomas would form by invagination of the cortex after accumulation of menstrual debris from bleeding of these surface endometrial implants adherent to the peritoneum. Brosens et al., based on ovarioscopy and *in situ* biopsies, confirmed that active endometrial implants are located at the site of cyst inversion.[4]

Sampson's original theory related to a possible role of ovarian follicles in the pathogenesis of endometriotic cysts[4] has been later supported by Nezhat et al. who observed that some large endometriomas had histological characteristics of luteal or follicular ovarian cysts.[4] More recently, Jain and Dalton showed, by serial transvaginal tracking of ovarian follicles, that a chocolate cyst can develop from an ovarian follicle.[4] In each of the cases reported by these authors, the diagnosis was successfully confirmed laparoscopically. Biological data demonstrating the ability of follicular fluid to stimulate endometrial cell growth support this etiopathogenetic model. Bahtiyar et al. reported that follicular fluid from patients with endometriosis was able to induce an increased cell proliferation when compared to follicular fluid from women without the disease.[4] In a subsequent study, our group demonstrated that, although both peritoneal and follicular fluids were able to stimulate endometrial and

endometriotic cell growth *in vitro*, this effect was much more evident using follicular fluid that, therefore, would represent an extremely favorable environment for cellular proliferation. This follicular fluid–mediated induction of endometrial cell growth could not be merely due to steroid hormones since the control media used in this study did actually contain a concentration of hormones similar to that present in the follicular fluids tested.[7]

On the other hand, several are the arguments in favor of the hypothesis that the mesothelium covering the ovary can invaginate into the ovarian cortex forming mesothelial inclusions and that the celomic metaplasia of these invaginated epithelial inclusions could be responsible for formation of endometriomas.[6] This hypothesis is based on the metaplastic potential of pelvic mesothelium and the arguments in favor are:

- Presence of epithelial invaginations in continuum with ectopic endometrial tissue;
- Endometriomas have been described in patients with Rokitansky-Kuster-Hauser syndrome, who do not have a uterus and, therefore, do not have retrograde menstruation;
- 12% of endometriomas are not fixed to the broad ligament and Hughesdon's theory cannot explain the formation of the endometriomas in these cases;
- It is not unusual to find multilocular endometriomas that could not be explained by the theory of adhesions and by the bleeding of active superficial implants adherent to the peritoneum;
- Primordial follicles are found surrounding the endometriotic cyst. When the mesothelium invaginates deep into the ovary, the follicles located at the invagination site are pushed concomitantly with the mesothelium.

It should, lastly, be considered the potential existence of different types of endometriomas with different histogenesis instead of a single entity.[6]

Two are the ethiopathogenetic hypotheses for the *deep forms of the disease:*

- An adenomyotic nodule originating from modifications of müllerian rests into endometriotic glands by a process of metaplasia;
- The natural evolution of peritoneal endometriosis of Douglas pouch as consequence of its secondary infiltration.

The major arguments in favor of the rectovaginal septal origin of the deep nodule by metaplasia are the histological characteristics of the lesions and the absence of evolution of the rectal lesion after the removing of the nodule. Indeed, histologically, endometriosis of rectovaginal septum has the features of an adenomyotic nodule since, like an adenomyoma, it consists essentially of a circumscribed nodular aggregate of smooth muscle, glandular epithelium and scanty stroma.[6] The fact that the stroma component in the rectovaginal septum endometriotic nodule is very poor would indicate that the nodule is different from peritoneal endometriosis, in which epithelial glands are surrounded systematically by endometrial-type stroma. Moreover, the absence of evolution of the rectal lesion after removal of the endometriotic glands would suggest that the lesion is not evolutive; indeed, the apparent invasiveness of the lesions would be essentially determined by a secondary proliferation of smooth cells induced by endometriotic cells rather than by the invasion from ectopic endometrial cells.

Contrasting the metaplasia theory, patients with endometriosis of rectovaginal septum have about a one-third reduction in depth of the Douglas pouch, an observation that should not be expected if the origin of the lesions would be located extraperitoneally.[6] Indeed, the rectovaginal septal origin of the deep nodule would imply a similar anatomic structure of the pouch of Douglas in women with and without deep endometriosis. Alternatively, if deep foci are a manifestation of an intraperitoneal disease, the pouch of Douglas should be partly or completely obliterated, which is actually the case. Adhesions consequent to the inflammation triggered by intraperitoneal endometriotic lesions would create a bottom in the pouch of Douglas that may give the false impression that nodules are subperitoneal.

Animal Studies

In general, animal models have added credence to the implantation model of endometriosis. Spontaneous endometriosis has been reported in the rhesus macaque (*Macaca mulatta*), the Japanese macaque (*Macaca fuscata*), the pig-tailed macaque (*Macaca nemestrima*), and the Kenya baboon (*Papio doguera*), leading researchers to evaluate the use of the non-human primate as a model to investigate endometriosis.[8-11] It was proposed that iatrogenically induced retrograde menstruation would result in the development of endometriosis, supporting the hypothesis of Sampson. Indeed, TeLinde and Scott conducted an experiment in monkeys by diverting menstrual flow to permit intraperitoneal menstruation. Five of 10 monkeys developed extensive pelvic adhesions and microscopic evidence of endometriosis.[12] Similarly, D'Hooghe *et al.*, demonstrated that the experimental induction of endometriosis by inoculation of endometrial currettings

into the peritoneal cavity produced both readily recognizable pelvic endometriotic lesions macroscopically similar to those seen in women with spontaneous endometriosis and an increased rate of infertility.[13] Endometriosis was experimentally induced in female *Papio anubis* baboons, with documented regular menstrual cycles, by intraperitoneal inoculation with menstrual endometrium on two consecutive menstrual cycles. The peritoneal cavity and reproductive organs were visualized by laparoscopy and the absence of any lesions or adhesions was documented by video recording. Under laparoscopic guidance, menstrual tissue was deposited from the Pipelle at four sites; the pouch of Douglas, the uterine fundus, the cul de sac, and the ovaries. At the subsequent menstruation, the animals underwent a second laparoscopy and endometrial reseeding at the same ectopic sites. Intraperitoneal inoculation resulted in the formation of endometriotic lesions with gross morphological characteristics similar to those seen in women. The development of these endometriotic lesions was observed in all 24 animals that have undergone intraperitoneal inoculation. The number and type of lesions ranged between animals but significantly more red lesions, which are thought to represent the most active site of disease, were observed three months following inoculation while at six months of disease significantly more blue endometriotic lesions were present. Thereafter similar levels of red, blue, chocolate, white, and mixed lesions were observed. Morphologically, 67% of the ectopic lesions harvested at the time of laparotomy contained both endometrial glands and stroma. In the context of animal models of endometriosis development, it cannot be disregarded data from a mutagenesis approach in genetically engineered mice.[14] According to this study, expression of oncogenic *K-ras* within the ovarian surface epithelium resulted in the development of benign ovarian and peritoneal lesions reminiscent of endometriosis with a typical endometrioid glandular morphology. The peritoneal lesions were present within the soft tissue surrounding the ovary, as well as widespread throughout the peritoneum, being associated with the surface of the oviduct, uterus, cervix, liver, intestine, spleen, pancreas. The development of this model of *de novo* endometriosis enabled the authors to gain some insight into the mechanism of endometriosis initiation in mouse models. Thus, the metaplastic theory of endometriosis development has been tested by delivering a recombinant adenoviral vector expressing *Cre* recombinase (AdCre) directly into the peritoneum through intraperitoneal injections. These mice harbored a transcriptionally silenced, oncogenic allele of *K-ras* that could be activated by the expression of *Cre* recombinase. Animals were killed approximately 8 months after AdCre injection and the entire peritoneum was carefully analyzed in all cases. Notably, all animals injected intraperitoneally, being either wild-type controls or harboring the *k-ras* mutation, showed a normal histomorphology and no signs of endometriosis. These results indicate that at least in this mouse system, peritoneal endometriosis does not originate through a process of metaplastic differentiation from the pelvic peritoneum. Alternatively, the endometriotic lesions could have arisen directly from the ovarian surface epithelium through a metaplastic differentiation process induced by oncogenic *K-ras*, and subsequently implanted onto peritoneal surfaces. To clarify this issue, the authors used the same method of intrabursal AdCre injection in *K-ras*-positive mice, followed 48 hours later by transplantation of the ovary under the ovarian bursa of non-infected mice. The transplanted mice were killed 5.5 months later. Although all of the mice showed ovarian endometriotic-like lesions, none of them had peritoneal endometriosis. These results obtained raise the possibility that the ovarian and peritoneal lesions mice may have distinct origins, with the ovarian lesions arising from the ovarian surface epithelium and the peritoneal lesions having a uterine or tubal origin. It has however, to be noted that, although the oncogenic activation of *K-ras* did result in the development of both peritoneal and ovarian lesions with endometrioid morphology, this mouse model is probably not perfect as a genocopy of endometriosis. Indeed, lesions in the ovary showed proliferations of glands but lack a surrounding endometrial-like stroma.[14]

"Anatomical Distribution" Studies

Investigating the anatomical distribution of endometriotic lesions may provide insights into the pathogenesis of the disease.[15] If ectopic endometrium is due to retrograde menstruation, the pattern of lesions should be determined mainly by anatomical and physiological variables, whereas if coelomic metaplasia is the cause of endometriosis, lesions should not be distributed in relation to factors influencing the spreading and implantation of endometrial cells.[16] A lateral asymmetry in the location of ovarian endometriotic cysts has been demonstrated. In the patients with unilateral endometriomas, the observed proportion of left cysts (63%; 95% confidence interval, 58% to 68%) was significantly different from the expected proportion of 50%, (p<0.001). Including also the bilateral endometriotic cysts gave a total of 57% left-sided endometriomas. Indeed, the two adnexal regions are different in terms of exposure to the pelvic milieu, the left one being protected by the sigmoid colon. Not only does this portion of the large bowel lean on the left tube and ovary but it is very often fixed to the pelvic brim by film adhesions which are so frequently observed as to be considered a paraphysiological finding. A microenvironment is established around the left adnexa and, as a consequence, endometrial cells regurgitated are not exposed to the clockwise peritoneal current that keeps the peritoneal fluid circulating and may partly protected from the macrophage disposal system. These factors may facilitate adhesion, implantation, and growth of endometrial cells. Therefore, the demonstration of a lateral asymmetry in the location of ovarian endometriotic cysts is compatible with the anatomical differences of the left and right hemipelvis and supports the menstrual reflux theory. Another study considered a large series of consecutive women undergoing surgery for benign ovarian non-endometriotic cysts and no significant differences was observed in the proportion of left- and right-sided lesions.[17] This is at odds with the finding of a significantly more frequent development of endometriomas on the left ovary. Probably, when the lesion has an intrinsic ovarian origin its lateral distribution is symmetric, whereas when the cause is extrinsic, as well as refluxed and implanted endometrial cells, the lesion distribution is influenced by anatomical factors able to determine the asymmetry observed in ovarian endometriosis. These findings suggest that the pathogenesis of endometriotic and non-endometriotic cysts is different, supporting the menstrual reflux theory of endometriosis.

The ureter is in anatomic contiguity with the lateral gonadal aspect.[18] Consequently, if ureteral endometriosis develops from ovarian implants or if both lesions have a common pathogenesis, asymmetry should be found also in the left- and right-handed distribution of ureteral foci. Actually, based on results of a large surgical series and of a systematic review of published cases it has been confirm that, similar to ovarian endometriosis, ureteral disease is observed more frequently on the left than the right side. Interestingly, the proportion of left-sided gonadal and ureteral lesions was remarkably similar (63% and 64%). In keeping with these results, a significant asymmetry in lesion distribution has been also demonstrated for the lower intestinal tract.[19] The left adnexal region is covered by the sigmoid colon that creates a sort of shelter facilitating implantation of regurgitated endometrial cells, whereas the cecum is more cranial and hence less prone to be involved. A strong right-distribution asymmetry, but again supporting the menstrual reflux theory, was conversely demonstrated for diaphragmatic and sciatic nerve lesions.[20,21] Explanations for these findings still involve the clockwise peritoneal fluid current and the close contiguity of the sigmoid colon to the ipsilateral tube. In the first case, the refluxed endometrial cells transported by the intra-abdominal current coming down from the left peritoneal gutter and flowing across the pelvic floor and up along the right peritoneal gutter, once reaching the right hypochondrium are stuck by the falciform ligament, a crescentic fold of peritoneum extending to the surface of the liver from the diaphragm and anterior abdominal wall. This is supposed to facilitate implantation on the right leaf of the diaphragmatic peritoneum. In the second case, the interposition of the sigmoid colon between the regurgitated endometrial cells implanted on the left posterolateral pelvic peritoneum seems to protect the left lumbosacral plexus and sciatic nerve. Therefore, in general, this asymmetric distribution constitutes indirect evidence against the coelomic metaplasia theory, which is more likely to be associated with equal distribution.

"Association" Studies

A particular attention deserves results from those studies that have evaluated the frequency of association between the different forms of the disease.[22] These studies are based on the assumption that if a specific form of the disease does not share a pathogenetic mechanism with another, the two forms should not be significantly associated. In other words, if a different and peculiar pathogenetic mechanism leading to a specific form of the disease exists, the frequency of the presence of other forms of endometriosis in patients affected by the peculiar form should be similar to that observed in the general population.[22] To clarify the pathogenesis of deep infiltrating endometriosis, the frequency of non-deep forms of the disease such as superficial implants, ovarian cysts and pelvic adhesions have been investigated among patients affected by the "deep" form. Ninety-three women with deep peritoneal endometriosis were identified. The presence of superficial endometriotic implants, endometriomas and pelvic adhesions was documented in 61.3% (95% CI 51.4-71.2%), 50.5% (95% CI 40.3-60.7%) and 74.2% (95% CI 65.3-83.1%) of patients with deep endometriotic nodules, respectively. Overall, deep peritoneal endometriosis was the only form of the disease in only 6.5% (95% CI 2.8-12.3%) of cases. Results obtained did not support the hypothesis that deep

endometriosis should be considered as a distinct entity of the disease. A similar study design has been used to evaluate the pathogenesis of bladder endometriosis.[23] Again, if endometriotic nodules of the bladder have a distinct ethiopathogenetic origin, the frequency of concomitant non-vesical endometriotic lesions should be similar to the prevalence of endometriosis in the general population. Fifty-eight patients were recruited. The presence of superficial peritoneal implants, ovarian endometriomas, adhesions, and extravesical deep peritoneal endometriosis was observed in 58.6% (95% confidence interval [CI]: 45.2-71.2), 44.8% (95% CI: 32.2-58.2), 81.0% (95% CI: 68.4-89.6), and 27.6% (95% CI: 16.7-40.8) of cases, respectively. The presence of at least one of them was documented in 87.9% of cases (95% CI: 76.7-94.3). Again, these results did not support the vision that bladder endometriotic nodules should be considered an independent form of the disease.

Basic Research

If endometrial tissue has to implant in the peritoneum, it must be able to adhere to the peritoneal surface, invade the basement membrane and extracellular matrix, acquire a blood supply and survive. Although this sequence cannot be studied in humans, it has been studied extensively in various model systems. The experiments *in vitro* performed by Witz et al have given further support to the "implantation theory", specifically demonstrating that endometrium, both stroma and epithelium, can easily and rapidly adhere to an intact mesothelium.[24] The experimental model consisted in plating explants of peritoneum and culturing them in presence of endometrium in form of cellular aggregates or isolated epithelial and stromal cells or menstruated fragments.[24] The attachment process was evaluated by transmission electron microscopy and confocal laser-scanning microscope. The results obtained indicate that endometrial attachment to an intact mesothelium occurs within 1 hour and transmesothelial invasion occurs between 1 and 18-24 hours. Thus, contrary to previous observations,[25] the intact mesothelium does not seem to constitute a defence barrier to the adhesion of endometrial fragments and traumas to the mesothelial lining are not a prerequisite for endometrial cell adhesion.

From a pathogenetic point of view, it is also important to underline that in the last few years, in patients with endometriosis, specific constitutive and/or acquired molecular alterations of eutopic and/or ectopic endometrium have been identified for each of the processes potentially involved in the sequence of events at the basis of "implantation" theory.[3] These alterations, which may affect the physiologic activity of endometrium, are thought to explain why only some women develop the disease. A reduction in the percentage of menstruated cells undergoing programmed death; an increase in the endometrial expression of the anti-apoptotic gene Bcl-2; the ability of regurgitated endometrial cells to escape peritoneal immunosurveillance by means of several antibody- and cell-mediated mechanisms; a deregulation in the endometrial cell E-cadherin system and in the expression pattern of integrins facilitating adhesion, matrix degradation and invasion; the endometrial expression of high levels of aromatase and basic fibroblast growth factor stimulating mitotic activity; the development of selective resistance of certain target genes to progesterone action; a disregulation of endometrial MMPs synthesis and secretion combined with aberrant amounts of TIMP-1 facilitating cell invasion; an increased peritoneal fluid levels of VEGF and IL-8 stimulating neoangiogenesis and vascularization of ectopic implants have all been recognized in women with endometriosis, adding substantial biological evidence to this theory.[5]

On the other hand, very recent findings by Gaetje et al have renovated the metaplastic theory by demonstrating molecular-genetic parallels between female genital development and endometriosis. Specifically, a higher peritoneal expression of genes playing a decisive role during the embryonic development of the female genital tract and the endometrium (*WNT7A, PAX8*) has been demonstrated in women affected by endometriosis compared to controls. The expression of these genes in the normal peritoneum suggests that endometriosis can arise through metaplasia by engaging those developmental steps that are involved in the oncogenesis of endometrium.[26]

In conclusion, although epidemiological, surgical, and pathological data tend to suggest that peritoneal, ovarian, and the so-called "deep" lesions constitute different expressions of a single disease with a unique pathogenetic mechanism, i.e. retrograde menstruation, this model is not able to explain the various aspects of endometriosis fully and at present cannot be recognized as the sole ultimately valid explanatory model.

References

1. Oral E, Arici A. Pathogenesis of endometriosis. Obstet Gynecol Clin North Am 1997;24: 219-33.

2. Matarese G, De Placido G, Nikas Y, et al. Pathogenesis of endometriosis: natural immunity dysfunction or autoimmune disease? Trends Mol Med 2003;9:223-28.

3. Sampson JA. Peritoneal endometriosis due to the menstrual dissemination of endometrial tissue into the peritoneal cavity. Am J Obstet Gynecol 1927;14:422-69.

4. Vignali M, Infantino M, Matrone R, et al. Endometriosis: novel etiopathogenetic concepts and clinical perspectives. Fertil Steril 2002;78:665-78.

5. Viganò P, Parazzini F, Somigliana E, et al..Endometriosis: epidemiology and aetiological factors. Best Pract Res Clin Obstet Gynaecol. 2004;18:177-200.

6. Nisolle M, Donnez J. Peritoneal endometriosis, ovarian endometriosis, and adenomyotic nodules of the rectovaginal septum are three different entities. Fertil Steril 1997;68:585-96.

7. Somigliana E, Vigano P, La Sala GB, et al. Follicular fluid as a favourable environment for endometrial and endometriotic cell growth in vitro. Hum Reprod 2001;16:1076-80.

8. McClure HM, Ridley JM, Graham CE, et al. Disseminated endometriosis in a rhesus monkey (Macaca mulatta). J Med Assoc Ga 1971;60:11-3.

9. Fanton JW, Hubbard GB. Spontaneous endometriosis in a Cynomolgus monkey. Lab Anim Sci 1983;33:597-99.

10. Digiacomo RF, Hooks JJ, Sulima MP, et al. Pelvic endometriosis and Simian Foamy Virus Infection in a pigtailed macaque. J Am Vet Med Assoc 1977;171:859-61.

11. Merrill JA. Spontaneous endometriosis in the Kenya baboon (Papio doguera). Am J Obstet Gynecol 1968;101: 569-70.

12. Te Linde RW, Scott RB. Experimental endometriosis. Am J Obstet Gynecol 1950; 60:1147-73.

13. D'Hooghe TM, Bambra CS, Raeymaekers SCM, et al. Intrapelvic injection of menstrual endometrium causes endometriosis in baboons (Papio cynocephalus and Papio anubis). Am J Obstet Gynecol 1995;173:125-34.

14. Dinulescu DM, Ince TA, Quade BJ, Shafer SA, et al. Role of K-ras and Pten in the development of mouse models of endometriosis and endometrioid ovarian cancer. Nat Med 2005;11:63-70.

15. Vercellini P, Busacca M, Aimi G, et al. Lateral distribution of recurrent ovarian endometriotic cysts. Fertil Steril 2002;77:848-49.

16. Vercellini P, Aimi G, De Giorgi O, et al. Is cystic ovarian endometriosis an asymmetric disease? Br J Obstet Gynaecol 1998;105:1018-21.

17. Vercellini P, Pisacreta A, Vicentini S, et al. Lateral distribution of nonendometriotic benign ovarian cysts. BJOG 2000;107:556-58.

18. Vercellini P, Pisacreta A, Pesole A, et al. Is ureteral endometriosis an asymmetric disease? BJOG 2000;107:559-61.

19. Vercellini P, Chapron C, Fedele L, et al. Evidence for asymmetric distribution of lower intestinal tract endometriosis. BJOG 2004;111:1213-17.

20. Vercellini P, Abbiati A, Viganò P, et al. Asymmetry in distribution of diaphragmatic endometriotic lesions: evidence in favour of the menstrual reflux theory. Hum Reprod 2007;22:2359-67.

21. Vercellini P, Chapron C, Fedele L, et al. Evidence for asymmetric distribution of sciatic nerve endometriosis. Obstet Gynecol 2003;102:383-87.

22. Somigliana E, Infantino M, Candiani M, et al. Association rate between deep peritoneal endometriosis and other forms of the disease: pathogenetic implications. Hum Reprod 2004;19:168-71.

23. Somigliana E, Vercellini P, Gattei U, et al. Bladder endometriosis: getting closer and closer to the unifying metastatic hypothesis. Fertil Steril 2007;87:1287-90.

24. Witz CA, Thomas MR, Montoya-Rodriguez IA, et al. Short-term culture of peritoneum explants confirms attachment of endometrium to intact peritoneal mesothelium. Fertil Steril 2001;75:385-90.

25. Groothius P, Koks CA, de Goeij AF, et al. Adhesion of human endometrial fragments to peritoneum in vitro. Fertil Steril 1999;71:1119-24.

26. Gaetje R, Holtrich U, Engels K, et al. Endometriosis may be generated by mimicking the ontogenetic development of the female genital tract. Fertil Steril 2007;87:651-56.

Makrigiannakis A, Karamouti M

Chapter 4

Role of Inflammation in the Pathogenesis of Endometriosis

Introduction

Despite the high frequency of endometriosis and the significant consequences for the patients and for the health systems also, the exact pathogenesis of the disease has not yet been deciphered. Many theories have been described to explain the presence of ectopic endometrial tissue, some of which are contradictory to each other. Today retrograde menstruation is a widely accepted mechanism for the presence of ectopic endometrial tissue **(Figure 4-1)** but it does not explain the fact that retrograted cells do not survive, attach and multiply in all women. More specifically, retrograde menstruation occurs in more than 90% of women, but only 15-20% of women suffer from endometriosis. The causative factor for endometriosis remains a mystery but there are indications that immunological - inflammatory factors participate in its pathogenesis. It is well established that in women with endometriosis peritoneal fluid (PF) is modestly increased and is abandoned from phagocytic macrophages-monocytes, natural killer (NK) cells, cytotoxic T lymphocytes, B cells and inflammatory mediators—complement and cytokines.[1-3] Whether inflammation is the cause rather than the result of endometriosis, has not been clarified yet and can not be studied in women since it is unethical. However, studies in baboon and mice indicate that inflammation is the result rather than the cause of endometriosis.[4,5] More specifically in baboon menstruation, has been associated with increased PF volume, reach in white blood cells and inflammatory cytokines, which seem to be even more elevated in baboon with spontaneous endometriosis.[5] Furthermore the percentage of CD4+ and IL2R+ cells has been correlated to the stage of endometriosis.[5] However induction of endometriosis in an inflammatory peritoneal cavity of thioglycolate medium-treated mice, negatively affected the development of endometriosis.[4]

Cellular Constituents

Macrophages constitute the basic cell population in the PF, representing the 85% of PF leucocytes and reaching their peak during the menses.[6] Macrophages are responsible for the withdrawal of endometrial debris, sperm and follicular cells from the peritoneal cavity. It has been noted that in cases of bilateral tubal occlusion macrophage's number does not increase during menses.

Macrophages are increased in number in PF of women with endometriosis and this has been attributed to the presence of chemotactic molecules in the PF from women with endometriosis, such as monocyte chemotactic protein-1 (MCP-1), RANTES (Regulated upon activation normal T-cells, expressed and secreted) and lyso-phosphatidylcholine. Furthermore macrophages are much more activated, which is expressed by a larger size, elevated C3 and C4 release, as well as lysosomal phospholipase used for the synthesis of prostaglandins.[2,7,8] CD14, HLA DQ and lysosomal enzymes are also expressed in higher level. However conflicting are the data concerning the macrophages concentration and activity in eutopic endometrium from women with endometriosis.[9]

Despite the fact that macrophages are part of the normal peritoneal "disposal system", they have been implicated with the pathogenesis of endometriosis.[2,8] This could be partially explained by the presence of more than one different polarized subclasses of macrophages. In particular, it seems that classically activated macrophages M1 produce cytokines and participate in the distraction of microorganisms and tumor cells, while M2 macrophages tune inflammatory responses, Th1 immunity, angiogenesis and tissue remodeling. The altered balance in M1/M2 ratio could be involved in the pathogenesis of endometriosis. Capping phenomenon is however a unique phenomenon described only in peritoneal macrophages from women

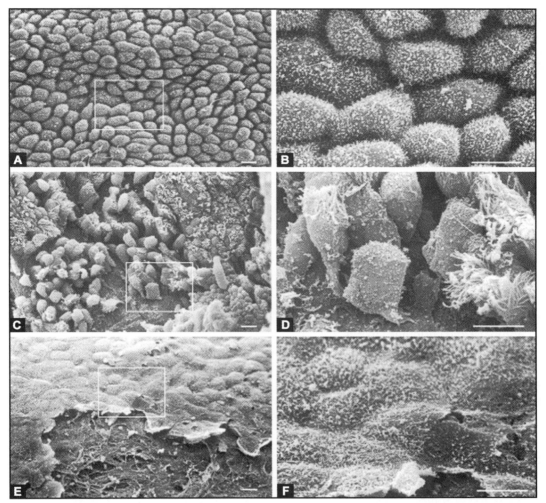

FIGURE 4-1: Reprinted from Trends in molecular endocrinology, Materese et al; 2003; Vol 9/ No 5; with permission from Elsevier. (A) Scanning electron micrograph of normal peritoneum. A complete sheath of mesothelial cells is covering the peritoneal surface. (B) Closer view of the boxed area in panel (A), showing that the mesothelial cells are covered with short and thick microvilli and have a cobblestone appearance. (C) Scanning electron micrograph of an active lesion, classified as a red-flamed spot (see Fig. 1B). In the upper left and right of the panel, epithelial implants of secretory and ciliated cells are present, forming a complete sheath. In the remaining areas, the cells are degenerating and detaching, exposing the underlying peritoneal surface. (D) Closer view of the boxed area in panel (C). Degenerative changes of the epithelial cells are evident, including rounding of their shape, loosening of their attachment to the substratum, an absence of microvilli, and decilliation. The substratum (the connective tissue of the peritoneum) appears covered with a fibrinous/amorphous material. (E) Scanning electron micrograph of a lesion classified as blue–black spot. Two distinct areas are visible: the upper and left parts of the panel show an area covered by a sheath of flattened mesothelial cells. In the lower right of the panel, the mesothelial cells are absent, exposing the underlying loose connective tissue, which appears to be covered with a fibrinous/ amorphous material, probably resulting from inflammatory reaction. (F) Closer view of the boxed area in panel (E). The mesothelial cells are flat and covered with amorphous material. The plasma membranes in some areas appear thinned. Scale bars in all panels represent 10 mm

The figure was reprinted from Trends in molecular medicine, Vol 9 /edition number 5, Giuseppe Materese, Giuseppe De Placido, Yorgos Nikas and Carlo Alviggi, Pathogenesis of endometriosis: natural immunity dysfunction or autoimmune disease?, Pages: 223-228, Copyright (2003), with permission from Elsevier; Licence number: 2130890960793 with endometriosis and describes the migration of antigen-antibody complexes (HLA class I and II antigens) towards a pole of the cell before internalization.[8]

Macrophages have been correlated with the initiation and the development of endometriosis through fibronectin, TNFα, cytokines and interleukin production.[2, 7, 10]

Fibronectin, apart from favoring the attachment of retrograded endometrial cells to the peritoneal cavity and organs, also induces the activity of the so called progression factors that promote the proliferation of retrograde endometrial cells, e.g. estradiol.[10] Activated macrophages secrete also TNFα, which enhances fibroplast proliferation and the synthesis of collagen, favoring the formation of adhesions, as well as cytokines that induce the proliferation of endometrial cells and the activation of T and B cells.[11] Macrophage's derived monocyte chemotactic protein 1 (MCP-1), vascular endothelial growth factor (VEGF) and macrophage-derived growth factor (MDGF) also enhance the proliferation of fibroblast and endometrial cells.

NK cells are lymphocytic cells and are also components of the "disposal system" of the peritoneum. NK cells express non-specific cytotoxicity, regulated by circulating cytokines. In endometriosis NK cells are defective in number and in function, in proportion to the stage of endometriosis.[2, 7, 12-14] Whether NK cytotoxicity defect is the primitive mechanism for the implantation and development of retrograded endometrial cells, or impaired NK cells cytotoxic function is the result of an imbalance in the immune response to a chronic antigen presentation – endometriotic cells- or to a previously initiated autoimmune event unrelated to endometriosis, is a matter of debate. However studies have revealed a resistance of endometrium in NK cytotoxicity in women with endometriosis, compared to healthy women and an elevated CD4/CD8 ratio and TGFβ level in PF, that inhibit NK cells cytotoxicity.[15] Under study is still the role of endorphin β and autoimmunity defects on NK cells, while well established is the role of steroids and in particular estradiol in the development of endometriosis.

T lymphocytes are significantly reduced in PF in women with endometriosis.[2, 7, 15, 16] In endometriosis, when endometrial cells, probably with altered characteristics fall in the peritoneal cavity, "defective" macrophages favor their implantation and growth. More specifically it has been found using RT-PCR studies that in women with endometriosis, peritoneal T cells, under the control of macrophage derived cytokines, express primarily Th2 cytokines, IL-4, IL-5, IL-6, IL-10 and IL-13, that activate B cells and induce cell-mediated immunity, while Th1 cytokines, interleukin 2 (IL-2), IL-12 and interferon γ, that activate cellular immunity, are in deficit.[7]

Cytokines

Cytokines are low molecular weight proteins or glycoproteins synthesized by peritoneal macrophages, lymphocytes, ectopic endometrial implants and mesothelial cells of the peritoneum. Cytokines have miscellaneously been implicated with the pathogenesis and progression of endometriosis, through the accumulation, induction or depletion of different cells actions, as well as the induction of other cytokines secretion.[2, 7, 12, 18] Data show that the microenvironment of peritoneum is characterized by the aberrant expression of cytokines that favor the implantation and development of endometrial cells, the angiogenesis and the formation of adhesions. Cytokines that have been identified in the PF form patients with endometriosis are IL-1, IL-4, IL-5, IL-6, IL-8, IL-10, IL-12, IL-13, interferon-γ, TNF-α, RANTES, MCP-1, MCSF (macrophage colony stimulating factor), TGF-β (transforming growth factor) and VEGF.

IL-1 has been found to be elevated in the PF of women with endometriosis, partly derived from macrophages of peritoneal cavity, which secrete higher levels of IL-1 in patient with endometriosis. IL-1 action is counterbalanced by IL-1ra (IL-1 receptor antagonist), the cellular receptor for IL-1.[19] It has been elucidated that in endometriotic cells, this regulatory mechanism is defective, due to different localization of IL-1ra, leading to enhanced levels of IL-1 in the PF. IL-1 also modulates IL-6 secretion by macrophages, and IL-2 by T cells and NK cells, induces the synthesis of prostaglandins, favors the formation of adhesions and fibrosis and stimulates B-cells proliferation and antibody production.[2] **IL-6** has also been implicated in the pathogenesis of endometrosis although its exact action has not been determined yet.[19] What arises from studies is that IL-6 in eutopic endometrium, inhibits stromal and glandular proliferation through IL-6 receptor, an action that is abolished in ectopic endometriotic lesions. **IL-8** is also secreted in higher amounts by peritoneal macrophages in women with endometriosis.[19] Endometrial cells can also produce IL-8 and in turn respond to its growth-promoting action. IL-8 has been implicated with the adherence and growth of endometriotic cells, neoangiosis, chemoattraction and activation of neutrophils.[20] **IL-10** and **IL-13** also enhances macrophage activation but their exact role remains to be clarified.

TNF-α is secreted by activated macrophages, fibroblasts, T and B cells and its concentration in PF has been positively related by some authors with the stage of endometriosis.[19] In vitro TNF-α induces endometrial cells proliferation as well as the formation of adhesions, through fibroblasts proliferation and collagen sedimentation. **RANTES** is another cytokine that is found to be elevated in the PF of women with endometriosis. It has been implicated in the pathogenesis of endometriosis probably through the activation of macrophages and T-lymphocytes, although its exact role remains obscure. **TGF-β** is also found to be elevated in the PF of patients with endometriosis and in proportion to the stage of disease. TGF-β probably intervenes in endometrial proliferation, angogenesis and inhibition of lymphocyte and NK cell.[21] **MCP 1** (Monocyte chemotactic protein) also induces endometrial cell proliferation as well as macrophages stimulation, while **VEGF** promotes angiogenesis. Both are elevated in PF in case of endometriosis and reduced after gonadotrophin treatment. Angiogenetic and mitogenic actions have also been attributed to platelet derived growth factor (**PDGF**). Finally intracellular adhesion molecule 1 (**ICAM-1**) is also a possible escape mechanism of the ectopic endometrium for NK cytotoxicity.

Endometriosis and Defective Immunity

Data show that endometriosis and chronic inflammatory reaction are linked by a defective immune system.[7, 12, 17, 22] More specifically it has been speculated that in women with endometriosis, endometrial cells in the PF avoid immunoreaction. There are contradictory data supporting the defective natural-innate immune response or the altered adaptive-specific immune response respectively, although it seems possible that a combination of disorders is the case. However, NK cells represent the key interface between the innate and adaptive response and participate in the fragile balance of immune tolerance. It seems that in endometriosis the altered cytokine secretion by NK cells leads to an altered T- and B- activation and/or to defective autoantigen presentation form macrophages and dendritic cells to autoreactive T cells. T cells malfunction could either be due to direct T cell cytotoxicity or the indirect adjustment of macrophages, NK cells and B cells function. As long as it concerns the humoral-mediated immune response, endometriosis has been linked to the presence of specific anti-endometrium antibodies in PF, in serum and in endometrium implants,[23, 24] as well as in the presence of some kind of atypical autoantibodies (Lupus anticoagulant, antinucleotide, antiphospholipids,

antihistones, antithyroids, etc.) in almost 85% of women suffering from endometriosis. Furthermore, recently an absence of humoral response against specific endometrial antigens has been recorded. In women with endometriosis Fas-Fas ligand (Fas-FasL) system could also be defective, since in endometriosis Garcia-Velasco et al[25] showed that macrophage conditioned media, stimulated Fas-FasL expression by endometrial cells, inducing the apoptosis of T-cells, the implantation and development of endometriosis.

HLA class I molecules are also enhanced in ectopic endometrial cells, probably secondary to local cytokine- and hormone-mediated mechanisms, and regulate endometrial sensitivity in NK lytic action.[26]

Conclusions

- Endometriosis is characterized by local sterile inflammation of peritoneal cavity.
- PF of women with endometriosis has different synthesis compared to normal women and is characterized by elevated levels of macrophages, cytokines, angiogenetic and growth factors.
- Macrophage derived cytokines, growth and adherence factors and NK cells dysfunction is probably the principal etiopathogenetic factors that enable the adherence and development of ectopic endometrial cells.
- Angiogenetic factors produced locally provide micro – neovascularization of endometriotic foci.
- New data implicate in the pathogenesis of endometriosis, inflammation, cellular and chemical immunological changes and hormonal factors. The way all these factors are combined remains to be clarified.

References

1. Halis G, Arici A. Endometriosis and inflammation in infertility. Ann N Y Acad Sci 2004; 1034: 300-15.
2. Gazvani R, Templeton A. Peritoneal environment, cytokines and angiogenesis in the pathophysiology of endometriosis. Reproduction 2002; 123: 217-26.
3. Ho HN, Wu MY, Yang YS. Peritoneal cellular immunity and endometriosis. Am J Reprod Immunol 1997; 38: 400-12.
4. Nowak NM, Fischer OM, Gust TC, Fuhrmann U, Habenicht UF, Schmidt A. Intraperitoneal inflammation decreases endometriosis in a mouse model. Hum Reprod 2008; 23: 2466-74.
5. D'Hooghe TM, Debrock S. Endometriosis, retrograde menstruation and peritoneal inflammation in women and in baboons. Hum Reprod Update 2002; 8: 84-88.

6. Van Furth R, Raeburn JA and Van Zwet TI. Characteristics of human mononuclear phagocytes. Blood 1979; 54: 485-500.

7. Vinatier D, Dufour P, Oosterlynck D. Immunological aspects of endometriosis. Hum Reprod Update 1996; 2: 371-84.

8. Halme J, Becker S and Wing R. Accentuated cyclic activation of peritoneal macrophages in patients with endometriosis. Am J Obstet Gynecol 1984; 148: 85–90.

9. Berbic M, Schulke L, Markham R, Tokushige N, Russell P, Fraser IS. Macrophage expression in endometrium of women with and without endometriosis. Hum Reprod 2009; 24: 325-32.

10. Kauma S, Clark MR, White C, Halme J. Production of fibronectin by peritoneal macrophages and concentration of fibronectin in peritoneal fluid from patients with or without endometriosis. Obstet Gynecol 1988; 72:13-18.

11. Rana N, Braun DP, House R, Gebel H, Rotman C, Dmowski WP. Basal and stimulated secretion of cytokines by peritoneal macrophages in women with endometriosis. Fertil Steril 1996; 65: 925-30.

12. Matarese G, De Placido G, Nikas Y, Alviggi C. Pathogenesis of endometriosis: natural immunity dysfunction or autoimmune disease? Trends Mol Med 2003; 9: 223-28.

13. Iwasaki K, Makino T, Maruyama T et al. Leukocyte subpopulations and natural killer activity in endometriosis. Int J Fertil 1993; 38: 229-34.

14. Garzetti G, Ciavattini A, Provinciali M, et al. Natural killer cell activity in endometriosis; correlation between serum estradiol levels and cytotoxicity. Obstet Gynecol 1993; 81: 665-58.

15. Hill JA, Faris HM, Schiff I and Anderson DJ. Characterization of leukocyte subpopulations in the peritoneal fluid of women with endometriosis. Fertil Steril 1988; 50: 216-22.

16. Cunningham DS, Hansen KA and Coddington CC. Changes in T cell regulation of responses to self antigens in women with pelvic endometriosis. Fertil Steril 1992; 58: 114-19.

17. Kyama CM, Debrock S, Mwenda JM, D'Hooghe TM. Potential involvement of the immune system in the development of endometriosis. Reprod Biol Endocrinol 2003; 1: 123.

18. Harada T, Iwabe T, Terakawa N. Role of cytokines in endometriosis. Fertil Steril 2001; 76: 1-10.

19. Wieser F, Fabjani G, Tempfer C, Schneeberger C, Zeillinger R, Huber JC, Wenzl R. Tumor necrosis factor-alpha promotor polymorphisms and endometriosis. J Soc Gynecol Investig 2002, 9: 313-18.

20. Arici A, Seli E, Zeyneloglu HB, Senturk LM, Oral E and Olive DL Interleukin 8 induces proliferation of endometrial stromal cells a potential autocrine growth factor. J Clin Endocrinol Metabolism 1998; 83: 1201-05.

21. Oral E, Olive DL and Arici A. The peritoneal environment in endometriosis Hum Reprod Update 1996; 2: 385–98.

22. Barrier BF, Kendall BS, Ryan CE, Sharpe-Timms KL. HLA-G is expressed by the glandular epithelium of peritoneal endometriosis but not in eutopic endometrium. Hum Reprod 2006; 21: 864-69.

23. Halme J and Mathur S. Local autoimmunity in infertile patients with endometriosis. Int J Fertil 1987; 32: 309–12.

24. Mathur S, Chihal HJ, Homm RJ Homm RJ, Garza DE, Rust PF, Williamson HO.Endometrial antigens involved in the autoimmunity of endometriosis. Fertil Steril 1988; 50: 860-63.

25. Garcia-Velasco JA, Arici A, Zreik T, Naftolin F, Mor G. Macrophage derived growth factors modulate Fas ligand expression in cultured endometrial stromal cells: a role in endometriosis. Mol Hum Reprod 1999; 5: 642-50.

26. Semino C, Semino A, Pietra G, Mingari MC, Barocci S, Venturini PL, Ragni N, Melioli G. Role of major histocompatibility complex class I expression and natural killer-like T cells in the genetic control of endometriosis. Fertil Steril 1995; 64: 909-16.

Sajal Gupta, Anjali Chandra, Shubhangi Kesavan
Deborah Eapen, Ashok Agarwal

Chapter 5

Oxidative Stress and the Pathogenesis of Endometriosis

Introduction

Endometriosis is a complicated disease with an ambiguous etiology. It affects 10% of all women in the general population and is an important causative factor in 40% of all cases of female infertility and in 60% of all cases of female chronic pelvic pain.[1]

Endometriosis occurs in women of reproductive age and in postmenopausal women secondary to the use of exogenous estrogen. Generally, the disease is characterized by the presence of endometrial glands and stroma outside the endometrium and uterine muscle. It is diagnosed primarily by laparoscopy, the current gold standard. Although laparoscopy attempts to diagnose endometriotic lesions at various stages, the procedure is unable to detect subtle endometriotic lesions and therefore cannot render an early diagnosis.[2] As a result, the current prevalence of endometriosis is most likely an underestimation. A nonsurgical method of diagnosing endometriosis would have many benefits, including the possibility of early diagnosis, sensitivity to a wider range of endometriotic stages, and the provision of a non-invasive option for treatment or prevention. The most anticipated noninvasive option for diagnosis is the analysis of serum and peritoneal markers. Of particular interest is the identification of markers that indicate elevated levels of oxidative stress (OS) and altered immune function in the follicular and peritoneal environments.

The relationship between endometriosis and reactive oxygen species (ROS) such as superoxide anions, hydrogen peroxide, and hydroxyl radicals is currently being evaluated as a possible source for serum and peritoneal fluid markers. Damage caused by ROS produces an inflammatory cascade that gives rise to a plethora of serum and peritoneal fluid markers such as interleukin 6 (IL-6), tumor necrosis factor alpha (TNF-α), interleukin 8

(IL-8), interleukin 1 (IL-1) beta, and serum paraoxonase-1 (PON-1). In this chapter, we will further discuss the influence of ROS on endometriosis as well as summarize what the latest research shows on the use of these markers as a noninvasive option for diagnosing endometriosis.

Endometriosis: Theories of Etiology

Although the etiology of endometriosis is uncertain, four main hypotheses have been circulated as plausible causes: (1) Sampson's theory of retrograde menstruation, (2) celomic metaplasia and induction theories (an extension of the celomic metaplasia theory), (3) the embryonic rest theory, and (4) lymphatic and vascular metastasis theories.[3] The most widely accepted hypothesis is the theory of implantation, also known as Sampson's theory. It proposes that the disorder arises due to retrograde menstruation of endometrial tissue into the peritoneal cavity through patent fallopian tubes.[4] Women with endometriosis have been found to have larger amounts of menstrual reflux of both blood and endometrial tissue than women without the disorder.[5] The anatomical distribution of endometriotic lesions supports the idea of retrograde reflux and subsequent peritoneal implantation. Flow of peritoneal fluid is arrested or repetitive in the peritoneal cavity in four main places: the pouch of Douglas at the rectosigmoid level, the cecum and ileocecal junction, the superior portion of the sigmoid mesocolon, and the right paracolic gutter.[6] These areas are consequently the main areas where ectopic endometriotic lesions are generally found.[6]

A number of animal studies support Sampson's theory, including one in which menstrual endometrium was injected into the retroperitoneal space of four baboons, all of which subsequently developed endometriosis.[7] In 1950 a study conducted by TeLinde and Scott also supported

Sampson's theory. The results of the study demonstrated that 50% of monkeys developed endometriosis after their menstrual flow was diverted into the peritoneal cavity.[8]

Sampson's theory provides and explains three requirements for the establishment of endometriosis.[4] The first requirement is retrograde menstruation through the fallopian tubes. In fact, 76% to 90% of all women with patent fallopian tubes have some degree of retrograde menstruation;[3] however, not all develop endometriosis. The second requirement is the presence of viable refluxed cells in the peritoneal cavity. Mungyer *et al* found endometrial cells in peritoneal fluid of women with endometriosis after performing endometrial lavage, and the cells stayed viable in culture for up to two months.[9] The third requirement necessitates that refluxed endometrial cells adhere to the peritoneal epithelium where they implant and proliferate.[3] In order for the implant to survive, a blood supply must be established. Oxidative stress contributes to angiogenesis in ectopic endometrial implants by increasing VEGF production.[10] This effect is partially mediated by glycodelin—a glycoprotein with increased expression caused by OS. Glycodelin acts as an autocrine factor that augments VEGF expression within ectopic endometrial tissue.[10]

Some researchers believe that endometriosis also has a genetic component. This belief is based on the fact that women with first-degree relatives who have endometriosis have a high incidence of the disease themselves. This is especially true with maternal inheritance patterns. One of every 10 women with severe endometriosis has a first-degree relative with clinical manifestation of endometriosis.

Investigating Role of Oxidative Stress in Endometriosis

Oxidative stress is a cause of female infertility as it affects ovulation, fertilization, and embryo development and implantation. It occurs when there is an imbalance between levels of oxidants and antioxidants. Usually, OS is a product of ROS overproduction rather than low antioxidant levels, both of which have been found in women with endometriosis.[11, 12] Elevated ROS levels in oviductal fluid might have adverse effects, impairing oocyte and spermatozoa viability and fertilization and embryo transport within the oviduct. Oxidative stress is known to occur when neutrophils and macrophages become activated—as in pro-inflammatory states, for example—which further amplifies ROS production in the oviductal fluid.[13] A substantial increase in ROS produc-

tion might result in oxidative damage to sperm plasma and acrosomal membranes, impairing their motility and hindering the ability of spermatozoa to bind to and penetrate an oocyte. DNA damage secondary to OS may lead to failed fertilization, reduced embryo quality, failure of pregnancy, and spontaneous abortion.

To date, no true cause-and-effect relationship has been established between OS and endometriosis. Two studies determined a positive association,[11, 14] whereas others have reported no association.[15, 16] It is difficult to establish a definitive conclusion in regards to the association between OS and endometriosis based on these studies. Jackson *et al* investigated this relationship by evaluating women undergoing laparoscopy for suspected endometriosis. The serum from these women was measured for four biomarkers of OS and antioxidant levels. The biomarkers that were selected were presumed to measure the main targets in the biochemical pathways involved in OS: (i) thiobarbituric acid-reacting substances (TBARS), (ii) 8-F2-isoprostane, (iii) fat-soluble antioxidants, and (iv) paraoxonase activity. The study adjusted for the following potential confounding factors: age, body mass index, smoking status, hormone use in the past 12 months, gravidity, serum vitamin E levels, and serum estradiol and total serum lipid levels. The authors reported a weak association between TBARS, a measure of overall OS, and endometriosis. However, at the time of serum collection, no agent was added to prevent auto-oxidation (AO) from occurring. This may have altered the levels of oxidants and AO. Furthermore, the type of biospecimen used in this study (serum versus peritoneal fluid) served to further limit the study.

In the peritoneal fluid, OS is initiated in the inflammatory cells with cellular debris acting as a substrate, and products of OS are transported to the serum. Peritoneal fluid from patients with endometriosis has been shown to exhibit inadequate antioxidant defenses, including low total antioxidant capacity (TAC) and significantly reduced levels of individual antioxidant enzymes such as superoxide dismutase (SOD).[11, 17] Statistically, it has been found that infertile women with endometriosis have lower concentrations of SOD than fertile controls. Despite the various associations between OS in peritoneal fluid and endometriosis, many studies have failed to demonstrate a difference in ROS, nitric oxide (NO), lipid peroxide, and antioxidant levels in the peritoneal fluid of women with endometriosis and fertile controls.[16,18] This may be due to the fact that only stable enzymes and byproducts of OS have been observed at the time when endometriosis is diagnosed. Another possible explanation might be that focal OS is not great enough to increase total ROS levels in peritoneal fluid. On the other hand, a study done by Murphy et al demonstrated that peritoneal fluid has significantly lower levels of vitamin E, an antioxidant, than the serum. This suggests that the peritoneal cavity has less AO protection, resulting in more susceptibility to OS. This belief can be further supported by a 2007 study by Mier-Cabrera et al. They reported the effect of vitamin C and E supplementation on peripheral OS markers such as plasma levels of malondialdehyde (MDA) and lipid hydroperoxides (LOOHs) in women with endometriosis. The authors found that levels of MDA and LOOHs were significantly lower following therapeutic intervention with vitamin C and E supplementation, although supplementation with vitamin C and E did not have any effect on pregnancy rates after therapy.[19]

Researchers have noted that the mitochondrial gene in endometriotic tissue becomes rearranged after its deletion. Ectopic and eutopic endometrium have exhibited differential gene expression, including 904 differentially expressed genes and differential expression of the glutathione-S-transferase gene family, which is involved in glutathione antioxidant metabolism. Cell proliferation and angiogenesis are cellular responses to OS that also may be determined by differential gene expression.[20] Also, free radicals such as NO and hydrogen peroxide activate transcriptional factor, nuclear factor κβ, and activator protein 1, which mediate the expression of cell adhesion molecules involved in cell–cell and cell-tissue binding.[21] Expression of cell adhesion molecules is a very important phenomenon for the initiation and progression of the adhesion process between ectopic endometrial and mesothelium tissue.

ROS and Antioxidants

Reactive oxygen species such as superoxide anion, hydrogen peroxide, and the hydroxyl radical are types of oxidants that can attack biomolecules such as lipids, proteins, and nucleic acids. Antioxidants, on the other hand, can help prevent that damage. There are two types: enzymatic antioxidants such as catalase and SOD and non-enzymatic antioxidants such as vitamin C and glutathione.[22] Antioxidants stabilize ROS by donating electrons to oxygen-based free radicals.[23] In the follicular fluid of healthy patients, antioxidants protect oocytes from ROS damage. In endometriosis, ROS production increases due to stimulated peritoneal fluid mononuclear cells and macrophages.[24] In some instances, the peritoneal fluid in women with endometriosis contains increased concentrations of NO and inducible nitric oxide synthase (iNOS)

activity. Abnormally elevated NO concentrations, as generated by activated macrophages, can counteract fertility by altering: the composition of the peritoneal fluid environment, processes of ovulation, gamete transport, sperm oocyte interaction, fertilization, and early embryonic development.[25] It has been shown that the peritoneal fluid nitrite and nitrate content is higher in women with endometriosis. Interferon-alpha and interferon –gamma with lipopolysaccharide (LPS) can activate macrophages in the endometriotic peritoneal fluid and increase iNOS and NO production. Levels of oxidatively modified lipid–protein complexes, which are strong chemotaxins for monocytes and inducers of cytokine secretion in the peritoneal fluid of women with endometriosis, are also increased.[13]

Nitric oxide regulates endometrial stromal edema production, which is an important step for endometrial growth during the menstrual cycle, embryo implantation, and uterine contraction. In healthy fertile women, contractions in the subendometrial myometrium vary with the phases of menstrual cycle, but in women with endometriosis, uterine hyperperistalsis and dysperistalsis have been observed.[13] Excessive NO production might disturb uterine contractions and tubal function, impairing fertilization and implantation in the process, and lead to spontaneous abortion and compromised fecundity.

For uterine receptivity, integrin alpha V beta 3 is the best adhesive molecule marker. Its levels and those of eNOS have the same expression patterns throughout the menstrual cycle.[13] Both are located predominantly in endometrial glandular epithelium. In cases of endometriosis, however, when eNOS expression in glandular and luminal epithelium increases, integrin alpha V beta 3 expression decreases.[13] The prominent increase in eNOS during the mid-luteal phase and the decrease in integrin alpha V beta 3 lead to implantation difficulties in endometriosis. Since NO can induce endometrial cell apoptosis, high NO levels in the endometrium may also impair embryo implantation and development.[13]

The endometrium of women with endometriosis has been described to have elevated levels of NO and NOS[25] and increased expression of NOS. Altered NOS expression may affect endometrial receptivity and hinder embryo implantation. Deviations in endothelial NOS gene expression also may induce endometrial angiogenesis, thereby facilitating the development of endometriosis.[25]

Increased expression of manganese and copper/zinc SOD (defensive enzymes) has been seen in the endometrium of women with endometriosis and adenomyosis throughout the menstrual cycle.[13] In addition, aberrant expressions of glutathione peroxidase and xanthine oxidase have been found in both eutopic and ectopic endometrium.[13] This change in antioxidant enzyme levels may lead to significant OS in endometriosis.

Circulating levels of OS from other sources, such as the endometrium and ectopic endometrial implants, may also contribute to the pathogenesis of endometriosis. The endometria of patients with endometriosis have an increased lipid-protein complex modification resulting in high lipid peroxide concentrations.[11,17] The epitopes that are produced as a result of lipid peroxidation have been found in macrophage-enriched areas of both the endometrium and endometriosis implants.[26] One study showed that high levels of various antioxidants inhibit the proliferation of endometrial stromal cells and that moderate levels of OS promote endometrial stromal cell proliferation. It also was found that the highest tested level of OS inhibits proliferation. This can be attributed to the biphasic dose-response to OS in which only moderate doses of ROS instigate growth/proliferation, whereas higher doses cannot, due to direct cytotoxic effects and higher rates of apoptosis.[27]

Serum paraoxonase-1 is a high-density lipoprotein (HDL)-associated enzyme that prevents oxidative modification of low-density lipoprotein (LDL). A study conducted by Verit et al in 2008 compared serum PON-1 activity in women with endometriosis with that of healthy controls.[28] Serum PON-1 activity, LOOH levels, serum triglyceride (TG), total cholesterol (TC), HDL, and LDL levels were measured. PON-1 activity was significantly lower and LOOH levels were significantly higher in women with moderate to severe endometriosis than in women with mild endometriosis and controls. Also, lower PON-1 activity was observed in women with mild endometriosis compared with controls. A significant negative correlation was found between PON-1 activity and stage of the disease. PON-1 activity and HDL levels were decreased, whereas levels of LOOH, TG, TC, and LDL were higher in all women with endometriosis than in, controls. Reduced serum PON-1 activity and increased LOOH levels are pieces of evidence suggesting that OS plays a role in the pathophysiology of endometriosis. PON-1 activity can be used indirectly to detect endometriosis, but an official diagnosis requires histopathologic confirmation.

Role of Iron

Erythrocytes from retrograde menstruation yield the pro-inflammatory factors hemoglobin and heme, which contain the redox-generating iron molecule.[29] The presence of iron[12]—as well as macrophages[13] and environmental contaminants such as polychlorinated biphenyls[30]—may disrupt the balance between ROS and antioxidants in the peritoneal fluid. Iron-overload provokes iron-mediated damage, oxidative injury, and inflammation, leading to pathogenesis of endometriosis.

In the case of endometriosis, the source of iron overload in the pelvic cavity is a result of pelvic erythrocyte lysis. Under normal conditions; the pelvic cavity has protective mechanisms to counteract the reflux of erythrocytes. However, it has been suggested that women with endometriosis have strained peritoneal protective mechanisms due to one of two hypotheses: (1) abundance of reflux or (2) defective AO capacity. The result is iron accumulation. Studies indicate that blood from bleeding lesions in the ectopic endometrium contribute significantly to the abundant erythrocyte population.[5,31] Experimental mouse model studies mimicking retrograde menstruation conditions and lesion bleeding have confirmed the origin of iron overload in the pelvic cavity. In one study, endometriosis was induced in nude mice by injection. Iron deposits similar to those found in human endometriosis were observed in lesions that had been induced with injected menstrual effluent or endometrial cells with erythrocytes.[5,32,33] Peritoneal macrophages phagocytize a number of erythrocytes entering the pelvic cavity. Heme-oxygenase 1 (HO-1) metabolizes hemoglobin and releases iron. Iron is incorporated into the macrophages as ferritin or is released into peritoneal fluid where it binds with Tf, an iron transporter.

Defrere et al demonstrated that ectopic endometrial cells can incorporate Tf and metabolize it into ferritin.[32] This concept was further demonstrated by Mizuuchi et al. who studied the expression of transferrin receptor (TfR) by endometrial cells.[34] Numerous studies and murine endometriosis models all have observed the presence of iron conglomerates in endometriotic lesions. Additionally, ectopic lesions in the peritoneal cavity release Hp. Hemoglobin released by erythrocytes binds Hp to form Hb-Hp complex. This complex is endocytosed by macrophages, which become saturated with Hp, thereby signifying strain on peritoneal protective mechanisms.

In endometriosis, the number of peritoneal macrophages is increased and they are also more highly activated, resulting in chronic inflammation. Oxidative injury occurs when iron is continuously delivered to peritoneal macrophages, preventing ferritin from storing and sequestering iron. Consequently, iron generates free radicals and disrupts the balance between ROS production and antioxidant defense, and OS ensues.

In 2003, Wagener et al studied the HO-1 detoxification system to demonstrate the association between iron overload and subsequent OS contributing to endometriosis. Heme plays a critical role in a wide variety of enzymes and also enhances gene expression. In respect to endometriosis, the concentration of HO-1, a heme-degrading enzyme, is low due to poor expression by macrophages and mesothelial cells. HO-1 functions to degrade heme and generate CO, bilirubin, and ferritin. These degradation products serve as a defense mechanism by detoxifying and protecting against adverse effects of oxidative stress. Consequently, low HO-1 concentrations seen in endometriosis result in an impaired detoxifying system and subsequent OS.

Oxidative stress might cause local damage to the peritoneal mesothelium.[30, 35] Normally, the mesothelium lining serves as a protective barrier to the adhesion of menstrual endometrial fragments. However, because of its fragile state, the mesothelium can easily be disrupted in the presence of OS, resulting in adhesion sites on the surface. Demir et al showed that the menstrual effluent factor iron-binding protein Hb is harmful to mesothelium.[36] This supports the above theory since iron is a known factor that induces OS, causing macromolecular oxidative damage, tissue injury, and chronic inflammation.[37]

Iron overload further contributes to the development of endometriosis by promoting epithelial cell proliferation. Defere et al created a murine endometriosis model to study the effect of iron overload on ectopic endometrium.[32] The study demonstrated how an erythrocyte injection increased the proliferative activity of epithelial cells in endometriotic lesion whereas desferrioxamine (DFO) administration drastically inhibited it.

Reactive oxygen species affect the regulation of the transcriptional factor, NF-kB.[38] NF-kB is responsible for the expression of proinflammatory cytokines, growth factor, angiogenic factor, adhesion molecules, and inducible enzymes iNOS and COX-2.[39] These products all play a role in the development of endometriosis by inducing endometrial fragment adhesion, proliferation, and neovascularization.[40] A study by Lousse *et al* found that NF-kB activity in peritoneal macrophages from patients with endometriosis was significantly higher than that in controls **(Figure 5-1)**.[41]

Role of TNF-α in Pathogenesis of Endometriosis

Tumor necrosis factor-alpha (TNF-α), a pleiotropic cytokine, is produced and activated by a number of cell types including, but not limited to, neutrophils,

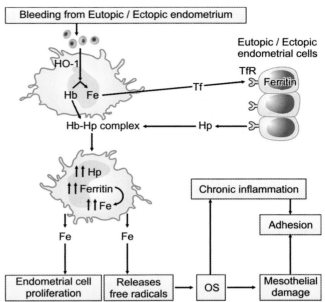

FIGURE 5-1: Chronic inflammation and adhesions in endometriosis. Bleeding from eutopic and ectopic endometrium causes release of erythrocytes into the peritoneal cavity. Peritoneal macrophages phagocytose erythrocytes. HO-1 metabolizes Hb component of erythrocytes and subsequently releases Fe. Fe is transported via Tf to bind TfR on eutopic and ectopic endometrial cells. Once bound, it is incorporated into ferritin. Eutopic and ectopic endometrial cells synthesize Hp. Hb is released from the peritoneal macropahge to bind Hp, forming the Hb-Hp complex. Macrophages phagocytose the Hb-Hp complex to become saturated, thereby impairing the peritoneal protective mechanism, resulting in increased Hp, ferritin and Fe. The consequent release of Fe from saturated macrophages results in chronic inflammation and OS, ultimately leading to adhesions. HO-1: heme oxygenase-1; Hb: hemoglobing; Fe: iron; Tf: transferrin; TfR: transferrin receptor; Hp: haptoglobin; Hb-Hp complex: hemoglobin-haptoglobin complex; OS: oxidative stress

lymphocytes, and macrophages. TNF-α is a major pro-inflammatory cytokine known to impair glutathione (GSH) production by several mechanisms, creating an environment conducive to the development of OS. This pathogenic cycle of GSH disturbances and enhanced TNF-α production may be active in the female reproductive tract in endometriosis. An *in vitro* study investigating endometriosis-associated infertility has shown that spermatozoa quality decreases following incubation with TNF-α in a dose- and time-dependent manner.[42]

The actions of TNF-α include the activation of Th cells,[43] upregulation of metallomatrix proteins in concert with IL-1,[44] instigation of angiogenic and cytotoxic effects on targets in concert with IL-1 and IL-6, attraction of neutrophils and stimulation of neutrophil adhesion to endothelial cells, and the production of IL-1, oxidants and PGE2.[44] Tumor necrosis factor-alpha secretion is stimulated by IL-1 and bacterial endotoxin.[44] When mediated by IL-8, TNF-α has been known to promote the growth of endometriotic cells.[45] Elevated levels of peritoneal fluid TNF-α have been associated with endometriosis.[46-49]in comparison with women who do not have the disease or women with idiopathic infertility.[44] Higher concentrations of TNF-α receptors (TNFR), both sTNFR-1 and sTNFR-II, have been found in the peritoneal fluid of endometriotic patients as well.[44] Tumor necrosis factor-alpha has not been associated with the severity or stage of the disease.[50] However, a lower frequency of TNF-α 1031 c polymorphism in the promoter region of the TNF-α gene was found in the most severe cases of endometriosis in a Japanese study, suggesting that the polymorphism has a protective mechanism.[51] Peritoneal fluid TNF-α, along with IL-6, was found by Bedaiwy and colleagues to be both a sensitive and specific marker for diagnosing individuals with and without the disease—at a level of 15 pg/mL, the sensitivity was 100% and the specificity was 89%; at a level of 20 pg/mL, the sensitivity was 96% and the specificity was 95%.[50]

Interleukin 6

Interleukin 6 (IL-6) not only regulates cytokine secretion, but also plays an important role in implantation events and endometrial cell growth regulation.[43] Interleukin 6 is produced in monocytes, macrophages, endothelial cells, vascular smooth-muscle cells, and endometrial epithelial stromal cells.[52] IL-6 and other inflammatory cytokines have been suggested to contribute to the maintenance of peritoneal endometriosis.[53]

A study conducted by Sharpe-Timms et al sought to demonstrate the relationship between IL-6 and endometriosis. Endometriotic tissue is a biochemically active tissue that secretes and synthesizes numerous proteins. Of interest are the endometriosis proteins (Endo), in particular Endo-I, which is a unique form of haptoglobin requiring IL-6 for maximal expression. Haptoglobin (Hp) is predominantly synthesized by the liver in response to inflammation or injury;[54] however, a variety of other tissues have been demonstrated to synthesize Hp,[55-63] including endometriotic lesions. Endo-I differentiates itself from hepatic Hp in that it is secreted in a glycosylated form.[55] The alteration in the pattern of protein glycosylation initiates the phagocytic process and allows Endo-I to bind to peritoneal macrophages,[64] thereby initiating the immune response seen in women with endometriosis. When bound

to peritoneal macrophages, Endo-I blocks macrophage phagocytic capacity by interfering with adherence. Altered macrophage function elicits production of inflammatory mediators, such as IL-1, IL-6, and TNF-alpha.[65-67] In turn, these cytokines function to upregulate the expression of Endo-I, creating a positive feed-forward loop between endometriotic haptoglobin and IL-6.[68] Interleukin 1 (IL-1) in peritoneal fluid instigates IL-6 production, and therefore exacerbates the inflammatory effects of IL-6.[44] The concentration of IL-6 in peritoneal fluid was found to be significantly higher in women with endometriosis than in control subjects[69] and could be used to differentiate between women with and without the disease with a high specificity (67%) and sensitivity (90%).[50] Levels of IL-6 are also significantly higher in women with a large number of implants.[70] Interleukin 6 has also been found to be elevated in the serum of women with endometriosis,[71] as IL-6 is produced by both eutopic and ectopic endometrium. However, using serum levels as an independent tool has limited value in predicting the disease.[72]

Role of Leptin in Endometriosis

Leptin is considered a class I cytokine due to its role in cell growth and maturation.[73] It is produced mainly in adipose tissue, but also in human ovarian follicles (both granulosa and cumulus cells), placenta, stomach, and skeletal muscle. Leptin receptors are found in a plethora of tissues including endothelial cells,[74] T cells,[75] and endometrium.[76] Leptin expression is inhibited by testosterone and increased by ovarian sex steroids.[77]

Although leptin helps regulate food intake and plays a role in energy balance and hematopoesis, peritoneal fluid levels have been positively correlated with stage III and IV endometriosis[73] and chronic co-morbid pelvic pain.[72] However, no correlation was found with leptin levels and infertility associated with endometriosis[72] or ovarian endometriosis.[73] A possible explanation of the difference is that leptin is free to diffuse into the peritoneal fluid in peritoneal endometriosis, whereas it is sequestrated in the cystic fluid of ovarian endometriomata.[78] Leptin has been found to promote neoangiogenic activity by up-regulation of VEGF.[79] The cytokine also promotes the invasion of the extracellular matrix by ectopic endometriotic stromal cells via increased expression of matrix metalloproteinases,[77] bcl2, and intercellular adhesion molecule.[77] Leptin is produced during the acute phase inflammatory response and acts as a c reactive protein and IL-1 beta during systemic inflammation and fever.[80] Furthermore, levels of leptin significantly increase in response to acute infection and sepsis and have an instigating effect on CD4+ T cell lymphocyte proliferation, macrophage phagocytosis, and IL-1 and TNF-α (both inflammatory cytokines) secretion.[77] Hypoxia inducible factor-1α (HIF-1α), working in conjunction with pro-inflammatory cytokines such as IL-1β and prostaglandins, increases levels of leptin in ectopic endometriotic stromal cells due to hypoxic stress (<1% O_2) in the peritoneal cavity.[81]

Conclusion

Oxidative stress plays an integral role in the pathogenesis of endometriosis resulting from increased free radical generation and/or decreased levels of scavenging antioxidants. Whether there is a cause–effect relationship between free radical excess and the pathophysiology of these conditions or a temporal one remains to be demonstrated. Regardless, it appears reasonable to investigate the role of antioxidant agents in both the prevention and treatment of endometriosis. They may help ameliorate the extent of lesions and help reduce the severity of symptoms and any subsequent complications that develop. Thus, the identification of OS markers or markers of altered immune function such as IL-6, TNF-alpha, IL-8, IL-1 beta and PON-1 in the serum and peritoneal fluid as a noninvasive option for diagnosing the disease and gauging its severity is important but is still investigational. Further, iron overload contributes to the development of endometriosis by promoting epithelial cell proliferation, and the role DFO plays in inhibiting lesion growth represents an exciting new avenue of research.

References

1. Eltabbakh GH, Bower NA. Laparoscopic surgery in endometriosis. Minerva Ginecol. 2008;60:323-30.
2. Falcone T, Mascha E. The elusive diagnostic test for endometriosis. Fertil Steril. 2003;80:886-88.
3. Seli E, Berkkanoglu M, Arici A. Pathogenesis of endometriosis. Obstet Gynecol Clin North Am. 2003;30:41-61.
4. Giudice LC, Kao LC. Endometriosis. Lancet. 2004;364:1789-99.
5. Halme J, Hammond MG, Hulka JF, Raj SG, Talbert LM. Retrograde menstruation in healthy women and in patients with endometriosis. Obstet Gynecol. 1984;64:151-54.
6. Chapron C, Chopin N, Borghese B, Foulot H, Dousset B, Vacher-Lavenu MC, et al. Deeply infiltrating endometriosis: pathogenetic implications of the anatomical distribution. Hum Reprod. 2006;21:1839-45.
7. D'Hooghe TM, Bambra CS, Raeymaekers BM, De Jonge I, Lauweryns JM, Koninckx PR. Intrapelvic injection of menstrual endometrium causes endometriosis in baboons (Papio cynocephalus and Papio anubis). Am J Obstet Gynecol. 1995;173:125-34.
8. Te LR, Scott RB. Experimental endometriosis. Am J Obstet Gynecol. 1950;60:1147-73.
9. Mungyer G, Willemsen WN, Rolland R, Vemer HM, Ramaekers FC, Jap PH, et al. Cell of the mucous membrane of the female genital tract in culture: a comparative study with regard to the histogenesis of endometriosis. In Vitro Cell Dev Biol. 1987;23:111-17.
10. Park JK, Song M, Dominguez CE, Walter MF, Santanam N, Parthasarathy S, et al. Glycodelin mediates the increase in vascular endothelial growth factor in response to oxidative stress in the endometrium. Am J Obstet Gynecol. 2006;195:1772-77.
11. Szczepanska M, Kozlik J, Skrzypczak J, Mikolajczyk M. Oxidative stress may be a piece in the endometriosis puzzle. Fertil Steril. 2003;79:1288-93.
12. Agarwal A, Allamaneni SS. Role of free radicals in female reproductive diseases and assisted reproduction. Reprod Biomed Online. 2004;9:338-47.
13. Alpay Z, Saed GM, Diamond MP. Female infertility and free radicals: potential role in adhesions and endometriosis. J Soc Gynecol Investig. 2006;13:390-98.
14. Shanti A, Santanam N, Morales AJ, Parthasarathy S, Murphy AA. Autoantibodies to markers of oxidative stress are elevated in women with endometriosis. Fertil Steril. 1999;71:1115-18.
15. Arumugam K, Dip YC. Endometriosis and infertility: the role of exogenous lipid peroxides in the peritoneal fluid. Fertil Steril 1995;63:198-99.
16. Wang Y, Sharma RK, Falcone T, Goldberg J, Agarwal A. Importance of reactive oxygen species in the peritoneal fluid of women with endometriosis or idiopathic infertility. Fertil Steril. 1997;68:826-30.
17. Polak G, Koziol-Montewka M, Niedzwiadek J, Tarkowski R, Sidor-Wojtowicz A, Kotarski J. [Lipid peroxides, tumor necrosis factor alpha (TNF-alpha) and interferon gamma (IFN-gamma) in peritoneal fluid from infertile women with minimal and mild endometriosis]. Ginekol Pol. 2001;72:422-26.
18. Ho HN, Wu MY, Chen SU, Chao KH, Chen CD, Yang YS. Total antioxidant status and nitric oxide do not increase in peritoneal fluids from women with endometriosis. Hum Reprod. 1997;12:2810-15.
19. Mier-Cabrera J, Genera-Garcia M, De la Jara-Diaz J, Perichart-Perera O, Vadillo-Ortega F, Hernandez-Guerrero C. Effect of vitamins C and E supplementation on peripheral oxidative stress markers and pregnancy rate in women with endometriosis. Int J Gynaecol Obstet. 2008;100:252-56.
20. Wu Y, Kajdacsy-Balla A, Strawn E, Basir Z, Halverson G, Jailwala P, et al. Transcriptional characterizations of differences between eutopic and ectopic endometrium. Endocrinology. 2006;147:232-46.
21. Defrere S, Donnez J, Moulin P, Befahy P, Gonzalez-Ramos R, Lousse JC, et al. Expression of intercellular adhesion molecule-1 and vascular cell adhesion molecule-1 in human endometrial stromal and epithelial cells is regulated by interferon-gamma but not iron. Gynecol Obstet Invest. 2008;65:145-54.

22. Sikka SC. Role of oxidative stress and antioxidants in andrology and assisted reproductive technology. J Androl. 2004;25:5-18.

23. Gupta S, Agarwal A, Krajcir N, Alvarez JG. Role of oxidative stress in endometriosis. Reprod Biomed Online. 2006;13:126-34.

24. Zeller JM, Henig I, Radwanska E, Dmowski WP. Enhancement of human monocyte and peritoneal macrophage chemiluminescence activities in women with endometriosis. Am J Reprod Immunol Microbiol. 1987;13:78-82.

25. Gupta S, Agarwal A, Agarwal R, Loret de Mola JR. Impact of ovarian endometrioma on assisted reproduction outcomes. Reprod Biomed Online. 2006;13:349-60.

26. Murphy AA, Santanam N, Parthasarathy S. Endometriosis: a disease of oxidative stress? Semin Reprod Endocrinol. 1998;16:263-73.

27. Foyozi N, Berkkanoglu M, Arici A, Kwintkiewicz J, Izquierdo D, Duleba AJ. Effects of oxidants and antioxidants on proliferation of endometrial stromal cells. Fertil Steril 2004;82 Suppl 3: 1019-22.

28. Verit FF, Erel O, Celik N. Serum paraoxonase-1 activity in women with endometriosis and its relationship with the stage of the disease. Hum Reprod. 2008 ;23:100-04.

29. Reubinoff B, Shushan A. Preimplantation diagnosis in older patients, To biopsy or not to biopsy? Hum Reprod. 1996;11:2071-75.

30. Van Langendonckt A, Casanas-Roux F, Donnez J. Oxidative stress and peritoneal endometriosis. Fertil Steril. 2002;77:861-70.

31. D'Hooghe TM, Debrock S. Endometriosis, retrograde menstruation and peritoneal inflammation in women and in baboons. Hum Reprod Update. 2002;8:84-88.

32. Defrere S, Van Langendonckt A, Vaesen S, Jouret M, Gonzalez Ramos R, Gonzalez D, et al. Iron overload enhances epithelial cell proliferation in endometriotic lesions induced in a murine model. Hum Reprod. 2006;21:2810-16.

33. Van Langendonckt A, Casanas-Roux F, Eggermont J, Donnez J. Characterization of iron deposition in endometriotic lesions induced in the nude mouse model. Hum Reprod. 2004;19:1265-71.

34. Mizuuchi H, Kudo R, Tamura H, Tsukahara K, Tsumura N, Kumai K, et al. Identification of transferrin receptor in cervical and endometrial tissues. Gynecol Oncol. 1988;31:292-300.

35. Arumugam K, Yip YC. De novo formation of adhesions in endometriosis: the role of iron and free radical reactions. Fertil Steril. 1995;64:62-64.

36. Demir AY, Demol H, Puype M, de Goeij AF, Dunselman GA, Herrler A, et al. Proteome analysis of human mesothelial cells during epithelial to mesenchymal transitions induced by shed menstrual effluent. Proteomics. 2004;4:2608-23.

37. Hippeli S, Elstner EF. Transition metal ion-catalyzed oxygen activation during pathogenic processes. FEBS Lett. 1999;443:1-7.

38. Dalton TP, Shertzer HG, Puga A. Regulation of gene expression by reactive oxygen. Annu Rev Pharmacol Toxicol. 1999;39:67-101.

39. Viatour P, Merville MP, Bours V, Chariot A. Phosphorylation of NF-kappaB and IkappaB proteins: implications in cancer and inflammation. Trends Biochem Sci. 2005; 30(1):43-52.

40. Lebovic DI, Mueller MD, Taylor RN. Immunobiology of endometriosis. Fertil Steril. 2001;75:1-10.

41. Lousse JC, Defrere S, Van Langendonckt A, Gras J, Gonzalez-Ramos R, Colette S, et al. Iron storage is significantly increased in peritoneal macrophages of endometriosis patients and correlates with iron overload in peritoneal fluid. Fertil Steril. 2008

42. Said TM, Agarwal A, Falcone T, Sharma RK, Bedaiwy MA, Li L. Infliximab may reverse the toxic effects induced by tumor necrosis factor alpha in human spermatozoa: an in vitro model. Fertil Steril. 2005;83:1665-73.

43. Siristatidis C, Nissotakis C, Chrelias C, Iacovidou H, Salamalekis E. Immunological factors and their role in the genesis and development of endometriosis. J Obstet Gynaecol Res. 2006;32:162-70.

44. Gupta S, Agarwal A, Sekhon L, Krajcir N, Cocuzza M, Falcone T. Serum and peritoneal abnormalities in endometriosis: potential use as diagnostic markers. Minerva Ginecol. 2006;58:527-51.

45. Iwabe T, Harada T, Tsudo T, Nagano Y, Yoshida S, Tanikawa M, et al. Tumor necrosis factor-alpha promotes proliferation of endometriotic stromal cells by inducing interleukin-8 gene and protein expression. J Clin Endocrinol Metab. 2000;85:824-29.

46. Eisermann J, Gast MJ, Pineda J, Odem RR, Collins JL. Tumor necrosis factor in peritoneal fluid of women undergoing laparoscopic surgery. Fertil Steril. 1988;50: 573-79.

47. Overton C, Fernandez-Shaw S, Hicks B, Barlow D, Starkey P. Peritoneal fluid cytokines and the relationship with endometriosis and pain. Hum Reprod. 1996 ;11:380-86.

48. Taketani Y, Kuo TM, Mizuno M. Comparison of cytokine levels and embryo toxicity in peritoneal fluid in infertile women with untreated or treated endometriosis. Am J Obstet Gynecol. 1992;167:265-70.

49. Mori H, Sawairi M, Nakagawa M, Itoh N, Wada K, Tamaya T. Peritoneal fluid interleukin-1 beta and tumor necrosis factor in patients with benign gynecologic disease. Am J Reprod Immunol. 1991;26:62-67.

50. Bedaiwy MA, Falcone T, Sharma RK, Goldberg JM, Attaran M, Nelson DR, et al. Prediction of endometriosis with serum and peritoneal fluid markers: a prospective controlled trial. Hum Reprod. 2002;17:426-31.

51. Asghar T, Yoshida S, Kennedy S, Negoro K, Zhuo W, Hamana S, et al. The tumor necrosis factor-alpha promoter -1031C polymorphism is associated with decreased risk of endometriosis in a Japanese population. Hum Reprod. 2004;19:2509-14.

52. Laird SM, Li TC, Bolton AE. The production of placental protein 14 and interleukin 6 by human endometrial cells in culture. Hum Reprod. 1993;6:793-98.

53. Rier SE, Zarmakoupis PN, Hu X, Becker JL. Dysregulation of interleukin-6 responses in ectopic endometrial stromal cells: correlation with decreased soluble receptor levels in peritoneal fluid of women with endometriosis. J Clin Endocrinol Metab. 1995;80:1431-37.

54. Pos O, van Dijk W, Ladiges N, Linthorst C, Sala M, van Tiel D, et al. Glycosylation of four acute-phase glyco-proteins secreted by rat liver cells in vivo and in vitro. Effects of inflammation and dexamethasone. Eur J Cell Biol. 1988;46:121-28.

55. Sharpe-Timms KL, Piva M, Ricke EA, Surewicz K, Zhang YL, Zimmer RL. Endometriotic lesions synthesize and secrete a haptoglobin-like protein. Biol Reprod. 1998;58:988-94.

56. Pelletier N, Boudreau F, Yu SJ, Zannoni S, Boulanger V, Asselin C. Activation of haptoglobin gene expression by cAMP involves CCAAT/enhancer-binding protein isoforms in intestinal epithelial cells. FEBS Lett. 1998;439:275-80.

57. D'Armiento J, Dalal SS, Chada K. Tissue, temporal and inducible expression pattern of haptoglobin in mice. Gene. 1997;195:19-27.

58. Olson GE, Winfrey VP, Matrisian PE, Melner MH, Hoffman LH. Specific expression of haptoglobin mRNA in implantation-stage rabbit uterine epithelium. J Endocrinol. 1997;152:69-80.

59. O'Bryan MK, Grima J, Mruk D, Cheng CY. Haptoglobin is a Sertoli cell product in the rat seminiferous epithelium: its purification and regulation. J Androl. 1997;18:637-45.

60. Hoffman LH, Winfrey VP, Blaeuer GL, Olson GE. A haptoglobin-like glycoprotein is produced by implantation-stage rabbit endometrium. Biol Reprod. 1996;55:176-84.

61. Kliffen M, de Jong PT, Luider TM. Protein analysis of human maculae in relation to age-related maculopathy. Lab Invest. 1995;73:267-72.

62. Friedrichs WE, Navarijo-Ashbaugh AL, Bowman BH, Yang F. Expression and inflammatory regulation of haptoglobin gene in adipocytes. Biochem Biophys Res Commun. 1995;209:250-56.

63. Yang F, Friedrichs WE, Navarijo-Ashbaugh AL, deGraffenried LA, Bowman BH, Coalson JJ. Cell type-specific and inflammatory-induced expression of haptoglobin gene in lung. Lab Invest. 1995;73:433-40.

64. Aderem A, Underhill DM. Mechanisms of phagocytosis in macrophages. Annu Rev Immunol. 1999;17:593-623.

65. Oh SK, Ross S, Walker J, Zeisel S. Role of a SER immune suppressor in immune surveillance. Immunology. 1988;64:73-79.

66. Yong K, Khwaja A. Leucocyte cellular adhesion molecules. Blood Rev. 1990;4:211-25.

67. Fan ST, Edgington TS. Integrin regulation of leukocyte inflammatory functions. CD11b/CD18 enhancement of the tumor necrosis factor-alpha responses of monocytes. J Immunol. 1993;150:2972-80.

68. Piva M, Horowitz GM, Sharpe-Timms KL. Interleukin-6 differentially stimulates haptoglobin production by peritoneal and endometriotic cells in vitro: a model for endometrial-peritoneal interaction in endometriosis. J Clin Endocrinol Metab. 2001;86:2553-61.

69. Punnonen J, Teisala K, Ranta H, Bennett B, Punnonen R. Increased levels of interleukin-6 and interleukin-10 in the peritoneal fluid of patients with endometriosis. Am J Obstet Gynecol. 1996;174:1522-26.

70. Mahnke JL, Dawood MY, Huang JC. Vascular endothelial growth factor and interleukin-6 in peritoneal fluid of women with endometriosis. Fertil Steril. 2000;73:166-70.

71. Seeber B, Sammel MD, Fan X, Gerton GL, Shaunik A, Chittams J, et al. Panel of markers can accurately predict endometriosis in a subset of patients. Fertil Steril. 2008;89:1073-81.

72. Bedaiwy MA, Falcone T, Goldberg JM, Sharma RK, Nelson DR, Agarwal A. Peritoneal fluid leptin is associated with chronic pelvic pain but not infertility in endometriosis patients. Hum Reprod. 2006;21:788-91.

73. Wertel I, Gogacz M, Polak G, Jakowicki J, Kotarski J. Leptin is not involved in the pathophysiology of endometriosis-related infertility. Eur J Obstet Gynecol Reprod Biol. 2005;119:206-09.

74. Sierra-Honigmann MR, Nath AK, Murakami C, Garcia-Cardena G, Papapetropoulos A, Sessa WC, et al. Biological action of leptin as an angiogenic factor. Science. 1998;281:1683-86.

75. Lord GM, Matarese G, Howard JK, Baker RJ, Bloom SR, Lechler RI. Leptin modulates the T-cell immune response and reverses starvation-induced immunosuppression. Nature. 1998;394:897-901.

76. Kitawaki J, Koshiba H, Ishihara H, Kusuki I, Tsukamoto K, Honjo H. Expression of leptin receptor in human endometrium and fluctuation during the menstrual cycle. J Clin Endocrinol Metab. 2000;85:1946-50.

77. La Cava A, Alviggi C, Matarese G. Unraveling the multiple roles of leptin in inflammation and autoimmunity. J Mol Med. 2004;82:4-11.

78. De Placido G, Alviggi C, Carravetta C, Pisaturo ML, Sanna V, Wilding M, et al. The peritoneal fluid concentration of leptin is increased in women with peritoneal but not ovarian endometriosis. Hum Reprod. 2001;16:1251-54.

79. Styer AK, Sullivan BT, Puder M, Arsenault D, Petrozza JC, Serikawa T, et al. Ablation of leptin signaling disrupts the establishment, development, and maintenance of endometriosis-like lesions in a murine model. Endocrinology. 2008;149:506-14.

80. Matarese G, Alviggi C, Sanna V, Howard JK, Lord GM, Carravetta C, et al. Increased leptin levels in serum and peritoneal fluid of patients with pelvic endometriosis. J Clin Endocrinol Metab. 2000;85:2483-87.

81. Wu MH, Chen KF, Lin SC, Lgu CW, Tsai SJ. Aberrant expression of leptin in human endometriotic stromal cells is induced by elevated levels of hypoxia inducible factor-1alpha. Am J Pathol. 2007;170:590-98.

Sun-Wei Guo

Chapter 6

Relevance of Genetics to Endometriosis

Summary

There is a burgeoning interest in the identification of susceptibility genes or DNA variants that predispose women to endometriosis. However, progress has been painfully slow. In this article, I shall examine premises and assumptions behind the endeavor to hunt endometriosis susceptibility genes, expose complexities in the genotype-phenotype relationship in endometriosis, and discuss the relevance of genetic research in endometriosis.

Introduction

In the 2002 American Society of Reproductive Medicine annual meeting held in Seattle, a rather confident prediction was made that within about five years, at least one endometriosis susceptibility gene will be identified. Seven years have since passed mercilessly, yet so far not a single gene has ever been or is close to be identified. This failed prediction seems to echo Niels Bohr's famous quote: "Prediction is very difficult, especially about the future".

Difficulty in predicting future aside, for an enigmatic disease such as endometriosis for which etiology is poorly understood and, consequently, there is a pressing need for novel efficacious therapeutics with low side-effects profile, an interesting issue is why the prediction failed to materialize in the first place, or whether this prediction will ever, albeit belatedly, be materialized at all. Indeed, there is a burgeoning interest in the identification of genes or DNA variants that predispose women to endometriosis. A PubMed search with the words "endometriosis" and "polymorphism" showed that, starting from 1996, in which the first report on genetic association of endometriosis with GSTM1 polymorphism was published,[1] the number of publication has since grown roughly exponentially **(Figure 6-1)**.

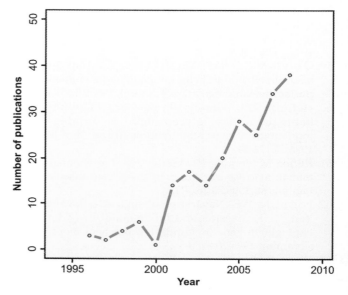

FIGURE 6-1: Growth of publications on endometriosis and polymorphisms. The number in 2008 was projected based on the number of publications indexed in PubMed in the first half of 2008 and doubled it.

Has any headway been made in the identification of endometriosis susceptibility genes ever since? Has the genetic research of endometriosis helped better understand the pathogenesis of endometriosis in any way as promised? What prevented the materialization of the ill-fated prediction? What is the relevance of genetics to endometriosis research? These issues are obviously relevant to endometriosis research. In this paper, I will go over these issues.

Appeals of Identification of Endometriosis Susceptibility Genes

Endometriosis is believed to be a polygenic disease, and, as such, genes or genetic variants that predispose women to endometriosis can be identified through genetic linkage or association studies.[2] Once a major gene or genes are identified, the characterization of their functions would in theory not only help better understand genotype-phenotype interactions but also enhance the development of specific therapies and/or preventative measures and identification of those women at increased risk of developing endometriosis.[2] It is also hoped that once the risk of particular combinations of genotype and environmental exposure is known, medical interventions such as change in lifestyle, could then be instituted to target high-risk groups or individuals, with the aim of preventing the disease.[3]

Conceptually, the identification of endometriosis susceptibility genes is rather straightforward, although its successful execution does require a careful study design, meticulous genotyping, and rigorous statistical analysis,[4] and would demand substantial resources upfront. Linkage studies identify genes of interest through DNA markers physically linked with the putative genes in pedigree data.[5] The association studies, on the other hand, identify genes of interest through identification of correlations between genetic variants and phenotypic differences on a population scale, often through the detection of differential genotypic frequencies in cases and controls.[6]

With rapid advances in genomic technology, both the speed and throughput of genotyping have been greatly improved while the cost of genotyping per sample has decreased substantially. This, along with the conceptual simplicity and the promised huge payoff, makes the genetic approach to endometriosis a very attractive one to many investigators who are dissatisfied with the slow progress in endometriosis research.

A Reality Check: Much Ado about too Little?

The conceptual simplicity, coupled with readily available technologies, apparently buoyed up increasing interests, enthusiasms, and confidence in hunting down endometriosis susceptibility genes, and could well be the basis of the 2002 prediction.

However, the success or failure of either linkage or association studies hinges critically on the assumption that the disease of interest has a genetic, or, more precisely, *hereditary*, component. For complex diseases such as endometriosis in which both genes and environments may be involved, just to show, beyond reasonable doubts, that the disease has a hereditary component before, ironically, any genes are identified is not an easy task for outbred populations such as humans.

While some studies, through statistical modeling, confidently report that for a disease of interest a certain percentage of variation in a disease phenotype is due to genetic components and the rest to environmental counterpart, these assertions have little, if any, practical relevance since the statistical models employed often entail unchecked or simply unrealistic assumptions, such as no gene-environment interaction. Indeed, there is no such immutable law in nature that dictates that gene and environment should interact in additive or multiplicative fashion, or without any time-dependency.

In fact, Di and Guo recently questioned the strength of evidence that endometriosis has a hereditary component through the enumeration of deficiencies in familial and genetic epidemiological studies of endometriosis.[7] Not surprisingly, three meta-analyses on association of endometriosis and some genetic polymorphisms coding for dioxin detoxification enzymes and for sex steroid biosynthesis and their receptors found no evidence of association,[8-10] even though meta-analysis is known to have upward biases in risk estimates, especially the "winner's curse" of first reports.[11] A recent review of genetic association studies of endometriosis found little evidence that certain genetic polymorphisms are associated with increased risk of endometriosis.[12] Indeed, a careful review of PubMed publications would indicate that, for almost any polymorphism ever reported to be positively associated with endometriosis, sooner or later there would be one or more negative studies. Conflicting reports appear to be a hallmark of genetic association studies of endometriosis.

Against this foreground is the increasing awareness that the lack of replication is a perennial and serious problem in linkage and association studies of complex diseases such as endometriosis.[13-16] Thus, there has been a lot of heat, yet little, if at all, light has been shed on the pathogenesis of endometriosis.

So what is going on? Are these setbacks merely some inevitable potholes in the road to success, or the tip of an iceberg signaling some more serious issues?

Familial Aggregation, Heritability, and Genetics of Endometriosis: A Case Study

As Di and Guo[7] pointed out, the evidence that endometriosis has a hereditary component is far from watertight. Here, I dissect a fairly recent yet typical familial study and show some inherent challenges in demonstrating that endometriosis has a hereditary component.

Kashima et al reported a study that "demonstrate[s] a familial tendency for endometriosis and suggest that endometriosis has a genetic factor in the pathogenesis".[17] Specifically, "339 patients with endometriosis were questioned about endometriosis in their sisters". As control, 284 "healthy fertile women with no history of endometriosis" were questioned in a similar fashion. Of the 339 cases, 198 of them had a total of 251 sisters, of whom 22 had endometriosis (8.8%). In contrast, only 4 sisters were found to have endometriosis among 262 sisters of the control group (1.5%). Hence, "the relative risk of endometriosis in female siblings was 5.7", and thus the authors concluded that it suggests a genetic factor in the pathogenesis of endometriosis.[17]

While the result is certainly interesting, a closer inspection reveals that the choice of controls may not be entirely appropriate. Specifically, the cases were one generation younger than the controls (mean age of 32.3 vs. 56.3 years, a difference of 24 years). Since the prevalence of endometriosis appears to be rising worldwide,[18] the difference in prevalence among relatives of cases and controls may be attributable to, at least in part, the cohort effect, which was not adequately controlled for.

In fact, there is a telltale sign that this generation gap may be consequential: while each case had on average 251/339=0.74 sisters, her counterpart in the control group had 262/284=0.92 sisters, a difference that most likely reflects the declining birthrate in Japan. Since higher fertility is associated with younger were at first birth and higher number of births, both of which are reported to be protective against endometriosis,[19] the choice of controls is biased. The fact that all controls were fertile (e.g. parous) further underscores this point. Moreover, since symptomatic women may seek medical attention more readily if they have a relative with similar problems who had already consulted a physician, and since cases may be more diligent than controls in checking the disease status in their sisters, these may be additional biases unduly in favor of the authors' conclusion.[20]

Even if the familial aggregation of endometriosis is genuine, one important point that appears to have been often overlooked is that the familial aggregation does not necessarily suggest the existence of a susceptibility gene for endometriosis. Rather, it could be due to the familial aggregation of risk factors for endometriosis, since clustering of risk factors can also result in apparent aggregation of diseases.[21] In fact, younger age at menarche has been identified as a risk factor for endometriosis.[22] But ages at menarche in sisters have been shown to be highly correlated.[23] Body mass index, length of menstrual cycles, and the amount of menses have also been reported to be

risk factors for endometriosis but may, too, be familially correlated.[24] The most difficult challenge is to draw the inference that there is a hereditary component in the etiology of endometriosis before most, if not all, responsible genes and environmental factors are identified.

The reported heritability estimates also should be closely evaluated. For example, it is often stated that a certain percentage of variation in endometriosis prevalence is due to genetic components. However, all published heritability estimates hinge critically on rather simple mathematical models (mainly to ease computations and interpretations) that take no account of possible gene-environment interactions.[25] These models either become unidentifiable or are too complicated to be useful when gene-environment interactions are introduced, or demand data that are currently lacking.

It also should be noted that, at the molecular level, almost all diseases are genetic, in the sense that biochemical and pathological changes and ultimately clinical presentations are usually associated with structural or functional changes in genes. But these structural (e.g. genomic aberrations) or functional (e.g. expression) changes may not be hereditary and are thus not amenable for mapping or association studies.

The validity of future genetic epidemiologic study of endometriosis calls for methodological soundness and vigor that requires proper choice of controls, adjustment for ascertainment bias, and adjustment for familial aggregation of risk factors for endometriosis. As gene mapping/association studies are often an expensive undertaking, a carefully designed and meticulously executed study will save a lot of confusions in the long run.

There is also a possibility that a phenotype can be entirely genetic yet pinning down its causal genes can be practically difficult, if not impossible. This happens when the phenotype is a result of combined effects of *many* discretely segregating loci—each contributing a miniscule portion of individual effect yet collectively constituting the polygenes that contribute to the phenotype, a scenario originally depicted mathematically by RA Fisher. If this is the case, there is a perfect genetic correlation among relatives, yet identification of each individual locus would be a nightmare.

Causal Relationship between Genes and Endometriosis: Does it Exist?

There is a lingering uncertainty as whether the hereditary component, if any, is causal for the development of endometriosis. As pointed out by Noble,[26] although the word, gene, was coined by Wilhelm Johannsen in the beginning of the last century nearly a half century before the DNA structure was elucidated, the concept had existed for some time and was based on "the silent assumption [that] was made almost universally that there is a 1:1 relation between genetic factor (gene) and character".[27] In other words, it ("gene") refers to the *totality* of the inherited causes of the phenotype of interest. Yet the concept or even the definition of gene has since changed quite dramatically,[28] especially so when it comes to the issue of causation.[26] However, genes, as originally conceptualized, are not the same as the DNA sequences unless we adopt the view that the inheritance of all phenotypic variations originates exclusively from DNA sequences since genes are necessarily *the cause* of inheritable phenotypes.[26]

As extensive experiments have shown, virtually all cross-species clones do not develop into adults, suggesting that cellular machinery, besides genomic DNA, are also important to development. Indeed, what is transferred from parents to offspring is not just the DNA, egg cell machinery, for example, also is transferred. Hence it is plainly incorrect to exclude the non-DNA inheritance from this process of information transmission. It makes little sense to view the gene as operating without the rest of the cellular machinery.[26] Recall that only 1.1% of the human genome is spanned by exons, whereas 24% is in introns, with 75% of the genome being intergenic DNA.[29] There also exist multiple splice variants, multiple exons and introns, and various ways in which the DNA is folded in chromosomes. All these make the human genome structure very complex, and could be viewed as an efficient way of coding and transmitting the "real" causes of biological activity, i.e. proteins.[26] Indeed, the cell machinery does not just simply read the genomic code, it also imposes extensive patterns of marking and expression on the genome through epigenetic mechanisms.[30] Thus, looking for endometriosis susceptibility genes may overlook important sources of causality.

For genetic association studies, the purported susceptibility genes predisposing women to endometriosis are often identified through significant correlations between genetic variants and phenotypic differences on a population scale, often through the detection of differential genotypic frequencies in cases and controls.[6] However, the difference cannot completely reveal the *totality* of the functions of the identified gene(s) as we typically have little idea as what all the effects of the gene(s) are. Also, since many genetic modifications are buffered, there is a functional robustness at the organismal level.

Thus, as large numbers of genes are involved in each and every high-level function (such as in pain perception and fertility in women) and that, at that level, individual genes are also involved in many functions (e.g. progesterone receptors are expressed not only in uterus, but also in the breast and the brain), it is premature, at best, to assume that the first phenotype-genotype correlation we found for a given gene is its only or even its main function. This obviously raises some issues for the utility of an identified susceptibility gene, if any.

For complex diseases such as endometriosis, because of the likely polygenic involvement, a picture has now emerged showing that genes explain only a fraction of variation in a trait or a disease.[11] Frequently, it is found that the alleles at the putative "disease genes" often have low detectance and low penetrance, and are not necessary nor sufficient to cause disease.[11]

Complex Diseases: Emergent Properties of Molecular Networks

Research in the last few years has demonstrated that changes in DNA may not necessarily associate with the disease of interest *directly*.[31] Instead, DNA variants may act on intermediate, molecular phenotypes that in turn induce changes in the higher-order disease phenotypes.[31] Hence the key to the successful delineation of the genotype-phenotype relationship is to identify molecular phenotypes that vary in response to DNA variants that also associate with changes in disease phenotype, and this can provide the functional information necessary to not only identify and validate the susceptibility genes directly affected by DNA variants, but to understand as well the molecular networks in which such genes operate and how changes in these networks lead to changes in disease phenotypes.[31]

There is a converging view that complex diseases such as endometriosis are not simply a result of gene mutation or genetic polymorphisms. Rather, they are more likely to be emergent properties of molecular networks that are *modulated* by complex genetic loci and environmental and/or lifestyle factors.[32]

DNA variants associated with disease should be better viewed as perturbations to a biological system that ultimately result in alteration of the genomic, epigenetic, transcriptional, proteomic, and/or signaling networks in a way that increases susceptibility to disease.[33] Indeed, large-scale gene expression profiling studies have identified a large number of genes that are differentially expressed in ectopic and homologous eutopic endometrium[34] and in women with and without endometriosis.[35-37] These

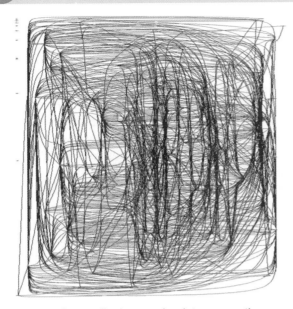

FIGURE 6-2: Astoundingly complex interconnections among 567 genes identified to be differentially expressed between ectopic and eutopic endometrium. The 567 genes were those with known names in the ~900 genes reported to be differentially expressed between ectopic and eutopic endometrium in Wu et al.[34] The network was constructed by Dr. Jonathan Wren (J Wren, Personal communication)

differentially expressed genes often form an astoundingly complex gene network **(Figure 6-2)**.

While not all these identified genes are causes of endometriosis, it is doubtful that there are only a few major susceptibility genes for endometriosis. With such a complex genetic network, it surely is a challenge to identify major susceptibility genes. Even when all these major genes are identified, the huge number of constellations of all possible genotype combinations would render risk assessment very difficult, let alone possible age-dependency, and gene-gene and gene-environment interactions. In other words, the genetic risk of developing endometriosis may be context-dependent, thus it is certainly a challenge to do personalized medicine or genotype-based interventions.

Since all functions/malfunctions in humans are system properties emerging from the network of interacting elements, the notion that there is a magic gene to cause homosexuality or endometriosis is thus questionable.

Endometriosis: An Ultimate Epigenetic Disease?

The neo-Darwinian concept of heredity dictates that the hereditary materials are written in DNA sequences and thus are impervious to lifestyle or environmental influences.

Yet as Theodosius Dobzhansky once said, "Heredity is not a status but a process". Indeed, "DNA in organisms with nuclei is in fact coated with at least an equal mass of protein, forming a complex called chromatin, which controls gene activity and the inheritance of traits".[38] "Like a puppet, DNA comes alive only when numerous proteins pull its 'strings'".[39] In eukaryotic cells, DNA is packaged into chromatin, which, together with histones, linker histones, and other functional proteins profoundly influences nuclear processes such as transcription, replication, repair and recombination.[40]

In the last decade, it became increasingly evident that the way the information is distributed along chromosomes is far more complex than previously thought.[28] As Kenneth Burke once said, "A way of seeing is also a way of not seeing—a focus upon Object A involves a neglect of Objective B."[41] The focus on sequence variation and its impact on disease risk could somehow distract our attention from other possible and perhaps more important causes, such as epigenetic aberration including methylation,[42] histone acetylation,[43] and other chromatin remodeling mechanisms.[38]

Given the wide spectrum of symptomology in endometriosis, it is unlikely one or few polymorphisms would account for all causes of endometriosis and for its variable age at onset. If susceptibility-conferring DNA variants do exist, they are either likely to be responsible for only a small portion of endometriosis, as in the case of BRCA1 to breast cancer, or are individually of small marginal importance and of high frequency, and are characterized by extensive heterogeneity. The small, likely marginal, individual effect of each of the variants will be difficult to justify for genotype-based interventions that are typically costly, difficult to execute, and uncertain in outcome.[44, 45] Hence, for majority of endometriosis cases, epigenetic aberrations are very likely the main culprit.

The curse of heterogeneity can be a blessing for epigenetic research since the hallmark of epigenetic effects on gene transcription is the variable expression of a gene in an isogenic population.[46] Since transgenerational epigenetic inheritance[47, 48] and epigenetic inheritance of environmentally induced phenotypes[49-52] have been discovered recently in mammals, including humans,[53, 54] it is likely that epigenetic aberrations may be responsible for most cases of endometriosis and for its familial aggregation.

Several lines of evidence support this notion. First, the highest estimated monozygote (MZ) concordance in affection status in endometriosis, even with a small sample size and thus potentially biased, is 75%.[55] The discordance in affection status in MZ may well be attributable to the age-dependent divergence in the epigenomes in the MZ twins.[56] Second, endometriosis displays remissions, relapses, and in some mild or superficial endometriosis even full recovery without any intervention.[57,58] This may be difficult to explain under the assumption of susceptibility-conferring DNA variants, but could be easily explained by the reversal of epigenetic changes. Third, the variable age at onset in endometriosis, while difficult to explain in genetics context, could be well explained by the age-dependent change in methylation.[59-61]

Recent studies indicate that endometriosis is an epigenetic disease, in that HOXA10 is aberrantly methylated in the endometrium of women with endometriosis,[62] that PR-B is aberrantly methylated in ectopic endometrium,[63] and that genes coding for DNA methyltransferases are aberrantly expressed in ectopic endometrium.[64] While these aberrations are indeed only associated with endometriosis, it is still possible that factors other than genetic result in epigenetic changes that eventually leads to endometriosis. One piece of evidence is the finding that in two genes that are not expressed in endometrium, significantly less methylation is observed in multiparous women with three or more children and lean (BMI<24) vs. obese women,[65] indicating that lifestyle difference (parity or body weight) result in differential epigenetic changes, which ultimately result in overt endometriosis.

Genetic Association Hang-up

A gene or DNA variant is reported to be associated with increased risk of developing endometriosis. Now what?

As the proverb goes, one swallow doesn't make a summer. Since nowadays many genes are genotyped and then analyzed in a single study, the chance for false positive results increases dramatically, especially when no attempt is made for the adjustment for multiple testing. In addition, improper choice of cases and/or controls, selective reporting, and even genotyping errors may also yield rather impressive p-values. Therefore, independent replication is needed before such reports are taken seriously. Furthermore, functional and, preferably, mechanistic data should also be needed.

One interesting feature, as noted by Di and Guo,[7] of published genetic association studies of endometriosis is that a sizeable portion of these publications is produced by a handful of prolific research teams. When a research team has collected blood samples from cases and controls

and even immortalizes the peripheral blood monocytes for future DNA extraction, it is well positioned to hunt down endometriosis-predisposing DNA variants and can keep publishing their findings. However, if after publishing over a dozen or even more positive associations over a sizeable time span it still cannot capitalize on its findings to further understand the functional significance of the association, it would effectively become a genetic association hang-up and should raise some red-flags, especially if its reported finding cannot be independently replicated or is even refuted by other research teams.

Needless to say, a genetic quest for genomic polymorphisms that predispose women to endometriosis should not stop at the successful identification of certain polymorphisms. Ideally, it should further provide functional data that prove, at first, that such a causal relationship does exist, and, second, elucidate as why and how such causal relationship is there. At the very least, efforts should be made to explore the potential utility, if any, of the identified polymorphisms in diagnosis, screening, and prognosis.

Yet the realization of any diagnostic and/or prognostic value afforded by the genetic test would require accurate genetic risk estimation, which would be prospective in nature. Sample size and the demand for resources and time aside, quantification of nongenetic contribution would be a great challenge. Even for undisputed mutations such as BRCA1 and BRCA2 that are associated with breast and ovarian cancer risk, their estimated risk may differ by as much as about twofold when birth cohort effect is accounted for.[66,67] Presumably, for a disease that is less serious yet displays more heterogeneities than breast cancer such as endometriosis, nongenetic factors may well be more pronounced.

Will Genetics Revolutionize the Diagnosis and Treatment of Endometriosis?

Even if certain DNA variants can be identified that increase disease risk, there are critics who believe that it is likely to be of limited benefit to health.[44,45,68-70] One area of debate concerns the proportion of cases of a given common disease that might be avoided by targeting environmental or lifestyle interventions at those at high genomic risk. Known genetic risk factors have to date shown limited utility in this respect.[71]

Grandiose promises would inevitably elicit unrealistically high expectations and, ultimately, disappointment in the public, although they may help attract funding support initially. We should be realistic about delivering promises since unrealistic promises may backlash, diminishing the public's trust on genetic research. Hence in the long run grandiose promises would hurt endometriosis research.

We also should be aware that even if a genetic polymorphism that predisposes women to endometriosis has been consistently and conclusively identified, it may take years, if not decades, before therapeutics can be developed. The genetic basis of sickle-cell anemia was known well over a half century ago, yet so far no gene-based treatment has been available.

Historical Lessons

History has taught us a few valuable lessons regarding genetic association studies. In assessing published genetic association studies, one should also resist the temptation to take authors' conclusions at their face value.

When the genetic association between male homo-sexuality and Xq28 was reported in early 1990s, it surprised everyone, generated a great deal of excitement and concern in scientists and laymen, galvanized the nature-versus-nurture debate, and led to intense speculation about what can really be inherited in complex traits as human sexuality. Yet the excitement and concern gradually subsided, after failed replication[72] and, above all, failed cloning of the putative gene(s). Surprisingly or not, similar examples abound. Manic depression, bipolar disorder, and myopia, to name just a few, had more or less similar situation.[73]

In assessing published genetic association studies, one should look beyond "shock-and-awe" and critically scrutinize the data before an independent conclusion is made. While a p-value of 0.00001 or smaller may sound impressive, we should keep in mind that after all the evidence for the reported association is largely statistical, and there are many factors that could tint statistical evidence: wrong choice of cases or controls or both, selective reporting (e.g. selecting a subset of cases/controls/pedigrees), multiple testing without proper adjustment, genotyping errors, among other things. "In Lord we trust", as in genetic association studies, should really have been "In evidence we trust". Therefore, independent replication is indispensible to separate the wheat from the chaff. In addition, results from association studies are "association", not necessarily a causal relationship. The firm establishment of a causal relationship should await for the cloning of the putative gene(s), and at least the proof that with the putative genotypes or DNA polymorphisms have increased risk of devloping endometriosis prospectively.

Conclusions

Although conceptually the identification of endometriosis susceptibility genes is rather straightforward and the genotyping technology is fast and affordable, the presumption that major susceptibility genes exist for endometriosis still needs to be carefully scrutinized. With the emergent view that complex diseases are emergent properties of molecular networks that are modulated by complex genetic loci and environmental and/or lifestyle factors, such a presumption may seem somewhat over-simplified. For endometriosis in which age-dependency, phenotypic and genetic heterogeneity, environmental/life-style factors, gene-environment interactions, and gene-gene interactions all seem to be present, there are seemingly insurmountable methodological difficulties. All these could have contributed to the failure of the prediction made in 2002.

Even if a susceptibility gene for endometriosis is identified, we also should be reminded that, while a gene-based diagnostics may be developed rather quickly, its utility may still need careful evaluation. In addition, the gene-derived therapeutics may still be decades away.

All these sobering thoughts and cautions are not meant to discourage, disparage, dismiss or discount the efforts to hunt for endometriosis-susceptibility genes. On the contrary, they are meant to help interested investigators view things in perspective and understand the goals, scopes, strengths as well as limitations of genetic association/mapping studies. The better we understand these issues and challenges, the better we will be prepared. In addition, a realistic assessment of the field would prevent us from making unrealistic promises that ultimately may result in backlashes from the public.

For a young aspiring scientist contemplating to work in this area, his/her decision also needs to be carefully weighted against, besides other options, the reality of an initial requirement for resources (a large sample of cases and controls), a roller-coaster experience of "Eureka" moments followed by subsequent letdown of failed replication, a demand for keen quantitative/analytical skills or at least appreciation, and the ability to clone the gene(s) and to elucidate its/their functions and roles in the pathogenesis of endometriosis. It is certainly not fun to work in an area where replication can be so difficult.

As in any scientific endeavor, of course, no one can be absolutely sure that the project he is about to embark on will surely succeed. Surprises do occur. There are successful stories of cloning genes for complex diseases such as breast cancer. It is also possible that some mutations or polymor-phisms may be responsible for a small portion of endometriotic cases, similar to BRCA1. Yet, once we understand the rationales behind the genetic research of endometriosis, and after weighing pros and cons of such research, it should help us make rationale and sensible decisions as which directions to pursue, and increase our chance to bring tangible benefits to better patient care ultimately.

Even monogenic Mendelian diseases are now known to be "complex, context-dependent entities"[74] to which the genes make a necessary, but only partial, contribution.[75] Between seemingly simple genotype and apparently complex phenotype (endometriosis included), there are many, hierarchical levels of control with each being defined by a dynamic system,[74, 76] which may be modulated by complex genetic loci and environmental and/or lifestyle factors.[32] Epigenetics may also play a vital role in the pathogenesis of endometriosis. Thus, when huge resources and possibly a career are at stake, one necessarily needs to critically scrutinize all the evidence, hidden assumptions, the strengths and limitations of genetic approach to endometriosis. Even though the approach is conceptually simple and all the technologies are there, there are still serious conceptual and methodological challenges ahead. Given the past history of rather rocky journey in genetics of complex diseases, the road to the identification of endometriosis susceptibility genes is not going to be a smooth ride, even though the payoff may be great.

Acknowledgment

This work was supported in part by a grant from the Shanghai Science and Technology Commission (074119517) and a grant from the National Science Foundation (30872759).

References

1. Baranov VS, Ivaschenko T, Bakay B, et al. Proportion of the GSTM1 0/0 genotype in some Slavic populations and its correlation with cystic fibrosis and some multifactorial diseases. Hum Genet 1996; 97:516-20.
2. Bischoff FZ, Simpson JL. Heritability and molecular genetic studies of endometriosis. Hum Reprod Update 2000; 6:37-44.
3. Collins FS, McKusick VA. Implications of the Human Genome Project for medical science. Jama 2001; 285:540-4.
4. Hattersley AT, McCarthy MI. What makes a good genetic association study? Lancet 2005;366:1315-23.
5. Ott J. Analysis of Human Genetic Linkage. 3rd Ed. ed. Baltimore: The John Hopkins University Press.; 1999.
6. Zondervan KT, Cardon LR, Kennedy SH. The genetic basis of endometriosis. Curr Opin Obstet Gynecol 2001; 13: 309-14.
7. Di W, Guo SW. The search for genetic variants predisposing women to endometriosis. Curr Opin Obstet Gynecol 2007; 19:395-401.
8. Guo SW. Glutathione S-transferases M1 (GSTM1)/T1 (GSTT1)Gene Polymorphisms and Endometriosis: A Meta-Analysis of Genetic Association Studies. Molecular Human Reproduction 2005; 11:729-43.
9. Guo SW. Association of Endometriosis Risk and Genetic Polymorphisms Involving Sex Steroid Biosynthesis and Their Receptors: A Meta-Analysis. Gynecol Obstet Invest 2005; 61:90-105.
10. Guo SW (2005). The association of endometriosis risk and genetic polymorphisms involving dioxin detoxification enzymes: a systemic review. Eur J Obstet Gynecol Reprod Biol 2006 Feb 1;124(2):134-43.
11. Weiss KM. Tilting at quixotic trait loci (QTL): an evolutionary perspective on genetic causation. Genetics 2008; 179:1741-56.
12. Falconer H, D'Hooghe T, Fried G. Endometriosis and genetic polymorphisms. Obstet Gynecol Surv 2007; 62:616-28.
13. Altmuller J, Palmer LJ, Fischer G, et al. Wjst M. Genome-wide scans of complex human diseases: true linkage is hard to find. Am J Hum Genet 2001;69:936-50.
14. Hirschhorn JN, Lohmueller K, Byrne E, et al. Comprehensive review of genetic association studies. Genet Med 2002; 4:45-61.
15. Ioannidis JP, Ntzani EE, Trikalinos TA. Contopoulos-Ioannidis DG. Replication validity of genetic association studies. Nat Genet 2001; 29:306-09.
16. Chanock SJ, Manolio T, Boehnke M, et al. Replicating genotype-phenotype associations. Nature 2007; 447:655-60.
17. Kashima K, Ishimaru T, Okamura H, et al. Familial risk among Japanese patients with endometriosis. Int J Gynaecol Obstet 2004; 84:61-64.
18. Koninckx PR, Braet P, Kennedy SH, et al. Dioxin pollution and endometriosis in Belgium. Hum Reprod 1994; 9: 1001-2.
19. Parazzini F, Ferraroni M, Fedele L, et al. Pelvic endometriosis: reproductive and menstrual risk factors at different stages in Lombardy, northern Italy. J Epidemiol Community Health 1995; 49:61-64.
20. Guo SW. Inflation of sibling recurrence-risk ratio, due to ascertainment bias and/or overreporting. Am J Hum Genet 1998; 63:252-58.
21. Guo SW. Familial aggregation of environmental risk factors and familial aggregation of disease. Am J Epidemiol 2000; 151:1121-31.
22. Moen MH, Schei B. Epidemiology of endometriosis in a Norwegian county. Acta Obstet Gynecol Scand 1997; 76:559-62.
23. Salces I, Rebato EM, Susanne C, et al. Familial resemblance for the age at menarche in Basque population. Ann Hum Biol 2001; 28:143-56.
24. Salces I, Rebato E, Slachmuylder JL, et al. Genetic and environmental sources on familial transmission in Basque families. II. Stature, weight and body mass index. Ann Hum Biol 2003; 30:176-90.

25. Guo SW. Gene-environment interaction and the mapping of complex traits: some statistical models and their implications. Hum Hered 2000; 50:286-303.

26. Noble D. Genes and causation. Philos Transact A Math Phys Eng Sci 2008; 366:3001-15.

27. Mayr E. The growth of biological thought. Cambridge, MA: Harvard University Press. 1982.

28. Pearson H. Genetics: what is a gene? Nature 2006; 44:398-401.

29. Venter JC, Adams MD, Myers EW, et al. The sequence of the human genome. Science 2001; 29:1304-51.

30. Qiu J. Epigenetics: unfinished symphony. Nature 2006; 441:143-45.

31. Schadt EE, Molony C, Chudin E, et al. Mapping the genetic architecture of gene expression in human liver. PLoS Biol 2008; 6:e107.

32. Chen Y, Zhu J, Lum PY, et al. Variations in DNA elucidate molecular networks that cause disease. Nature 2008; 452:429-35.

33. Schadt EE. Novel integrative genomics strategies to identify genes for complex traits. Anim Genet 2006; 37 1:18-23.

34. Wu Y, Kajdacsy-Balla A, Strawn E, et al. Transcriptional characterizations of differences between eutopic and ectopic endometrium. Endocrinology 2006; 147:232-46.

35. Kao LC, Germeyer A, Tulac S, et al. Expression profiling of endometrium from women with endometriosis reveals candidate genes for disease-based implantation failure and infertility. Endocrinology 2003; 144:2870-81.

36. Burney RO, Talbi S, Hamilton AE, et al. Gene expression analysis of endometrium reveals progesterone resistance and candidate susceptibility genes in women with endometriosis. Endocrinology 2007; 148:3814-26.

37. Giudice LC. Microarray expression profiling reveals candidate genes for human uterine receptivity. Am J Pharmacogenomics 2004; 4:299-312.

38. Felsenfeld G, Groudine M. Controlling the double helix. Nature 2003; 42:448-53.

39. Aleem F, Pennisi J, Zeitoun K, et al. The role of color Doppler in diagnosis of endometriomas. Ultrasound Obstet Gynecol 1995; 5:51-54.

40. Luger K. Dynamic nucleosomes. Chromosome Res 2006; 14:5-16.

41. Burke K. Permanence and Change: An Anatomy of Purpose. 3rd. Ed. ed. Berkeley: University of California Press.; 1984.

42. Robertson KD, Wolffe AP. DNA methylation in health and disease. Nat Rev Genet 2000; 1:11-19.

43. Huang C, Sloan EA, Boerkoel CF. Chromatin remodeling and human disease. Curr Opin Genet Dev 2003; 13:246-52.

44. Cooper RS, Psaty BM. Genomics and medicine: distraction, incremental progress, or the dawn of a new age? Ann Intern Med 2003; 138:576-80.

45. Baird P. The Human Genome Project, genetics and health. Community Genet 2001; 4:77-80.

46. Whitelaw E, Martin DI. Retrotransposons as epigenetic mediators of phenotypic variation in mammals. Nat Genet 2001; 27:361-65.

47. Morgante G, Ditto A, La Marca A, et al. Low-dose danazol after combined surgical and medical therapy reduces the incidence of pelvic pain in women with moderate and severe endometriosis. Hum Reprod 1999; 14:2371-74.

48. Rakyan VK, Chong S, Champ ME, et al. Transgenerational inheritance of epigenetic states at the murine Axin(Fu) allele occurs after maternal and paternal transmission. Proc Natl Acad Sci USA 2003; 100:2538-43.

49. Weaver IC, Cervoni N, Champagne FA, et al. Epigenetic programming by maternal behavior. Nat Neurosci 2004; 7:847-54.

50. Weaver IC, Champagne FA, Brown SE, et al. Reversal of maternal programming of stress responses in adult offspring through methyl supplementation: altering epigenetic marking later in life. J Neurosci 2005; 25:11045-54.

51. Szyfelbein WM, Baker PM, Bell DA. Superficial endometriosis of the cervix: A source of abnormal glandular cells on cervicovaginal smears. Diagn Cytopathol 2004; 30:88-91.

52. Anway MD, Cupp AS, Uzumcu M, et al. Epigenetic transgenerational actions of endocrine disruptors and male fertility. Science 2005; 308:1466-69.

53. Suter CM, Martin DI, Ward RL. Germline epimutation of MLH1 in individuals with multiple cancers. Nat Genet 2004; 36:497-501.

54. Hitchins M, Williams R, Cheong K, et al. MLH1 germline epimutations as a factor in hereditary nonpolyposis colorectal cancer. Gastroenterology 2005; 129:1392-99.

55. Moen MH. Endometriosis in monozygotic twins. Acta Obstet Gynecol Scand 1994; 73:59-62.

56. Fraga MF, Ballestar E, Paz MF. Epigenetic differences arise during the lifetime of monozygotic twins. Proc Natl Acad Sci U S A 2005; 102:10604-09.

57. Hoshiai H, Ishikawa M, Sawatari Y, et al. Laparoscopic evaluation of the onset and progression of endometriosis. Am J Obstet Gynecol 1993; 169:714-19.

58. Koninckx PR. Is mild endometriosis a condition occurring intermittently in all women? Hum Reprod 1994; 9:2202-05.

59. Boggi U, del Chiaro M, Pietrabissa A, et al. Extrapelvic endometriosis associated with occult groin hernias. Can J Surg 2001; 44:224.

60. Issa JP. Age-related epigenetic changes and the immune system. Clin Immunol 2003; 109:103-08.

61. Bennett-Baker PE, Wilkowski J, Burke DT. Age-associated activation of epigenetically repressed genes in the mouse. Genetics 2003; 165:2055-62.

62. Wu Y, Halverson G, Basir Z, et al. Aberrant methylation at HOXA10 may be responsible for Its aberrant expression in the endometrium of patients with endometriosis. Am J Obstet Gynecol 2005; 192.

63. Wu Y, Strawn E, Basir Z, et al. Promoter hypermethylation of progesterone receptor isoform B (PR-B) in endometriosis. Epigenetics 2006; 1:106-11.

64. Wu Y, Strawn E, Basir Z, et al. Aberrant expression of deoxyribonucleic acid methyltransferases DNMT1, DNMT3A and DNMT3B in women with endometriosis. Fertil Steril 2006.

65. Kim JY, Tavare S, Shibata D. Counting human somatic cell replications: methylation mirrors endometrial stem cell divisions. Proc Natl Acad Sci U S A 2005; 102:17739-44.

66. Chen S, Iversen ES, Friebel T, et al. Characterization of BRCA1 and BRCA2 mutations in a large United States sample. J Clin Oncol 2006; 24:863-71.

67. King MC, Marks JH, Mandell JB. Breast and ovarian cancer risks due to inherited mutations in BRCA1 and BRCA2. Science 2003; 302:643-46.

68. Strohman RC. The coming Kuhnian revolution in biology. Nat Biotechnol 1997; 15:194-200.

69. Harris RD, Holtzman SR, Poppe AM. Clinical outcome in female patients with pelvic pain and normal pelvic US findings. Radiology 2000; 216:440-43.

70. Vineis P, Schulte P, McMichael AJ. Misconceptions about the use of genetic tests in populations. Lancet 2001; 357:709-12.

71. Vineis P, Ahsan H, Parker M. Genetic screening and occupational and environmental exposures. Occup Environ Med 2005; 62:657-62, 597.

72. Rice G, Anderson C, Risch N, Ebers G. Male homosexuality: absence of linkage to microsatellite markers at Xq28. Science 1999; 284:665-67.

73. Risch N, Botstein D. A manic depressive history. Nat Genet 1996;12:351-53.

74. Strohman R. Maneuvering in the complex path from genotype to phenotype. Science 2002; 296:701-03.

75. Weatherall DJ. Phenotype-genotype relationships in monogenic disease: lessons from the thalassaemias. Nat Rev Genet 2001; 2:245-55.

76. Schadt EE, Lum PY. Thematic review series: systems biology approaches to metabolic and cardiovascular disorders. Reverse engineering gene networks to identify key drivers of complex disease phenotypes. J Lipid Res 2006; 47:2601-13.

Dominique de Ziegler, Isabelle Streuli, Bruno Borghese
Marina Bellavia, Ioannis Vasilopulos, Charles Chapron

Chapter 7 *Tuning of Endometriosis: Review of Environmental Effects on a Disease of Unknown Origin*

Introduction

Common gynecological wisdom holds that endometriosis is a disease of unknown origin that causes pelvic pain and infertility. The link between endometriosis and pelvic pain is a straightforward one that is rooted in the anatomical development of the disease in the very area where clinical soreness develops.[1] The corollary is that surgical removal of disease implants offers reprieve from symptoms, even if recurrence may occur. Endometriosis and infertility is more of a loose-canon fraternity however, in which the nature and hierarchy of mechanisms by which endometriosis interferes with reproduction are still the source of fierce debates. At the heart of these enduring powwows, 2 effects of endometriosis strike out as mainstay paradigms by which endometriosis causes infertility: (i) Pelvic inflammation interferes with sperm-oocyte interaction and thus, hampers *in vivo* – but not *in vitro* fertilization (IVF). (ii) Alterations of the eutopic endometrium encountered in case of endometriosis interfere to various extents with embryo implantation, an effect particularly preeminent in IVF.

Amongst the scores of candidate factors – spanning from genetic[2] to immunological ones[3] – purported as causing or facilitating endometriosis, the role played by the environment is an emerging domain with mushrooming implications of public health relevance.[4] The recent years have indeed unveiled that chemicals in our environment can affect reproduction and reproductive hormones related disorders such as endometriosis by mimicking hormones and/or interacting with hormone receptors and/or modify gene expression by DNA-methylation. One putative mechanism put forth for explaining these disruptions of reproductive-hormone related functions is altered gene expression mediated by inappropriate activation or deactivation of hormone receptors that act as transcription factors.[5] The aim of this review is to determine whether and to which extent environmental factors may be associated with, let alone cause endometriosis and/or partake in its impact on female fecundity by compounding any of the disease's effects on human reproduction.

Environmental Estrogens

Endometriosis being an estrogen-driven process, one must rightfully query whether the disturbing escalade in the amounts of environmental estrogens that humans are likely to be exposed to may impact on the incidence and extent of the disease. Bisphenol-A (BPA) is a hormonally active chemical used in plastics and various resins, which has been documented to leech from food[6] and beverage containers[7,8] with documented possible contamination of tap water[9] and presence identified in a variety of bodily fluids.[10] In spite of these serious grounds for concern if not fear of an outright of risks, the U.S. Environmental Protection Agency (EPA) is still to provide guidance for determining a dose-related scale for carcinogenic and transplacental risks. To this date therefore, there is no clear indication from available data that the BPA doses normally consumed by humans – as per findings made in tap water for example – pose an increased risk for immunologic or neurologic disease or conversely, are free of such risks.[11] The possibility that toxic exposure to endocrine-disrupting chemicals (EDC) and specifically, larger doses of BPA that are inadvertently caused by industrial pollution is shockingly real however. This possibility has been abruptly reminded to us by the dreadful recount of reproductive disruption in fish encountered downstream from a waste water effluent.[12]

In experimental conditions *in utero* exposure to BPA led to anatomical alterations of the genital track in offspring mice that were ultimately revealed in adulthood with decreased wet weight of the vagina, decreased volume of the endometrial lamina propria and increased expression of estrogen receptor-α (ERα) and progesterone receptor (PR).[10] Because BPAs have estrogenic properties that are several orders of magnitude inferior to those of E2, the possibility has been propounded that BPA acts by mechanisms not mediated by ERs. Alternatively, the reports of genital track alterations following fairly limited BPA exposure may speak for the great sensibility of the developing organism to environmental estrogen exposure with the consequences of *in utero* BPA exposure resulting from an ER-mediated effect.[11] As discussed below in the section on epigenetic modulation of hormonal effects, these anatomical and physiological alterations may cause functional disruptions of the endometrial cells that in turn lead to the development of endometriosis.

Environmental Dioxins and Endometriosis

Several lines of evidence have suggested that exposure to 2,3,7,8-tetrachlorodibenzo-p-dioxin (dioxin) and dioxin-like products may lead to the development of endometriosis. The dioxin family of products includes dibenzo-p-dioxins (PCDDs) dibenzofurans, (PCDFs) and biphenyls (PCBs). TCDD, PCDDs and PCDFs are produced as unwanted byproducts of many industrial processes. PCBs, which are used in various commercial products, account for approximately 85% of the dioxin exposure that is encountered practically. Dioxin and several dioxin-like products constitute a family of molecules that share a common mechanism of action whereby these products' effects are mediated by binding to the well characterized aryl-hydrocarbon receptor (AhR).[14] Following ligand binding, the ligand-receptor complex is translocated to the nucleus where transcriptional activation takes place with target genes including cytochrome P-450 and differentiation and inflammation related genes.[15]

The first link between dioxin exposure and endometriosis was reported in the monkey.[16] These authors' data indicated that 4-year treatment with increasing doses of the dioxin-like product TCDD led to a dose-dependant development of endometriosis. Moreover, serum concentration of dioxin-like products confirmed the actual exposure to the toxic.[17]

Worrisomely, the concentrations of dioxin and dioxin-like products commonly encountered in human equal if not surpass those artificially created in monkeys that induce the spontaneous appearance of endometriosis.[18] This therefore underscores the possibility that exposure to these chemicals is a concern of wide public health dimension. Japanese authors stressed the fact that current regulatory standards fail to guarantee proper protection for the average citizens against the risk of developing environment-related endometriosis and other environment-related diseases such as notably, certain cancers.[19]

Concerns about possible links between the development of endometriosis in humans and exposure to dioxin and dioxin-related products was amplified in Belgium because of the high incidence of endometriosis reported in infertile women in this country and the high dioxin concentrations reported in various reports including in breast milk.[20] Since then, some studies confirmed while others failed to verify the existence of a link between exposure to dioxin and dioxin-like products and the development of endometriosis.[21]

Food and Endometriosis

The possibility that hormone related diseases – endometriosis among them – might be influenced by the constituents of food has been entertained for the past 2 decades.[22, 23] In 2 case-control studies conducted in Northen Italy, Parazzini et al[24] performed unconditional multiple logistic regression, with maximum likelihood fitting, to obtain the odds ratios (OR) of endometriosis for various food diets. With this approach as investigative paradigm, the authors observed that a significant reduction in risk of endometriosis emerged for high intake of green vegetables (OR ¼ 0.3) and fresh fruit (OR ¼ 0.6) whereas, an increased risk was associated with beef and other red meat (OR ¼ 2.0) and ham (OR ¼1.8) consumption. Using multiple logistic regression, these authors determined OR (95% CI) that were 1.0 (0.7-1.4) and 1.8 (1.3-2.5) for intermediate and high level of consumption of beef and other red meat, respectively and 0.5 (0.3-0.9) and 0.3 (0.1-0.5) for intermediate and high consumption of vegetables, respectively. Socio-economic status, level of education and body mass index (BMI), which stand as possible confounding factors, did not appear to explain by themselves the observed differences.

Parallel findings were made for other estrogen dependant ailments. For example, there was a direct association between the frequency of consumption of red meat and ham and the incidence of endometrial and ovarian cancer and fibroids in the Northern Italy population.[25] The mechanism put forth is that a diet rich in fat increases circulating estrogens.[26] Conversely, high consumption of vegetable and fruits conferred some degree of protection.[26, 27] Likewise Levi et al,[28] looking at the population leaving in Switzerland and Northern Italy, observed that aside of the predictable adverse effects of being overweight, the intake of animal proteins and fat was directly associated with the risk of endometrial cancer. On the contrary, the regular consumption of fresh fruit, vegetables and fibers were protective for endometrial cancer.[28] It has been propounded that, by extension, the same is valid for endometriosis.

In a study conducted in Japanese women, Tsuchiya et al[29] observed that dietary isoflavones may reduce the risk of endometriosis. In a university hospital in Tokyo, these authors studied 138 women diagnosed with endometriosis by laparoscopy. These women were divided in 3 groups according to whether they had no endometriosis (control), mild-moderate (AFS I-II) or severe endometriosis (AFS III-IV). The urinary levels of genistein and daidzein – taken as markers for dietary intake of soy isoflavones – showed an inverse correlation with the risk of severe endometriosis **(Figure 7-1)**. For advanced endometriosis, the adjusted odd ratios for the highest quartile group was 0.21 (95% confidence interval = 0.06-0.76) for genistein and 0.29 (0.08-1.03) for daidzein, when compared with the lowest group.[29]

Aside of the possible exposure to hormonally active compounds described above, food may also be the source of toxic contaminants, which may alter the expression of crucial genes through DNA-demethylation related activation of key promoters as described in the following section. In a cross-sectional study performed on 80 Japanese women, aged 26-43 years, who consume fish frequently, Tsukino et al[30] observed that a variety of organochlorines accumulated in the bodies of these individuals.

The data reported above establish grounds for concern that diets constituents may favor the development of endometriosis, a disease whose social toll is considerable in terms of the health care costs generated through pelvic pain and infertility and their costly treatments. Further work is therefore warranted for confirming these findings and diffusing the information to the general population and particularly, the individuals at higher risk as for example young women suffering from dysmenorrhea.

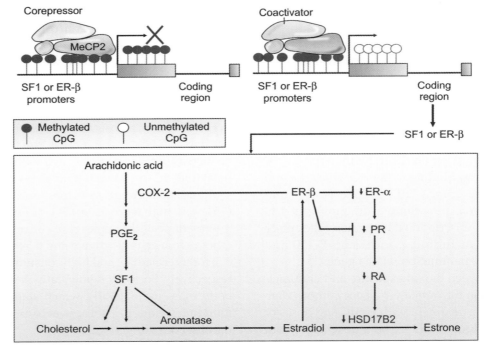

FIGURE 7-1: Epigenetic changes in endometriosis tissue. The promoters of steroidogenic factor 1 (SF1) and estrogen receptor β (ER-β) are normally silenced through heavy methylation. DNA-demethylation – possibly as a result of exposure to environmental contaminants – leads to promoter activation and pathologic over-expression of SF1 and ER-β. SF1 triggers prostaglandin E2 dependant activation of the SYP-19 aromatase gene and in turn local production of estrogen. ER-β suppresses ER-α and progesterone receptors (PRs) expression. *(From: Bulun SE. Endometriosis N Engl J Med 2009;360: 268-79, with permission)*

Epigenetic Modulation of Local Production and Metabolism of E2 and Progesterone

A number of lines of evidence lend support to Sampson's theory[31] that first put the role of retrograde menstruation in the limelight of the scientific debate, proposing this mechanism as responsible for the genesis of endometriosis. An emerging concept in this already old theory, which we started to propose in 2002, is the fact the regurgitated endometrial cells acquire an enhanced invasiveness in endometriosis, which is instrumental in the genesis of this disease.[32] The observed alterations that affect endometrial cells and the change of function that result in enhancing the tendency of the shed cells to adhere and invade the pelvic cavity probably directly stem from the functional changes that are cast in the uterus itself[33] and the pelvic cavity as a whole.[34]

In the normal endometrium, the orphan nuclear receptor SF1 is not expressed as a result of DNA-methylation and silencing of the transcription factor binding domain.[35] A lack of promoter methylation as encountered as a result of exposure to various environmental toxics leads to the stimulatory factor 2 binding to the unmethylated SF1 promoter and activating it.[36] This leads to over-expression of ER-α and under-expression of ER-β and in turn the down regulation of the PR expression particularly, in stromal cells. Hyper-expression of ER-β leads to inactivating 17OH-steroid dehydrogenase, which normally inactivates E2 into the lesser active estrogen, E1, thus further contributing to the hyper-estrogenization of the endometrium (and endometriotic implants) encountered in endometriosis.[36]

Changes in DNA-methylation patterns may be encountered in case of exposure to certain toxics or result from effects of the parental diet on fetal DNA-methylation pattern.[37,38] One interesting mode of gene alteration is the inheritance of methylation patterns by which the parent's acquired alterations in DNA-methylation are passed on to offspring. For example, exposure of male rats to a fungicide with antiandrogenic properties, vinclozolin, or an estrogenic organochlorine insecticide, methoxyclor, during the time of gonadal sex determination resulted in reduced sperm count and increased risk in infertility in adulthood.[39] Remarkably, the impairment of fertility was passed to the next 4 generations who all displayed altered sperm characteristics. This mechanism is proposed for the transmission of consequences of exposure to toxic substances such as DES to the next generation and possibly that of putative toxic exposures, which might confer an enhanced susceptibility to develop endometriosis in the daughter generation.

Environmental Perspectives for Endometriosis Treatment: The Medicinal Plants

The flip side of the fact that environmental contaminants generate the development of endometriosis by direct estrogenic effects of environmental BPAs or through an epigenic effects of toxics such dioxin is the possibility of using the environment through medicinal plants for treatment. Indeed our emerging understanding of how the environment may under certain circumstances interact with and at times alter gene expression through DNA-methylation and demethylation processes sheds new lights for explaining some of the claimed benefits of traditional herbal medicine.

Certain traditional Chinese herbal medicines such as YWN – a mixture of several plants – have been positively tested for preventing the post-surgical recurrence of endometriosis,[40] yet leaving us at a loss for outlining an alleged mechanism of action. Compounding the problem for obtaining evidence-based proof of efficacy of herbal products stems from the fact that concentrations of constituents of herbal mixtures are inherently variable. New perspectives for understanding the potential benefits of these traditional medicaments should guide the further research notably, in the direction of determining whether some medicinal products may actually dampen the pervasive and disruptive properties of certain environment contaminants.

Conclusion

By the mechanism of DNA-methylation, exposure to toxic environmental substances and/or alteration in the parental diet may lead to alterations of genital tract organs and specifically, lead to the development of endometriosis. An emerging understanding of this mechanism of action whereby environmental substances may durably affect gene expression possibly in ways that it is passed on to the future generations should be grounds for arising the awareness about environmental pollutants. Government bodies should tighten the span and content of the regulatory blue print that should draw the rules for testing, setting limits in levels measured and if need be, deploy corrective measures for restraining exposure to possibly dangerous environmental hazards.

Likewise, efforts should aim at setting and validating non-invasive methods for diagnosing endometriosis and assessing its progression or regression in response to changes in environmental contaminant exposure.

Candidates for surrogate markers of endometriosis include blood-born parameters such as CA-125 and particularly, the amplitude of changes in CA-125 levels observed in relation with menses. Alternate options for findings non-invasive markers of endometriosis include the array of alterations described in the eutopic endometrium in case of endometriosis, albeit the latter admittedly requires an endometrial biopsy for detection, procedure not as handily available as serum samples. Finally the emerging science of DNA-methylation and epigenetic alteration of gene expression may lead to new diagnostic tools as well as prognostic factors and markers of recurrence, which may orient the treatment of endometriosis related infertility. Moreover this field may lead the way toward new forms of therapy of endometriosis as epigenetic alterations of gene expression contrary to mutations are reversible.[41] Indeed, there are prospects for developing in some near future, directed epigenetic-specific therapies with the use of transcription factors that target particular gene promoters.

References

1. Fauconnier A, Chapron C, Dubuisson JB, Vieira M, Dousset B, Bréart G. Relation between pain symptoms and the anatomic location of deep infiltrating endometriosis. Fertil Steril. 2002;78:719-26.

2. Borghese B, Mondon F, Noël JC, Fayt I, Mignot TM, Vaiman D, Chapron C. Gene expression profile for ectopic versus eutopic endometrium provides new insights into endometriosis oncogenic potential. Mol Endocrinol 2008;22:2557-62.

3. Ulukus M, Arici A. Immunology of endometriosis. Minerva Ginecol. 2005;57:237-48.

4. Ryer S, Foster W. Environmental dioxins and endometriosis. Toxicological Sciences 2002;70:161-70.

5. Edwards TM, Myers JP. Environmental exposures and gene regulation in disease etiology. Environ Health Perspect. 2007;115:1264-70.

6. Villalobos M, Olea N, Brotons JA, Olea-Serrano MF, Ruiz de Almodovar JM, Pedraza V. The E-screen assay: a comparison of different MCF7 cell stocks. Environ Health Perspect. 1995;103:844-50.

7. Biles JE, White KD, McNeal TP, Begley TH. Determination of the diglycidyl ether of bisphenol A and its derivatives in canned foods. J Agric Food Chem. 1999;47:1965-69.

8. Mariscal-Arcas M, Rivas A, Granada A, Monteagudo C, Murcia MA, Olea-Serrano F. Dietary exposure assessment of pregnant women to bisphenol-A from cans and microwave containers in Southern Spain. Food Chem Toxicol. 2009;47:506-10.

9. Willhite CC, Ball GL, McLellan CJ. Derivation of a bisphenol A oral reference dose (RfD) and drinking-water equivalent concentration. J Toxicol Environ Health B Crit Rev. 2008;11:69-146.

10. Markey CM, Wadia PR, Rubin BS, Sonnenschein C, Soto AM. Long-term effects of fetal exposure to low doses of the xenoestrogen bisphenol-A in the female mouse genital tract. Biol Reprod. 2005;72:1344-51.

11. Nagel SC, vom Saal FS, Welshons WV. Developmental effects of estrogenic chemicals are predicted by an in vitro assay incorporating modification of cell uptake by serum. J Steroid Biochem Mol Biol. 1999;69:343-57.

12. Vajda AM, Barber LB, Gray JL, Lopez EM, Woodling JD, Norris DO. Reproductive disruption in fish downstream from an estrogenic wastewater effluent. Environ Sci Technol. 2008;42:3407-14.

13. Rier S, Foster WG. Environmental dioxins and endometriosis. Toxicol Sci. 2002;70:161-70.

14. Safe SH. Polychlorinated biphenyls (PCBs): environmental impact, biochemical and toxic responses, and implications for risk assessment. Crit Rev Toxicol. 1994;24:87-149.

15. Wen LP, Koeiman N, Whitlock JP Jr. Dioxin-inducible, Ah receptor-dependent transcription in vitro. Proc Natl Acad Sci U S A. 1990;87:8545-9. ; Whitlock JP Jr. Genetic and molecular aspects of 2,3,7,8-tetrachlorodibenzo-p-dioxin action. Annu Rev Pharmacol Toxicol. 1990;30:251-77.

16. Rier SE, Martin DC, Bowman RE, Dmowski WP, Becker JL. Endometriosis in rhesus monkeys (*Macaca mulatta*) following chronic exposure to 2,3,7,8-tetrachlorodibenzo-p-dioxin. Fundam Appl Toxicol. 1993;21:433-41.

17. Rier SE, Turner WE, Martin DC, Morris R, Lucier GW, Clark GC. Serum levels of TCDD and dioxin-like chemicals in Rhesus monkeys chronically exposed to dioxin: correlation of increased serum PCB levels with endometriosis. Toxicol Sci. 2001;59:147-59.

18. Kahn PC, Gochfeld M, Nygren M, Hansson M, Rappe C, Velez H, Ghent-Guenther T, Wilson WP. Dioxins and dibenzofurans in blood and adipose tissue of Agent Orange-exposed Vietnam veterans and matched controls. JAMA. 1988;259:1661-67.

19. Yoshida K, Ikeda S, Nakanishi J. Assessment of human health risk of dioxins in Japan. Chemosphere. 2000;40:177-85.

20. Koninckx PR, Braet P, Kennedy SH, Barlow DH. Dioxin pollution and endometriosis in Belgium. Hum Reprod. 1995;10:1274.

21. Mayani A, Barel S, Soback S, Almagor M. Dioxin concentrations in women with endometriosis. Hum Reprod. 1997;12:373-75.

22. Ingram DM, Bennett FC, Willcox D, de Klerk N. Effect of low-fat diet on female sex hormone levels. J Natl Cancer Inst. 1987;79:1225-29.

23. Bennett FC, Ingram DM. Diet and female sex hormone concentrations: an intervention study for the type of fat consumed. Am J Clin Nutr. 1990;52:808-12.

24. Parazzini F, Chiaffarino F, Surace M, Chatenoud L, Cipriani S, Chiantera V, et al. Selected food intake and risk of endometriosis. Hum Reprod. 2004;19:1755-59.

25. Bosetti C, Negri E, Franceschi S, Pelucchi C, Talamini R, Montella M, et al. Diet and ovarian cancer risk: a case-control study in Italy. Int J Cancer. 2001;93: 911-15.

26. Gorbach SL, Goldin BR. Diet and the excretion and enterohepatic cycling of estrogens. Prev Med. 1987;16:525-31.

27. Chiaffarino F, Parazzini F, La Vecchia C, Chatenoud L, Di Cintio E, Marsico S Diet and uterine myomas. Obstet Gynecol 1999;94:395–98.

28. Levi F, Franceschi S, Negri E, La Vecchia C. Dietary factors and the risk of endometrial cancer. Cancer. 1993 Jun 1;71:3575-81.

29. Tsuchiya M, Miura T, Hanaoka T, Iwasaki M, Sasaki H, Tanaka T, et al. Effect of soy isoflavones on endometriosis: interaction with estrogen receptor 2 gene polymorphism. Epidemiology. 2007;18:402-08.

30. Tsukino H, Hanaoka T, Sasaki H, Motoyama H, Hiroshima M, Tanaka T, et al. Fish intake and serum levels of organochlorines among Japanese women. Sci Total Environ. 2006;359:90-100.

31. Sampson JA, peritoneal endometriosis due to menstrual dissemination of endometrial tissue into the peritoneal cavity. Am J Obstet Gynecol 1927;14:422-69.

32. Bulletti C, De Ziegler D, Polli V, Del Ferro E, Palini S, Flamigni C. Characteristics of uterine contractility during menses in women with mild to moderate endometriosis. Fertil Steril. 2002;77:1156-61.

33. Wei Q, St Clair JB, Fu T, Stratton P, Nieman LK. Reduced expression of biomarkers associated with the implantation window in women with endometriosis. Fertil Steril. 2008;29.

34. Weinberg JB, Haney AF, Xu FJ, Ramakrishnan S. Peritoneal fluid and plasma levels of human macrophage colony-stimulating factor in relation to peritoneal fluid macrophage content. Blood. 1991;78:513-16.

35. Yin P, Lin Z, Cheng YH, Marsh EE, Utsunomiya H, Ishikawa H, et al. Progesterone receptor regulates Bcl-2 gene expression through direct binding to its promoter region in uterine leiomyoma cells. J Clin Endocrinol Metab. 2007;92:4459-66.

36. Xue Q, Lin Z, Cheng YH, Huang CC, Marsh E, Yin P, et al. Promoter methylation regulates estrogen receptor 2 in human endometrium and endometriosis. Biol Reprod. 2007;77:681-87.

37. Dolinoy DC, Weidman JR, Jirtle RL. Epigenetic gene regulation: linking early developmental environment to adult disease. Reprod Toxicol. 2007;23:297-307.

38. Dolinoy DC, Das R, Weidman JR, Jirtle RL. Metastable epialleles, imprinting, and the fetal origins of adult diseases. Pediatr Res. 2007;61:30-37.

39. Anway MD, Cupp AS, Uzumcu M, Skinner MK. Epigenetic transgenerational actions of endocrine disruptors and male fertility. Science. 2005;308:1466-69.

40. Wieser F, Cohen M, Gaeddert A, Yu J, Burks-Wicks C, Berga SL, et al. Evolution of medical treatment for endometriosis: back to the roots? Hum Reprod Update. 2007;13:487-99.

41. Moore M, Ullman C. Recent developments in the engineering of zinc finger proteins. Brief Funct Genomic Proteomic 2003;1:342-55.

Andrew Prentice, Alka Prakash

Chapter 8

Role of Endogenous Hormones in Endometriosis

Introduction

Endometriosis is defined as the presence of endometrial tissue at ectopic sites. Histologically endometriosis is the growth of the endometrium outside the uterine cavity; this endometrium undergoes cyclical changes under the influence of endogenous hormones very much like the functionalis layer of the eutopic endometrium. The commonest theory for the displacement of endometrial tissue in the peritoneal cavity is retrograde menstruation. However genetic studies suggest that there is an inherent abnormality in the endometrium of women who develop endometriosis. This is related to increased survival and reduced clearance of the refluxed cells into the peritoneal cavity.[1] Endometriosis is present in 7-10% of women in the general population.[2] True prevalence is difficult to identify as surgery is the only reliable way of diagnosing this condition and not performed in women who are asymptomatic. Asymptomatic endometriosis was identified in 4% of women undergoing elective surgical sterilization.[3] Various epidemiological studies agree to a general prevalence rate of 3-10% in the reproductive age group. Studies have suggested that the ectopic endometrial tissue responds to endogenous and exogenous hormones very much like the eutopic endometrium. Hence, the endometrial fragments in the peritoneal cavity are responsive to ovarian hormone regulation.

Roles of Various Endogenous Hormones

The pathogenesis of endometriosis therefore would require the adherence of the endometrial fragments on the peritoneal surfaces followed by extensive remodelling of the peritoneal mesothelial layers; this requires activation of MMPs (matrix metalloproteinases). MMPs mediate endometrial breakdown and help with new growth of endometrium under stimulation of estrogen. Abnormal expression of MMPs has been suggested to confer invasive potential to refluxed endometrium and thereby helping in proliferation of endometriosis.[4]

Studies have now shown that estrogen production and metabolism are altered in endometriosis in a way that promotes the disease pathology.[5] These alterations vary from reduced anti-proliferative and differentiative effects of progesterone on endometriosis tissue compared with endometrium to abnormalities in the expression of aromatase in endometriosis tissue. As with eutopic endometrial tissue, endometriotic deposits require continuous supply of estrogen for growth and therefore seem to regress in estrogen deficient conditions which may be natural or iatrogenically created. In this chapter we will elucidate the role of endogenous hormones in endometriosis and hence their role in treatment of this condition **(Table 8-1)**.

In the natural state it is rare to find endometriosis in childhood unless they have been exposed to exogenous hormones. After birth, effects of maternal hormones resolve within 1-2 months of postnatal life and there is little or no hormonal stimulation during childhood. This leads to a small uterus with corpus being smaller than cervix. There is one published case report of pre-menarcheal endometriosis.[6] In this series authors suggested a pathophysiology which is likely to be different to adult theory of retrograde menstruation. They found laparoscopically seen lesions suggestive of endometriosis in 5 girls of which 2 went on to have histological proof on repeat laparoscopy post-menarche. Whether the initial lesions were endometriotic or not is debatable as there was no histological diagnosis made in the premenarcheal stage. The celomic metaplasia theory would explain endometriosis in unusual situations and age groups. This suggests that the mesothelial cells

Table 8-1: Evidence supporting the endocrine basis of endometriosis

- It requires estrogen exposure (rare in childhood and after menopause)
- Exceptional in Turner or Kallman syndrome or ovarian dysgenesis (Swyer syndrome), with abnormal reduction in estrogen production
- Hyperprogestogenic (pregnancy)/hypoestrogenic (lactation) states seem beneficial
- Observed in the menstrual phase of life (cyclical effect of estrogen and progesterone)
- Non-existent in men, unless exogenous estrogen administered
- Endometrial and endometriotic tissue express estrogen and progesterone receptors
- Beneficial effect of inhibiting estrogen production (aromatase inhibitor, GnRH agonists and antagonists) or opposing its effects (progestins)

undergo metaplasia either spontaneously or under the influence of some irritant such as refluxed menstrual blood but in the absence of specific proof remains just a theory.

Looking into the next sequential natural state which is relatively hyper progestogenic but also estrogenic namely pregnancy and in contrast the relatively hypoestrogenic state that is lactation. Both these varying states tend to have beneficial effect on endometriosis. Pregnancy causes decidualization of the endometrium leading to reduction of symptoms. Decidual cells are derived from stromal cells of the endometrium under the stimulation of progesterone; these cells are characterized by accumulation of glycogen droplets and the endometrium in turn becomes thin and atrophic. These progestogenic effects require prior estrogen priming as the progesterone receptor has been shown to be a estrogen dependent protein. Therefore, the suppressive effects of progesterone is due to decidualization and endometrial atrophy[7] over a period of time and also the inhibition of ovulation leading to amenorrhea. In theory preventing further development of endometriosis and potentially leading to natural resolution of disease. However various studies in animal models have shown contradictory results, D'Hooghe et al in 1997[8] did not show any improvement in stage of endometriosis in baboon models in first and second trimester of pregnancy. In contrast the murine model showed a significant reduction of endometriotic lesions in pregnancy.[9] However, the mouse model is unique in the sense that it does not have spontaneous endometriosis and extrapolating this data to humans requires caution. In humans, it is often stated that endometriosis improves in pregnancy. Whether this is an effect of pregnancy *per se* or the prolonged amenorrhea or the hypo-estrogenic state of breastfeeding is unclear.

Studies have shown a significant effect on progesterone receptor expression during pregnancy in both eutopic and ectopic endometrium[10] and this may form the basis of progestagen therapy in endometriosis.

The reproductive / menstruating phase of life on the other hand will be the classical model to study endometriosis as this is the time when there is cyclical effect of estrogen and progesterone on the endometrium. Ovarian steroids have profound effect on endometrial differentiation and function; this is likely to be similar in the ectopic endometrium. As retrograde menstruation is one of the theories behind development of endometriosis, it is easy to understand that endometriosis is commonly seen in the menstruating phase of life. Although there is no conclusive evidence that endometrium regurgitated through the fallopian tubes at menstruation implants at ectopic sites, the circumstantial evidence is compelling. This includes studies that confirm the viability of shed endometrium and potential to implant at ectopic sites in both animal and human models. However it perhaps should be considered that retrograde menstruation is one of many mechanisms by which endometrium will reach sites outside the uterine cavity and give rise to endometriosis rather than promote retrograde menstruation—the sole mechanism in the pathogenesis of endometriosis.

Another concept that helps us in understanding the endocrine basis of endometriosis is that estrogen and progesterone both of which are present in the menstruating women leads to growth and differentiation of tissue that express their receptors. The presence of these receptors has been confirmed in both endometrial and endometriotic tissue and this is used in the treatment of endometriosis as will be discussed later. These receptors have not been observed in tissue derived from celomic epithelium.

Menopause is the next natural stage in life where endometriosis is unlikely or infrequently seen. Most women report an improvement of symptoms after menopause. Those that have active endometriosis at this stage of life are usually exposed to exogenous hormones. Occasionally this may be seen in the absence of hormonal therapy but such patients are more likely to have other hormone dependent conditions seen commonly in the obese such as endometrial and breast cancer, again reinforcing the role of endogenous hormones, which may be extra-ovarian in origin.[11] Hence although it is a hypogonadal state some amount of hormonal stimulation can occur and may therefore explain the presence of endometriosis albeit rarely in postmenopausal women. Doubts have been raised in the past that pathophysiology of postmenopausal endometriosis is different to premenopausal disease. However a recent study[12] confirmed similar immunohistochemical profile in the two situations and inferred that it is the same process which has the potential to reactivate given the appropriate stimulation.

In contrast to the above situations in a normal human life where circulating estrogen is at its lowest, leading to inhibition of endometriosis, there are conditions where there is an abnormal reduction of estrogen production or effect such as ovarian failure or dysgenesis.

Turner's syndrome leads to accelerated germ cell atresia and presence streak ovaries with early loss of ovarian function. Such patients usually have primary amenorrhea due to hypo-estrogenic state. The reported cases of endometriosis with Turner's syndrome were all associated with exogenous hormone administration.[13] Another disorder leading to hypo-gonadotrophic hypogonadism is Kallman syndrome and again there are no reported cases of endometriosis in such a group further reinforcing the role of endogenous estrogens in endometriosis. Gonadal dysgenesis such as Swyer's syndrome present with primary amenorrhea and lack of secondary sex characteristics usually associated with mutations of SRY gene or deletions of short arm of Y. They usually have streak gonads, raised FSH and are hypo-estrogenic and again are unlikely candidates for endometriosis. The few reported case of endometriosis in Swyer's syndrome had exposure to cyclical HRT.

With estrogen playing an important part in the etiopathogenesis of endometriosis, it is unlikely to present in individuals with XY karyotype, this may be complete androgen insensitivity syndrome (CAIS) or normal men. In the former (CAIS), patients have XY functional gonads in the form of testes, and due to the action of MIF (Müllerian inhibiting factor) from Sertoli cells, there is a blind-ending vagina, absent uterus and tubes. Estrogen may be produced from testes and peripheral aromatization of testosterone, and there is no reported case of endometriosis in this subgroup.

Moving to the endometriosis in men, case reports so far include men who have received exogenous estrogen treatment for prostate cancer. There is only one case arising in a Müllerian duct remnant in a man. These remnants found in 1% of men which may be due to *in utero* hormone exposure. The prostatic cancer cases and the Müllerian duct remnant case all arise in Müllerian derived tissue. The prostatic cancer is from the prostatic utricle (derived from Müllerian duct) and gave rise to endometroid carcinoma of the prostate.

The development of endometriosis requires the trophic effect of estrogens which may be endogenous or exogenous on derivatives of the Müllerian duct. Estrogen action results in endometrial proliferation and menstruation. In the absence of regular endometrial shedding endometriosis does not appear to occur. Common strategies to minimize these consequences may therefore be useful in developing preventative strategies. Hence epidemiological evidence is strong enough to confirm the role of hormones especially estrogen in the pathogenesis of endometriosis.

The role of endogenous hormones has played a part in developing the preventive/treatment strategies for endometriosis. Animal models have shown the transcription of steroid hormone receptors, and estrogen converting enzymes (dehydrogenase, sulphatase, aromatase) in ectopic endometrial tissue, furthermore the application of progestagens and danazol significantly inhibited aromatase transcription leading to a parallel decrease in endometrial proliferation.[14] In essence the principle behind the study is the same that is used in studying the role of endogenous hormones in endometriosis. At a histological level, there appears to be unpredictable response of endometriotic implants to cyclic endogenous hormones and therapy. This may be explained by the architectural relationships between the cellular elements such as stromal implants appear to be more synchronous with eutopic endometrium and implants with fibrosis appear to be relatively under-responsive to hormones.[15]

Estrogen has been shown to play a significant role in development and proliferation of endometriosis. This may be due to the activation of various biochemical pathways in the endometrial tissue. The extensive regulation, remodelling and cyclical shedding of endometrial tissue requires the activation of MMPs which may play an important part in the development of endometriosis. Most MMPs are under the influence of estrogen and are up regulated with estrogen and down regulated with progesterone.[16] In a recent study, EMMPRIN which is a glycosalated transmembrane protein regulates the production of MMPs and is expressed by eutopic endometrial and the peritoneal mesothelial cells in endometriotic lesions.[16] Furthermore, the expression of EMMPRIN is strongest during the proliferative phase when ER and PR are maximally expressed in these tissues.[17] This expression of EMMPRIN may be involved in stimulating MMP production at the site of invasion into the peritoneal surfaces and hence the initiation of endometriosis.

The key role of estrogen in the etiopathogenesis can also be studied in a reverse manner by investigating the role of aromatase inhibitors in treatment of endometriosis. Aromatase p-450 is the key enzyme for extraovarian estrogen biosynthesis and acts by catalyzing the conversion of androstenedione and testosterone to estrone and estradiol. Studies have reported aromatase expression in eutopic and ectopic endometrial tissue in women with endometriosis and no aromatase activity in healthy eutopic endometrial tissue.[18] It is therefore logical to consider the use of aromatase inhibitors in patients with endometriosis. However with reduction of extra-ovarian estrogen, there may set up a positive feedback for ovarian estrogen synthesis and hence negate the effect on endometriosis. Hence for patients with endometriosis these may be used in combination with standard regimes that reduce ovarian estrogen synthesis. A recent systematic review of studies using aromatase inhibitors in treatment of endometriosis appear to alleviate pain, lesion size and improve the quality of life.[19] However, larger trials are required to confirm these trends. Most of the studies included in the systematic review used a combination of aromatase inhibitor with either GnRH analog or progesterone. Endometriotic implants contains both ER (estrogen receptor) and PR (progesterone receptor) in both glandular epithelium and stroma but are more hetero- geneous and showed unpredictable response to cyclic hormone milieu, but respond to hormonal suppression over prolonged period.[20]

The role of gonadotrophin releasing hormone agonists (GnRH) in endometriosis further supports the key role of estrogen in the pathogenesis and proliferation of endo- metriosis. GnRH suppress ovarian estrogen synthesis by suppressing the pituitary ovarian axis but have no effect on extra-ovarian synthesis of estrogens as it does not effect aromatase activity and the peripheral aromatization and production of estrogen continues. Studies have also shown these to exert anti-proliferative and apoptotic effect on cultured endometriotic cells.[21] Another form of GnRH (GnRH II) which has a more potent anti-proliferative effect than GnRH I on human endometrial cells is widely distributed in the central nervous system and peripheral tissues of the female reproductive tract and endometrium and ovarian granulosa cells.[22] GnRH II exerts its effect dually by GnRH receptor (GnRHr) pathway as well as independent of GnRHr. Recent studies suggest that expression of GnRH II are lower in endometrial tissues and in endometriotic tissues of women with endometriosis compared with those of women without the disease. There is growing evidence that even eutopic endometrium from women with endometriosis has aberrant properties compared with that from women without the disease, and

that this may be a key in the pathophysiology of the disease.[23] A recent study showed that the expression of GnRH II was significantly decreased in eutopic endometrium of women with endometriosis. Furthermore, as GnRH II has antiproliferative and anti-inflammatory effect on endometriotic cells, these findings support the view that endometrial cells in women with endometriosis have enhanced proliferative activities.[24]

In parallel to the above findings suppression of gonadotrophins can also be done by gonadotrophin releasing hormone antagonist. Gonadotrophin releasing hormone antagonist is currently licensed for use only in advanced prostatic cancer or to prevent premature luteinizing hormone surge in certain types of controlled ovarian stimulation for IVF. As the name suggest, they antagonize the action of gonadotrophin releasing hor- mones and have the advantage of a more rapid suppres- sion of gonadotrophins without any initial flare which is seen with GnRH agonists.[25] However the net result is still a pituitary suppression leading to a hypoestrogenic state, again reiterating the role of estrogens in endometriosis.

Progesterone plays an important part in the normal menstrual cycle. Progestagens induce secretory activity in endometrial glands and decidual reaction in the endo- metrial stroma thereby creating a pseudopregnancy like state. Progestagens (progestational drugs) have been and are still widely used for the treatment of endometriosis. They help by reducing pain and somatic symptoms in majority of women with endometriosis.[26] The principle behind their use is the opposition of estrogenic effect on the endometrium by down regulating estrogen receptors. The physiological effects of progesterone are mediated by progesterone receptors A and B, unfortunately 9 % of women do not respond to progestagen therapy. Progestagens appears to down regulate PR-B but not PR- A receptors in endometriosis. This is due to the inability to hypermethylate the promoter region of PR-A receptor in endometriotic tissue.[27] Hence it has been suggested that endometriosis may have an epigenetic basis for its pathophysiology. Whatever the basis of disease process it is obvious that the endocrinological milieu plays an important role in the manifestation and treatment of this condition. Progestagens may be derivatives of progesterone or 19 nortestosterone, the latter being able to exert effect via the androgenic receptors. Furthermore progesterone appears to have a suppressive effect on MMPs which appears to mediate endometriosis.[28] *In vitro* studies have reported a down regulation of endometrial RANTES (Regulated on activation, normal T cell expressed and secreted) gene transcription by prolonged progestin exposure.[29] RANTES is a chemokine expressed by eutopic and ectopic endometrial stromal cells and appears to be elevated in peritoneal fluid of women with endometriosis.[30] Hence the suppression of pelvic pain associated with endometriosis by progestagens may be explained by suppression of inflammatory markers via inhibition of RANTES gene expression.

The role of androgen, androgen receptors and 5α reductase activity in the endometrium is still unclear. Recent study has confirmed the presence of 5α reductase gene expression in both ectopic and eutopic endometrium suggesting a role of local and systemic androgens on endometriotic cells.[31] This may suggest the conversion of testosterone to 5 hydroxy-testosterone within the endometrium which is a very potent androgen. Androgens can have two very different effects, *per se* androgens inhibit proliferation[32] and hence the presence of 5α reductase activity may be a regulatory mechanism on the other hand it may stimulate the aromatase activity leading to increased local estrogen and hence have a stimulatory effect. From epidemiology so far it is likely that the former action far outweighs the latter and a hyperandrogenic environment tends to cause endometrial atrophy and suppresses endometriosis. Danazol is a synthetic androgen (isoxazol derivative of 19 alpha ethinyl testosterone) that inhibits luteinizing hormone and follicle-stimulating hormone, leading to a chronic anovulatory state producing a relatively hypoestrogenic state and endometrial atrophy. Side effects particularly androgenic effects such as acne, hirsuitism, edema, weight gain, and voice changes have greatly restricted its use in clinical medicine.[33] Furthermore, danazol appears to inhibit aromatase activity in endometriosis-derived stromal cells without affecting either the mRNA or protein levels of aromatase and hence the efficacy of local application of danazol to endometriotic lesions. New approaches such as the use of vaginal danazol for symptomatic relief in recurrent deeply infiltrative lesions may be considered as an alternative.[34] Gestrinone is a 19 –nortestosterone which has androgenic and anti-estrogenic property and is used to suppress endometriosis. This further highlights the role of estrogens and androgens in endometriosis.

Endogenous hormones not only have a direct impact on endometriosis by affecting the growth of endometrium but may even have an indirect impact by altering the immune system. Systemic immune alterations have been suggested as a possible etiopathogenic factor for endo-metriosis. This has been suggested due to dysregulation of cytokine production.[35] To what extent and how the endogenous and exogenous hormones regulate the immune function (altered macrophage and cytokine function) and thereby exert their effect at the biochemical level remains to be seen. Altered secretion of cytokines and growth factors appear to stimulate the ectopic endometrium and down regulate the scavenging action of macrophages.[36] These tend to promote the adhesion of ectopic endometrium and the angiogenic factors stimulate angiogenesis and proliferation. However estrogenic toxicants such has dioxin have shown to alter leukocyte production of inflammatory mediators which is also seen in endometriosis[37] lending further support that endo-metriosis is characterized by systemic immune alteration which may be influenced by the hormonal milieu of the body.

Conclusion

To conclude, it is easy to see how endometriosis can be labeled as an endocrine disease in view of the role of endogenous hormones in its pathophysiology, develop-ment and treatment options. Endometriosis is a steroid dependent condition which histologically is similar to the endometrium. However quantitative differences exist between endometriosis and endometrium in response to hormonal environment, this may be due to the variations in expression of steroid receptors. Although finer details of pathogenesis and treatment remain to be studied and are continually being updated, the two essential components which are estrogen and endometrium have been proven beyond doubt to be the main components of endometriosis.

References

1. Garcia-Velasco JA, Arici A. Apoptosis and the pathogenesis of endometriosis. Semin Reprod Med 2003;21:165-72.
2. Kjerulff KH, Erickson BA, Langenberg PW. Chronic gynecological conditions reported by US women: findings from the National Health Interview Survey, 1984 to 1992. Am J Public Health 1996;86:195-99.
3. Mahmood TA, Templeton A. Prevalence and genesis of endometriosis. Hum Reprod 1991;6:544-49.
4. Osteen KG, Yeaman GR, Bruner-Tran KL. Matrix metalloproteinases and endometriosis. Semin Reprod Med 2003;21:155-64.
5. Gurates B, Bulun SE. Endometriosis: the ultimate hormonal disease. Semin Reprod Med 2003;21:125-34.
6. Marsh EE, Laufer MR. Endometriosis in premenarcheal girls who do not have an associated obstructive anomaly. Fertil Steril 2005;83:758-60.
7. Song JY, Fraser IS. Effects of progestogens on human endometrium. Obstet Gynecol Surv 1995;50:385-94.

8. D'Hooghe TM, Bambra CS, De Jonge I, et al. The effect of pregnancy on endometriosis in baboons (Papio anubis, Papio cynocephalus). Arch Gynecol Obstet 1997;261: 15-19.

9. Cummings AM, Metcalf JL. Effect of surgically induced endometriosis on pregnancy and effect of pregnancy and lactation on endometriosis in mice. Proc Soc Exp Biol Med 1996;212:332-37.

10. Dunselman GA, Willebrand D, Evers JL. Immuno-histochemical analysis of oestrogen and progesterone receptors of eutopic and ectopic endometrium in the rabbit model of endometriosis: the effect of pregnancy. Hum Reprod 1992;7:73-75.

11. Punnonen R, Klemi PJ, Nikkanen V. Postmenopausal endometriosis. Eur J Obstet Gynecol Reprod Biol 1980; 11:195-200.

12. Cumiskey J, Whyte P, Kelehan P, Gibbons D. A detailed morphologic and immunohistochemical comparison of pre- and postmenopausal endometriosis. J Clin Pathol 2008;61:455-59.

13. Tazuke SI, Milki AA. Endometrioma of uterine serosa in a woman with mosaic Turner's syndrome receiving hormone replacement therapy: case report. Hum Reprod 2002;17:2977-80.

14. Fechner S, Husen B, Thole H, et al. Expression and regulation of estrogen-converting enzymes in ectopic human endometrial tissue. Fertil Steril 2007;88:1029-38.

15. Metzger DA, Szpak CA, Haney AF. Histologic features associated with hormonal responsiveness of ectopic endometrium. Fertil Steril 1993;59:83-88.

16. Braundmeier AG, Fazleabas AT, Lessey BA, et al. Extracellular matrix metalloproteinase inducer regulates metalloproteinases in human uterine endometrium. J Clin Endocrinol Metab 2006;91:2358-65.

17. Lessey BA, Killam AP, Metzger DA, et al. Immuno-histochemical analysis of human uterine estrogen and progesterone receptors throughout the menstrual cycle. J Clin Endocrinol Metab 1988;67:334-40.

18. Bulun SE, Fang Z, Imir G, et al. Aromatase and endometriosis. Semin Reprod Med 2004;22:45-50.

19. Patwardhan S, Nawathe A, Yates D, Harrison GR, Khan KS. Systematic review of the effects of aromatase inhibitors on pain associated with endometriosis. Bjog 2008;115:818-22.

20. Lessey BA, Metzger DA, Haney AF, McCarty KS, Jr. Immunohistochemical analysis of estrogen and proges-terone receptors in endometriosis: comparison with normal endometrium during the menstrual cycle and the effect of medical therapy. Fertil Steril 1989;51:409-15.

21. Borroni R, Di Blasio AM, Gaffuri B, et al. Expression of GnRH receptor gene in human ectopic endometrial cells and inhibition of their proliferation by leuprolide acetate. Mol Cell Endocrinol 2000;159:37-43.

22. Khosravi S, Leung PC. Differential regulation of gonadotropin-releasing hormone (GnRH)I and GnRHII

messenger ribonucleic acid by gonadal steroids in human granulosa luteal cells. J Clin Endocrinol Metab 2003;88: 663-72.

23. Sharpe-Timms KL. Endometrial anomalies in women with endometriosis. Ann N Y Acad Sci 2001;943:131-47.

24. Morimoto C, Osuga Y, Yano T, et al. GnRH II as a possible cytostatic regulator in the development of endometriosis. Hum Reprod 2005;20:3212-18.

25. Griesinger G, Felberbaum R, Diedrich K. GnRH-antagonists in reproductive medicine. Arch Gynecol Obstet 2005;273:71-78.

26. Goldman MB, Cramer DW. The epidemiology of endometriosis. Prog Clin Biol Res 1990;323:15-31.

27. Wu Y, Strawn E, Basir Z, Halverson G, Guo SW. Promoter hypermethylation of progesterone receptor isoform B (PR-B) in endometriosis. Epigenetics 2006;1:106-11.

28. Bruner KL, Eisenberg E, Gorstein F, Osteen KG. Progesterone and transforming growth factor-beta coordinately regulate suppression of endometrial matrix metalloproteinases in a model of experimental endo-metriosis. Steroids 1999;64:648-53.

29. Zhao D, Lebovic DI, Taylor RN. Long-term progestin treatment inhibits RANTES (regulated on activation, normal T cell expressed and secreted) gene expression in human endometrial stromal cells. J Clin Endocrinol Metab 2002;87:2514-19.

30. Hornung D, Bentzien F, Wallwiener D, Kiesel L, Taylor RN. Chemokine bioactivity of RANTES in endometriotic and normal endometrial stromal cells and peritoneal fluid. Mol Hum Reprod 2001;7:163-68.

31. Carneiro MM, Morsch DM, Camargos AF, Reis FM, Spritzer PM. Androgen receptor and 5 alpha-reductase are expressed in pelvic endometriosis. Bjog 2008;115: 113-17.

32. Rose GL, Dowsett M, Mudge JE, White JO, Jeffcoate SL. The inhibitory effects of danazol, danazol metabolites, gestrinone, and testosterone on the growth of human endometrial cells in vitro. Fertil Steril 1988;49:224-28.

33. Selak V, Farquhar C, Prentice A, Singla A. Danazol for pelvic pain associated with endometriosis. Cochrane Database Syst Rev 2007:CD000068.

34. Razzi S, Luisi S, Calonaci F, et al. Efficacy of vaginal danazol treatment in women with recurrent deeply infiltrating endometriosis. Fertil Steril 2007;88:789-94.

35. Halme J, Becker S, Haskill S. Altered maturation and function of peritoneal macrophages: possible role in patho-genesis of endometriosis. Am J Obstet Gynecol 1987;156: 783-89.

36. Lebovic DI, Mueller MD, Taylor RN. Immunobiology of endometriosis. Fertil Steril 2001;75:1-10.

37. Rier SE, Martin DC, Bowman RE, Becker JL. Immuno-responsiveness in endometriosis: implications of estrogenic toxicants. Environ Health Perspect 1995;103:151-56.

W Paul Dmowski, Donald P Braun

Chapter 9

Immunology and Endometriosis: Is there a Link?

Introduction

For almost a century endometriosis, like no other disease of the female reproductive system, has been the subject of extensive clinical and experimental research. Yet our knowledge of its etiology and pathogenesis remains unclear, and we cannot easily identify susceptible individuals, nor effectively diagnose, treat or cure women with this condition. Endometriosis histologically is a benign disease without atypical cellular changes, but it shares many characteristics with cancer. It originates from the female reproductive system but can spread and metastasize like a cancer into any tissue or organ. Although under the control of reproductive hormones of ovarian origin, endometriosis acquires the ability to produce these hormones as well as secrete a variety of factors which in turn stimulate in the auto- or paracrine fashion its autonomous growth. Like cancer, endometriotic cells produce a variety of substances which suppress the immune response, permit escape from immune surveillance and allow endometriotic cell invasion. Numerous studies have been published since the early 1980s demonstrating alterations in the immune system or the immune response in endometriosis. Interestingly, however, most of these alterations were observed only to some degree and only in some subjects with the disease. Furthermore, not all studies could be reproduced with consistency. Contributing to the problem is the fact that endometriosis varies significantly in the extent, location and appearance, that it is associated with a variable extent of local tissue reaction and that visual appearance of the lesions may be deceiving contributing to diagnostic errors. Furthermore, it is unclear to what extent findings from experimental endometriosis induced in laboratory animals can be extrapolated to women. Numerous theories have been proposed to explain the role of the immune system in the pathogenesis of endometriosis. However, it remains unclear which alterations of immune function are predisposing to, and which are the result of, ectopic endometrial growth.

In this chapter, we will discuss evidence provided by the literature as well as pertinent results from our own published studies which suggest a link between endometriosis and the immune system. Our approach to this topic comes from a theoretical perspective and, therefore, we do not cite exhaustively the full complement of relevant literature. Instead, the reader is directed towards the many excellent reviews, chapters and textbooks devoted to this subject. Our goal is to invite the reader to examine, ponder, and speculate what the evidence obtained from almost four decades of investigation tells us about this fundamental question: does the immune system cause endometriosis?

Immune System and its Function

To the Reader: The concepts presented in this section are included to provide a context in which to consider how the immune system might play a role in endometriosis development and pathogenesis. The reader is directed to Parham, Peter. *The Immune System, 2nd Ed*. New York, NY, Garland Science, 2005 for a more comprehensive treatment of this subject. Please note that we do not claim credit for the concepts discussed although we are responsible for the narrative. We do, however, indicate with italics our view on how different immunologic concepts and mechanisms, whether first described by ourselves or others, are relevant to the etiology and pathogenesis of endometriosis.

Innate and Adaptive Specific Immune Responses

The past three decades of investigation have seen a remarkable increase in our understanding of the immune response and its role in different pathologic conditions. Much of this work has been aimed at understanding how immunologic reactions of the innate and adaptive-specific immune system contribute to pathologic processes characteristic of different disease states. Immunologic reactions provoked by a broad spectrum of conditions (e.g. infections, trauma, mutations) elicit inflammatory responses mediated by the cells (e.g. neutrophils, macrophages, NK cells) and cytokines (e.g. IL1, TNFα, TGFβ) of the innate immune system. Activation of the innate immune system is fundamental to the survival of the host. Therefore, these reactions are stimulated almost immediately by infectious or traumatic triggering events via induction of rapid activating signals (e.g. chemokines, pattern recognition receptors) that have been maintained and refined throughout the phylogenesis of the species. These reactions lead to destruction of the targeted organism, tissue or cell, followed by the recruitment of antigen-processing cells (e.g. macrophages, dendritic cells) to the site, and subsequent activation of adaptive (antigen-specific) immunity. These reactions link innate and adaptive immune responses leading to durable, long-term sensitization of the host. An important by-product of these host defense reactions that may occur, however, is the destruction of normal bystander cells and tissues.

In some individuals, the destruction of normal tissues by inflammatory reactions results in the loss of self-tolerance. This is manifested by the development of reactions mediated by T cells and B cells, against normal or quasi-normal tissue epitopes. Once these reactions have developed, continuous exposure of the sensitized immune system to self antigens produces chronic, cyclical stimulation of T cell and B cell clones, accompanied by amplification of the tissue destructive response through recruitment and activation of additional inflammatory cells. As this cycle is repeated, the condition becomes chronic with continuous tissue damage and destruction characteristic of the pathophysiology associated with an individual disease or condition. *This sequence of events provides a useful paradigm to explain many of the relationships that appear to operate in the immunologic reactions observed in women with endometriosis.*

Humoral and Cell-mediated Immunity

The adaptive specific immune system was once viewed as a relatively simple system that could be separated into reactions mediated by antibodies (humoral immunity) or cells (cellular immunity). We now recognize that the immune system is a complex, integrated and coordinated physiologic process that functions in a tightly-regulated manner. Its functions are critical for host defense, maintenance of homeostasis, and control of multiple cellular and metabolic processes. Except for a select few locations classified as "immunologically priviledged", the immune system is present and operational in all compartments and spaces in the body; it functions in all physiologic environments; and effects and is affected by the environment in which it operates. Thus, immunologic reactions of the innate and adaptive immune system have the capacity to influence the behavior of cells in virtually any anatomic compartment or tissue.

Rather than viewing the effector arm of the immune response in terms of singular events or reactions, we now recognize these reactions are mediated by multiple cellular and biochemical effectors. Such reactions are elicited by a series of cellular and biochemical processes that yield mediators (both cellular and humoral) capable of exerting potent biologic effects that may be beneficial or detrimental to the host. Furthermore, immune responses evolve in terms of the magnitude and affinity (specificity) for those immunogens eliciting the response. Induction of antibody synthesis or T cell activation are familiar, well-studied examples of immune responses where this more complex view of the system is useful.

We also recognize that stimulation of an immune response elicits a cascade of "regulatory" responses capable of controlling innate and adaptive immunity. During the afferent (activation) stage of the adaptive immune response, regulatory mechanisms determine the type of lymphocyte populations stimulated (i.e. B cell predominant vs T cell predominant). During the amplification stage of the response, other regulatory mechanisms determine the magnitude and specificity of the responding lymphocyte pool. And during the efferent stage of the response, additional regulatory mechanisms determine duration of the response. Thus, we recognize that cytokines of "helper" CD4+ T cells responsible for induction of humoral immunity are distinguishable from cytokines responsible for induction of cell-mediated immunity. Type 1 cytokines (typified by gamma interferon) induce cellular immunity and Type 2 cytokines (typified by IL4) induce humoral immunity. Not surprisingly, the balance between Type 1 and Type 2 cytokines determines the type of immune response elicited (i.e. cell-mediated predominant or antibody-mediated predominant) as well as its overall "tone" or "polarity".

And it is the polarity of the immune response which oftentimes determines the pathogenesis of a disease as well as its outcome in terms of host survival. For example, a Type 1 predominant response to an infection with *Mycobacterium leprae* leads to activation of macrophages including those that harbor the bacillus. These activated macrophages are able to suppress the bacilli resulting in low level infectivity and non-lethal infections termed Tuberculoid leprosy. In contrast, a Type 2 predominant response to the same organism produces antibodies which are inaccessible to the bacilli. This response fails to activate infected macrophages, producing a disease with high infectivity and a sometimes fatal condition termed Lepromatous leprosy.

Another important regulatory mechanism elicited during an immune response is mediated by another subset of the CD4+ "helper" subpopulation. Although helper T cells were traditionally understood to be activated by antigen-presenting cells and subsequently activating CD8+ T cells, macrophages, or B cells to elicit and amplify cell-mediated and humoral immunity, the CD4+ T cells termed T regulatory (Treg) cells have been shown to suppress the immune response. Activation of Treg cells prevents perpetuating the response after elimination of the triggering stimulus and are critical for determining magnitude and duration of the immune response. Treg cells accomplish this by expressing a receptor (designated CTLA4) competitive with an early-acting co-stimulatory receptor expressed on "helper" T cells (designated CD28) that enables T cell activation by antigen presenting cells. The capacity of the immune system to produce effectors (humoral and cellular) for host defense against deleterious organisms or cells is constantly balanced by regulatory systems that prevent perpetuating responses indefinitely and overwhelming normal homeostasis. *These concepts concerning immune system activation and regulation are useful when examining the evidence for a role of the immune system in development and pathogenesis of endometriosis.*

Elimination of Senescent, Misplaced or Ectopic Cells

The view that the immune response is devoted primarily to elimination of "foreign" material or "non-self" antigens has been replaced by an expanded view recognizing the critical role of this system in elimination of abnormal cells or tissues derived from the host. This view accommodates an expanded repertoire of immunogens capable of provoking reactions against senescent cells; misplaced (ectopic) cells; damaged cells; stressed cells; and mutated cells. Thus, a principal function of the system is

maintenance of normal homeostasis through a spectrum of "housekeeping" functions in virtually all physiologic compartments. For example, macrophages are largely responsible for phagocytosis and elimination of senescent red blood cells that express phosphatidyl serine residues normally restricted to the inner leaflet of the red cell membrane until senescence. Homeostatic elimination of senescent red cells by macrophages is essential for host survival.

Other immune functions participate in tissue repair and tissue remodeling. Some of these operate during the menstrual cycle as endometrial cells in the uterine cavity undergo cyclic proliferation, apoptosis, shedding, expulsion and regeneration. *Moreover, whenever endometrial cells become misplaced into ectopic locations during menses, it is reasonable to postulate that homeostatic functions of the immune system are critical for elimination of these misplaced cells. It can also be postulated, therefore, that failure of the immune system to perform these functions correctly could contribute to the development of endometriosis.*

These possibilities would be strengthened if it could be shown that there are endometrial factors or functions that signal the immune system during the menstrual cycle. Thus, studies showing the synthesis of various chemokines and cytokines by endometrial cells, as well as the presence of endometrial macrophages and other immune cells which fluctuate during the menstrual cycle argues for a role of the immune system in normal endometrial growth, apoptosis, and regeneration/remodeling.

Recognition of Self, Non-self, and Altered-self

One of the most significant advances in our knowledge of the immune system has been a greater understanding of antigen recognition, processing, and presentation. From these studies, we have learnt a great deal about how the immune system is programmed to tolerate "self" and recognize "non-self". There are two pathways to process and display antigens: one in association with Class II MHC molecules and the other in association with Class I MHC molecules. Antigens display in association with Class II molecules is primarily a function of professional antigen-presenting cells and leads to activation of adaptive specific immunity. The display of "self" antigens on MHC Class I molecules occurs on all nucleated cells of the body and is essential for maintenance of "self-tolerance" and prevention of autoimmunity.

Significantly, the concept of "non-self" as the primary requirement for immunogenicity has been expanded to include the concept of "modified-self" or "altered-self". In this context, normal "self"antigens altered through various means (e.g. oxidative stress; senescence, mutation) express epitopes capable of stimulating anti-"modified-self" immune reactions. This concept has been very useful in the study of antigens expressed by malignant cells derived from normal "self" antigens, a situation that challenges the immune system to recognize epitopes on cells and tissues that should normally be tolerated. "Self-modification" comes about through multiple mechanisms occurring at either the genomic level (e.g. deletion mutations), the expression level (e.g. post-translational modifications) or through epigenetic changes and may occur in any somatic cell exposed to stress through oxidative and other processes ubiquitous during inflammatory reactions.

One of the most common modifications of "self" antigens seen on malignant tissues results from reduced glycosylation of mucinous glycopeptides. Not only is the glycosylated portion of the glycoprotein modified, reduced glycosylation also exposes cryptic epitopes on the core peptide that are normally sequestered from the immune system. Thus, at least 2 immunogenic epitopes are expressed by "self-modification" of normal cellular glycopeptides as a consequence of mutational events in malignant cells. These so called "Muc-1" epitopes are expressed on a variety of human cancers (e.g. breast, lung, ovary, pancreas) and are currently under investigation as components of human cancer vaccines.

With respect to endometriosis, it is reasonable to speculate that endometrial cells from some women might express "modified-self" epitopes capable of stimulating the immune system. Furthermore, if the immune response fails to eliminate these "modified-self" cells, their persistence would be expected to produce chronic inflammation, damage to bystander cells, possible sensitization against normal "self" antigens, and eventual immunologic suppression. This model explains some of the features of the endometriosis:immune system relationship in terms of disease establishment, pathogenesis, clinical chronicity and cyclicity.

Is Altered Immune Response a Cause or a Consequence of Endometriosis?

Association between endometriosis and alterations in the immune system has been recognized since the early 1980s and has been the subject of numerous comprehensive reviews that are updated regularly.[1, 2] But while there is universal acknowledgement that these changes are temporally associated with endometriosis, there is no definitive evidence that these immune abnormalities are the cause of the disease.

This conundrum is not restricted to the problem of endometriosis, but remains a fundamental issue for many diseases associated with immunologic disturbances. Failure of the immune system to recognize and eliminate malignantly transformed cells has long been postulated as a critical factor for cancer development and is supported by studies showing an increased incidence of cancer in humans with immune deficiency or in carcinogenesis models in which the host is subjected to immunologic suppression. *Thus, it is reasonable to postulate that either an acquired immune deficiency or intentional immune suppression might be associated with an increased incidence of endometriosis.*

How Might Disturbances in Cellular Immunity Contribute to Endometriosis?

As described above, destruction of an inciting stimulus, followed by antigen processing, leading to expression of epitopes that stimulate CD4+ helper cells, which in turn, activate antigen-specific B or T lymphocytes, are critical steps in the development of adaptive immunity. The outcome of these events for a type 1 response is the production of activated, antigen-specific CD4+ and CD8+ T cell populations capable of mediating a broad spectrum of effector reactions upon a subsequent encounter with antigen, including: (i) direct attack against antigen positive cells; (ii) mobilization and activation of macrophages; (iii) heightened activation of NK cells; and, (iv) stimulated synthesis and secretion of soluble mediators with pluripotent effects against virtually all cell types known to participate in endometriosis development.

Mechanisms for Disruption of Cellular Immunity in Endometriosis

If T cell activation and induction of cellular immunity is triggered normally in response to aberrant endometrial-associated antigens, it is reasonable to speculate that disruption of these processes could allow persistence of abnormal endometrial cells. Multiple types of disruption are feasible and could result in either or both defective immunity to endometrial cells and generalized immunologic disturbance. This may explain why some, but not all women with endometriosis show significant suppression of general cell-mediated immunity.

The evidence for disturbed cellular immunity in endometriosis comes from studies showing that endometriotic cells produce immunosuppressive substances detectable in the circulation, peritoneal fluids, or culture media from endometriotic cells. Substances such as: haptoblobin, sKIR (soluble form of Killer Inhibitory Receptors), cadherins, sICAM-1, or RCAS1 (receptor binding cancer antigen) have all been documented in these sorts of studies. RCAS1, according to recent reports, appears to be expressed in the ectopic and eutopic endometrium, decidua and tubal and cervical mucosa; it is also expressed by gynecologic cancer cells and postulated to contribute to escape from host immunological surveillance.[3] It inhibits NK and cytotoxic T cell activity by stimulating apoptosis in these cells. Abnormal RCAS1 expression in eutopic endometrium of women with endometriosis is associated with increased soluble RCAS1 levels in the circulation and correlated with immune suppression. Similarly, immune suppression may be mediated by endometriotic cells expressing FAS ligand capable of inducing apoptosis of T cells and NK cells.[4, 5]

How Might NK Cells Participate in Endometriosis Causation or Pathogenesis?

NK cells mediate cellular destruction of susceptible targets; respond to and synthesize type 1 cytokines such as gamma interferon, IL12, and TNFα; and collaborate with antibodies to mediate antibody-dependent, cellular cytotoxicity (ADCC). Their recognition and activation functions are regulated by families of membrane receptors that transduce activating signals (known collectively as Killer Cell Activating Receptors (KARs) and inhibiting signals (known collectively as Killer Cell Inhibitory Receptors (KIRs). These receptor families interact with cognate ligands on potential target cell surfaces, the outcome of which is either inhibition of NK activation (a state of non-responsiveness) or promotion of activation. It should be appreciated that normal somatic cells express both inhibiting and activating ligands and it is the balance between activating and inhibiting receptor engagement that determines whether the NK cell is activated or remains quiescent.

Inhibiting receptors on NK cells engage inhibiting ligands expressed by normal cells, most predominantly epitopes on MHC Class I molecules. Thus, normal cells of the host which express Class I "self" molecules engage the inhibitory ligands on NK cells which do not react to "self". However, loss or aberrant expression of Class I molecules on cells, events commonly seen in viral infections or malignant diseases, results in decreased engagement of the inhibitory receptors on NK cells. This situation quantitatively favors engagement of the activating ligands on the target cell resulting in NK activation and target cell lysis. These mechanisms are the subject of numerous excellent reviews which are updated regularly.[6]

If endometrial cells transported to ectopic locations during menstruation express stress-related epitopes or downregulate Class I molecules or other KIRs on their membrane, NK cells in the ectopic environment should participate in elimination of these endometrial cells. If that is so, it is logical to postulate that endometriosis development might be associated with failure of NK cells to perform this function. This might occur through different mechanisms related to the NK cells or the endometrial cells, resulting in either failure of NK recognition, activation, or target cell destruction.

Different studies have shown deficient NK killing of reference target cells and endometrial cells in women with endometriosis.[7] To date, there is no definitive evidence to suggest a deficiency in NK cell numbers in either the circulation or peritoneal fluids of patients. Similarly, there are no reports that show loss of activating ligands or increased numbers of inhibiting ligands on the endometrial cells of women with endometriosis.

What has been reported, however, is an increase in the number of the KIR family of killer cell inhibitory receptors on both circulating and peritoneal NK cells in women with endometriosis.[8-10] For example, over expression of killer inhibitory receptor CD-158A on NK cells was demonstrated in women with endometriosis and apparently was not affected by either surgical or medical treatment. These CD-158A+ NK cells were over a thousand times more abundant in peripheral blood than peritoneal fluid suggesting a genetic predisposition to the development of endometriosis and immune tolerance of misplaced endometrial cells.

A number of investigators have also provided evidence that soluble factors from endometrial stromal cell cultures have an inhibitory effect on NK killing.[11-13] Soluble ICAM-1 and the p40 subunit of the IL12 receptor (note: IL12 is a potent NK activating cytokine) are both found in increased levels in the peritoneal fluid of women with endometriosis suggesting yet another mechanism whereby NK destruction of ectopic endometrial cells may be inhibited in women with the disease. Taken together, these results suggest that disturbances in NK cell activation and cytolytic function lead to defective NK killing of ectopic endometrial cells in women with endometriosis. The implication of these findings on endometriosis establishment and persistence is substantial but has not, to date, led to controlled clinical trials with NK cell stimulators in endometriosis patients.

How Might T Cells Play a Role in Endometriosis Causation or Pathogenesis?

T lymphocytes responsible for induction and expression of adaptive cellular immunity include CD4 cells which express a Type 1 cytokine profile (i.e. TH1 CD4+ T cells) along with CD8+ T cells. Studies from the past decade also show induction of CD4+ T regulatory cells (Tregs) that control the magnitude and duration of the response. Notably, all of these T cells express antigen-specific receptors for stimulating epitopes.

The requirement for antigen-specific receptors on T cells raises the provocative question of whether T cell receptors bind endometrial cell epitopes. Unfortunately, there are no definitive data demonstrating this. Several reports from the early 1980s provide indirect evidence for recognition of autologous endometrial cells by lymphocytes with functional assays considered to be mediated by T cells.[14] But many of these studies failed to test antigenic specificity with endometrial cells from unrelated donors and more rigorous investigation of T cell receptor rearrangement consistent with antigenic specificity on clonally expanded T cells in women with endometriosis have not been performed. Significantly, none of the studies reported that the (presumed) T cell reactivity was restricted to the presence of endometriosis.

For example, delayed type hypersensitivity reactions to intradermal injection of autologous endometrial cells, and lymphocyte proliferation in response to these cells was reported to be reduced in monkeys with spontaneous endometriosis compared to normal controls.[14] Similarly, peripheral blood lymphocytes from women with endometriosis were reported to mediate less cytotoxicity against autologous endometrial cells than control subjects using an *in vitro* 51-chromium release assay.[15] The conclusion suggested by these results is that T cell recognition of autologous endometrial cell antigens is not directed against epitopes uniquely expressed on endometrium of women with endometriosis.

Recent studies have investigated the state of T cell immunity in women with endometriosis by determining cytokine profiles in CD4 populations based on the aforementioned roles of Type 1 and Type 2 cells in inducing cellular and humoral immunity respectively. *Assuming that the cytokine content of a CD4+ T cell population will be evoked by antigen-specific stimulation through antigen presenting cells, the balance between TH1 and TH2 cells should reflect the polarity of the T cell response in terms of cellular vs humoral immunity. Moreover, this can be assessed without knowing the antigenic specificities involved.*

It is notable that the majority of such studies show TH1:TH2 ratios which favor induction of humoral immunity in women with endometriosis.[16] This has been found with circulating and peritoneal T cells and differs from results in control subjects without endometriosis wherein the majority of CD4+ cells are of the TH1 phenotype. Some studies have also assessed TH1 and TH2 populations with cells recovered from ectopic endometrium of women with endometriosis.[17] Once again, the results indicate that T cell reactivity favors induction of humoral immunity in women with endometriosis. *Nevertheless, without evidence of clonally expanded T cells capable of binding to endometrial cells through rearranged receptors specific for endometrial antigens, the existence and importance of adaptive specific T cell immunity in endometriosis remains unproven.*

How Might Macrophages Play a Role in Endometriosis Causation or Pathogenesis?

Cells of the mononuclear phagocyte system, i.e. macrophages, are perhaps the most widely-studied leukocyte population in women with endometriosis. Macrophage lineage cells serve multiple roles in both the innate and adaptive immune system. They are derived from monocytes produced by the bone marrow, which normally circulate in the periphery for 2-3 days and then traffic to organs and tissues where they undergo further differentiation in response to factors in the resident microenvironment. When activated, macrophages synthesize and secrete dozens of different mediators that function as chemokines, cytokines, inflammatory mediators, growth factors, angiogenesis factors, differentiation factors, cytolytic factors, and other functions too numerous to discuss.

In acute inflammatory conditions, monocyte production in the bone marrow is substantially increased with subsequent mobilization and activation at the site of the inciting stimulus. The events which ensue can involve phagocytosis and/or neutralization of the stimulus; degradation, processing and display of antigenic epitopes; T cell activation; and generation of adaptive specific immunity. This system is highly efficient for rapidly responding to infectious or traumatic events and is essential for host defense.

In chronic inflammatory conditions, however, it may not be possible to eliminate the inciting stimulus successfully such that some form of persistent stimulation occurs. In this case, monocyte/macrophage numbers and functional status fluctuate overtime in ways that are not rigorously coordinated and predictable in terms of timing, magnitude, and duration. This is the situation presented by endometriosis.

In women with endometriosis, monocytes and macrophages in the circulation, the peritoneal and pelvic cavities, and the endometrium have been the subject of extensive study for close to 4 decades. The overwhelming majority of studies demonstrate that macrophage numbers and activation status are increased in women with the disease. The same can be said for virtually all chronic inflammatory conditions including those in which the fundamental defect responsible for the condition has been identified. It has been seen that the presence of the disease causes changes in macrophage number and function which in turn, influence the clinical course and severity of the disease. But without identification of a fundamental defect responsible for endometriosis development, the importance of macrophage changes for endometriosis causation is not clear. What is clear, however, is that the changes in macrophages seen in women with endometriosis have a profound capacity to influence endometriosis pathogenesis and clinical course.

The list of macrophage functional changes in the circulation, peritoneal and pelvic cavities, and the eutopic endometrium of women with endometriosis is extensive, continues to grow, and beyond the scope of this chapter. Suffice it to say that these changes have been reported by our group and others to have the potential for facilitating the establishment, growth, neovascularization, and spread of ectopic endometrial lesions characteristic of endometriosis. This is attributable to the fact that activated macrophages are producers of a large number of diverse and pluripotent mediators. Moreover, many of these factors participate in and across different physiologic systems such as the inflammatory, immunologic, and neurologic. The significance of this for endometriosis can be appreciated by considering what we and others have reported for the cytokine, TNFα, which is described in some detail below. *When one appreciates the multiplicity of effects that can be elicited by a single macrophage-derived cytokine among the many cytokines shown to be altered in women with endometriosis, it can be stated that the importance of macrophage changes in women with endometriosis are as profound as they are complex.*

Chronic Inflammation as a Mediator and Modulator of Endometriosis

Mononuclear and polymorphonuclear leukocytes (e.g. macrophages and neutrophils) that participate as part of the innate immune system are principal sources of oxidized lipids, superoxides, hydrogen peroxide, prostaglandins, and other mediators that serve to perpetuate the inflammatory component of endometriosis. Along with inflammatory cytokines and chemokines, these oxygenated molecular species are some of the most potent biologic mediators known. They have a profound capacity to mediate cellular stress that can contribute to endometriosis symptoms in multiple ways. More recently, the capacity of these inflammatory mediators to function as growth modulators, differentiation factors, angiogenesis factors, coagulation factors, and mediators of metastasis has also been shown.

It is significant, therefore, that increased levels of diverse inflammatory mediators have been detected in peritoneal fluids of women with endometriosis.[18-20] Because of their extreme potency for biological systems, these mediators are tightly regulated with extremely short half-lives. It is not surprising, therefore, that their levels fluctuate continuously. Nevertheless, the effects elicited on bystander cells and tissues including other cells of the immune system are more long lived. For example, a mediator such as prostaglandin E2 has the capacity to suppress the cytotoxic function of NK cells, T cells and macrophages.[21] This may be one mechanism responsible for suppression of immune cells that would otherwise eliminate ectopic endometrial cells in women with endometriosis. Appreciation for the presence of increased levels of oxygenated inflammatory mediators in women with endometriosis has prompted clinical trials of cyclooxygenase inhibitors or antioxidants in such patients. To date, the results are interesting but not definitive and more investigation is clearly needed.

Endometriosis and Immune Suppression: Is there a Relationship?

If deficiency in cellular immunity is a factor in the development of endometriosis, we would expect either an increased incidence or more rapid progression of the disease in the presence of immune suppression or deficiency. Indeed, Wood, et al[22] reported in 1983 that Rhesus monkeys 7 to 10 years after systemic exposure to a single dose proton irradiation had advanced endometriosis twice as often as controls. Similarly, Campbell, et al[23] and Rier, et al[24] reported aggressive endometriosis involving bowel in monkeys several years after chronic exposure to polychlorinated biphenyls (PCBs) or dioxin. PCBs and dioxin are organochlorides with immunotoxic effects, common contaminants of the environment.

While the goal of the studies was to investigate the pathologic consequences of dioxin exposure on multiple physiologic processes, the striking dose-dependent increase in incidence and severity of endometriosis in these animals makes it difficult to avoid the conclusion that agents which disturb normal immune physiology promote development of endometriosis. Still, it should be appreciated that dioxin is a mutagen whose activity, like many carcinogenic agents, can produce genetic or epigenetic changes in endometrial cells. Such changes may be critical for endometrial cells to acquire the characteristics or apoptotic resistance and ability to grow in ectopic locations that we have come to associate with endo-metriosis. *Dioxin exposure sufficient to produce genetic or epigenetic changes in endometrium, while disrupting immunologic surveillance mechanisms that would normally eliminate these cells, may be dual requirements for the induction of endometriosis in these monkeys.*

In a prospective experimental study D'Hooghe et al[25] were unable to demonstrate development of endometriosis after three months of immunosuppression in baboons with normal pelvis physiology. However, immunosuppressed baboons with spontaneous endometriosis in that study had a significantly higher number and larger surface area of endometriotic lesions after treatment than non-treated animals. It is possible that the period of immunosuppression in that study was too short to demonstrate new cases of endometriosis in previously healthy animals while acceleration of the existing process of the disease was feasible. This would be consistent with our current under-standing of disease pathogenesis as a slow gradual process.

Polychlorinated biphenyls, including Dioxin, bind to estrogen receptors acting as anti-estrogens and induce adverse effects on the reproductive system. They have been referred to as "endocrine disruptors". Recent reports indicate that estradiol beta receptor, unlike alpha receptor, modulates also the immune response and may be preferentially activated by endocrine disruptors. Dioxin has also been demonstrated in animals as a suppressor of cell mediated and humoral immunity.[26] In rats and mice exposed to Dioxin prior to and after induction of experi-mental endometriosis there was a dose related increase in the size of endometriotic lesions.[27] Interestingly, this effect was also observed in mice following *in utero* exposure to Dioxin.[28] It needs to be considered, however, that "experimental endometriosis" induced in laboratory rodents, while sharing some features of endometriosis, is not truly replicative of the disease in humans.

These animal studies, combined with reports indicating the greatest incidence of endometriosis in countries with the highest Dioxin pollution, suggest a causal relationship between industrial pollution and endometriosis.

Unfortunately, there are no prospective studies on the frequency of endometriosis in immunosuppressed women. Such studies would be difficult, if not impossible, considering the protracted time frame required for disease development coupled with the need for invasive techniques for diagnosis. This would make the relationship between disease onset and the beginning of immunosuppression difficult to establish.

Individual case reports of endometriosis diagnosed in women on immunosuppression after organ transplant provide little, if any, information on causality. Similarly, there are no convincing epidemiological data linking exposure to immunotoxicants with increased frequency of endometriosis in humans. Prospective studies following industrial accidents were unable to demonstrate a significant increase in the risk of endometriosis in women exposed to Dioxin, and there have been no convincing epidemiological studies linking endometriosis to environmental immunotoxicants.[29, 30] On the other hand, blood and fat tissue concentrations of PCB's seem to be higher in women with endometriosis than in controls.[31] In a recent study, higher concentrations of immunoto-xicants in the serum of women with endometriosis were associated with impaired NK cell mediated cytotoxicity and a decrease in IL-1β and IL-12 production by peripheral blood monocytes.[32] A similar down regulation of NK cytotoxicity and IL-1β and IL-12 production were observed when normal human monocytes were pulsed with these substances.

It is possible that immunotoxicant induced immune suppression predisposes to the development of endometriosis as suggested by these studies, but a long delay period is required. However, impaired cellular immunity in endometriosis was observed without evidence of immunotoxicant exposure or increase in the blood/tissue concentrations of these substances. *We interpret the findings to suggest that increased incidence of endometriosis in subjects exposed at sufficient levels for sufficient duration is explicable by induction of genetic or epigenetic modifications of endometrial cells, whose survival is enhanced by the immunosuppressive effects of the agent on immunologic control mechanisms.*

Changes in Endometrial Cell Proliferation/ Apoptosis; Implications for Immunologic Resistance and Promotion of Endometriosis

Uterine endometrium under cyclic stimulation by Estradiol and Progesterone undergoes cyclic, proliferative and secretory changes and then a breakdown and shedding associated with the withdrawal of these hormones. In a normal menstrual cycle proliferative changes peak around the time of ovulation; and if there is no pregnancy, endometrial cell apoptosis begins during the secretory phase and peaks during the time of menstrual shedding. Retrograde dissemination of the endometrial cells to ectopic locations occurs during menses in all women. Yet ectopic implantation and development of endometriosis is limited to not more than 10% of the female population.

We speculate that immunologic disturbances are critical factors which determine the fate of ectopic endometrial cells and thus, the predisposition for developing endometriosis. Further, we postulate that disturbances in the following functions are likely to be significant: (a) recognition of non-self or altered-self; (b) elimination of abnormal cells or substances; (c) production of mediators that promote cell growth; (d) production of mediators that promote cell death; (e) production of angiogenesis factors; (f) production of chemokines; and (g) production of regulatory and cellular differentiation factors. It should also be appreciated that either or both qualitative or quantitative disturbances in any of these functions could create conditions that favor the survival and growth of misplaced endometrial cells that could ultimately form ectopic sites of endometrial tissues that are the hallmark of endometriosis.

In women with endometriosis, there is solid evidence for disturbances in many of these immunologic functions including the production of mediators that modulate cell growth, cell death, angiogenesis, and the attraction of other cells capable of contributing to endometriosis pathogenesis. What has not been demonstrated convincingly to date is the existence of endometriosis-associated antigens, whether altered-self or unique. And because of this, it has also not been possible to convincingly show patient sensitization against abnormal endometrium in women with the disease. The fact that the search for such antigens and the immune reactions provoked by them has gone on for decades without obtaining definitive proof is daunting. Furthermore, while there is definitive evidence for increased amounts of different growth regulating and angiogenic factors in women with endometriosis, their presence does not invariably correlate with the severity of the disease or its clinical course.

In 1998, we proposed that endometriosis is a manifestation of the dual phenomena of an abnormal endometrium combined with a dysfunctional immune response.[33] We came to that conclusion based on our earlier demonstration that eutopic and ectopic endometrial cells from women with endometriosis are significantly more resistant

to apoptosis than endometrium from controls.[34, 35] One of the key findings from those early investigations showed that in endometriosis in the eutopic endometrium there is less cyclicity in proliferation/apoptosis and a significant overall decrease in apoptosis. In the ectopic endometrium apoptosis is even further decreased. Based on these findings, we proposed that apoptotic changes in the shedding endometrium normally lead to the programmed death of endometrial cells at the end of the cycle preventing their implantation if misplaced into the ectopic locations.[36] We went on to demonstrate correlation between endometrial apoptotic bodies and the concentration of endometrial monocytes/macrophages both in women with endometriosis and in healthy controls.[37]

The other arm of this dual mechanistic model, namely that of a dysfunctional immune response to ectopic endometrial cells, was provided at about the same time by our demonstration of the resistance of eutopic and ectopic endometrial target cells from women with endometriosis to killing by circulating monocytes and peritoneal macrophages.[38] This led to our subsequent studies examining the implications of the resistance of ectopic endometrial cells to the products of activated macrophages, focusing especially on TNFα. We and others had reported previously that TNF-α, a major secretory product of the activated monocytes/macrophages, is synthesized in increased amounts in both circulating monocytes and peritoneal macrophages of women with endometriosis.[39,40] Our subsequent studies showed in women with and without endometriosis a differential response of endometrial cells to the proliferation/apoptosis modulating effects of TNFα. In the healthy endometrium TNF-α stimulates endometrial cell apoptosis. In the endometriotic endometrium, both eutopic and ectopic, TNF-α stimulates cell proliferation. It is well recognized that TNFα signal transduction through the TNF-α 1 or 2 receptors leads to the sphingomyelinase mediated breakdown of sphingomyelin in a cascade towards either cell proliferation/inflammation or apoptosis. The switch in the signaling pathway appears to be at the level of ceramide. Recent studies seem to suggest an abnormal signaling pathway from ceramide to apoptosis in both eutopic and ectopic endometrial cells in women with endometriosis.

The evidence is compelling that cell cycle events, i.e. proliferation/apoptosis, in the endometrial cells are controlled by monocytes/macrophages and their product TNF-α. Significantly, the effect differs depending on the origin of the endometrial cells. In the healthy endometrium, monocytes/macrophages and TNF-α suppress endometrial cell proliferation and stimulate apoptosis. In endometriosis in eutopic and ectopic endometrial cells, monocytes/macrophages and TNF-α stimulate cell proliferation and decrease apoptosis resulting in survival of these cells. This differential response was observed, not only with autologous monocytes/macrophages,[41] but also with peritoneal fluids from women with endometriosis as well as with recombinant TNF-α. Furthermore, the stimulatory effects of peritoneal fluids on endometrial cell proliferation were abolished by TNF-α blockers.[42] *Thus, the evidence supporting a role for TNF-alpha, a cytokine that functions as a mediator of both innate and adaptive specific immunity, in contributing to key functions relevant to the establishment of endometriosis is reasonably solid.*

There is no question that the interaction between endometrial and immune cells is reciprocal. As indicated above, immune cells can induce proliferation/apoptosis in the endometrial cells. But endometrial cells can also stimulate apoptosis and presumably proliferation of the immune cells. Endometrial glandular and stromal cells express FAS ligand and its receptor FAS. IL-8 and other factors produced by activated macrophages and present in increased concentrations in the endometriotic peritoneal fluid increase expression of FAS ligand and upregulate apoptosis of T-lymphocytes.[4, 5] It was also found that the levels of FAS ligand were greatest in stromal cells obtained from the eutopic endometrium of women with endometriosis compared to normal controls. Finally, evidence for increased levels of soluble FAS ligand in the endometriotic peripheral blood and peritoneal fluid was provided by Garcia-Velasco, et al.[43] This effect was most pronounced in women with moderate to severe disease with serum and peritoneal fluid levels being comparable in those patients. Both T cells and NK cells express FAS ligand, as well as FAS. The attack by a T cell or NK cell against endometriotic cells can therefore be subverted resulting in inhibition of cell mediated killing and apoptosis of the immune cells.

Does Genetic/Epigenetic Immune Modulation Play a Role in Endometriosis?

Genetic predisposition to the development of endometriosis is an attractive concept considering there is an increased prevalence of endometriosis in first degree relatives. Interestingly, both genetic and epigenetic alterations have been reported. For instance, recent studies suggest polymorphisms in the TNF-α- promoter region as a factor determining genetic susceptibility to endometriosis in some populations.[44, 45] This finding is of interest given the central role played by this inflammatory, immuno-

modulatory, growth modulating, and proangiogenic cytokine to list only some of its pluripotent effects that we and others have demonstrated. Similarly, overexpression of KIR on NK cells and KIR polymorphism resulting in decreased NK cell cytotoxicity may confer predisposition to endometriosis, at least in some women.[10-12] Hever, et al[46] using genome wide transcriptional profiling recently reported in endometriosis a gene expression signature consistent with an underlying autoimmune mechanism. Altogether, these data argue for genetically modified immune response as a causal factor in endometriosis. On the other hand, Wu Yan and Associates[47] recently reported that immortalized human endometrial stromal cells stimulated *in vitro* with TNF-α for 30 days exhibited partial methylation of the promoter region of progesterone receptor Isoform B (PR-B) with concomitant reduction of PR-B expression. The authors previously reported hypermethylation of PR-B in women with endometriosis indicating that PR-B down regulation may block the action of progesterone resulting in progesterone resistance in endometriosis. Furthermore, immunotoxicants as discussed previously may induce epigenetic changes in both endometriotic and/or immune cells modifying, on one hand, the endometrial cell cycle and on the other, cell mediated immunity. Impaired NK cytotoxicity and increased TNF-α production were reported in Rhesus monkeys 13 years after termination of Dioxin treatment and also in women with endometriosis and high blood concentrations of PCBs.[32, 48] Interestingly, in one of these studies normal monocytes when pulsed with immuno-toxicants showed a significant down-regulation of NK cytotoxicity.

Are Changes in the Immune Response a Result of Ectopic Endometrial Growth?

Ectopic implantation of endometrial cells unquestionably stimulates the immune system and results in an inflammatory immune response. Some reactions participate directly in controlling the growth of ectopic endometrial tissues, either positively or negatively. Nevertheless, there are no data that establish a direct causative link between growth promotion or growth reduction of endometriotic lesions for any immunologic reaction studied to date in women with endometriosis. *The possibility of a causative link between the immune system and endometriosis would be strengthened if it can be shown that ectopic endometriotic lesions are physically associated with functional immune cells of either the innate or adaptive specific immune system.* While there are numerous studies that have reported increased numbers of different immunologic cells in the peritoneal cavity and fluids of women with endometriosis, immune cell infiltration in intimate association with exophytic lesions or in close proximity to other forms of ectopic endometrium has not been investigated adequately. If, however, a physical association of immune cells with endometriotic tissues is a frequent occurrence in endometriosis, a critical next step will be to determine the types of cells comprising the infiltrates, their functionality, and ultimately, their effect on the behavior of endometrial cells *in vitro* and *in vivo*. While it is unlikely that we can elucidate the sequence of immunologic events associated with immune recognition of ectopic endometrial lesions during the initial onset of endometriosis (especially without a suitable animal model), it should be possible to determine this sequence during disease recurrence.

As a corollary to the question of immune cell proximity or infiltration of endometriotic lesions, the recognition mechanisms for endometrial cells employed by innate and adaptive specific immune cells must be defined. Are there differences in the recognition of normal eutopic endometrium vs. eutopic endometrium from women with endometriosis? Are there differences in reactivity between eutopic and ectopic endometrium? What is the nature of the epitopes seen by the immune system on endometriotic cells (e.g. altered-self, stress-related, completely unique)? And are there resistance mechanisms that render ectopic endometrial tissues insensitive to immunologically mediated destruction? It is significant that all of these issues have been the subject of intense investigation in patients with cancer, but have not been well studied in women with endometriosis.

Humoral Immunity in Endometriosis: What can this tell us about Endometrial Cell Antigenicity?

Some of the earliest evidence documenting the presence of immune reactions that might be directed against "modified-self" epitopes expressed by endometriotic tissues came from studies of autoantibodies in endometriosis patients. The presence of these autoantibodies was reminiscent of autoimmunity in other conditions and lead many investigators to conclude that endometriosis must be related to a loss of self-tolerance with subsequent development of anti-self reactivity. The demonstration of increased auto-antibodies in the circulation of endometriosis patients was one of the seminal findings that promulgated this view, even though it was not possible to show that the autoantibodies produced in patients were uniquely reactive against endometriotic antigens.

Abnormal autoantibody production and increased autoantibody concentrations in the peripheral circulation, peritoneal and other body fluids has been repeatedly observed in endometriosis by a number of investigators. This includes anti-endometrial, anti-endothelial, anti-ovarian, anti-thyroid and other tissue and organ specific antibodies, as well as antibodies against substances integral to the cell structure such as phospholipids, DNA, histones and autoantibodies against oxidatively modified lipoproteins, markers of the oxidative stress. Polyclonal activation of B cells and elevation of all three isotypes of immunoglobulins were reported. In this respect, endometriosis shares multiple characteristics with autoimmune diseases with which it is frequently associated. A recent study demonstrated in the endometriotic lesions, high concentrations of activated macrophages producing BLyS protein which stimulates B-lymphocytes along with a high concentration of antibody producing plasma cells which respond to BLyS.[46] BLyS is a member of the TNF super family implicated in autoimmune diseases. It binds to BCMA receptor which is expressed by plasma cells and is strongly up regulated in endometriotic lesions. BLyS seems to be also elevated in the peripheral circulation in women with endometriosis.

The presence of abnormal autoantibodies in endometriosis seems highly variable, and some investigators were unable to demonstrate a difference in this respect between endometriosis and controls. Part of the problem may be related to the technology used as well as diagnostic challenges which sometimes make differentiation between women with and without endometriosis difficult. Recently, Bohler, et al[49] used a different technique for autoantibody measurement. They analyzed antigenic protein targets recognized by patient derived IgG, a technique used in identifying autoantigen markers for ovarian cancer. They report that, while variability was observed, all patients with endometriosis exhibited a significant level of autoantibodies unlike control subjects. Furthermore, the authors demonstrated a gradual but significant increase in the level of immunoreactivity against ovarian, as well as endometrial cell membrane derived antigens according to the stage of the disease.

Altogether, these data suggest that appearance of a primary endometriotic lesion precedes the activation of humoral immunity. The lesion is then invaded by monocytes/macrophages and then plasma cells which produce autoantibodies. The concentration of the autoantibodies and the number of autoantigens involved appear to increase with the stage of the disease. Under this concept activation of humoral immunity and development of autoantibodies would be secondary to ectopic implantation of misplaced endometrial cells and may represent a defense mechanism aimed at limiting the size and number of the lesions. Variability in the number and concentration of the antibodies would also be controlled by the individual's immune response.

Conclusions

The immune response can best be viewed as an organ system that functions as a principal control mechanism for numerous, diverse, physiologic and pathologic events through a complex but well coordinated group of specialized cells and their products. The immune system continuously reacts in response to changes in both the external and internal environments in order to maintain homeostasis and facilitate survival of the individual. Traditional concepts depicting the immune response as devoted predominantly towards elimination of invading microorganisms have been replaced by the more comprehensive view of a multifaceted, complex, and highly regulated system designed for preservation of the individual rather than the species. There is overwhelming evidence that the healthy immune system not only fights foreign pathogens, but also serves as the principal defense mechanism to detect, neutralize and remove self-antigens/cells that have been modified, mutated, stressed, and/or misplaced in ways that potentially are deleterious to the well being of the host. These "housekeeping" functions of the immune system prevent development of neoplasia, diseases such as endometriosis and premature aging.

In our view, it is these immune system "housekeeping" functions that are most relevant to the development, maintenance and progression of endometriosis. The hallmark of this condition is the ectopic growth of misplaced endometrial cells. These cells share many of the characteristics of normal endometrium, but they also differ in critically important ways. *It is our contention that the most significant behavioral differences between misplaced endometrial cells that can establish endometriosis and those that can't are the dual abilities to circumvent immunologic destruction and to avoid apoptosis.*

The wide-ranging and ever-increasing number of studies showing alteration of different immune functions in women with endometriosis, while potentially useful for understanding different aspects of endometriosis clinical behavior have failed to elucidate whether these alterations are primarily a cause or a consequence of this disease. The concepts presented here suggest that both mechanisms may be operative. Specifically, some

immunologic alterations may be highly influential on endometriosis development (e.g. failure to recognize and react to altered-self antigens displayed on misplaced endometrial cells; over-expression of NK inhibitory receptors), while others may be elicited following establishment or progression of the disease (e.g. development of autoantibodies; hyperactivation of macrophages or inflammation).

We propose that the development of endometriosis is the result of the altered balance between immune system capacity to eliminate misplaced cells and alteration(s) in the endometrial cells facilitating their survival. Both immune system and endometrial alterations in endometriosis may be the result of independent factors, or possibly one factor could contribute to both.

One possible scenario may involve the effect of industrial immunotoxicants. At the level of the uterine endometrium, they are able to modify TNF-α signal transduction resulting in decreased cell apoptosis and increased proliferation/inflammation. At the same time women with elevated blood levels of these substances have been shown to have a decrease in cellular immunity. Under this scenario misplaced abnormal endometrial cells would survive in ectopic locations and would not be eliminated from these locations because of suppressed cellular immunity. Another scenario may involve polymorphism in the TNF-α gene resulting, on one hand, in the decrease of endometrial cell apoptosis and increased survival; and on the other hand, suppression of cellular immunity. The dynamic process of resolution of some lesions and simultaneous development of new ones demonstrated in baboons and in women with endometriosis is consistent with this concept. Furthermore, it suggests that the dynamic balance between the ectopic growth and its elimination may be shifted just slightly in one or the other direction, resulting in progression or spontaneous resolution of the disease.

We also propose that increased local and systemic inflammatory reactions associated with endometriosis are most likely a consequence of endometriotic growth and not sufficient to cause the disease. Similarly, autoantibody production is most likely a secondary response to the evolving endometriotic implants and perhaps aimed at limiting their growth.

In conclusion, we propose that there are genetic, epigenetic and functional factors, that are subject to forces in the external and internal environments of the human female, that can shift the balance of the immune system and the endometrium resulting in either establishment and progression or inhibition and spontaneous resolution of endometriosis.

References

1. Arulkumaran S, Brosen I (Editors). Best practice in Research. London: Elsevier, Ltd; 2004. (vol 18, number 2).

2. Carr BR, Arici A (Editors). Research Seminars in Reproductive Medicine. New York: Thieme; 2003. (vol 21, number 2).

3. Wicherek, L. Alterations in RCAS1 serum concentration levels during the normal menstrual cycle and the lack of analogical changes in ovarian endometriosis. Am J Reprod Immunol 2008; 59:535-44.

4. Selam B, Kayisli UA, Garcia-Velasco JA, Akbas GE, Arici A. Regulation of fas ligand expression by IL-8 in human endometrium. J Clin Endocrinol Metab 2002; 87: 3921-27.

5. Selam B, Kayisli UA, Akbas GE, Basar M, Arici A. Regulation of FAS ligand expression by chemokine ligand 2 in human endometrial cells. Biol of Reprod 2006; 75: 203-09.

6. Terme M, Ullrich E, Delahaye NF, Chaput N, and Zitvogel L. Natural killer cell-directed therapies: moving from unexpected results to successful strategies. Nature Immunol 2008; 9: 486-94.

7. Vinatier D, Dufour P and Oosterlynck D. Immunological aspects of endometriosis. Human Repro 1996; 2(5): 371-84.

8. Wu M, Yang J, Chao K. Increase in the expression of killer cell inhibitory receptors on peritoneal natural killer cells in women with endometriosis. Fertil Steril 2000; 74: 1187-91.

9. Maeda N, Izumiya C, Kusum T, Masumoto T, Yamashita C, Yamamoto Y, et al. Killer inhibitory receptor CD158a overexpression among natural killer cells in women with endometriosis is undiminished by laparoscopic surgery and gonadotropin releasing hormone agonist treatment. Am J Reprod Immunol 2004; 51:364-72.

10. Matsuoka S, Maeda N, Izumiya C, Yamashita C, Nishimori Y, Fukaya T. Expression of inhibitory-motif killer immunoglobulin-like receptor, KIR2DL1, is increased in natural killer cells from women with pelvic endometriosis. Am J Reprod Immunol 2005; 53:249-54.

11. Kitawaki J, Xu B, Ishihara H, Fukui M, Hasegawa G, Nakamura N, et al. Association of killer cell immuno-globulin-like receptor genotypes with susceptibility to endometriosis. Am J Reprod Immunol 2007; 58:481-86.

12. Finas D, Huszar M, Agic A, Dogan S, Kiefel H, Riedle S, et al. L1 cell adhesion molecule (L1CAM) as a pathogenetic factor in endometriosis. Human Reprod 2008; 23(5): 1053-62.

13. Maeda N, Izumiya C, Oguri H, Kusume T, Yamamoto Y, Fukaya T. Aberrant expression of intercellular adhesion molecule-1 and killer inhibitory receptors induces immune tolerance in women with pelvic endometriosis. Fertil and Steril 2002; 77(4):679-83.

14. Dmowski WP, Steele RW, Baker GF. Deficient cellular immunity in endometriosis. Am J of Obstetrics and Gynecology 1981;141(4):377-83.

15. Steele RW, Dmowski WP, Marmer DJ. Immunologic aspects of human endometriosis. Am J Reprod Immunol 1984; 6:33-36.

16. Podgaec S, Abrao MS, Dias Jr. JA, Rizzo LV, deOliveira RM, and Baracat EC. Endometriosis: An inflammatory disease with a TH2 immune response component. Human Repro. 2007; 22, 1373-79.

17. Antsiferova YS, Sotnikova NY, Posiseeva LV, Shor AL. Changes in the T-helper cytokine profile and in lymphocyte activation at the systemic and local levels in women with endometriosis. Fertil Steril 2005; 84: 1705-11.

18. Santanam N, Song M, Rong R, Murphy AA, Parthasarathy S. Atherosclerosis, oxidation and endometriosis. Free radical research 2002;36(12):1315-21.

19. Rong R, Ramachandran S, Santanam N, Murphy AA, and Parthasarathy S. Fertil Steril 2002; 78: 834-38.

20. Slater M, Quagliotto G, Cooper M, Murphy CR. Endomet-riotic cells exhibit metaplastic change and oxidative DNA damage as well as decreased function, compared to normal endometrium. J Molec Histol 2005; 4: 257-63.

21. Braun DP, Harris JE. The impact of prostaglandins on cancer patient immunity: in Prostaglandin Inhibitors in Tumor Immunology and Immunotherapy. CRC Press; Boca Raton, 1994; 109-29.

22. Wood DH, Yochmowitz MG, Salom YL, Eason RL, Boster RA. Proton irradiation and endometriosis. Aviation, Space and Environmental Medicine 1983; 54:718-24.

23. Campbell JS, Wong J, Tryphonas H, Arnold DL, Nera E, Cross B, et al. Is simian endometriosis an effect of immuno-toxicity? Presented at the Annual Meeting, Ontario Association of Pathologists, London, Ontario, 1985.

24. Rier SE, Martin DC, Bowman RE, Dmowski WP, Becker JL. Endometriosis in rhesus monkeys (Macaca mulatta) following chronic exposure to 2,3,7,8-tetrachlorodilbenzo-p-dioxin. Fundamental Application of Toxicology 1993; 21:433-41.

25. D'Hooghe TM, Bambra CS, Raeymaekers BM, De Jonge I, Hill JA, Koninckx PR. The effects of immunosuppression on development and progression of endometriosis in baboons (Papio anubis). Fertil Steril 1995;64(1):172-78.

26. Holsapple MP, Snyder NK, Wood SC, Morris DL. A review of 2,3,7,8-tetrachlorodibenzo-p-dioxon-induced changes in immunocompetence: 1991 update. Toxicology 69:219-55.

27. Cummings AM, Metcalf JL, Birnbaum L. Promotion of endometriosis by 2,3,7,8-tetrachlorodibenzo-p-dioxon in rats and mice: Time-dose dependence and species comparison. Toxicol Appl Pharmacol 1996; 138:131-39.

28. Cummings AM, Hedge JM, Birnbaum LS. Effect of prenatal exposure to TCDD on the promotion of endometriotic lesion growth by TCDD in adult female rats and mice. Toxicol Sciences 1999; 52:45-49

29. Pauwels A, Schepens PJ, D'Hooghe T, Delbeke L, Dhont M, Brouwer A, Weyler J. The risks of endometriosis and exposure to dioxins and polychlorinated biophenyls: a case-controlled study of infertile women. Hum Reprod 2001; 16:2050-55.

30. Eskenazi B, Mocarelli P, Warner M, Samuels S, Vercellini P, Olive D, et al. Serum dioxin concentrations and endometriosis: a cohort study in Seveso, Italy. Environ Health Perspect 2002; 110:629-34.

31. Porpora MG, Ingelido AM, di Domenico A, Ferro A, Crobu M, Pallante D, et al. Increased levels of polychlorobiphenyls in Italian women with endometriosis. Chemosphere 2006; 63:1361-67.

32. Quaranta MG, Porpora MG, Mattioli B, Giordani L, Libri I, Ingelido, AM, et al. Impaired NK-cell-mediated cytotoxic activity and cytokine production in patients with endometriosis: a possible role for PCBs and DDE. Life Sciences 2006; 79:491-98.

33. Braun DP, Dmowski WP. Endometriosis: Abnormal endometrium and dysfunctional immune response. Current Opinion in Obstetrics and Gynecology. 1998;10: 365-69.

34. Gebel HG, Braun DP, Frame D, Tambur A, Rana N, Dmowski WP. Spontaneous apoptosis in eutopic and ectopic endometrium from women with endometriosis. Fertil Steril 1998; 69:1042-47.

35. Braun D, Ding J, Shaheen F, Willey J, Rana N, Dmowski WP. Quantitative expression of apoptosis-regulating genes in endometrium from women with and without endometriosis. Fertil Steril 2007;87:263-68.

36. Dmowski WP, Ding J, Shen J, Rana N, Fernandez BB, and Braun DP. Apoptosis in endometrial glandular and stromal cells in women with and without endomeriosis. Human Reprod 2001; 16: 1802-07.

37. Braun DP, Ding J, Shen J, Rana N, Fernandez BB and Dmowski WP. Relationship of apoptosis and macrophage numbers in eutopic endometrium of women with and without endometriosis. Fertil Steril 2002; 78: 830-35.

38. Braun DP, Gebel HG, Rana N, Dmowski WP. Cytolysis of eutopic and ectopic endometrial cells by peripheral blood monocytes and peritoneal macrophages in women with endometriosis. Fertil and Steril 1998; 69: 1103-08.

39. Rana N, Braun DP, Rotman C, Gebel HM, Dmowski WP. Cytokine Synthesis by peritoneal macrophages in patients with endometriosis. Fertil Steril 1996; 65:925-31.

40. Braun DP, House R, Gebel HG, Rana N, and Dmowski WP. Cytokine synthesis by peripheral blood monocytes of patients with endometriosis. Fertil Steril 1996; 65: 1125-29.

41. Braun DP, Muriana M, Gebel HG, Rotman C, Rana N, Dmowski WP. Monocyte-mediated enhanced of endometrial cell proliferation in women with endometriosis. Ferti Steril 1994; 61: 78-85.

42. Braun DP, Ding J, Dmowski WP. Peritoneal fluid-mediated enhancement of eutopic and ectopic endometrial cell proliferation is dependent on TNF-alpha in women with endometriosis. Fertl Steril 2002;78:727-32.

43. Garcia-Velasco JA, Mulayim N, Kayisli, UA, Arici A. Elevated soluble Fas ligand levels may suggest a role for apoptosis in women with endometriosis. Fertil Steril 2002; 78:855-59.

44. Lee GH, Choi YM, Kim SH, Hong MA, Oh ST, Lim YT, et al. Association of tumor necrosis factor-α gene polymorphisms with advanced stage endometriosis. Hum Reprod 2008; 23(4):977-81.

45. Teramoto M, Kitawaki J, Koshiba H, Kitaoka Y, Obayashi H, Hasegawa G, et al. Genetic contribution of tumor necrosis factor (TNF)-α gene promoter (-1031, -863 and -857) and TNF receptor 2 gene polymorphisms in endometriosis susceptibility. Am J Reprod Immunol 2004; 51: 352-57.

46. Hever A, Roth RB, Hevezi P, Marin ME, Acosta JA, Acosta H, et al. Human endometriosis is associated with plasma cells and overexpression of B lymphocyte stimulator. PNAS 2007; 104(30):12451-56.

47. Wu Y, Starzinski-Powitz A, Guo SW. Prolonged stimulation with tumor necrosis factor-a induced partial methylation at PR-B promoter in immortalized epithelial-like endometriotic cells. Fertil Steril 2008; 90(1):234-37.

48. Rier SE, Coe CL, Lemieux AM, Martin DC, Morris R, Lucier GW, et al. Increased tumor necrosis factor-alpha production by peripheral blood leukocytes from TCDD-exposed rhesus monkeys. Toxicol Sci 2001; 60:327-37.

49. Bohler HC, Gercel-Taylor C, Lessey BA, Taylor DD. Endometriosis markers: immunologic alterations as diagnostic indicators for endometriosis. Reproductive Sciences 2007; 14(6):595-04.

David Redwine

Chapter 10
Sampson Revisited: A Critical Review of the Development of Sampson's Theory of Origin of Endometriosis

Introduction

The origin of any disease is important to know as precisely as possible, because rational, effective treatment can then be developed. The origin of endometriosis continues to be debated against a background of confusion. This suggests that some fundamental concepts about the disease might be wrong. For example, two decades ago it was learnt that most visual manifestations of endometriosis had long been overlooked, which should have led to re-evaluation or disposal of existing concepts about endometriosis, including its origin. Instead, this new information was patched onto existing thought, which only amplified confusion about the disease.

Could Sampson have been wrong? A critical appraisal of the development of his theory of origin of endometriosis might illuminate errors of thought which persist to this day, allowing us to discard what is wrong so that we may see what is correct.

Certain steps must occur during the development of a theory of origin of a disease, from the first descriptions to a robust, profound understanding of origin and effective therapy **(Table 10-1)**.

Table 10-1: Steps in developing a theory of disease origin
1. Accurate initial observations
2. Confirmation and expansion of observations
3. Development of a theory of origin
4. Comparing theory with old and new facts
5. Adjusting or discarding theory to accommodate all facts and observations
6. Emergence of the correct pathogenesis

The efficiency with which these necessary repetitive steps of observation and introspection are taken may vary with the scientific era: initial observations in a technologically unsophisticated era may result in a slower and less efficient development and dissemination of knowledge than first descriptions in a modern era with the advantages of advanced technology and instant communication of thoughts. However, modern instantaneous electronic communications of incorrect thoughts may do harm more quickly. Repeated and robust confirmation of initial observations is important since anecdotal reports or small series may not be representative of the entire spectrum of a disease.

The rate of development of valid information about a disease is also important in defining a theory of origin. Intellectual voids left by slowly developing knowledge will be filled with myths, nonsense, or "herd wisdom", a consensus whereby physician-scientists act on their mutually supported beliefs rather than on science. Near-truths or outright mistakes, if repeated by the "herd" often enough, will seem to masquerade as scientific fact, although the supporting evidence can never quite be pinned down. Progress in identifying a correct theory of origin will be delayed, and the resultant persistent ignorance will result in frustrating confusion, especially among patients. More importantly, an incorrect theory of origin necessarily results in misdirected treatment which may harm patients and waste resources.

Eliminating scientific confusion about the origin of endometriosis does not necessarily require a laboratory but can be combated by examining how closely the steps in **Table 10-1** were followed. If the steps were not followed rigorously, errors of thought will occur, and confusion will continue. The history of endometriosis is littered with unfortunate examples of departures from the required steps of developing a correct theory of origin, which perfectly explains the confusion so prevalent today. A portion of this history will be discussed by examining the original works of Dr. Sampson.

Development of Sampson's Theory of Origin of Endometriosis

As an historical note regarding nomenclature, the term "endometriosis" did not exist when Sampson began writing about the disease. Severe manifestations of a disease are frequently the first to be described, since they are more clinically obvious, and this was true with endometriosis. Reports by Lockyer in 1913,[1] Cullen in 1914[2] and then Sampson focused on what would today be described as severe or deeply invasive disease, usually with ovarian chocolate cysts and frequently with complete cul de sac obliteration with rectal and vaginal involvement. The histology of these deeply invasive lesions of the uterosacral ligaments and other pelvic sites was characterized by small deposits of glands and stroma resembling eutopic endometrium, surrounded by fibromuscular metaplasia. Since this resembled adenomyosis of the uterus, these invasive pelvic lesions located away from the uterus were called "adenomyomas" and could involve nodules of the rectovaginal septum, uterosacral ligaments, inguinal canal and bowel wall. Sampson often referred to invasive disease of the pelvic floor as "implantation adenomyoma of endometrial type" or "implantation adenomas". He also recognized that early, superficial peritoneal lesions also existed and these were also called "implantation adenomas". He often referred to ovarian chocolate cysts as "cysts of endometrial type".

Sampson began his publishing career in a radiological lab,[3] performing transcervical injections of gelatinized bismuth or barium into surgically removed uteri which were then X-rayed. He noted that if the endometrium were intact, no injected medium would flow out of the stumps of the uterine arteries or veins. If menstruation was occurring at the time of hysterectomy, or if the endometrium had been disrupted by curettage, the study medium could flow out of the open vascular stumps along each side of the uterus, since receiving veins underneath the endometrium were exposed. He also noted that the study material would flow out the fallopian tubes. Although not directed at the question of endometriosis, this paper clearly was important in focusing his attention on the consequences of retrograde flow out the fallopian tubes, as he warned that ascending pelvic infections might occur from intrauterine injections. Although not mentioned in the paper, he later noted[4] that this study taught him that the diameter of the fallopian tubes in resected uteri could be variable, and that this might facilitate retrograde tubal flow of menstruum or material injected transcervically. Although one might wonder if evidence collected on resected surgical specimens would transfer seamlessly to other clinical interpretations, Sampson had no such difficulty. In 1925[5] he borrowed these findings to infer that in menstruating women, endometrium sloughing into uterine veins could cause adenomyosis and disease beyond the pelvis.

In an often-cited paper,[6] Sampson in 1921 wrote of 23 patients with chocolate ovarian cysts, only 9 of whom had histologically proved ovarian cysts of "endometrial type". Other cysts had flat, cuboidal linings while others appeared to be corpora lutea. His extremely detailed observations led him to believe that endometrial cysts formed by downgrowth of endometrium from the ovarian cortex into a ruptured ovarian cyst, including follicle and corpus luteum cysts. Since many of these patients had what today would be called deeply invasive endometriosis of pelvic surfaces, by the fourth page of the paper he postulated that chocolate fluid leaking out of these ruptured cysts would carry endometrial cells which implanted on the pelvic surfaces, eventually becoming implantation adenomas, in a process resembling spread of ovarian cancer. He tentatively began thinking that some endometrial cells might reflux out of the fallopian tubes to cause the peritoneal disease he occasionally saw in women without ovarian involvement. On the basis of only his beliefs, he specifically rejected reactive metaplasia due to irritation of refluxed menstrual blood as the origin of peritoneal disease. He had only operated on two women under 30 years of age with such cysts, while the oldest was 47. Seven of 16 (44%) married patients had been pregnant, in an era when the "normal" pregnancy rate was believed to approach 100% and knowledge of other factors contributing to infertility was scant. He thus initiated the thought that pregnancy was protective against endometriosis. Succeeding generations of readers have assumed that this was a seminal paper on endometriosis, but the accuracy of this initial paper with respect to ovarian endometrioma cysts was manifestly low if most of the patients did not have cysts of endometrial type. We see in this paper the origins of several long-held beliefs regarding endometriosis. To Sampson, it appeared to be a disease of older women with reduced fertility; it appeared to spread throughout the pelvis by mechanical dispersion of sloughed endometrial fragments, similar to the presumed mode of spread of ovarian cancer or transtubal infection. It appeared to be a disease which usually involved the ovary as perhaps the most common site of occurrence. Yet we also see in this paper departures from the requisite steps toward the truth: even in modern tertiary referral centers dealing with endometriosis, most women do not have the severe disease described in this early paper, so Sampson's observations were obviously skewed by selection bias. Therefore, any demographic conclusions or theory of origin cannot necessarily be applied to all women with the disease. While this paper is illustrated with a multitude of excellent illustrations and photomicrographs, no photomicrograph was offered of either initial attachment of endometrial cells or tissue fragments to peritoneal surfaces or secondary proliferation and invasion of tissue by those cells. Immediately out of the gate, he presented a partially-evolved theory as a proven fact without supporting scientific evidence. This is most clearly illustrated by one of his conclusions: "The fact that material escaping from the ovarian hematomas may give rise to . . . adenomas of endometrial type . . . is further proof that these hematomas contain endometrial tissue." He presented no supporting evidence for this statement and this proactive mixing of "factual" statements supported only by adverbs or subjunctive verb forms was to become a foundation for "proof" of his theory in subsequent publications as he sought to expand and defend it.

In 1922, in an example[7] of what today would be regarded as duplicate publication, he republished the information and many of the line drawings of his 1921 paper.[6] He continued to focus on seeding of the ovary by endometrial cells refluxing out of the adjacent fallopian tubes (which he found always to be patent), with superficial lesions or deeper-lying ovarian chocolate cysts forming. He believed that rupture of these cysts would later seed further disease throughout the pelvis, reinforcing a concept of geographic disease spread. One figure illustrated an endometrial polyp in a lymph vessel. No photomicrograph of initial attachment or secondary proliferation and invasion is shown.

The first sentence of a paper published in 1922[8] states that reflux menstruation is the cause of implantation adenomas (endometriosis). Thus, in just over 1 year, observations in a few dozen patients, many without proven endometriosis, had transformed into a theory which he now pronounced correct. Heavily illustrated like his previous articles, this paper made much of pelvic microanatomy: differences of fallopian tube lengths of just a few millimeters was taken as evidence to explain why superficial ovarian implants were found on the lateral or mesial side of the ovary. This began to introduce the concept of regulation of flow of reflux menstruation by the pelvic environment. He continued to champion the ovary as a site of common occurrence of disease since it lay adjacent to the fimbriae. Sampson was not particular about

where endometrial-like tissue might come from, stating that it might have "escaped either from the tubes . . . or from the perforating hematoma of the ovary, or probably from both. " Since his earlier thoughts had convinced him that the ovaries were key in the development of "implantation adenomas", he was reluctant to drop the ovaries from the origin equation. He believed that ovarian cysts of endometrial type and implantation adenomas were simply misplaced tissue which originally came from the eutopic endometrium. Once this tissue fell on suitable "soil", it could attach, multiply and invade, and subsequently respond by menstruating like eutopic endometrium. In the ovary, he postulated that if the entire cyst lining sloughed and shed, the cyst would regress completely, although he thought it was more common for incomplete shedding to occur, with resultant persistence of such a cyst. In the audience discussion, it is apparent that his hard work and enthusiasm had won devoted adherents. Dr. JW Williams said "I do not hesitate to tell you that I believe that everything Dr. Sampson has said is entirely justified . . . I have no hesitation in endorsing everything Dr. Sampson has said . . ."

By the autumn of 1922,[9] Sampson's experience with hemorrhagic ovarian cysts was up to 49 patients. He had begun to understand that implantation adenomas could exist on pelvic surfaces without ovarian disease as an intermediary. To account for the occurrence of superficial or deeply invasive peritoneal disease in some women without ovarian endometrial cysts, he postulated that endometrial and tubal epithelium refluxing out the fimbriated end of the fallopian tube might attach and implant on peritoneal surfaces without having to attach to the ovary first, especially in the cul de sac where he envisioned gravity directing the refluxed tissue. Without supporting evidence, he again stated that peritoneal implantations arose from perforation and leakage of ovarian hematomas. His evidence consisted of numerous line drawings, photomicrographs of established superficial disease resembling eutopic endometrium, as well as tangential cuts across uterine adenomyosis and arrangement of the resulting pictures to make it appear that the disease began on the uterine serosa and then invaded the muscularis. Once again there were no photomicrographs of initial attachment of endometrial cells or tissue fragments to peritoneal or ovarian surfaces, nor were there photomicrographs of secondary proliferation and invasion of these cells. Using a scientific argument supported only by adverbs, he noted implantation adenomas on the sigmoid, rectum, terminal ileum and appendix and observed that these sites were in close proximity to the ipsilateral ovary, from which the intestinal disease "usually (possibly always)" came. Pathoconsertive relationships observed at surgery were thus taken literally as cause-and-effect relationships. He dismissed the possibility of a developmental origin because he had only once seen ovarian hematomas of endometrial type in woman younger than 30 and thought that this manifestation of endometriosis should be present in the early teenage years if it were developmental. This was another example of conclusions reached from a small number of observations skewed toward older age groups and women with severe disease. Unbeknownst to Sampson, an entire unidentified reservoir of other disease morphologies was present, but by focusing on the minority of patients with severe disease and by repeating observations as causal fact, errors in understanding were simply reinforced. Severe disease does not just appear overnight but must have early, subtle morphologies.

In 1924,[10] Sampson discussed benign implantation adenomas and peritoneal metastases of endometrial cancer to illustrate his belief that both conditions could arise from reflux of endometrial tissue from the fallopian tubes. The ovarian tumors described are benign endometrial cysts and are included in the paper somewhat tangentially since he had focused previously on the ovaries as the initial site of implantation adenomas. Soon thereafter,[11] he united the concept of reflux menstruation and ovarian endometrioid carcinoma, which no doubt pleased him greatly since it reinforced his belief that the mode of spread of cancer was identical to the mode of spread of endometriosis. Sampson's belief that refluxed endometrial cancer cells could mimic implantation adenomas arising from reflux menstruation caused him to recommend ligation of the fallopian tubes before hysterectomy for endometrial carcinoma. He also wondered whether vigorous bimanual examination might force malignant cells out of the uterus and postulated that uterine retroversion, polyps, or fibroid tumors might augment reflux menstruation. Sampson stated that most evidence that he and others had provided for reflux menstruation as the cause of implantation adenomas has been only circumstantial. He indicated that the one solid proof that endometrium could implant and grow ectopically was that of endometriosis of a surgical scar. He did not consider the profound difference between intact peritoneum and an open incision, instead borrowing scar endometriosis as further proof of reflux menstruation as the cause of pelvic endometriosis. He also did not consider that Iwanoff's serosal theory of peritoneal totipotentiality might be too restrictive but could extend to totipotentiality

of more far-ranging areas of the body, including the lower anterior abdominal wall in the path of surgical incisions. In such areas, substrate tissue might exist which could be susceptible to metaplasia into endometriosis, aided and abetted by the growth factors of wound healing. By this time Sampson had more experience with the varied morphologies that could be displayed by implantation adenomas, using terms such as "red/purple raspberry" and "blueberry", which would delight a later generation of morphologists.

In 1925,[12] Sampson first introduced the term "endometriosis", although he was not quite comfortable with discarding the term "implantation adenomyoma", which he occasionally used as well. Also notable are depictions of lesions of various colors, including white. Photomicrographs of superficial endometriosis of the uterus and ovarian cortex are supplied, but none of initial attachment of endometrial cells or tissue fragments to pelvic surfaces, or of secondary proliferation and invasion.

Sampson stated[13] that during menstruation, pregnancy and menopause, endometriosis was identical in structure and function to eutopic endometrium, a notion that was finally discarded in the 21st century when the dozens of differences noted between endometriosis and native endometrium[14] multiplied into hundreds.[15] He asserted without biochemical evidence that refluxed menstrual blood was far more irritating to the pelvis than normal blood, and this was what led to the formation of significant adhesions in some patients. The possibility never crossed his mind that endometrial glands are biologically active and might secrete some paracrine substance which is the actual cause of inflammation, hemorrhage and adhesions. He continued to offer as evidence for his theory that if surgery were done during menstruation, blood could occasionally be seen coming from the fimbriated ends of the tubes, although Novak commented that in all the surgeries that he had done during menstruation, he had never seen blood exiting the fimbriae. Further "evidence" of repeated monthly seedings was the observation that in an individual patient, different morphologies could be seen. To him, this indicated different stages of development resulting from different episodes of implantation. He did not consider that different areas of endometriosis in the same pelvis might have innately different potentials for both biologic activity and virulence which could result in different morphologies. Scar endometriosis following surgeries where the uterus was not opened was explained by unseen refluxed endometrial cells which were present in the peritoneal cavity and which implanted in the fresh surgical incision, again not considering the possibility that tissue near the pelvis might have some potential for Mullerian metaplasia promoted by growth factors of healing. On the basis of his radiological work published in 1918,[3] he postulated that adenomyosis of the uterus was caused by venous emboli of endometrium.

Sampson firmly believed that endometriosis presents the same structural variations as eutopic endometrium and is often governed by the same hormonal events regardless of location.[16] He continued to cobble together circumstantial evidence to define menstruum as a never-dying super-tissue: experimental autotransplantation of endometrium in non-menstruating animals mirrored the finding of post-cesarean section scar endometriosis; endometrium had occasionally been observed in the lumen of the fallopian tube during menses and might escape from the fimbriated end; menstrual blood possibly could cause reactive peritoneal metaplasia into endometriosis; monkey endometrium scattered in the peritoneal cavity could result in implantation; endometrium can be found in lymphatics and venous channels.

In a nascent mixing of two competing theories of origin, (reflux menstruation and coelomic metaplasia), he stated that menstrual blood might, "in some magical and mysterious way" convert the peritoneum into endometriosis. He postulates a solid element in refluxed menstrual blood acting as a specific irritant, or "there are scattered throughout the pelvic peritoneum areas of potential mullerian tissue which under the specific action of menstrual blood develop into endometrial tissue."

He postulated gravity as the reason for the most common areas of involvement by virtue of reflux menstruation, ignoring the pathways of fetal organogenesis across the posterior coelomic cavity which might lay down the tracts of potential mullerian tissue which he had previously rejected as a possible cause of endometriosis.

Without any proof whatsoever, he stated that "Menstrual blood undoubtedly irritates the peritoneum causing inflammatory exudation, granulation tissue, adhesions and peritoneal inclusions... the very conditions which would favor the retention and growth of any epithelium or other tissue present in this blood, just as similar peritoneal reactions make possible the retention and growth of fragments of cancer escaping into the peritoneal cavity. While menstrual blood may be very injurious to the mesothelium the fragments of uterine tissue in it might remain alive for a longer time, being more accustomed to its presence." This fanciful notion of reflux menstruation inciting such florid peritoneal reaction is belied, of course, by the rather bland morphologies and clear peritoneal fluid which can commonly be seen with early stage disease. Again, his focus on severe disease led

him to "borrow" findings in that uncommon morphology as an explanation for the origin of the disease.

Having experience with only 101 patients with ovarian endometriosis[17] by 1929 he continued to be heavily dependent on qualifying verb forms to support his argument rather than hard science, including "might, suggested, could have, probably, may, at least suggest, it is natural to assume,..." as well as definitive unsupported adverbial statements such as "undoubtedly,..." He also was quick to come to scientific conclusions without supporting evidence, such as peritonitis due to refluxed menstrual blood allowing enhanced attachment of endometrium to peritoneal surfaces.

In 1932,[18] Sampson studied peritoneal spread of ovarian cancer, implying that evidence of possible metastases could be borrowed to explain peritoneal endometriosis **(Figure 10-1).**

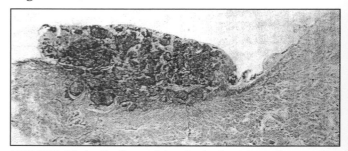

FIGURE 10-1: Peritoneal implant of metastatic ovarian carcinoma.[18] Such lesions were used as ancillary "proof" of Sampson's theory. Reproduced by permission of the American Society for Investigative Pathology.

By 1932[19] Sampson must have been feeling pressure from objections to his theory of reflux menstruation. He reluctantly agreed that peritoneal metaplasia might cause some cases of peritoneal endometriosis, especially when there was no ovarian endometriosis to blame for spread to the peritoneum. However, since most patients with endometriosis had patent tubes, he was unwilling to let go of a possible contribution of reflux menstruation as a specific irritant to the peritoneum which might result in reactive metaplasia of peritoneum into endometriosis. Straining ever-more-mightily to protect his theory, he stated (without direct evidence) that irritative cellular detritus (menstruum) or perhaps nuclei extruded from secretory endometrial cells escaping the fimbriated ends of the fallopian tubes incited irritative reactive metaplasia of the peritoneum into endometriosis just like cellular detritus escaping the tubes during pregnancy incited decidual reaction in similar locations of the pelvic peritoneum. Progesterone as a cause of decidual reaction was apparently unknown to him. He thought some type of cellular or nuclear debris was important because he had never seen endometriosis in women who had a previous ruptured tubal pregnancy, his thought being that tubal pregnancy would 'soil' the peritoneum with pure blood rather than any cellular debris. The validity of this thought is questionable given that with a ruptured tubal pregnancy, embryonic, fetal and placental tissue could conceivably provide cellular detritus to the peritoneum. Giving his power of free association unfettered but somewhat confusing reign, and without direct evidence, he posed that if Müllerian epithelial tissue could stimulate mesenchymal tissue into Müllerian stroma, then why couldn't Müllerian tissue stimulate epithelial tissue into epithelial stroma? He went on to show in elegant photomicrographs that tubal endometriosis could arise *de novo* beneath the normal tubal epithelium (independent of reflux menstruation), and posited that preceding inflammation and repair of the tube had resulted in metaplasia into endometriosis, similar to the process by which endosalpingiosis can affect tubal stumps.[20] He then suggested that these deposits of new endometriosis would undergo sloughing due to menstruation (no photomicrographic evidence was ever shown), and implant in the pelvis causing peritoneal or ovarian endometriosis. Sampson repeatedly asks scientific questions and supplies his own answers based on rhetorical logic. It is clear that he depended on rote repetition of what he had stated in previous publications, reinforced by copious photomicrographs illustrating his thoughts only up to a point, but never delivered robust photomicrograph proof of menstruating endometriosis, attachment of endometrial tissue to peritoneal surfaces, or secondary proliferation and invasion.

In a summation of his career,[21] he focused on peritoneal disease, stating that endometriosis occurred because of reflux menstruation and that peritoneal implants would menstruate and thus create new implants, causing the disease to spread, similar to ovarian cancer. He admitted that there was no positive proof that endometrial tissue from ovarian cysts is shed and becomes implanted on the peritoneum to become endometriosis, but he suggested that the evidence was very strong. In a preternatural defense of his theory, he stated "If bits of Müllerian mucosa carried by menstrual blood escaping into the peritoneal cavity are always dead, the implantation theory . . . also is dead and should be buried and forgotten. If some of these bits are even occasionally alive, the implantation theory also is alive."

Sampson's great strengths as a researcher included his unbounded curiosity and enthusiasm for studying endometriosis, as well as an active imagination which continually sought to mold clinical observations to his fervently-held theory instead of the opposite way around. His papers were long, averaging over 35 pages with the longest being 88 pages. His works were copiously and elegantly illustrated with surgical photographs, line drawings, and photomicrographs, all of which would be very impressive to any reader and which would lend an air of supreme authority to his work which would be difficult to question.

Much of Sampson's work would be found unsuitable for publication today.

In retrospect, the weaknesses of his arguments outnumbered the strengths. His papers included numbing repetition of the same thoughts, supported by very detailed speculations and by frequent use of qualifying words such as "might", "probably", "possibly", "could", etc. His beliefs were little altered by the passage of time or new findings such as discovery of more subtle disease morphologies which might shed a new perspective on the origin of disease. He tried to characterize objections or exceptions to his theory as uncommon outliers which really had no effect on the veracity of his beliefs, instead of attempting to modify his theory to explain all instances of observations. There seemed to be few of his peers who were willing to challenge his strongly held convictions, and this allowed his thoughts to reign unchecked over several generations of gynecologists. His clinical experience with endometriosis appears to have been limited only to perhaps a few hundred patients, skewed toward the minority of patients with advanced disease. This inexperience would necessarily result in his having an incomplete view of the disease which would make incorrect conclusions more likely in that era. How could he possibly have come up with the correct theory of origin with all of these limitations?

His strong conviction that he was correct, combined with illustrations and scholarly repetition, served as proxies for what was lacking: he never published a photomicrograph of endometriosis menstruating, and published only one photomicrograph of alleged initial attachment and none of secondary proliferation and invasion of endometrial cells or tissue fragments. Since he did not do serial sections of the rare examples of alleged initial attachment to peritoneal surfaces of what he assumed was refluxed endometrium we don't know whether there might have been evidence that such tissue might have originated in the peritoneum without the need for reflux menstruation. He never discussed the origin of the fibromuscular metaplasia surrounding deeply invasive disease. Perhaps he considered that reconciling this finding with reflux menstruation would require either postulating that myometrium also sloughs and sheds by reflux menstruation or that the theory of reflux menstruation was not the origin of implantation adenomyomas, in which case he never would have proposed the theory in the first place.

Reflux menstruation as the origin of endometriosis requires that endometriosis be a surgically incurable, progressively spreading, autotransplant disease. Yet all of these features have been disproved.[22] The high prevalence of endometriosis and the frequency of surgical diagnosis should have resulted in robust photomicrographic confirmation of Sampson's allegations of initial attachment of refluxed tissue, as well as of proliferation and invasion, yet investigators looking for this have never found it. Initial attachment and secondary proliferation and invasion remain unexplained miracles.

Despite these fatal flaws, some authors still make efforts to support this theory, the latest being the peritoneal circulation modification of Sampson's theory.[23] This inventive model attempts to explain the slightly increased frequency of involvement of the ovary and uterosacral ligament on the left side of the pelvis compared to their paired twins on the right. Supporters of this modification propose that there is a natural clockwise (as one views the patient) circulation of the peritoneal fluid, but that the pelvic portion of the sigmoid colon diverts the circulation toward the midline and away from the left pelvic region. This "protected" area on the left side of the pelvis theoretically allows refluxed endometrial tissue from the left tube to lay alongside the peritoneum longer, thus facilitating attachment compared to the right side of the pelvis, where the peritoneal current sweeps refluxed cells away from the pelvis. Lacking their own supporting evidence, the authors relied entirely on work published by Meyers in 1970,[24] in which radiological dye was injected into the peritoneal cavity of male and female adults suffering from peritoneal cancer, effusions, abscesses, and adhesions. The position of the patients was altered on a tilt table, and radiographs taken during position changes. A schematic diagram was published **(Figure 10-2)**, indicating that dye could travel virtually anywhere in the abdominal cavity depending on the tilt of the table. Beyond the obvious objection that such work is unphysiologic and unrelated to the question of reflux menstruation lies a more serious concern. To support their argument, the author took the figure published by Meyers and altered it to fit their arguments, erasing or adding arrows to fabricate supportive "evidence" for the circulation they propose. **(Figure 10-3)**. By further alteration, Meyers' original figure could also be shown to "prove" that only a counterclockwise circulation exists **(Figure 10-4)**.

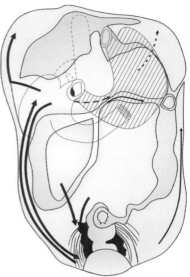

FIGURE 10-2: The original figure published by Meyers.[24] Notice there are strong arrows running up and down the right colonic gutter, with flow toward Morrison's pouch, and a weak arrow toward the right hepatic margin, with another strong arrow from Morrison's pouch to the subphrenic space. *Reproduced by permission of the Radiological Society of North America.*

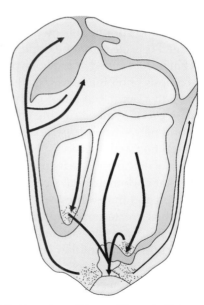

FIGURE 10-3: Alteration of Meyers' figure by Bricou et al.[23] Notice Meyers' strong arrow going caudad down the right colonic gutter has been deleted and his weak arrow shaft going past the right hepatic margin has been replaced by a strong arrow which is continuous with the pelvis. Meyers' strong arrow from Morrison's pouch to the right subphrenic space has been deleted. Bricou et al don't discuss the effects on the distribution of endometriosis of the weak arrow ascending the left colonic gutter – there should be frequent deposition of disease near the spleen (although disease in this area is extremely rare or unreported). *Reproduced from reference 23 by permission of Elsevier.*

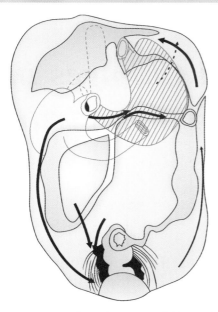

FIGURE 10-4: Hypothetical alteration of Meyers' figure. All arrows which depict a clockwise path have been deleted, and a strong arrow added around the spleen, giving the impression of a counter-clockwise peritoneal circulation, thus "proof" that a clockwise circulation does not exist.

Conclusion

Sampson's theory and ineffective medical or superficial surgical treatment of endometriosis have an unholy symbiosis. Sampson's theory predicts failure of all treatment modalities while ineffective treatments provide that failure. Physicians don't have to blame ineffective treatment for therapeutic failures, because "it's the nature of the disease. It always comes back." Sampson's theory has guided thought on endometriosis for too long and women are being physically harmed by its continued acceptance, since repeated surgeries and rounds of medical therapy are the unfortunate hallmarks of modern therapy. Supporters of this theory have failed to address its fatal flaws and now are creating "evidence" out of thin air. If Sampson's theory is finally discarded, we will be free to imagine another, possibly more correct theory of origin which will be helpful both to science and to patients.

References

1. Lockyer C, Proc Roy: Soc Med 1913: 6.
2. Cullen TS. Adenomyoma of the rectovaginal septum. JAMA 1914; 14:835.
3. Sampson JA. The escape of foreign material from the uterine cavity into the uterine veins. Am J Obstet, August, 1918;78:161-75.
4. Sampson JA. Benign and malignant endometrial implants in the peritoneal cavity, and their relation to certain ovarian tumors. Surg Gynecol Obstet, March, 1924;38:286-311.
5. Sampson JA. Heterotopic or misplaced endometrial tissue. Am J Obstet Gynecol 1925;10:649-64.
6. Sampson JA. Perforating hemorrhagic (chocolate) cysts of the ovary. Arch Surg Sept 1921;3:245-323.
7. Sampson JA. Ovarian hematomas of endometrial type (perforating hemorrhagic cysts of the ovary) and implantation adenomas of endometrial type. Boston Med Surg J April, 1922;180;445-56.
8. Sampson JA. The life history of ovarian hematomas (hemorrhagic cysts) of endometrial (Mullerian) type. Am J Obstet Gynecol November, 1922; 4:451-512. (Discussion pp. 561-63).
9. Sampson JA. Intestinal adenomas of endometrial type. Arch Surg Sept 1922; 5:217-80.
10. Sampson JA. Benign and malignant endometrial implants in the peritoneal cavity, and their relation to certain ovarian tumors. Surg Gynecol Obstet March, 1924;38:286-311.
11. Sampson JA. Endometrial carcinoma of the ovary, arising in endometrial tissue in that organ. Arch Surg January, 1925; 10:1-72.
12. Sampson JA. Inguinal endometriosis (often reported as endmetrial tissue in the groin, adeomyoma in the groin, and adenomyoma of the round ligament) Am J Obstet Gynecol 1925;10:462-503.
13. Sampson JA. Heterotopic or misplaced endometrial tissue. Am J Obstet Gynecol 1925;10:649-64.
14. Redwine DB. Was Sampson wrong? Fertil Steril, 2002;78:686-93.
15. Eyster KM, Klinkova O, Kennedy V, Hansen KA. Whole genome deoxyribonucleic acid microarray analysis of gene expression in ectopic versus eutopic endometrium. Fertil Steril 2007;88(6):1505-33.
16. Sampson JA. Endometriosis of the sac of a right inguinal hernia, associated with a pelvic peritoneal endometriosis and an endometrial cyst of the ovary. Am J Obstet Gynecol 1926:459-83.
17. Sampson JA. Infected endometrial cysts of the ovaries. Am J Obstet Gynecol 1929;18:1-16.
18. Sampson JA. Implantation peritoneal carcinomatosis of ovarian origin. Am J Path 1931; 7(5):423-44.
19. Sampson JA. Pelvic endometriosis and tubal fimbriae Am J Obstet Gynecol 1932;24:497-542.
20. Sampson JA. Endometriosis following salpingectomy. Am J Obstet Gynecol 1928;16:461-99.
21. Sampson JA. The development of the implantation theory for the origin of peritoneal endometriosis. Am J Obstet Gynecol 1940;40:549-557.
22. Redwine DB. Was Sampson wrong? In: Redwine DB (Ed): Surgical Management of Endometriosis. New York, Martin Dunitz, Taylor and Francis Group, 2004.
23. Bricou A, Batt RE, Chapron C. Peritoneal fluid flow influences anatomical distribution of endometriotic lesions: why Sampson seems to be right. Eur J Obstet Gynecol Reprod Biol 2008; 138:127-34.
24. Meyers MA. The spread and localization of acute intraperitoneal effusions. Radiology 1970 95:547-54.

Luciano G Nardo, Carolyn JP Jones

Chapter 11

Endometrial Changes in Women with Endometriosis

Introduction

Implantation is a complex and crucial step in the establishment of pregnancy. As with the molecular signalling pathways, the ultrastructural changes governing endometrial receptivity are only partially known. Asynchronous development of the endometrium in some subfertile women may account for the failure of the embryo to implant during the highly controlled implantation window. An abnormal hormonal milieu, such as the one resulting from controlled ovarian hyperstimulation or an underlying disease like endometriosis, may alter the mechanisms involved in implantation and early pregnancy.

Endometriosis, one of the most common causes of infertility and chronic pelvic pain, affects about 10% of women in the reproductive-age group,[1] with this number increasing to 30% in patients with infertility and up to 45% in patients with chronic pelvic pain.[2] It is defined as the extrauterine growth of endometrial glandular epithelial and stromal cells, with the lesions developing on pelvic peritoneal and visceral surfaces. The mechanisms by which endometriosis impairs fertility are varied, from distortion of pelvic anatomy to negative effects on implantation. Postulated mediating factors include local paracrine action of cytokines, alteration in inflammatory responses and/or autoimmune influences. Owing to the increased prevalence of endometriosis in subfertile women, many studies have focused on the development, growth and structure of these lesions. But, to date, little is known about the structural changes that might be present in the eutopic endometrium of women with this disease. Here, we describe the current literature pertaining to such anomalies and also describe findings from our own recently published investigations on endometrial ultrastructure and glycosylation in women with endometriosis.[3,4]

Endometrial Histology, Ultrastructure and Glycosylation in Endometriosis

Amongst the current reviews on endometrial changes in women with endometriosis only two studies reporting structural changes in the endometrial have been cited.[5,6] One reported the presence of a thinner endometrium in women with endometriosis[7] while the other examined tissue from the endometriotic endometrium by transmission and scanning electron microscopy and also by using morphometric techniques on histological sections.[8] In the latter series, only preovulatory women were selected, and the histology of the endometrium appeared to be normal. However, morphometry showed that the number of mitoses in both glands and stroma, and the presence of subnuclear vacuolation were less in the affected cases, while ultrastructural examination showed heterogeneity of the surface epithelium and an irregular distribution of the gland openings; ciliogenesis was also found to be incomplete. Transmission electron microscopy revealed the height of gland cells to be reduced, though not significantly so, and cilia and microvilli to be poorly developed. Other studies by the same authors, reporting the effects of various treatments on endometriosis, described the eutopic endometrium as being as either normal in its ultrastructure or mentioned only the presence of normal features such as finely granular nuclear chromatin, well-developed Golgi apparatus, small mitochondria and a fine rough endoplasmic reticulum in the ultrastructural examination of eutopic endometrium from affected women.[9-12] However, the information provided was scanty and illustrations inadequate for a meaningful assessment.

In our recent investigation of eutopic endometrium from 24 women with endometriosis matched with 14 healthy controls, we found the most significant changes to occur

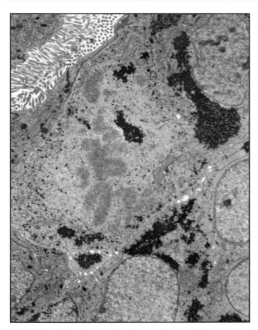

FIGURE 11-1A: Endometriotic endometrium on day 24 showing a mitotic figure with darkly stained intracellular aggregates of glycogen. Adjacent cells also show large glycogen aggregates as well as dispersed foci. Original screen mag: x2,600.

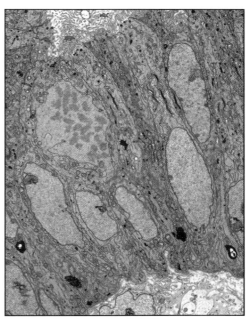

FIGURE 11-1B: Normal proliferative endometrium on day 9 showing a mitotic figure and cells with only occasional, small foci of glycogen, mainly basally situated. Original screen mag: x 2,600.

in the mid- to late- secretory phase of the cycle, both with respect to ultrastructure and also to the expression of glycans bound by the lectin *Dolichos biflorus* agglutinin (DBA).[3,4] No specific ultrastructural abnormalities were found compared to tissue from normal women but in the second part of the menstrual cycle features normally confined to particular stages of the cycle appeared over a much wider period of time. Mitotic figures, which are usually rare after days 14-16 of the cycle, were found in three cases of days 17, 22 and 24, and in two of those (days 17 and 24) the dividing cells contained aggregates of glycogen **(Figure 11-1A)**, a feature never seen in the control tissue **(Figure 11-1B)**. Under normal circumstances, the process of cell division is separated chronologically from glycogenesis and the two are not observed together. Glycogen deposits, normally diminishing from day 17, were found to be more prominent later in the cycle **(Figure 11-2A)** as were giant mitochondria and nucleolar channel systems **(Figure 11-2B)**. In control tissues there are generally changes in the appearance of nuclei as the secretory phase develops, with chromatin aggregation producing very heterochromatic nuclei in the late secretory phase **(Figure 11-3A)**. This feature was absent in some cases, the nuclei remaining relatively euchromatic throughout the cycle **(Figure 11-3B)**. In contrast, some specimens showed accelerated maturation, with features normally found

towards the end of the secretory phase (shorter cells, heterochromatic nuclei, increased complexity of lateral membrane interdigitation) appearing much earlier, for instance, on day 15 **(Figure 11-4A)**, while controls around that time have heavy deposits of glycogen, giant mitochondria and nucleolar channel systems **(Figure 11-4B)**. Great heterogeneity in the appearance of glands from the same specimen was often found, but this can also be seen in normal secretory phase tissue. Such variations in ultrastructure were seen between specimens obtained on the same day of the cycle, with some showing more advanced features for their date, and others showing a delay in maturation. This heterogeneity was a striking feature of the study overall. A detailed study by Metzger and colleagues comparing the hormonal responsiveness of ectopic with eutopic endometrium, noted that 83% of eutopic samples dated as secretory were in phase but only within 5 days, which also implies that some variation from the normal endometrium was observed.[13]

Cell Cycling Abnormalities in Eutopic Endometriotic Endometrium

The maintenance of a proliferative-type profile into the secretory phase is consistent with the findings of Burney and collaborators who suggested that, in women with endometriosis, pathways governing the transition from

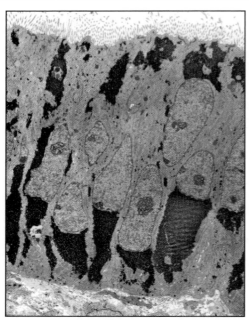

FIGURE 11-2A: Late secretory endometriotic endometrium on day 24 of the cycle showing features of an earlier stage with heavy deposits of subnuclear and apical glycogen. Original screen mag x 2,600.

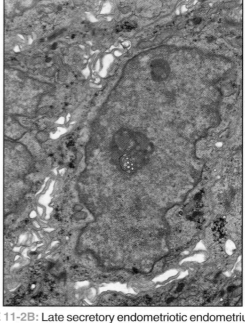

FIGURE 11-2B: Late secretory endometriotic endometrium from day 25 with a nucleolar channel system, normally found between days 17-20. Other features are more in keeping with the dates such as lateral membrane interdigitation, intercellular spaces and dispersed foci of glycogen. Original screen mag x 10,500.

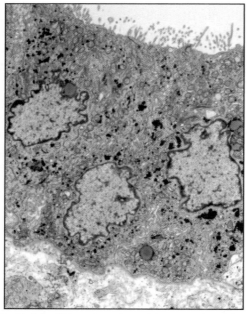

FIGURE 11-3A: Normal endometrium at day 22 showing crenated, somewhat heterochromatin nuclei, dispersed glycogen, a basal, homogeneous fat droplet and lateral membrane interdigitation. Mitochondria are small and round. Original screen mag x 2,600.

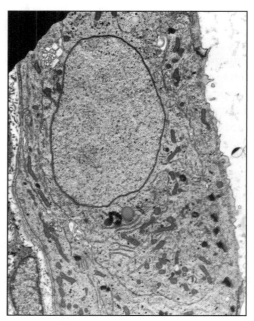

FIGURE 11-3B: Endometriotic endometrium from day 27 of the cycle, showing a very smooth, euchromatic nucleus, and sparse organelles. Original screen mag x 5,800.

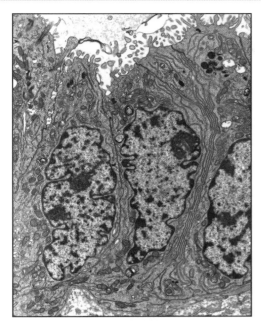

FIGURE 11-4A: Endometriotic endometrium from day 15 showing unusual features for that time in the cycle; nuclei are heterochromatic, there is no glycogen and lateral membranes show interdigitation. Original screen mag x 4,600.

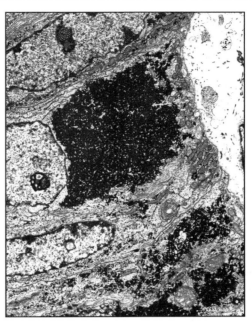

FIGURE 11-4B: Normal endometrium at the early secretory phase (day 17) showing characteristic subnuclear aggregates of glycogen, a nucleolar channel system in the uppermost nucleus, and some enlarged basal mitochondria (on the right-hand side of the image). Original screen mag x 2,600.

the proliferative to the differentiated state were dysfunctional, with an attenuated progesterone response.[14] Some researchers have shown the dysregulation of cell cycle genes GOS2 and SALP (Sam68-like phosphotyrosine protein α) in endometriosis, and these may affect mitotic activity.[15] Other reports of decreased apoptosis in the endometrium are also consistent with this finding, both using tissue sections and single cell suspensions.[16-19] Ki67 expression, indicative of dividing cells, has been reported to be higher in the proliferative, early- and mid- secretory phases of the endometrium in cases of endometriosis, while in the same study TGF-β1 failed to show the increased levels found in normal glands.[20] Furthermore, it has been suggested that such an abnormal survival of cells may result in their continuing growth in ectopic locations.[16,20]

Altered Glycosylation in Eutopic Endometriotic Endometrium

Another interesting feature of the eutopic endometrium found in our study was the complete absence of glycans bound by DBA in gland secretions in tissue from women with severe (stage IV) endometriosis, and from two of the three cases from the mid-to-late secretory phase. Gland surface staining was also reduced in many instances.[3,4] We have previously demonstrated that these glycans are normally expressed in the endometrium from the mid-secretory phase onwards[21] and their absence in these specimens is in keeping with the delayed maturation seen morphologically. The glands also tended to have a proliferative phase phenotype, being tubular and with nuclei situated basally. Endometria from women with stages I to III endometriosis generally, but not always, showed normal or even enhanced expression of the DBA-binding glycans, though one case at day 22 of the cycle with stage II disease had negligible binding of DBA which was associated with the presence of mitotic figures. Thus, the abnormal transition from proliferative to secretory phase in moderate to severe disease appears to be associated with an inability of progesterone to down-regulate cell proliferation and may reflect the attenuated progesterone response with dysregulation of progesterone target genes which has been reported in women with pelvic endometriosis.[14,15] Glycodelin, for instance, was down-regulated by 51.5-fold in such endometrial compared to normal tissue. The dysregulation would lead to the development of an inhospitable environment for embryo implantation and influence the fertility potential of affected women.

Genomic Alterations in Endometriosis

As well as an observed failure to express glycans associated with the window of implantation,[3] genomic alterations have been identified in the eutopic endometrium of women with endometriosis.[15,22] There is currently a wide range of proteins that show different gene expression,[5,6] detailed discussion of which is beyond the scope of this chapter. Both HOXA10 and 11 have been shown to be aberrant.[23] It is known that these homeobox genes regulate endometrial development during the course of the menstrual cycle and are essential for embryo implantation, and the lack of a mid-luteal rise may contribute to the etiology of endometriosis-associated infertility. Successful embryo implantation may also be compromised by differences in integrin expression on the endometrium of women with endometriosis. Of note, the β3-subunit, normally expressed after days 19-20 of the cycle, was found to be lacking in endometria from affected women, even despite the presence of in-phase histological features.[24,25] Sharpe-Timms and co-workers found that αvβ3 integrin forms a complex with matrix metalloproteinases (MMPs) on the luminal surface of eutopic endometrium, which may coordinate functions such as embryo adhesion, migration and invasion and so facilitate implantation.[26] The lack of αvβ3 expression may also affect fertility by this indirect mechanism. Aromatase activity, which catalyses the conversion of C_{19} steroids to estrogens, has been found to be elevated in eutopic endometrium from women with endometriosis,[27,28] though not to such high levels as has been found in the endometriotic lesions. The resulting localized estrogen production may be one of the factors that help to sustain endometriotic lesions. It has been suggested that examination of aromatase cytochrome P450 expression in endometrial biopsies might be used as an initial screening at outpatient infertility clinics to discriminate between the presence and absence of endometriosis.[27]

Peritoneal Fluid Abnormalities

Other factors affecting fertility performance may emanate from the maternal environment as it has been shown that alterations in peritoneal fluid involving growth factors, inflammatory mediators and immune cells may adversely affect gamete function and transport, fertilization and embryo implantation.[29,30] There are *in vitro* indications that eutopic endometriotic stromal cell decidualization may also be affected by peritoneal TNF-α, levels of which are increased in women with endometriosis.[31] Whether these changes are predisposed to, or are a consequence of endometriosis, has yet to be determined.

Effects of Medical Treatment of Endometriosis on the Endometrium

Although both medical and surgical management of endometriosis have been associated with an improvement of symptoms, the effect on fertility potential is still a matter of much debate, thus requiring further research. *In vitro* fertilization (IVF) offers the highest chance of pregnancy and is often used to treat women with endometriosis-associated infertility, nevertheless, patients with this disease have lower pregnancy rates compared with that of women with other indications for IVF. Additionally, it appears that the IVF success rate is poorer with an increase in severity of endometriosis.[32]

Medical treatment for endometriosis includes hormonal drugs, which use different doses and route of administration, and have different untoward effects. Amongst all the therapeutic compounds, gonadotrophin releasing hormone analogues (GnRH-a) seem to be the most commonly used in women trying to conceive in recent years. It is recognized that hormonal therapy does not treat endometriosis but helps manage the symptoms, primarily by switching off ovarian function. It may be debated whether medical therapy prior to IVF has beneficial direct and indirect effects on the endometrial environment of subfertile women with pelvic endometriosis, leading to an improvement of pregnancy outcome. On the other hand, there is enough evidence to demonstrate that medical treatment is not effective for infertility associated with minimal to mild endometriosis, and is responsible for a further delay in conception.[33]

Luteinized unruptured follicle (LUF) syndrome, luteal phase dysfunction and premature as well as multiple luteinizing hormone (LH) surges, which all contribute to normal endometrial function, have been associated with endometriosis.[34] These data lend credence to the speculation that GnRH-a treatment prior to IVF may control the endocrine abnormalities associated with endometriosis and which may cause subfertility.

Some authors have demonstrated that, in women with severe endometriosis, long-term treatment with GnRH-a before initiation of an IVF cycle may improve the stimulation outcome, pregnancy potential and reduce early pregnancy losses.[35,36] Meta-analytical pooling of three randomized controlled trials came to the conclusion that the administration of GnRH-a for a period of 3-6 consecutive months in women with endometriosis waiting for IVF increases the clinical pregnancy rate fourfold.[37] Furthermore, the number of oocytes retrieved was significantly higher following medical treatment. Notwithstanding the limitations of this analysis, the overall results suggest that prolonged periods of pre-treatment with GnRH-a prior to IVF may have beneficial effects. Whether these depend on the embryo (as more oocytes are collected) or are mainly at the level of the endometrium remain to be established by future randomized trials. It is plausible to speculate that treatment with GnRH-a in this group of women may account for a better follicular recruitment and may allow the endometrium to be "reset in-phase".

References

1. Eskenazi B, Warner ML. Epidemiology of endometriosis. Obstet Gynecol Clin North Am 1997; 24:235-58.

2. Gruppo italiano per lo studio dell'endometriosi. Prevalence and anatomical distribution of endometriosis in women with selected gynecological conditions: results from a multicentric Italian study. Hum Reprod 1994; 9:1158-62.

3. Jones CJP, Nardo LG, Litta P, et al. Peritoneal lesions from women with endometriosis show abnormalities in progesterone-dependent glycan expression. Fertil Steril (in press) DOI:10.10.16/j.fertnstert.2008.11.032.

4. Jones CJP, Inuwa IM, Nardo LG, et al. Eutopic endometrium from women with endometriosis shows altered ultrastructure and glycosylation compared to that from healthy controls—a pilot observational study. Reprod Sci 2009, in press.

5. Sharpe-Timms KL. Endometrial anomalies in women with endometriosis. Ann NY Acad Sci 2001; 943:131-47.

6. Ulukus M, Cakmak H, Arici A. The role of endometrium in endometriosis.J Soc Gynecol Investig 2006; 13:467-76.

7. Shapiro DB, Walsh SJ, Algert C, et al. Endometrial thickness in women with endometriosis or unexplained infertility undergoing superovulation with intrauterine insemination. The 42nd Annual Meeting of the Soc Gynecol Invest, March 15 - 18, 1995, Chicago, IL. J Soc Gynecol Invest 1995; **2:**367.

8. Fedele L, Marchini M, Bianchi S, et al. Structural and ultrastructural defects in pre-ovulatory endometrium of normo-ovulating infertile women with minimal or mild endometriosis. Fertil Steril 1990; 53:989-93.

9. Fedele L, Marchini M, Bianchi S, et al. Endometrial patterns during Danazol and Buserelin therapy for endometriosis: comparative structural and ultrastructural study. Obstet Gynecol 1990; 76:79-84.

10. Fedele L, Marchini M, Baglioni A, et al. Evaluation of histological and ultrastructural aspects of endometrium during treatment with Gestrinone in women with amenorrhea or spotting. Acta Obstet Gynecol Scand 1990; 69:143-46.

11. Marchini M, Fedele L, Bianchi S, et al. Endometrial patterns during therapy with danazol and cyproterone acetate treatment for endometriosis: structural and ultrastructural study. Eur J Obstet Reprod Biol 1991; 40:137-43.

12. Marchini M, Fedele L, Bianchi S, et al. Endometrial patterns during therapy with danazol or gestrinone for endometriosis: structural and ultrastructural study. Hum Pathol 1992; 23:51-56.

13. Metzger DA, Olive DL, Haney AF. Limited hormonal responsiveness of ectopic endometrium: histologic correlation with intrauterine endometrium. Hum Pathol 1988; 19:1417-24.

14. Burney RO, Talbi S, Hamilton AE, et al. Gene expression analysis of endometrium reveals progesterone resistance and candidate susceptibility genes in women with endometriosis. Endocrinology 2007; 148:3814-26.

15. Kao LC, Germeyer A, Tulac S, et al. Expression profiling of endometrium from women with endometriosis reveals candidate genes for disease-based implantation failure and infertility. Endocrinology 2003; 144:2870-81.

16. Meresman GF, Vighi S, Buquet RA, et al. Apoptosis and expression of bcl-2 and bax in eutopic endometrium from women with endometriosis. Fertil Steril 2000; 74:760-66.

17. Dmowski WP, Ding J, Shen J, et al. Apoptosis in endometrial glandular and stromal cells in women with and without endometriosis. Hum Reprod 2001; 16:1802-08.

18. Szymanowski K. Apoptosis pattern in human endometrium in women with pelvic endometriosis. Eur J Obstet Gynecol Reprod Biol 2007; 132:107-10.

19. Gebel HM, Braun DP, Tambur A, et al. Spontaneous apoptosis of endometrial tissue is impaired in women with endometriosis. Fertil Steril 1998; 69:1042-47.

20. Johnson MC, Torres M, Alves A, et al. Augmented cell survival in eutopic endometrium from women with endometriosis: expression of c-myc, TGF-beta1 and bax genes. Reprod Biol Endocrinol 2005; 3:45.

21. Jones CJP, Fazleabas AT, McGinlay PB, et al. Cyclic modulation of epithelial glycosylation in human and baboon (*Papio anubis*) endometrium demonstrated by the binding of the agglutinin from *Dolichos biflorus* (DBA). Biol Reprod 1998; 58: 20-27.

22. Wu Y, Strawn E, Basir Z, et al. Genomic alterations in ectopic and eutopic endometria of women with endometriosis. Gynecol Obstet Invest 2006; 62:148-59.

23. Taylor HS, Bagot C, Kardana A, et al. HOX gene expression is altered in the endometrium of women with endometriosis. Hum Reprod 1999; 14:1328-31.

24. Nardo LG, Bartoloni G, Di Mercurio S, Nardo F. Expression of avβ3 and a4β1 integrins throughout the putative window of implantation in a cohort of healthy fertile women. Acta Obstet Gynecol Scand 2002; 81:753-58.

25. Lessey BA, Castelbaum AJ, Sawin SW, et al. Aberrant integrin expression in the endometrium of women with endometriosis. J Clin Endocrinol Metab 1994; 79:643-49.

26. Sharpe-Timms KL, Cox KE, Ray B, et al. Localization of matrix metalloproteinase (MMP) enzymes, MMP-2 and MMP-3, to luminal endometrial epithelia by interaction with avβ3 and avβ5 integrins during the window of implantation. 33rd Annual Meeting Soc Study Reprod, Madison WI. Biol Reprod 2000; 62 (Suppl 1): 282, 447.

27. Kitawaki J, Kusuki I, Koshiba H, et al. Detection of aromatase cytochrome P-450 in endometrial biopsy specimens as a diagnostic test for endometriosis. Fertil Steril 1999; 72:1100-06.

28. Hudelist G, Czerwenka K, Keckstein J, et al. Expression of aromatase and estrogen sulfotransferase in eutopic and ectopic endometrium: evidence for unbalanced estradiol production in endometriosis. Reprod Sci 2007; 14:798-805.

29. Oral E, Olive DL, Arici A. The peritoneal environment in endometriosis. Hum Reprod Update 1996; 2:385-98.

30. Gazvani R, Templeton A. Peritoneal environment, cytokines and angiogenesis in the pathophysiology of endometriosis. Reproduction 2002; 123:217-26.

31. Minici F, Tiberi F, Tropea A, et al. Endometriosis and human infertility: a new investigation into the role of eutopic endometrium. Hum Reprod 2008; 23: 530-37.

32. Barnhart K, Dunsmoor-Su R, Coutifaris C. Effect of endometriosis on in vitro fertilization. Fertil Steril 2002; 77:1148-55.

33. Kennedy S, Bergqvist A, Chapron C, et al. ESHRE guideline for the diagnosis and treatment of endometriosis. Hum Reprod 2005; 20:2698-704.

34. Schenken RS, Asch RH, Williams RF, Hodgen GD. Etiology of infertility in monkeys with endometriosis: luteinized unruptured follicles, luteal phase defects, pelvic adhesions and spontaneous abortions. Fertil Steril 1984; 41:122-30.

35. Dicker D, Goldman JA, Levy T, Feldberg D, Ashkenazi J. The impact of long-term gonadotropin-releasing hormone analogue treatment on preclinical abortions in patients with severe endometriosis undergoing *in vitro* fertilization-embryo transfer. Fertil Steril 1992; 57:597-600.

36. Surrey ES, Silverberg KM, Surrey MW, Schoolcraft WB. Effect of prolonged gonadotrophin-releasing hormone agonist therapy on the outcome of in vitro fertilization-embryo transfer in patients with endometriosis. Fertil Steril 2002; 78:699-704.

37. Sallam HN, Garcia-Velasco JA, Dias A, Arici A. Long-term pituitary down-regulation before in vitro fertilization (IVF) for women with endometriosis. The Cochrane Database of Systematic Reviews 2006, Issue 1, CD004635. pub.2.

Diagnostic Dilemmas

Gareth C Weston, Peter AW Rogers

Chapter 12

Diagnosis of Endometriosis: Pitfalls of Current Methods

Introduction

Endometriosis is a common benign gynecological condition defined by the presence of endometrial tissue outside of the confines of the uterus, most typically in the lining of the pelvis, the ovaries, or the rectovaginal pouch, but occasionally in more distant sites. Its prevalence is estimated as 6-10% of the general female population, but rises to 35-50% in women with pelvic pain or infertility.[1] While a benign condition, 70-75% of women with endometriosis suffer from some degree of chronic pelvic pain, and 30-50% suffer from some degree of infertility.[2] In the USA alone, it has been estimated that the annual cost of endometriosis, both direct and indirect, is US$15 billion per year, with a significant part of that cost due to the current expensive diagnostic procedure of diagnostic laparoscopy.[2]

The 'gold standard' for diagnosis of endometriosis is visualization of the peritoneal cavity by laparoscopy. However, not only is the procedure costly, but there are operative risks associated, such as damage to the bowel, bladder, and hemorrhage if large blood vessels are damaged. The lack of a reliable non-invasive diagnostic test is one of the factors that contribute to an average 7-12 year delay between the onset of a woman's symptoms from endometriosis and its diagnosis.[3]

This chapter will review non-invasive tests which have been studied in the past, and the current diagnostic tests available for endometriosis. It will also deal with some of the current attempts by researchers in the field to develop new less invasive tests for endometriosis.

Symptoms

The common symptoms associated with endometriosis are dysmenorrhea, pelvic pain at other times of the menstrual cycle, and dyspareunia. The presence of these symptoms is usually used as a screening test to identify patients requiring the 'gold standard' diagnostic test of a laparoscopy. However, many different gynecological conditions cause pelvic pain, meaning that many laparoscopies in such women may find no endometriosis, or only minimal endometriosis which may not be sufficient to explain the woman's pain symptoms. Unnecessarily excessive use of diagnostic laparoscopy is not only a financially costly exercise, but entails health risks for the women concerned. Laparoscopy is associated with a 1 in 10,000 mortality risk, as well as a risk of damage to bowel, bladder, or major blood vessels of approximately 2.4 in 10,000 – a complication often requiring a laparotomy for surgical repair.[4]

In a recent systematic review,[4] the accuracy of pain symptoms in diagnosing endometriosis was assessed. Nineteen studies involving a total of 4540 patients met the investigators' inclusion criteria. The weighted positive predictive value for a pain history suggestive of endometriosis was only 41%. When examining individual symptoms (chronic pelvic pain, dysmenorrhea, and dyspareunia), the best performing symptom with regards to sensitivity and specificity was dysmenorrhea. However, with a sensitivity and specificity of only 65% and 70% respectively, it could not be recommended as an acceptable diagnostic or screening test.

While these pain symptoms are associated with endometriosis, they are clearly of little value in diagnosing the condition. The primary care clinician is thus left with the difficult decision of providing many unnecessary laparoscopies, or of attempting empirical treatments in the absence of a definitive diagnosis. Clearly, there is an urgent need for more accurate non-invasive diagnostic tests for this common and often debilitating condition.

Serum Markers

CA125 is a high molecular weight glycoprotein, originally discovered from use of a monoclonal antibody (OC125) raised against an ovarian cancer cell line. Although best known as a marker for epithelial ovarian cancer, it is expressed in most tissues derived from coelomic epithelium, including those of Mullerian origin, as well as peritoneal, pericardial and pleural membranes. Due to its wide distribution, particularly in the female pelvis, it has elevated serum levels in a variety of benign and malignant disorders, particularly gynecological conditions. These conditions include endometriosis, uterine fibroids, adenomyosis, and pelvic inflammatory disease.

The cut-off level above which endometriosis should be suspected was initially set arbitrarily at 35U/ml, based on testing for ovarian tumors.[5] However, at this level, it has a poor sensitivity and specificity as a test for endometriosis. Attempts have been made to improve the sensitivity and specificity of the test by altering the upper and lower levels of 'normal', with one group reporting a 78% negative predictive value with CA125 < 20U/ml, and 92.9% positive predictive value with CA125 > 30U/ml, but uncertainty about what to do with a value between 20-30U/ml.[6] Other attempts to improve the low utility of this test have included adding other concomitant markers, such as CA19.9, and inflammatory markers (IL-6, elevated neutrophil:lymphocyte ratio), all with only limited success. In a meta-analysis of 23 studies, CA-125 performs slightly better for severe endometriosis (stage III/IV; ovarian endometriomas) than for mild-moderate endometriosis[7] **(Figure 12-1)**. The highest level of CA125 reported for benign endometriosis was for a ruptured ovarian endometrioma (6,114U/ml).[8] CA-125 has been shown to have some limited use in the follow-up of recurrence in patients with advanced endometriosis and initially elevated CA-125 levels.[9] Despite this, the use of CA-125 and other currently-available serum markers for the diagnosis of endometriosis is of limited value.

Ultrasound

The only widely accepted use of ultrasound in diagnosing endometriosis is in the detection of ovarian endometriomas. An endometrioma, or 'chocolate cyst' may be unilateral or bilateral, and may be associated with reduced mobility of the ovary. Bilateral endometriomas may be stuck together behind the uterus as 'kissing ovaries'. The endometrioma is filled with old blood, giving a typical ground-glass appearance with low-level echoes

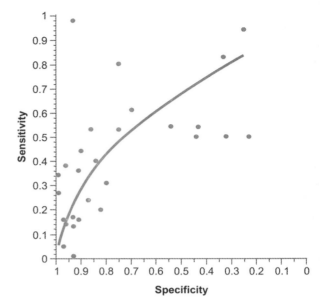

FIGURE 12-1: Summary ROC curve of serum CA-125 measurements in the diagnosis of any type of endometriosis. *Adapted from Mol et al, Fertil Steril 1998;70:1101-1108.*

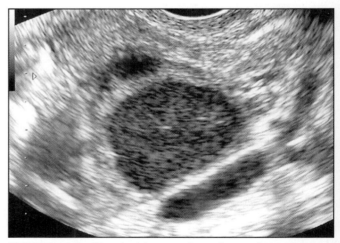

FIGURE 12-2: Classical image of ovarian endometrioma as seen by transvaginal sonography, where healthy ovarian tissue may be observed adjacent to the endometriotic cyst.

(Figure 12-2). The wall is usually thick and irregular in contrast to the thin wall of a hemorrhagic corpus luteum cyst (a common differential diagnosis). Ultrasound has a high sensitivity and specificity for diagnosing ovarian endometriomas, but has been relatively poor at diagnosing the more common peritoneal endometriosis. The detection of an ovarian endometrioma itself is poorly correlated with presence of peritoneal endometriosis.

Attempts have been made to improve the diagnostic utility of pelvic ultrasound for peritoneal endometriosis by use of soft markers, such as eliciting site-specific tenderness with the ultrasound probe, and examining the mobility of the ovaries.[10] While the negative predictive value with the addition of these soft markers was reported as 84%, the positive predictive value was poor, with many women finding ultrasound probing uncomfortable without having endometriosis. Others have reported the use of transvaginal ultrasound to detect hypoechoic nodularity in the uterosacral ligaments, as well as transrectal ultrasound combined with instillation of saline into the vagina to detect deep infiltrating rectovaginal endometriosis.[11] These types of imaging require considerable expertise not available in most centers, have subjective elements (i.e. eliciting of pain), or are technically difficult (i.e. vaginal saline instillation). Thus, ultrasound remains a poor test for endometriosis apart from the detection of endometriomas and large deep infiltrative deposits.

Computed Tomography (CT) Scans

While CT scanning is useful in diagnosing lung endometriomas and endometriomas in surgical scars in the abdominal wall, these are rare, and the exception rather than the rule. In diagnosis of more common ovarian endometriomas, the CT scan has little utility due to its poor ability to discriminate differences in soft tissue.[12] As for peritoneal endometriosis, it has no use at all at present. Most of the endometriosis lesions on the peritoneal surface are far too small to be detectable by CT scan.

There has been some interest in the use of CT scans in the diagnosis of deep infiltrating endometriosis of the rectovaginal septum, and of bowel endometriosis. One group[13] have described the 'virtual colonoscopy' technique, using a large obstetric tampon in the vagina and a Foley catheter insufflated with CO_2 in the rectum to demonstrate endometriosis in the rectovaginal space. Others have used colon distension with water to determine the presence and depth of endometriotic lesions causing constriction of the bowel. Nonetheless, there are few uses for CT scanning in diagnosing endometriosis at present.

Magnetic Resonance Imaging (MRI)

There is an increasing interest in the use of MRI to determine the location and depth of endometriotic lesions prior to considering surgery. If the exact spread and severity of endometriosis could be determined prior to laparoscopy, the patient would be able to be appropriately counselled regarding specific risks of required surgery (e.g. bowel involvement; involvement of ureters in deep

infiltrating disease). Also, the patients could be triaged to be operated on by surgeons with sufficient laparoscopic skills, and multi-disciplinary teams made available as required (e.g. laparoscopic colorectal surgeon, urologist, laparoscopic-trained gynecologist).

MRI scanning of the pelvis for endometriosis is best performed after day 8 of the cycle, due to the T1 hyperintensity of blood if performed earlier in the cycle.[14] A peristaltic inhibitor should be administered intramuscularly, and both T1 and T2-weighted images taken, with and without fat suppression in T1 weighted images, and before and after administration of gadolinium contrast.

In diagnosing ovarian endometriomas, ultrasound is the primary imaging modality of choice, but MRI is being promoted by some[14] as a second line investigation if the features of the ovarian mass on ultrasound are difficult to interpret. Irregularities of the cyst wall may lead to a suspicion of ovarian malignancy. MRI can detect endometriomas due to characteristic hyperintensity in both T1 and T2 weighted images (due to old blood in the 'chocolate cyst'), and use of fat-suppressed T1 images to differentiate it from a cystic teratoma. Sensitivities and specificities as high as 90% and 98% respectively have been reported for MRI diagnosis of endometriomas, although these outcomes can be highly operator-dependent.

There are many reports of the use of MRI to aid in the detection of rectovaginal endometriosis nodules and deep infiltrating endometriosis of the uterosacral ligaments. Owing to the poor ability of ultrasound to detect endometriosis in these locations, combined with relative difficulty in detection of subperitoneal lesions even with laparoscopy, there has been greater enthusiasm in using MRI in specific patients with symptoms suggestive of deep infiltrating lesions. While MRI, in expert hands, has been shown to have some use in detecting such lesions, the low predictive value of symptoms for actual presence of disease means that if MRI was employed for every patient with deep dyspareunia, it would be an extremely costly exercise. The problem with MRI is its high cost and low availability, combined with the need for considerable expertise in the interpretation of MRI scans of the female reproductive tract. MRI scanning may have a role in tertiary centers in planning surgery for suspected deep infiltrating disease diagnosed at laparoscopy.

Other Imaging Modalities

There have been some reports of the use of both immunoscintigraphy and positron emission tomography

(PET) in the detection of endometriotic lesions. Immuno-scintigraphy employing radiolabelled OC125 antibody binding to areas of CA125 expression proved to have only 33% specificity, due to the widespread expression of CA125 by benign gynecological pathology.[15] Increased uptake on PET scanning is more likely to be associated with inflammation than presence of endometriosis per se. While these kinds of tests merit further research, neither have any clinical role in diagnosing endometriosis at present.

Transvaginal Hydrolaparoscopy

This technique has been described in recent years as a possible alternative to diagnostic laparoscopy via the traditional umbilical route.[16] It has been proposed as an office procedure, with local anesthetic used in the posterior fornix prior to entry into the Pouch of Douglas with a Veress needle, a small incision, a 3 mm blunt trocar, followed by a 2.7 mm semi-rigid endoscope. Visualization of the ovaries, fallopian tubes, and Pouch of Douglas, including the uterosacral ligaments is possible with this technique using the instillation of warm saline. It has been proposed as a technique for visualizing endometriosis, as well as assessing the ovaries, and the patency of the tubes. While the technique avoids the need for a general anesthetic and permits visualization of the most common locations for endometriosis, there are several problems. It does not allow visualization of the entire pelvis, and may miss endometriosis at some sites (e.g. the uterovesical pouch). It is not possible to operate on any pathology found at the time without a subsequent anesthetic and a trans-abdominal laparoscopy. The rectum in particular is jeopardized during entry at the posterior fornix, and there is the risk of infection due to the vaginal route. In cases of endometriosis with rectovaginal nodules, this technique may be particularly dangerous, and patients should be examined prior to the procedure to rule out deep infiltrating disease between the vagina and the rectum. While many women may tolerate the procedure under a local anesthetic, others may not, forcing the procedure to be abandoned. Due to these problems, it has not proven to be popular, and has not replaced traditional laparoscopy as a diagnostic method for endometriosis.

Laparoscopic Visualization of the Pelvis

The earliest surgical method for diagnosing endometriosis was laparotomy. The use of laparoscopy in gynecology first gained popularity in the 1970s as a relatively non-invasive method for achieving tubal sterilization. It soon came to be used for diagnosing and treating a wide variety of gynecological conditions, including endometriosis.

Diagnostic laparoscopy is the 'gold standard' test for the diagnosis of endometriosis. This surgical procedure requires a general anesthetic for the patient, and provides a panoramic view of the pelvis from the umbilical port site after insufflation of the peritoneal cavity with CO_2 gas. No other currently available test comes close to its diagnostic accuracy, and endometriosis at all possible intraperitoneal sites cannot be excluded without visualizing the pelvis at laparoscopy. Simultaneously, the patency of the fallopian tubes can be examined by the retrograde passage of dye through the reproductive tract, an important test as many women with endometriosis present with the problem of infertility. Blocked tubes due to endometriotic adhesions are an indication for use of *in vitro* fertilization, rather than other forms of infertility treatment. Furthermore, laparoscopy enables the surgeon to employ the principle of 'see and treat' at the one operation, excising any visible endometriosis deposits at diagnosis, after the insertion of additional laparoscopic ports under vision. While this does have the disadvantage of uncertainty about the required surgery for a prior specific consent from the patient, it does enable the avoidance of a second procedure in most cases.

The revised American Fertility Society scoring system (1985) is the most widely accepted way of describing the location and severity of endometriosis in a standardized format. Such classification systems are essential for clinical trials comparing different treatments. A score is assigned to endometriotic lesions on the peritoneum and ovaries (based on size, location, and depth), to posterior cul-de-sac endometriosis (partial or complete obliteration), and to adhesions on the ovaries and tubes (based on whether adhesions are filmy or dense, and the proportion of the tube or ovary covered). Stage of disease is divided into:

Stage I (minimal)—score 1-5
Stage II (mild)—score 6-15
Stage III (moderate)—score 16-40
Stage IV (severe)—score > 40

While the revised AFS score provides a standardized reference point for different clinicians to communicate extent of endometriosis, there is a poor correlation between disease severity and symptoms. Some women have mild disease, but severe pain symptoms, while others have no symptoms despite severe disease.

The pathology of endometriosis lesion can vary widely.[17] It has been proposed that endometriotic lesions have different appearances depending on the stage of their life-cycle. Early lesions are 'red' lesions, comprising early active endometriosis, with much associated inflammation. The mature 'black' lesions are the classic 'chocolate cysts', composed of concentration of blood pigments from successive bleeds in response to cycling hormonal levels over time. The content of the cystic lesions becomes thick and tar-like, as the water content is absorbed, and the blood pigments remain. The final stage of the proposed life cycle of the endometriotic lesion is the 'white' lesion, old burnt-out endometriosis which has largely been replaced by collagen and scar tissue. On histopathology, the white lesions have only occasional pockets of endometrial glandular tissue, and are mainly comprised of connective tissue. The classification systems at present do not make distinctions between these different types of lesions. Nor have the different lesions stages been shown convincingly to display different symptomatology in patients. A patient with widespread white lesions can have the same or worse pain than the patient with active red lesions.

While many cases of endometriosis are obvious to the surgeon on laparoscopic visualization of the peritoneal cavity, the precise diagnosis of endometriosis still requires the skills of the pathologist. Endometriosis is defined as the presence of endometrial glands and stroma in ectopic extrauterine locations, which requires histopathological examination of the excised lesions.[17] The smaller the lesions, the less accurate the surgical diagnosis of endometriosis at specific locations. Often in our own research program, specimens that have been designated as 'endometriosis' by surgeons are found to have no demonstrable endometrial glands or stroma on histopathology. The accuracy of the surgical diagnosis appears to rely heavily on both the experience of the surgeon, and on the quality of the laparoscopic equipment.

There has been much discussion in the literature regarding invisible 'microscopic' endometriosis. Some surgeons believe that endometriotic lesions exist that are so small that they can still not be identified even under direct magnified vision with the laparoscope. A range of techniques have been described, including a thermocoagulation test (endometriosis-containing peritoneum turning brown rather than white with thermocoagulation due to the hemosiderin content), painting the endometrium with methylene blue dye, and laparoscopic spectral analysis with blue light, in order to detect and remove these otherwise invisible areas of endometriosis. The very existence of invisible 'microscopic' endometriosis has been questioned,[18] as lesions as small as 50 μm in diameter can be seen at laparoscopy, with sufficient experience and

magnification. Other authors have questioned whether such small lesions, whether visible or not, truly represent a disease state at all, or are just part of the spectrum of normality.[19] It is certainly controversial whether minimal endometriosis, much less invisible microscopic endometriosis, is responsible for patient symptoms.

As has already been mentioned, laparoscopy is not without its risks to the patient. The risks are magnified even further by women with established endometriosis, who often require several laparoscopies over the course of their reproductive life due to the high rate of recurrence despite surgical treatment. A non-invasive test to screen women with symptoms and determine which women require a laparoscopy, both for initial and recurrent disease, would be a great advance in the management of endometriosis. There are some promising areas of research into such tests at present.

Novel Diagnostic Tests

There has long been an understanding that the eutopic endometrium from women with endometriosis has molecular and cellular differences to that of women without endometriosis.[20] These differences may explain why 90% of women have retrograde flow of endometrial tissue through the fallopian tubes during menstruation, but only 8-10% of women develop the disease: characteristics of the retrogradely-shed endometrium make it more likely to implant, or more resistant to clearance by the immune system. Many aspects of endometrial function have been studied and found to differ in endometriosis – angiogenesis, immune function, cytokines, proliferative potential of cell populations, and inflammatory factors, amongst others. It is possible that a highly reproducible difference in eutopic endometrium between women with and without endometriosis could be exploited as a diagnostic test by pipelle sampling of the endometrium.

One such promising lead has been reported recently[21] by Professor Fraser's group in Sydney, Australia. They have reported the finding of small unmyelinated nerve fibers in the endometrium detected by staining with a rabbit polyclonal antibody to protein gene product 9.5 (PGP 9.5), a highly specific neuronal marker for unmyelinated nerve fibers. They were able to demonstrate nerve fibers in all 27 endometrial curettings from women with endometriosis, but in none of the 47 women without endometriosis, with all women undergoing a laparoscopy at the time of curettage to ensure correct classification of the patient. The existence of these nerve fibers has interesting implications in the understanding of the pain symptomatology of endometriosis. In addition, if translated into a clinical test for pelvic endometriosis prior to performing a laparoscopy, the test would have a 100% sensitivity and 100% specificity, albeit based on this small number of patients. Further work is clearly needed in this area.

Genomics is the study of gene expression patterns of large numbers of genes simultaneously, using tools such as gene expression microarrays. It is a technique that has been employed to examine differences in the eutopic endometrium between women with and without proven endometriosis.[22] Affymetrix microarrays have been used to compare gene expression profiles in endometrial biopsies obtained 6-8 days after the LH surge (the window of implantation). Of the genes studied, 91 were found to upregulated and 115 downregulated more than two-fold in the endometrial biopsies from women with endometriosis. One of the hopeful outcomes from such work is that molecular signatures particular to endometriosis may be discovered, enabling endometriosis in the peritoneal cavity to be diagnosed by molecular analysis of a small endometrial sample. Given the complexity and variability of endometrial tissue biology, this has yet to be accomplished, however. It may be that, given the variable nature of the disease, molecular signatures may need to be stratified into subsets. The obvious categories at present would be endometrioma, peritoneal and deep infiltrating, but could expand to include other lesion pathologies as well as patient symptoms.

There are an increasing number of reports of the use of proteomics[23] to examine differences in the protein profiles from uterine washings, serum, or eutopic endometrial biopsies from women with and without endometriosis. If any of these studies are able to discover a robust and reproducible difference in protein expression patterns between women with and without endometriosis, it will be possible to create a useful non-invasive test. It is hoped that this would lead to earlier detection of disease in women with symptoms.

Conclusion

Endometriosis is a common and often debilitating gynecological condition. The usually long delay in diagnosis is partially attributable to the fact that the only reliable diagnostic test at present involves an invasive and costly surgical procedure. While laparoscopy seems likely to maintain a central role in the treatment of the disease at present, via excision or ablation of endometriotic lesions, the development of non-invasive and less costly screening tests should be a priority in advancing the treatment of the disease.

Most of the currently available non-invasive diagnostic methods, including monitoring of symptoms, serum tests, and imaging techniques, have major flaws in diagnosing endometriosis. While several new lines of investigation are emerging with the application of genomic and proteomic profiling of eutopic endometrium, more work is urgently needed in this area.

References

1. Giudice L, Kao LC. Endometriosis. Lancet 2004; 364:1789-98.
2. Gao X, Outley J, Botteman M, et al. Economic burden of endometriosis. Fertil Steril 2006; 86:1561-72.
3. Sinaii N, Cleary SD, Ballweg ML, et al. High rates of autoimmune and endocrine disorders, fibromyalgia, chronic fatigue and atopic disease among women with endometriosis: a survey analysis. Hum Reprod 2002; 17: 2715-24.
4. Xu M, Vincent K, Kennedy S. Diagnosis of endometriosis. In: Rombauts L, Tsaltas J, Maher P, Healy D (Eds). Endometriosis 2008. Melbourne, Blackwell Publishing. 2008; 133-48.
5. Barbieri RL, Niloff JM, Bast RC, et al. Elevated serum concentrations of CA-125 in patients with advanced endometriosis. Fertil Steril 1986; 45: 630-34.
6. Kitawaki J, Ishihara H, Koshiba H, et al. Usefulness and limits of CA-125 in diagnosis of endometriosis without associated ovarian endometriomas. Hum Reprod 2005; 20:1999-2003.
7. Mol BW, Bayram N, Lijmer JG, et al. The performance of CA-125 measurement in the detection of endometriosis: a meta-analysis. Fertil Steril 1998; 70: 1101-08.
8. Kashyap R. Extremely elevated serum CA125 due to endometriosis. Austr N Zeal J Obstet Gynecol.1999; 39: 269-70.
9. Chen FP, Soong YK, Lee N, et al. The use of serum CA-125 as a marker for endometriosis in patients with dysmenorrhea for monitoring therapy and for recurrence of endometriosis. Acta Obstet Gynecol Scand. 1998; 77: 665-70.
10. Okaro E, Condous G, Khalid A, et al. Predictive value of transvaginal ultrasonography prior to diagnostic laparoscopy in women with chronic pelvic pain. Eur J Ultrasound 2002; 15:S11.
11. Okaro E, Condous G. Diagnostic and therapeutic capabilities of ultrasound in the management of pelvic pain. Curr Opin Obstet Gynecol 2005; 17:611-17.
12. Cody RF, Ascher SM. Diagnostic value of radiological tests in chronic pelvic pain. Baillieres Best Pract Res Clin Obstet Gynaecol 2000; 14:433-66.
13. Van der Wat J, Kaplan MD. Modified virtual colonoscopy: a non-invasive technique for diagnosis of rectovaginal septum and deep infiltrating pelvic endometriosis. J Minim Invasive Gynecol 2007; 14:638-43.
14. Kinkel K, Frei KA, Balleyguier C, et al. Diagnosis of endometriosis with imaging: a review. Eur Radiol 2006; 16:285-98.

15. Kennedy SH, Mojiminiyi OA, Soper ND, et al. Immuno-scintigraphy of endometriosis. Br J Obstet Gynaecol 1990; 97: 667-70.

16. Gordts S, Campo R, Rombauts L, et al. Transvaginal hydro-laparoscopy as an outpatient procedure for infertility investigation. Hum Reprod 1998; 13:99-103.

17. Clement PB. The pathology of endometriosis: a survey of the many faces of a common disease emphasizing diagnostic pitfalls and unusual and newly appreciated aspects. Adv Anat Pathol 2007; 14:241-60.

18. Redwine DB. 'Invisible' microscopic endometriosis: a review. Gynecol Obstet Invest 2003; 55:63-67.

19. Koninckx PR, Oosterlynck D, D'Hooghe T, et al. Deep infiltrating endometriosis is a disease whereas mild endometriosis could be considered a non-disease. Ann N Y Acad Sci 1994; 734: 333-41.

20. Matsuzaki S, Canis M, Pouly JL, et al. Endometrial dysfunction in endometriosis – Biochemical aspects. In: Rombauts L, Tsaltas J, Maher P, Healy D (Eds): Endometriosis 2008. Malden, Mass: Blackwell Publishing; 2008: 89-100.

21. Tokushige N, Markham R, Russell P, et al. High density of small nerve fibers in the functional layer of the endo-metrium in women with endometriosis. Hum Reprod 2006; 21:782-87.

22. Kao LC, Germeyer A, Tulac S, et al. Expression profiling of endometrium from women with endometriosis reveals candidate genes for disease-based implantation failure and infertility. Endocrinology 2003;144:2870-71.

23. Zhang H, Niu Y, Feng J, et al. Use of proteomic analysis of endometriosis to identify different protein expression in patients with endometriosis versus normal controls. Fertil Steril 2006; 86:274-82.

Francisco Domínguez, Carlos Simón

Chapter 13

Novel Non-invasive Diagnosis of Endometriosis

Introduction

Endometriosis is defined as the presence of endometrial tissue outside the uterus, a definition based on Sampson's concept that the disease is caused by peritoneal regurgitation and the implantation of viable endometrial cells in menstrual debris.[1] Consequently, the diagnosis of endometriosis is based on the histological identification of ectopic endometrial glands and stroma. Another typical component of endometriotic lesion is smooth muscle proliferation.[2,3] Deep endometriosis, located on the exterior of the mullerian tract, is mainly characterized by fibromuscular hyperplasia and the formation of an adenomyotic nodule and microendometriomas.[4,5] Peritoneal and ovarian endometriosis are characterized by chronic bleeding, leading to the formation of hemorrhagic blisters, fibrosis, adhesions, and ovarian endometriomas. Endometriosis is further distinguished by altered immune cell responses, inflammation, neoangiogenesis, and ovarian and uterine dysfunction.

Laparoscopy is the current gold standard for the diagnosis of endometriosis. However, it has many limitations, and novel non-invasive techniques are also used for screening and clinical purposes. There is an urgent need for precise non-invasive diagnostic techniques if the clinical management of women with endometriosis is to be more effective. Indeed it is now known that the younger the patient is when symptoms appear, the longer it takes before the diagnosis of endometriosis is made.

Transvaginal ultrasonography (TVU), magnetic resonance imaging (MRI) and endometrial and serum markers are the three main fields of study that may potentially improve diagnoses, and could be useful in patients' follow-ups. In the near future, however, new arising technologies, for instance transcriptomics and proteomics, could also be used for the non-invasive diagnosis of endometriosis. This review centers on recent studies which assess imaging and proteomic techniques, and describe the novel molecular markers currently being developed for the diagnosis of endometriosis.

Imaging Techniques

Imaging techniques are becoming more and more important to preoperatively determine the presence and extent of the surgical pathology. With the use of non-invasive techniques, the decision whether to operate or not should be based on the accurate preoperative diagnosis and the adequate assessment of the extent of the disease whenever possible. Last year, some publications contributed to an improved preoperative diagnosis of the various endometriosis stages.

Superficial Endometriosis and Endometriotic Adhesions

Currently, TVU does not detect superficial peritoneal endometriosis and ovarian surface implants. Additionally, MRI fails to detect subtle endometriotic lesions. Nonetheless, fat-saturated MRI improves the detection rate of small hemorrhagic lesions measuring less than 5 mm from 4% at conventional MRI to 50%.[6] Nowadays, the imaging technology available does not allow for a reliable classification or assessment of endometriotic adhesions.

Ovarian Endometrioma

Transvaginal ultrasonography has proven to be a useful tool for the detection and monitoring of ovarian endometriomas with a diameter exceeding 10 mm. Several authors have assessed TVU's accuracy for diagnosis purposes. The characteristic features are based mainly on the presence of diffuse, low-level internal echoes and hyperechoic foci in the wall. One main limitation of these studies is that the sonographic findings are yet to be correlated with the histological examination of *in situ* specimens or targeted biopsies. The pathologic significance of increased wall thickness, nodularity, and hyperechoic foci remains speculative. Other feasible discriminatory factors, such as location, lesion shape, and position, also remain to be assessed. Sonographic features of endometriomas may be present in hemorrhagic cysts, dermoid cysts, and occasionally in epithelial ovarian tumors. Repeat ultrasounds are highly recommended for cysts with low-level internal echoes but without wall nodularity or hyperechoic foci.[7] Should papillary structures protruding from the internal cyst wall be visualized, then ovarian malignancy, like endometroid adenocarcinoma, must be excluded.[8] Transvaginal ultrasonography combined with Doppler ultrasound, with the addition of color studies, has not been proven efficient for diagnosis purposes. Transvaginal ultrasonography may be applied in the transvaginal aspiration of endometriomas. Even though aspiration is not an effective treatment for ovarian endometrioma, it might prove useful for those patients who have previously undergone surgery and who present recurrences. Indeed, up to 73% of recurrent hemorrhagic cysts after surgery have actually been reported to be dysfunctional cysts.[9] The MRI features reported are almost exclusively based on the detection of chronic or recurrent bleeding in the endometrioma.

Deep Retroperitoneal Endometriosis

To date, few ultrasound studies have focused specifically on the detection of deep retroperitoneal endometriosis. With an ultrasonography, these endometriotic nodules may look like solid hypoechogenic lesions, ranging from 0.5 to 4 cm, which adhere to the anterior rectal wall. Normally, these characteristic lesions are more painful when examined during menstruation. Rectal endoscopic sonography has been employed to assess the thickness of the uterosacral ligaments and the presence of rectal infiltration in patients with deep endometriosis.[10] Recently, Chapron et al[11] detailed the MRI appearances of rectovaginal endometriotic nodules, which varied from 2.0 cm to 2.5 cm in eight affected patients. The nodules present an irregular contour and are indistinguishable from the uterovaginal structures. In some cases, a hyper-signal intensity transition zone may be identified between the rectum and the nodule, and this has been called the "safety margin".

In other cases, this "safety margin" is not observed; instead, a thickening of the rectum wall is noted. It is probable that the "safety margin" represents interposing fat tissue. The retraction among the torus uterinum, the endometriotic nodule, and the rectum results in an obliteration of the pouch of Douglas. This incident may give two false impressions: the lesion being located under the pouch, and the radiated infiltration of the perirectal space with a thickening and stiffness of the rectum wall. False-positive detection of endometriosis on MRI may be come about by misinterpreting normal anatomic structures, the MRI-related artifact, or previous surgery. One suggestion put forward was that the diagnostic efficiency of MRI in endometriosis could be improved by the regular use of phased-array coils and negative signal-reducing bowel contrast agents.[12]

Bladder Endometriosis

Nodular bladder endometriosis is not easily palpable during vaginal examinations. Typically, it is encountered in patients with dysmenorrhea and associated urinary symptoms, such as micturition frequency. TVU may reveal a solid nodule within the posterior bladder wall if the bladder is slightly filled. Color Doppler studies may detect low to moderate vascularity, and mild pressure with the vaginal probe often elicits focal pain. In a series of 12 patients with nodular bladder endometriosis, varying between 10 and 31 mm in diameter, TVU was normal in 4 patients, unlike MRI with the use of a body coil, which enabled the visualization of lesions in all the patients.[13] Using an endocavitary coil was seen to be an improvement over imaging with a body coil when determining the extent of infiltration of the bladder wall.[13]

Current imaging techniques do not enable an accurate staging of endometriosis as they lack the resolution required to visualize small superficial peritoneal and ovarian implants, and because they are unable to detect the presence or extent of adhesions. A key role that MRI plays, however, is to help visualize laparoscopic blind spots, such as the retroperitoneal space or lesions obscured by dense adhesions. Both TVU and MRI prove useful in assessing recurrence and response to treatment in patients with known disease. Early detection and the staging of disease are crucial in cancer. However, it is open to discussion whether a similar approach is required for benign diseases like endometriosis. There is absolutely no evidence that all the small endometriotic lesions necessarily progress or acquire a destructive invasive phenotype. Despite there being unequivocal evidence that endometriotic cells have invasive potential in invasion assays *in vivo*,[14] endometriosis neither invades the ovarian stroma nor the fat tissue in the retroperitoneal space. Nondestructive invasion is observed in structures with a fibromuscular or muscular wall. However, it seems feasible that the extent of invasion is primarily determined by changes in the local microenvironment, interstitial bleeding, inflammation, and the subsequent colonization by endometriotic cells. In clinical terms, a poor correlation is noted between lesion size and symptoms, e.g. infertility and pelvic pain. Finally, a surgical paradox reveals that surgery is more effective in pelvic pain and infertility in severe disease rather than in mild disease. Such reflections question the assumption that to be able to manage suspected cases of endometriosis means having to necessarily require an invasive procedure for meticulous staging and ablation of visible lesions, as with cancer. Instead, it seems reasonable to commence medical treatment in symptomatic patients who have presented ultrasound or MRI evidence of endometriosis if this is the preferred treatment option.

Endometriosis Serum Markers

Considerable interest has been shown in developing serum markers for endometriosis. Ideally, such markers should display the following features: high sensitivity and specificity, good prognostic value, and good correlation between serum levels and the severity of disease. Such markers might not only be used for diagnosing endometriosis but also for monitoring disease progression and responding to medical or surgical treatment. The peripheral blood levels of CA-125, placental protein-14 (glycodelin), and antiendometrial and anti-carbonic anhydrase antibodies have been investigated for their diagnostic potential in women with endometriosis. In clinical terms, CA-125, a high molecular-weight membrane glycoprotein, is the most widely used serum marker of endometriosis. This glycoprotein is expressed in all the tissues derived from embryonic coelomic epithelium, including endometrium, endocervix, fallopian tubes, peritoneum, pleura, and pericardium.[15] In patients with advanced endometriosis, CA-125 predominantly elevates during the first days of the menstrual cycle.[16] Although elevated serum concentrations of CA-125 are non-specific for endometriosis, they have been associated with many epithelial cancers and benign gynecologic and nongynecologic disorders, such as adnexitis, pancreatitis, peridontitis, pregnancy, and ovarian hyperstimulation syndrome. Combining CA-125 plasma levels with TVU does not merely result in a better

predictive capacity than TVU. One recent report suggested that the serum levels of interleukin-6, with a cut-off level of 2 pg/mL, could discriminate between patients with and without endometriosis.[17] Likewise, Matarese et al[18] recently reported marked increased leptin levels in serum and peritoneal fluid of patients with pelvic endometriosis. These authors suggested that the proinflammatory and neoangiogenic actions of this adipocyte-derived helical cytokine may contribute to the pathogenesis of endometriosis. Follow-up studies were unable to confirm an association between the presence of pelvic endometriosis and elevated serum leptin concentrations. Therefore, larger prospective studies are needed to determine the diagnostic potential of measuring circulating inflammatory cytokine levels in endometriosis.

Transcriptomics and Proteomic Analysis in Endometriosis

Various classical methodologies, which include suppression subtractive hybridization, differential display or reverse transcriptase PCR, have proven powerful in detecting and characterizing differentially expressed genes. Nonetheless, emerging "omics" technologies enable the simultaneous analysis of the expression of a large number of genes and proteins simultaneously. For instance, transcriptomics is the study of the transcriptome, that is, the complete set of RNA transcripts produced by the genome at any one time. With this approach, we can study the expression of all the genes of a cell, tissue or organism between two situations, in our case this would be the gene expression profile of a endometriotic endometrium and the eutopic endometrium.

With this technique, we have characterized the expression of genes, gene families, and signal transduction pathways, for example, during the implantation window in the human endometrium.[19] Eyster *et al*[20] used cDNA microarrays to identify differentially expressed genes between the eutopic and ectopic endometria, and they reported that the expression of eight genes from a total of 4133 genes on the microarray actually increased in endometriotic implants.

Proteomics focused on the global study of all the proteins present at a given time of the cell/organism (proteome) by using the technologies of large-scale protein separation and identification, and may be applied to tissue samples or body fluid. Proteome analysis is now widely accepted as a complementary technology to genetic profiling and, together, these two areas will lead to a better understanding of diseases and the development of new treatments in

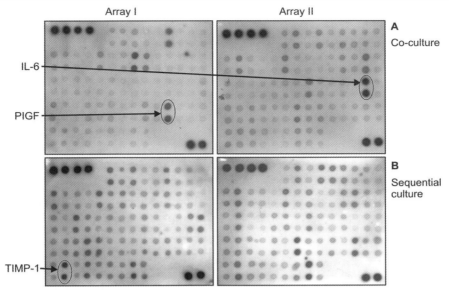

FIGURE 13-1: Protein array membranes including 120 proteins distributed into two membranes (I&II) showing the protein abundance in different culture situations. Each spot pair corresponds to one studied protein. Protein spot intensity correlates with higher protein abundance in the medium analyzed. Clear differences are shown in some proteins (see arrows and circles). (A) Protein profile of co-culture media, (B) protein profile of sequential media.

clinical medicine. Proteomic techniques are increasingly used in medical research in an attempt to identify proteins that are potential biomarkers of various disease states in the quest to develop a diagnostic test for the disease, as well as to improve the understanding of the specific pathways toward the formation of the disease. Protein arrays with antibodies **(Figure 13-1)** are also being developed as a new tool for the rapid measurement of protein expression, similarly to their use in human implantation research.[21] In this way, it is possible to screen thousands of proteins against one sample which, in the future, could measure the expression of multiple proteins to potentially reveal changes in their regulation and expression in disease states.

Classically, two-dimensional electrophoresis, based on a combination of isoelectric focusing and sodium dodecyl sulfate polyacrylamide gel electrophoresis, was the only method available to analyze the protein complement in a sample with a high resolution. The introduction of protein chips and mass spectrometry has vastly facilitated protein identification **(Figure 13-2)**. In particular, matrix-assisted laser desorption and ionization time-of-flight (MALDI) and surface-enhanced laser desorption and ionization time-of-flight (SELDI) are increasingly used for rapid protein profiling. As with microarrays, these protein profiles may contain thousands of data points, which in turn require a sophisticated bioanalysis.

A number of animal models, including baboons, rhesus monkeys, rats and mice, have been used in the past for endometriosis research. The drawback of using animal models is that many of the studied species have no menstrual cycle, and only primates develop endometriosis spontaneously.

Since the 1990s, two-dimensional electrophoresis has been used to investigate the molecules involved in the pathogenesis of endometriosis. More recently, Tabibzadeh et al compared the 2D-PAGE of PF of women with and without endometriosis; however, the gels exhibited a limited number of protein spots, and the identity of the majority of the protein spots with an abnormal expression in endometriosis was neither determined by either immunoblotting nor mass spectrometry.[22] Instead, they showed marked differences in the amount and type of the PF proteins present in six women with mild endometriosis, six women with severe endometriosis, six women with infertility and no endometriosis, and six fertile controls using 2-DE. The proteins observed in women with infertility and without endometriosis did not differ from those of healthy controls, and mild endometriosis was associated with only a mild reduction of proteins in the 35-40 kDa and pI 5.7-6.0 range compared with controls. In women with severe endometriosis, however, a more marked decrease in the same protein spots was observed, also with a two- to-four-fold increase in the amount of

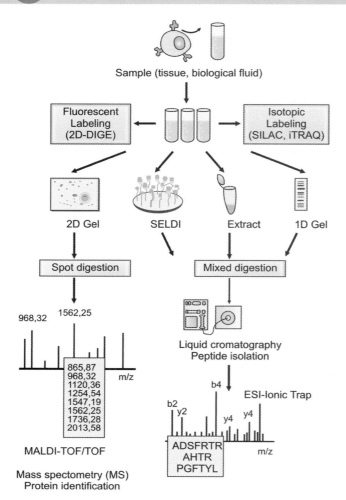

FIGURE 13-2: Different strategies for proteomic analysis. The proteins are extracted from different samples, and they are separated using different techniques. In gel-based methods (left), the separation is made by two-dimensional gels (2D) by taking into account their isoelectric point (IP), their molecular mass by identifying with the "peptide fingerprint" by MALDI mass spectrometry (MS). For the quantitative differential analysis between two samples, extracts are labeled with different fluorofores, separated in a unique gel, and their images are analyzed (2D-DIGE). Those proteins which are differentially expressed are identified by MALDI-MS.

In the methods based on chromotographic separation (right), proteins are enzimatically digested (trypsin, generally), and the peptide mix is separated by HPLC (high-pressure liquid chromatography). Generally, peptides are analyzed and identified as they appear from the HPLC column by electro-nebulization (ESI) coupled to an ionic trap. For the quantitative analysis, proteins or peptides could be previously labeled with different stable isotopes like the SILAC or iTRAQ techniques.

other numerous proteins seen in severe endometriosis if compared with controls.[22] With regard to the published literature, these protein differences have not been characterized, and these findings have not progressed to

the development of a diagnostic test for endometriosis to date. However, this is certainly an area with considerable potential that requires validation and exploration with further studies.

Fowler et al[23] investigated the effects of endometriosis on the proteome of the human eutopic endometrium by using 2D-PAGE and mass spectrometry **(Figure 13-3)**. Several dysregulated proteins were identified, including molecular chaperones, proteins involved in cellular redox state, molecules involved in protein and DNA formation/breakdown, and secreted proteins. In a similar study, Zhang et al[24] observed an abnormal expression of the proteins involved in the cell cycle, signal transduction, and the immunological function. The study of Zhang et al, published in 2006, was designed to search for endometriosis-specific proteins using 2-DE, Western blot, and mass spectrometry. Their first aim was to find a difference in the way serum and eutopic endometrial proteins were expressed in women with and without endometriosis. The authors were also interested in searching for endometriotic proteins, which were specifically recognized by sera from patients with endometriosis **(Table 13-1)**. The potential markers could lead to novel diagnostic, therapeutic, and prognostic methods to manage endometriosis, and may also improve our understanding of the pathogenic mechanism of endometriosis. The 2-DE profiles were very similar among six endometriosis sera samples. An average electrophoresis map of endometriosis sera was constructed by comparing the 2-DE maps from six endometriosis sera, which included 237 protein spots. Similarly, an average electrophoresis map of six normal sera was also established with 216 protein spots. The 2-DE protein patterns of the average gels of sera samples from women with and without endometriosis were compared and different protein spots were detected with a discrepancy which was at least three-fold. After the comparative proteomic study, the authors found 13 protein spots from serum correlated with 11 known proteins. These 11 proteins were correlated with 11 proteins which were differently expressed between women with and without endometriosis. While some of the matched proteins with a different expression may be cytoskeletons, others may be the regulatory proteins of the cell cycle, signal transduction, or the immunological function. Such proteins include the G antigen family B1 protein, actin-related protein 6, actinlike-7- anhydrase I, Dentin matrix acidic phosphoprotein I, CD166 antigen, cyclin A1, among others.[24]

Protein chip technology has also been recently applied to study the protein expressed by the endometrium,

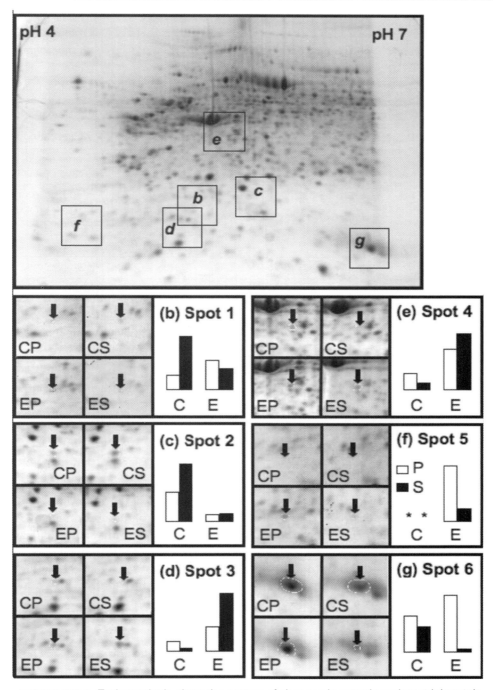

FIGURE 13-3: Endometriosis alters the pattern of changes in eutopic endometrial protein spot volumes between the proliferative and secretory phases of the menstrual cycle, as visualized by 2-DE using a 4–7 pH gradient: (a) representative 2-D gel showing zoom boxes (b–g), highlighting protein spots with endometriosis-related alterations in the pattern of changes in spot volumes during the menstrual cycle. Histograms show the average spot volumes during the proliferative (open boxes, P) and secretory (closed boxes, S) phases, which are separated according to whether the endometrial proteins were pooled from women with (E) or without (C) endometriosis.

Table 13-1: Differentially expressed proteins in serum from endometriosis and healthy patients							
Spot no.	Expression in endometriosis	Expression in normal	Ratio	Swiss-Prot accession no.	pI	MW	Protein name
1	0.898	0.042	21.24	O75459	4.15	16,130	G antigen family B$_1$ protein (Prostate-associated gene protein 1)
2	0.275	0.026	10.58	Q9GZN1	4.92	45,810	Actin-related protein 6
3	0.120	0.013	9.23	P08174	7.00	34,950	Complement decay-accelerating factor precursor (CD55 antigen)
4	0.293	0.035	8.37	Q16543	5.17	44,470	Hsp90 co-chaperone Cdc37 (Hsp90 chaperone protein kinase-targeting subunit)
5	5.028	1.299	3.87		3.62	81,820	?
6	0.673	0.220	3.06	Q08477	7.03	59,850	Cytochrome P450 4F3
7	0.086	0.289	3.36	P00915	6.63	28,740	Carbonic anhydrase 1
8	0.481	2.990	6.22		3.35	52,740	?
9	0.066	0.373	5.65	Q9UMQ3	6.37	28,250	Homeobox protein BarH-like 2
10	0.098	0.419	4.28	P53539	4.78	35,930	Protein fosB
11	0.370	0		O95400	4.49	37,650	CD2 antigen cytoplasmic tail-binding protein 2
12	0.493	0		Q9Y2V7	5.51	68,070	Conserved oligomeric Golgi complex component 6
13	0	1.17		Q13316	3.99	53,970	Dentin matrix acidic phosphoprotein 1

endometriotic tissues, and normal peritoneum obtained from women with and without endometriosis.[25]

Another recent study by Ametzazurra et al introduces another sample source to study the endometriosis that is endometrial fluid. Using the endometrial fluid from different stages of endometriosis patients they were able to find 31 proteins differentially expressed between endometriosis and controls. Among them, they were proteins related with cell signalling, cell death and cell movement, processes that can be involved in the onset and/or progression of the disease. Of all these proteins 14-3-3 and moesin were chosen for Western Blot validation.[26]

Finally, a new emerging "omic" technique has been used in different medicine fields to analyze the metabolic responses to drugs, environmental changes and diseases. Metabolomics (or metabonomics) is an extension of genomics (concerned with DNA) and proteomics (concerned with proteins). Following the heels of genomics and proteomics, metabolomics may lead to a more efficient drug discovery and to individualized patient treatment with drugs, among other things. In more technical terms,

metabonomics is the quantitative measurement of the dynamic multiparametric metabolic response of living systems to pathophysiological stimuli or genetic modification. In forthcoming years, this technique could prove most useful in the study of endometriosis or toward possible treatments for this disease.

Conclusion

The new imaging and "omics" techniques will be able to improve our understanding and early detection of endometriosis and the search for future candidates for endometriosis treatment. Once a gene/protein, or a small number of genes/proteins, has been shown to be differentially expressed in endometriosis, the next step will be to use this information in an attempt to develop a non-invasive diagnostic test for endometriosis. Ideally, this diagnostic test should display good sensitivity and specificity as well as satisfactory positive and negative predicative values for the detection of endometriosis, and should also be cost-effective and readily available.

References

1. Sampson JA. Peritoneal endometriosis due to the menstrual dissemination of endometrial tissues into the peritoneal cavity. Am J Obstet Gynecol 1927; 14:422-69.

2. Anaf V, Simon P, Fayt I, Noel J. Smooth muscles are frequent components of endometriotic lesions. Hum Reprod 2000; 15:767-71.

3. Cullen TS. The distribution of adenomyoma containing uterine mucosa. Arch Surg 1920; 1: 215-83.

4. Brosens IA. Classification of endometriosis revisited. Lancet 1993; 341:630.

5. Nisolle M, Donnez J. Peritoneal endometriosis, ovarian endometriosis, and adenomyotic nodules of the rectovaginal septum are three different entities. Fertil Steril 1997; 68:585-96.

6. Takahashi K, Okada M, Okada S, Kitao M, Imaoka I, Sugimura K. Studies on the detection of small endometrial implants by magnetic resonance imaging using a fat saturation technique. Gynecol Obstet Invest 1996; 41:203-06.

7. Patel MD, Feldstein VA, Chen DC, Lipson SD, Filly RA. Endometriomas: diagnostic performance of US. Radiology 1999; 210:739-45.

8. Timmerman D, Bourne TH, Tailor A, Collins WP, Verrelst H, Vandenberghe K, et al. A comparison of methods for preoperative discrimination between malignant and benign adnexal masses: the development of a new logistic regression model. Am J Obstet Gynecol 1999;181: 57-65.

9. Brosens IA, Puttemans PJ, Deprest J. The endoscopic localization of endometrial implants in the ovarian chocolate cyst. Fertil Steril 1994; 61:1034-08.

10. Ohba T, Mizutani H, Maeda T, Matsuura K, Okamura H. Evaluation of endometriosis in uterosacral ligaments by transrectal ultrasonography. Hum Reprod 1996; 11: 2014-17

11. Chapron C, Liaras E, Fayet P, Hoeffel C, Fauconnier A, Viera M, et al. Magnetic resonance imaging and endometriosis: deeply infiltrating endometriosis does not originate from the rectovaginal septum. Gynecol Obstet Invest 2002; 53:204-08.

12. Bis KG, Vrachliotis TG, Agrawal R, Shetty AN, Maximovich A, Hricak H. Pelvic endometriosis: MR imaging spectrum with laparoscopic correlation and diagnostic pitfalls. Radiographics 1997 ; 17 :639-55.

13. Balleyguier C, Chapron C, Dubuisson JB, Kinkel K, Fauconnier A, Vieira M, et al. Comparison of magnetic resonance imaging and transvaginal ultrasonography in diagnosing bladder endometriosis. J Am Assoc Gynecol Laparosc 2002; 9:15-23.

14. Gaetje R, Kotzian S, Herrmann G, Baumann R, Starzinski-Powitz A. Invasiveness of endometriotic cells in vitro. Lancet 1995; 346:1463-64.

15. Verheijen RH, von Mensdorff-Pouilly S, van Kamp GJ, Kenemans P. CA 125: fundamental and clinical aspects. Semin Cancer Biol 1999; 9:117-24.

16. Pittaway DE. Serum markers of endometrium and endometriosis. In: Diamond MP, Osteen KG, (Eds). Endometrium and Endometriosis. London: Blackwell Science; 1997;31-41.

17. Bedaiwy MA, Falcone T, Sharma RK, Goldberg JM, Attaran M, Nelson DR, et al. Prediction of endometriosis with serum and peritoneal fluid markers: a prospective controlled trial. Hum Reprod 2002;17:426-31.

18. Matarese G, Alviggi C, Sanna V, Howard JK, Lord GM, Carravetta C, et al. Increased leptin levels in serum and peritoneal fluid of patients with pelvic endometriosis. J Clin Endocrinol Metab 2000;85:2483-87.

19. Horcajadas JA, Pellicer A, Simón C. Wide genomic analysis of human endometrial receptivity: new times, new opportunities. Hum Reprod Update. 2007;13:77-86.

20. Eyster KM, Boles AL, Brannian JD, Hansen KA. DNA microarray analysis of gene expression markers of endometriosis. Fertil Steril 2002;77:38-42.

21. Domínguez F, Gadea B, Esteban FJ, Horcajadas JA, Pellicer A, Simón C.Comparative protein-profile analysis of implanted versus non-implanted human blastocysts. Hum Reprod. 2008;23:1993-2000.

22. Tabibzadeh S, Becker JL, Parsons AK. Endometriosis is associated with alterations in the relative abundance of proteins and IL-10 in the peritoneal fluid. Front Biosci. 2003 1;8:70-78.

23. Fowler PA, Tattum J, Bhattacharya S, Klonisch T, Hombach-Klonisch S, Gazvani R, Lea RG, Miller I, Simpson WG, Cash P. An investigation of the effects of endometriosis on the proteome of human eutopic endometrium: a heterogeneous tissue with a complex disease. Proteomics. 2007;7:130-42.

24. Zhang H, Niu Y, Feng J, Guo H, Ye X, Cui H. Use of proteomic analysis of endometriosis to identify different protein expression in patients with endometriosis versus normal controls. Fertil Steril. 2006;86:274-82.

25. Kyama CM, T'Jampens D, Mihalyi A, Simsa P, Debrock S, Waelkens E, Landuyt B, Meuleman C, Fulop V, Mwenda JM, D'Hooghe TM. ProteinChip technology is a useful method in the pathogenesis and diagnosis of endometriosis: a preliminary study. Fertil Steril. 2006; 86: 203-09.

26. Ametzazurra A, Matorras R, García-Velasco JA, Prieto B, Simon L, Martinez M, Nagore D. Endometril fluid is a specific and non-invasive biological sample for protein biomarker identification in endometriosis. Hum Reprod. 2009;1:1-12.

Section **4**

Clinical Relevance
and
Treatment Options

Andrea G Edlow, Marc R Laufer

Chapter 14

Endometriosis in Adolescents

Introduction

Dysmenorrhea and pelvic pain are frequent complaints among adolescents. After an evaluation, NSAIDs and hormone therapy (cyclic or continuous) are the first line treatment for pelvic pain in adolescents. For those whose pain is refractory to medical therapy, endometriosis should be considered as part of the differential diagnosis. While endometriosis is commonly associated with cyclic pelvic pain in adults, it may manifest as either cyclic or acyclic pelvic pain in adolescents. This pain may hamper or curtail participation in social activities and/or sports teams, and can lead to frequent or prolonged absence from school. Although it was previously assumed that endometriosis presented only after years of menstruation, there have been reports of the disorder prior to menarche,[1-3] and one and five months after menarche.[4,5]

Endometriosis is the presence of endometrial glands and stroma outside the uterine cavity and uterine musculature. While ectopic endometrial implants are most often located in the pelvis, they can occur anywhere in the body. Chronic pelvic pain is typically defined as 3-6 months of pain, and has a prevalence of 3.8% in women aged 15 to 73.[6] Endometriosis is the most common pathologic condition in adolescents with chronic pelvic pain, and has been reported in 25-38% of adolescents with chronic pelvic pain.[7,8] The prevalence of endometriosis among adolescents undergoing laparoscopy for pelvic pain refractory to medical therapy has been reported to be 50-70%.[9-11] Our experience with rates of diagnosis of endometriosis at the time of laparoscopy suggest that with the visual acuity afforded by advances in laparoscopic technology, and a surgeon experienced in intraoperative identification of endometriosis lesions, the prevalence may be even higher.

Because many providers (including pediatricians, family practitioners, nurse practitioners, and gynecologists) may not be aware of the symptoms of endometriosis in young women, there is often a significant time between presentation with symptoms and diagnosis. Data from the Endometriosis Association has shown that the delay between onset of symptoms and actual diagnosis of disease was 9.28 years.[12] The consequences of delayed diagnosis are physical, emotional, and social.[13] Endometriosis is known to be a progressive disease, and delayed surgical diagnosis has been shown to be associated with advanced disease at the time of surgery.[14] In addition, endometriosis has been shown to place a considerable economic burden on patients and society.[15] In this chapter, we hope to raise awareness of the typical presentation of endometriosis in adolescents, provide health care providers with a straightforward diagnostic and therapeutic approach, and in so doing, facilitate early diagnosis and intervention. Early diagnosis and intervention are critical in ameliorating the long-term effects of endometriosis (pain and suffering, masses and infertility), reducing economic burden from long-term advanced disease, and improving affected young women's quality of life.

Pathogenesis of Endometriosis

The observation that 6.9% of first degree female relatives of patients with endometriosis are affected, compared to 1% of relatives of controls, suggests that there may be a genetic predisposition to developing endometriosis.[16] Many theories have been proposed to explain the etiology of endometriosis; the origin of the disease is likely multifactorial and no one theory can account for all presentations.

In 1909, Meyer proposed that the coelomic (peritoneal) cavity contains undifferentiated cells, or cells capable of dedifferentiating into endometrial tissue.[17] This is also called the coelomic metaplasia theory, and may help explain the presence of endometriosis in premenarcheal girls with some breast development.[1-3]

In 1927, Sampson proposed that endometrial tissue seeds the pelvis via retrograde menstruation through the fallopian tubes.[18] Evidence supporting this theory includes:

1. Endometriosis is most common in the dependent portion of the pelvis.
2. Obstructive anomalies of the female genital tract that enhances retrograde flow have been associated with endometriosis in the adolescent population.[5,19,20]
3. Repair of obstructive anomalies of the reproductive tract has been associated with resolution of endometriosis.[20]

In 1924, Halban proposed that endometriosis may metastasize through lymphatic and vascular channels.[21] This theory helps explain endometriosis in locations remote from the pelvis such as the lung, brain, and skin. The most recently proposed theory, the cellular immunity theory, posits that deficient cellular immunity allows the proliferation of ectopic endometrial tissue.[22-24]

Diagnosis of Endometriosis

Evaluation of Pelvic Pain

Endometriosis in adult women may present as chronic pelvic pain, dysmenorrhea, dyspareunia, infertility, or a complex pelvic mass. In adolescents, endometriosis may present with more prominent bowel (rectal pain, constipation, painful defecation that may be cyclic, rectal bleeding) and bladder (dysuria, urgency, hematuria) symptoms; the pelvic pain may be both cyclic and acyclic.[11] Ovarian endometriomas and infertility are rare in adolescents.

We have developed an algorithm for evaluation of the adolescent with suspected endometriosis **(Figure 14-1)**.[25-26] This algorithm has been adapted by the American College of Obstetricians and Gynecologists for the Committee Opinion on Adolescent Endometriosis.[27]

History

A thorough history is a key component of the initial evaluation of an adolescent with pelvic pain. Questions that should be addressed by the initial history include:

1. Characteristics of the pain, including location, onset, magnitude, timing, quality, radiation, precipitating factors, alleviating factors, and duration.

2. Associated symptoms, including dysuria, urinary frequency, nausea, vomiting, chills, fever, backache/musculoskeletal pain, and changes in bowel habits.
3. Past medical and surgical history, with special attention to symptoms suspicious for, diagnosis of, or therapy for: endometriosis, pelvic inflammatory disease, gastrointestinal/genitourologic conditions, infection, musculoskeletal conditions, psychiatric conditions. Patients should also be queried about prior diagnostic tests or treatments for pain.
4. Menstrual, contraceptive, sexual, and gynecologic history
5. Family history of endometriosis and other relevant clinical conditions
6. Does pain interfere with daily activities?[28]

As described previously, a family history of endometriosis, particularly in first degree relatives, is correlated with a higher likelihood of endometriosis in the patient.[16] A history of sexual abuse or physical abuse may also be associated with chronic pelvic pain,[29] but should not preclude further evaluation. The patient should keep a pain diary documenting frequency and character of pain, and its relation to bowel/bladder function. Complaints of difficulty participating in normal activities, missing school or avoiding extracurricular and/or social activities secondary to pain suggests that intervention is appropriate.

Normalization of Symptoms and Delay in Diagnosis

It is very common for both adolescents and family physicians to "normalize symptoms", which can lead to a delay in diagnosis, and may damage the therapeutic bond between physician and patient. Ballard et al conducted a qualitative study of women's experiences reaching a diagnosis of endometriosis in the UK, and found that the normalization of symptoms by both women and family doctors, as well as the suppression of symptoms through hormones, led to significant delay in diagnosis.[13] This study found that women suffered at a physical, emotional, and social level when diagnosis was delayed. They benefited from being diagnosed with endometriosis, in that the diagnosis provided them a language with which to discuss their condition, offered them management strategies specific to their condition, provided reassurance that their symptoms were not due to cancer, and legitimized work absences and difficulty meeting social obligations. In addition, diagnosis also facilitated women's access to social support. Data from both New Zealand and the United Kingdom suggest women with chronic pelvic pain are dissatisfied with their interactions with physicians

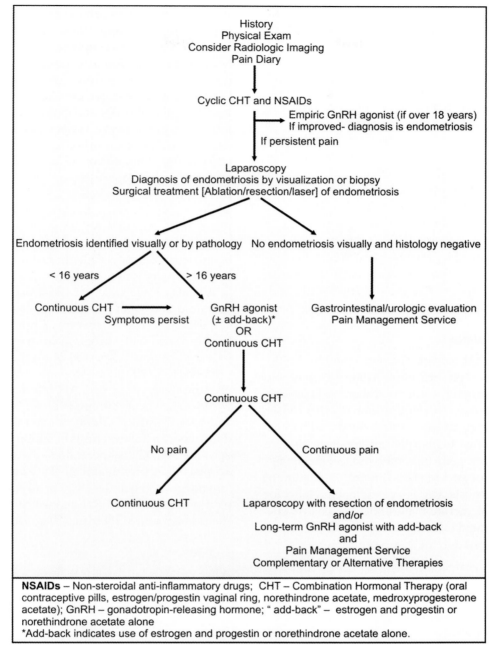

FIGURE 14-1: Protocol for evaluation and treatment of Adolescent Pelvic Pain/ endometriosis. (Adapted from Laufer MR, Sanfilippo J, Rose G. Adolescent endometriosis: diagnosis and treatment approaches. *J Pediatr Adolesc Gynecol* 2003:16:S3-S11).

and their experiences interfacing with the health care system.[30,31] Patients report difficulty communicating with their doctors, inadequate explanation/information provided to them, inadequate reassurance, and inappropriate treatment of their pain. In both studies, women reported that doctors negated their own experience of the pain, and that they often felt dismissed. Data from a research registry of 4000 women with endometriosis compiled by the Endometriosis Association found that 47% of women with endometriosis saw a doctor five or more times before being diagnosed or referred.[12] Women who had onset of symptoms before age 15 were more likely to see more physicians (average 4.2) before endometriosis was diagnosed. Data from this registry suggests that the average delay between onset of symptoms and diagnosis of disease was 9.28 years (women averaged 4.67 years with symptoms before presenting to a physician, and physicians averaged 4.61 years to diagnosis after women presented).

Women whose diagnosis was delayed were significantly more likely to have a subsequent hysterectomy.

Physical Examination

Although important, the gynecological pelvic examination should not be the cornerstone of the evaluation of adolescent pelvic pain and persistent dysmenorrhea. In adolescents who are not sexually active, a recto-abdominal exam to evaluate for any congenital anomalies may be better tolerated than a traditional bimanual pelvic exam. Additionally, a Q tip may be inserted into the vagina to exclude congenital obstructive or partially obstructive anomalies. Genital tract anomalies are present in approximately 5% of patients with endometriosis.[27] If a bimanual exam is possible, it is important to keep in mind that, unlike adults, adolescents rarely have uterosacral nodularity, and that adnexal enlargement with endometrioma is also rare in adolescents.

Radiologic Examination

A pelvic ultrasound should also be performed to supplement the often-limited physical examination; this may help determine if a pelvic mass or structural anomaly is present. Ultrasound may also aid in identification of other causes of pelvic pain including ovarian cysts, torsion, and tumors. CT scan with contrast helps rule out appendicitis as a source of acute pelvic pain, but otherwise is typically not revealing and is not part of the standard evaluation of suspected endometriosis. MRI is an excellent modality for evaluation of genital tract anomalies, but is expensive. MRI has been demonstrated to have poor sensitivity for detecting peritoneal lesions and for staging endometriosis.[32-34]

Laboratory Evaluation

Lab tests that may be ordered include:
1. CBC and ESR, to evaluate for acute or chronic inflammatory process.
2. Urinalysis and urine culture to investigate pain with a urinary tract component.
3. Pregnancy test and tests for gonorrhea and chlamydia, when appropriate.

Treatment

Initiating Empiric Treatment

If initial evaluation suggests a non-acute gynecological source of pain such as primary dysmenorrhea or endometriosis, a trial of non-steroidal anti-inflammatory drugs (NSAIDs) is recommended. If possible, NSAIDs should be started before the expected onset of severe pain. NSAIDs may be used alone, or in conjunction with a lowdose oral contraceptive pill (OCP) to suppress hormonal stimulation associated with ovulation, and to decrease menstrual flow. The American College of Obstetrics and Gynecology (ACOG) recommends a 3-month trial of NSAIDs and cyclic OCPs; if pain does not resolve at this time, further evaluation is necessary to determine if endometriosis is the etiology of pain.[27] If pain persists after 3 months of cyclic OCPs, it is reasonable to offer the patient laparoscopy to rule out endometriosis. Data collected in the early 1990s found that 69% of adolescents with pelvic pain not responding to conventional medical therapy had endometriosis at laparoscopy.[11] Given advancements in optical resolution in laparoscopy, the rate of identification of endometriosis at time of surgery is now likely much higher.

It is also reasonable, for those patients who are ≥ 18 years old and wish to avoid surgery, to offer a trial of empiric GnRH agonist therapy. Empiric depot leuprolide has been used with success in adult women with chronic pelvic pain and suspected endometriosis.[28,35] If pain responds to GnRH agonist therapy, endometriosis may be presumptively diagnosed. At Children's Hospital Boston, we do not advocate the empiric use of GnRH agonist with add-back therapy for those younger than 18 years of age, due to concern for the effects of the GnRH agonist on bone density.[36] ACOG does not endorse the use of empiric GnRH agonist therapy for treatment of presumed endometriosis for young women under 18.[27] For all young women whose pain persists after GnRH agonist therapy, laparoscopy should be pursued for visual diagnosis.

Laparoscopy

When patients fail empiric therapy, a definitive diagnosis should be established before proceeding with further treatment.[27] Laparoscopy is the gold standard for diagnosis of endometriosis. If a gynecologist is to perform the laparoscopy, he or she should have experience operating on patients in the age range in question, and therefore be in a position to perform not only diagnostic, but therapeutic laparoscopy. Otherwise, it is appropriate to refer adolescents with endometriosis to a pediatric gynecologist or pediatric surgeon for a combined diagnostic and therapeutic procedure, to avoid placing the patient at undue risk from two administrations of anesthesia. Cosmetic considerations are particularly important in young patients. We recommend placing a laparoscopic trocar through a 5 mm vertical incision directly in the umbilicus, with additional operative ports placed symmetrically 1 to 2 cm above the pubic symphysis, to minimize visible scarring.

Endometriotic implants in adolescents are most commonly clear, red, and white, as described in the revised American Society of Reproductive Medicine (ASRM) Classification of Endometriosis.[37] There is some evidence that endometriosis may have a slightly different appearance in adolescents at the time of laparoscopy compared to adults. Peritoneal Alan-Masters windows are more common in adolescents than adults, and are diagnostic of endometriosis. Endometriotic lesions may be subtle, appearing as clear, shiny peritoneal vesicles. These clear endometriotic lesions may be best visualized through a liquid medium such as saline, which may be suctioned after lesions have been identified to facilitate fulguration.[38] A series comparing the appearance of endometriotic lesions in adolescents to those found in adults concluded that red flame lesions were more common in adolescents, while powder-burn lesions (which may represent older implants) were more common in adults.[39] There is some evidence to suggest that clear and red lesions may be more painful than other endometriotic lesions.[40]

Ablation of endometriotic lesions using electrocautery, endocoagulation, or laser should be performed at the time of diagnostic laparoscopy.[41] A randomized, controlled study of 24 patients with Stage I or II endometriosis demonstrated that destruction of endometriotic lesions is as effective as excision for relief of pelvic pain.[42] Lysis of adhesions should also be performed at the time of surgery, and can be accomplished with electrocautery and scissors. While endometriomas are rare in adolescents, if large ovarian cysts are identified, cystectomy should be performed, taking care to preserve ovarian tissue. Reduction in pain from endometriosis was noted in 38 to 100% of adult women after surgical treatment.[43,44] Similar studies have not been performed in adolescents.

Staging should be performed at the time of laparoscopy according to the revised ASRM Classification of Endometriosis, to facilitate comparison if future surgery is performed.[37] If there is no evidence of endometriosis at the time of laparoscopy, a cul-de-sac biopsy may be performed to exclude the presence of microscopic disease. Evidence on the utility of non-directed biopsies is inconclusive; a low prevalence of microscopic endometriosis (1 in 55 patients) was found in one study,[45] while another reported a 6% rate of microscopic endometriosis on uterosacral ligament biopsy in patients with no gross evidence of endometriosis.[46] Both studies were performed in adults. Our experience at Children's Hospital Boston suggests a 3% prevalence of microscopic endometriosis in adolescents with a visually normal pelvis.[11] It is important to remember for postoperative counseling that the extent of disease does not correlate with severity of symptoms.[47]

Treatment of Laparoscopically-Proven Endometriosis

Medical Management

Surgical ablation or resection alone is not adequate treatment for endometriosis; microscopic residual disease may remain, and must be suppressed with medical therapy.[28] The return of symptoms in as many as 50% of adult women who receive surgical therapy only is well-documented.[28,44,49,50] Adolescents with endometriosis confirmed by laparoscopy should receive medical treatment until childbearing is complete or fertility is no longer desired.[27] The goal of treatment is to maximize pain relief and promote participation in school, social activities, and sports. Suppression of ovulation with continuous OCPs or GnRH agonists is the most effective method of achieving pain control. In addition, continuous hormone therapy (menstrual suppression) has the potential to prevent or slow the progression of disease by inhibiting ovulation and inducing decidalization and subsequent atrophy of endometrial tissue.[50,51] While numerous options for medical treatment of endometriosis have been described,[9,25] at Children's Hospital Boston, continuous OCPs for menstrual suppression are typically first-line therapy. If pain persists on continuous OCPs and the patient is 16 or older, GnRH agonists with Aygestin add-back therapy are an excellent option.[52] GnRH agonist with add-back therapy is not routinely used for those younger than 16 years of age, due to the potential of GnRH agonists to adversely affect the formation of normal bones and decrease bone density.

Oral Contraceptive Pills

Continuous hormonal therapy is typically well-tolerated, and appears to be safe and effective,[51,53] although long-term utilization data is lacking. In choosing a hormonal pill, a monophasic progestin-dominant OCP will induce amenorrhea most effectively. It is important to stress to patients the importance of taking the pill at exactly the same time each day. Patients may expect an average of 4 breakthrough bleeding events per year. If irregular bleeding more than four times a year persists, a switch can be made to a different monophasic progestin-dominant pill. NuvaRing may also be used continuously (i.e. replacing the ring every 3 weeks) to achieve anovulation and amenorrhea.

GnRH Agonist Therapy

If a patient is unable to achieve an acceptable degree of pain control or continues to have intolerable bleeding with combination OCPs and wishes to pursue GnRH agonist therapy, we typically prescribe depot leuprolide acetate

11.25 mg IM every 3 months. After 2 doses, greater than 90% of patients will become amenorrheic.[54] After 6 months of therapy, the patient may decide whether she wishes to return to continuous combination OCPs or NuvaRing, or continue on the GnRH agonist with add-back therapy. If the patient wishes to continue on the GnRH agonist, a baseline bone density assessment should be obtained after the initial 6-9 months of therapy and, if normal, repeated every 2 years while the patient is maintained on GnRH agonist therapy. Patients are instructed to take 1200 mg calcium and vitamin D daily in addition to their add-back therapy. The preservation of bone density in the setting of long-term GnRH agonist use, in conjunction with add-back therapy, calcium and vitamin D, has been documented in the literature.[55]

Nafarelin is an alternative GnRH agonist; the dosing is one puff twice daily intranasally. However, compliance with a nasal spray is often unpredictable in the adolescent population. The most common side effects of GnRH agonist therapy that affect the adolescent population include hot flashes, headaches, and difficulty in sleeping. The utilization of add-back therapy can help alleviate these side effects without reducing efficacy, provided the add-back regimen does not include high doses of estrogen.[56] Options for add-back therapy extrapolated from literature about the adult population include norethindrone acetate (5 mg daily), or conjugated equine estrogen (0.625 mg), plus either norethindrone acetate (5 mg) or medroxyprogesterone acetate (5 mg) daily.[57,58] Norethindrone acetate add-back therapy is associated with higher patient satisfaction compared to other regimens.[57]

Progestins

There is conflicting data on the effectiveness of progestins in the treatment of endometriosis.[59,60] Regimens include norethindrone acetate 15 mg daily, medroxyprogesterone acetate (MPA) 30-50 mg by mouth daily, or depot MPA 150 mg intramuscularly every 1-3 months.[59-61] The high dosages of progestins required to suppress ovulation are not well tolerated.[62] The most common side effects in adolescents include weight gain, bloating, acne, headaches, fluid retention, emotional lability, and irregular menses. Due to the poor side effect profile, progestin-only therapy is reserved for those who cannot tolerate continuous combination hormone therapy, or have contraindication to its use. It is advisable to start oral progestin therapy prior to initiating intramuscular injections so that side effects may be identified and the therapy may be discontinued if necessary. Long-term utilization of depot MPA has been shown to cause a decrease in bone density,

so monitoring of bone density in patients on this regimen is advised.[63,64]

Danazol

Danazol is a derivative of 17-α-ethinyl testosterone. Multiple studies have documented its efficacy in treating endometriosis to be equivalent to a variety of GnRH agonists.[65-70] Despite danazol's proven efficacy in the treatment of endometriosis, we do not prescribe it for adolescents due to its unacceptable side effect profile. The significant androgenic side effects are due to the increase in free testosterone. In a series of 220 patients on danazol therapy, common complaints included weight gain, depression, muscle cramps, decreased breast size, flushing, oily skin and hair, acne, hirsutism, irreversible deepening of the voice, and skin rash.[71] In fact, 7% of patients in this series discontinued the drug secondary to intolerable side effects. Patients using GnRH agonists report a better quality of life than patients using danazol.[72] In addition, danazol is associated with an unfavorable metabolic profile including decreased high-density lipoprotein cholesterol and increased insulin resistance.

Key Points

1. Evaluation of chronic pelvic pain in adolescents should begin with a complete history and physical exam, a pain diary, a pelvic ultrasound, and also may include laboratory evaluation.
2. Empiric treatment of pelvic pain and dysmenorrhea in adolescents includes a 3-month trial of nonsteroidal antiinflammatory drugs and cyclic oral contraceptive agents.
3. Definitive diagnosis of adolescent endometriosis is made by laparoscopy. Sixty-nine percent of adolescents with chronic pelvic pain will have endometriotic lesions at the time of laparoscopy.
4. In adolescents, the laparoscopic appearance of endometriosis may be subtle, with red flame lesions, clear shiny peritoneal vesicles, and peritoneal windows.
5. Surgical management involves diagnosis of endometriosis and destruction/ablation of lesions.
6. Medical management of endometriosis in adolescents after definitive diagnosis includes continuous hormonal suppression using continuous oral contraceptives, gonadotropin-releasing hormone agonists, or other medications. Medical therapy should be continued until the time fertility is desired, and between pregnancies as long as fertility is desired.

7. Long-term follow up studies of adolescents with endo-metriosis are needed to determine if early intervention improves quality of life and future reproductive outcomes.

References

1. Laufer MR. Premenarcheal endometriosis without an associated obstructive anomaly: presentation, diagnosis, and treatment. Fertil Steril 2000; 74: S15.

2. Marsh E, Laufer MR. Endometriosis in premenarcheal girls who do not have an associated reproductive anomaly. Fertil Steril 2005; 83:758-60.

3. Batt RE, Mitwally MF. Endometriosis from thelarche to midteens: pathogenesis and prognosis, prevention and pedagogy. J Pediatr Adolesc Gynecol 2003; 16:337.

4. Yamamoto K, Mitsuhashi Y, Takaike T, et al. Tubal endometriosis diagnosed within one month after menarche: a case report. Tohoku J Exp Med 1997; 181: 385.

5. Goldstein DP, deCholnoky C, Leventhal JM, Emans SJ. New insights into the old problem of chronic pelvic pain. J Pediatr Surg 1979; 14:65.

6. Zondervan KT, Yudkin PL, Vessey MP, et al. Prevalence and incidence in primary care of chronic pelvic pain in women: Evidence from a national general practice database. Br J Obstet Gynaecol 1999; 106:1149.

7. Vercellini P, Fedele L, Arcaini L, et al. Laparoscopy in the diagnosis of chronic pelvic pain in adolescent women. J Reprod Med 1989; 34:827.

8. Kontoravdis A, Hassan E, Hassiakos D, et al. Laparoscopic evaluation and management of chronic pelvic pain during adolescence. Clin Exp Obstet Gynecol 1999; 26:76.

9. Laufer MR, Goldstein DP. "Gynecological pain: Dysmenorrhea, acute and chronic pelvic pain, endomet-riosis, and premenstrual syndrome." In: Emans SJ, Laufer MR, Goldstein DP. Pediatric and Adolescent Gynecology (Fifth Edition), Philadelphia: Lippincott Williams & Wilkins Publishing Company, 2005;417-76.

10. Reese KA, Reddy S, Rock JA. Endometriosis in an adolescent population: The Emory experience. J Pediatr Adolesc Gynecol 1996; 9:125-28.

11. Laufer MR, Goitein L, Bush M, Cramer DW, Emans SJ. Prevalence of endometriosis in adolescent women with chronic pelvic pain not responding to conventional therapy. J Pediatr Adolesc Gynecol 1997;10:199-202.

12. Ballweg ML. Big picture of endometriosis helps provide guidance on approach to teens: Comparative historical data show endo starting younger, is more severe. J Pediatr Adolesc Gynecol 2003;16:S21-S26.

13. Ballard K, Lowton K, Wright J. What's the delay? A qualitative study of women's experiences of reaching a diagnosis of endometriosis. Fertil Steril 2006;86:1296-1301.

14. Matsuzaki S, Cainis M, et al. Relationship between delay of surgical diagnosis and severity of disease in patients with symptomatic deep infiltrating endometriosis. Fertil Steril 2006;86:1314-16.

15. Gao X, Outley J, et al. Economic burden of endometriosis. Fertil Steril 2006; 86:1561-72.

16. Simpson JL, Elias S, Malinak LR, Buttram VC. Heritable aspects of endometriosis. Am J Obstet Gynecol 1980; 137: 327-31.

17. Meyer R. Uber entzundliche neterope epithelwucherungen im weiblichen Genetalgebiet und uber eine bis in die Wurzel des Mesocolon ausgedehnte benigne Wucherung des Dar mepithel. Virch Arch Pathol Anat 1909; 195:487.

18. Sampson JA. Peritoneal endometriosis due to the menstrual dissemination of endometrial tissue into the peritoneal cavity. Am J Obstet Gynecol 1927; 14:422-69.

19. Schifrin BS, Erez S, Moore JG. Teenage endometriosis. Am J Obstet Gynecol 1973; 116:973-80.

20. Sanfilippo JS, Wakim NG, Schikler KN, Yussman MA. Endometriosis in association with uterine anomaly. Am J Obstet Gynecol 1986; 154: 39-43.

21. Halban J. Hysteroadenosis metastica. Wien Klin Wochenschr 1924; 37:1205-28.

22. Gleicher N, el-Roeiy A, Confino E, Friberg J. Is endometriosis an autoimmune disease? Obstet Gynecol 1987; 70:115.

23. Dmowski W, Braun d, Gebel H. Endometriosis: Genetic and immunologic aspects. Prog Clin Biol Res 1990; 323:99-122.

24. Nothnick WB. Treating endometriosis as an autoimmune disease. Fertil Steril 2001; 76: 223.

25. Propst AM, Laufer MR. Endometriosis in adolescents. Incidence, diagnosis and treatment. J Reprod Med 1999; 44:751-58.

26. Laufer MR, Sanfilippo J, Rose G. Adolescent endometriosis: Diagnosis and treatment approaches. J Pediatr Adolesc Gynecol 2003; 16:3-11.

27. American College of Obstetricians and Gynecologists. Endometriosis in adolescents. ACOG Committee Opinion No. 310. Obstet Gynecol 2005;105:921-27.

28. Gambone JC, Mittman BS, Munro MG, et al. Consensus statement for the management of chronic pelvic pain and endometriosis: proceedings of an expert-panel consensus process. Fertil Steril 2002; 78:961.

29. Walling MK, Reiter RC, et al. Abuse history and chronic pain in women: I. prevalences of sexual abuse and physical abuse. Obstet Gynecol 1994; 84:193-99.

30. Grace VM. Problems of communication, diagnosis and treatment experienced by women using the New Zealand health services for chronic pelvic pain: a quantitative analysis. Health Care Women Int 1995; 16:521-35.

31. Price J, Farmer G, Harris J, Hope T, Kennedy S, Mayou R. Attitudes of women with chronic pelvic pain to the gynaecological consultation: a qualitative study. BJOG 2006; 113: 446-52.

32. Stratton P, Winkel C, Premkmar A, et al. Diagnostic accuracy of laparoscopy, magnetic resonance imaging, and histopathologic examination for the detection of endometriosis. Fertil Steril 2003; 79:1078.

33. Tanaka YO, Itai Y, Anno I, et al. MR staging of pelvic endometriosis: role of fat suppression T1-weighted images. Radiat Med 1996; 14:111.

34. Ha HK, Lim YT, Kim HS, et al. Diagnosis of pelvic endometriosis fat-suppressed T1-weighted vs conventional MR images. Am J Roentgenol 1994; 163:127.

35. Ling FW. Randomized controlled trial of depot leuprolide in patients with chronic pelvic pain and clinically suspected endometriosis. Obstet Gynecol 1999; 93:51.

36. Propst AM, Laufer MR. Endometriosis in adolescents. Incidence, diagnosis, and treatment. J Reprod Med 1999; 44: 751.

37. Revised American Society for Reproductive Medicine classification of endometriosis: 1996. Fertil Steril 1997; 67: 817.

38. Laufer MR. Identification of clear vesicular lesions of atypical endometriosis: a new technique. Fertil Steril 1997; 68: 739.

39. Davis GD, Thillet E, Lindemann J. Clinical characteristics of adolescent endometriosis. J Adolesc Health 1993; 14:362.

40. Demco L. Mapping the source and character of pain due to endometriosis by patient-assisted laparoscopy. J Am Assoc Gynecol Laparosc 1998; 5:241.

41. Cook AS, Rock JA. Role of laparoscopy in the treatment of endometriosis. Fertil Steril 1991; 55:663-749.

42. Wright J, Lotfallah H, Jones K. A randomized trial of excision versus ablation for mild endometriosis. Fertil Steril 2005; 83:1830-36.

43. Redwine DB. Treatment of endometriosis-associated pain. Infertil Reprod Med Clin North Am 1993; 3:697.

44. Sutton CJ, Ewen SP, Whitelaw N, Haines P. Prospective, randomized double-blind, controlled trial of laser laparoscopy in the treatment of pelvic pain associated with minimal, mild, and moderate endometriosis. Fertil Steril 1994; 62: 696.

45. Redwine DB, Yocom LB. A serial section study of visually normal pelvic peritoneum in patients with endometriosis. Fertil Steril 1990; 54:648.

46. Nisolle M, Paindaveine B, Bourdon A, et al. Histologic study of peritoneal endometriosis in infertile women. Fertil Steril 1990; 53:984.

47. Fedele L, Parazzini F, et al. Stage and localization of pelvic endometriosis and pain. Fertil Steril 1990; 53:155-58.

48. Redwine DB. Conservative laparoscopic excision of endometriosis by sharp dissection: life table analysis of reoperation and persistent or recurrent disease. Fertil Steril 1991; 56:628.

49. Sutton CJ, Pooley AS, Ewen SP, Haines P. Follow-up report on randomized controlled trial of laser laparoscopy in the treatment of pelvic pain associated with minimal to moderate endometriosis. Fertil Steril 1997; 68:1070.

50. Kistner RW. Treatment of endometriosis by inducing pseudo-pregnancy with ovarian hormones. Feril Steril 1959; 10:539.

51. Vercellini P, Frontino G, DeGiorgi O, et al. Continuous use of an oral contraceptive for endometriosis-associated recurrent dymenorrhea that does not respond to a cyclic pill regimen. Fertil Steril 2003; 80:560.

52. Lubianca JN, Gordon CM, Laufer MR. "Add-back" therapy for endometriosis in adolescents. J Reprod Med 1998; 43:164.

53. Miller L, Notter KM. Menstrual reduction with extended use of combination oral contraceptive pills: randomized controlled trial. Obstet Gynecol 2001; 98: 771.

54. Barbieri RL. Treatment of endometriosis with the GnRH agonists. In Gonadotropin Releasing Hormone Analogs: Applications in Gynecology. Edited by Barbieri RL, Friedman AJ. New York: Elsevier Science 1991;63-76.

55. DiVasta A, Laufer MR, Gordon C. Bone density in adolescents treated with a GnRH agonist and add-back therapy for endometriosis. J Pediatr Adolesc Gynecol 2007; 20:293-97.

56. Hornstein MD, Surre ES, Weisberg GW, Casino LA. Leuprolide acetate depo and hormonal add-back in endometriosis: a 12-monh study. Lupron Add-Back Study Group Obstet Gynecol 1998; 91:16.

57. Surrey ES, Hornstein MD. Prolonged GnRH agonist and add-back therapy for symptomatic endometriosis: long-term follow-up. Obstet Gynecol 2002; 99:709.

58. Kiesel L, Schweppe KW, Sillem M, Siebzehnrubl E. Should add-back therapy for endometriosis be deferred for optimal results? Br J Obstet Gynecol 1996; 103 Suppl 14: 15.

59. Moghissi KS, Boyce CR. Management of endometriosis with oral medroxyprogesterone acetate. Obstet Gynecol 1976; 47:265.

60. Luciano AA, Turksoy N, Carleo J. Evaluation of oral med-roxyprogesterone acetate in the treatment of endometriosis. Obstet Gynecol 1988; 72:323.

61. Vercellini P, DeGiorgio, Oldani S, et al. Depot medroxyprogesterone acetate versus an oral contraceptive combined with very low-dose danazol for long-term treatment of pelvic pain associated with endometriosis. Am J Obstet Gynecol 1996; 175:396.

62. Ballweg ML. Tips on treating teens with endometriosis. J Pediatr Adolesc Gynecol 2003; 163:27.

63. Cromer BA, Blair JM, Mahan JD. A prospective comparison of bone density in adolescent girls receiving depo-medroxyprogeserone acetate (Depo-Provera), levonor-gestreal (Norplant), or oral contraceptives. J Pediatr 1996; 129:671.

64. Berenson AB, Radecki C, Grady JJ. A prospective, controlled study of the effects of hormonal contraception on bone mineral density. Obstet Gynecol 2001; 98: 576.

65. Wheeler JM, Knittle JD, Miller JD. Depot leuprolide acetate versus danazol in the treatment of women with symptomatic endometriosis: a multicenter, doubleblind randomized clinical trial. II. assessment of safety. The Lupron Endometriosis Study Group. Am J Obstet Gynecol 1993; 169:26-33.

66. Rock JA, Truglia JA, Caplan RJ. Zoladex (goserelin acetate implant) in the treatment of endometriosis: a randomized comparison with danazol. The Zoladex Endometriosis Study Group. Obstet Gynecol 1993; 82:198-205.

67. Nafarelin for endometriosis: a largescale, danazolcontrolled trial of efficacy and safety, with 1 year followup. The Nafarelin European Endometriosis Trial Group (NEET). Fertil Steril 1992; 57:514-22.

68. Leuprorelin acetate depot vs danazol in the treatment of endometriosis: results of an open multicentre trial. Clin Therap 1992; 14A:29-36.

69. Shaw RW. An open randomized comparative study of the effect of goserelin depot and danazol in the treatment of endometriosis. Zoladex endometriosis study team. Fertil Steril 1992; 58:265-72.

70. Shaw RW. Nafarelin in the treatment of pelvic pain caused by endometriosis. Am J Obstet Gynecol 1990; 162:574-76.

71. Buttram VC, Reiter RC, Ward S. Treatment of endometriosis with danazol: report of a 6-year prospective study. Fertil Steril 1985; 43:353-60.

72. Burry KA. Nafarelin in the management of endometriosis: quality of life assessment. Am J Obstet Gynecol 1992; 166: 735-39.

Antoine Watrelot

Chapter 15
Asymptomatic Endometriosis in Infertile Patients

Introduction

Endometriosis is accepted as cause of infertility when the disease is severe. It is more controversial when endometriosis is mild or moderate. Some studies suggest an interest to treat even minimal endometriosis. The Canadian study, showed interest to treat laparoscopically minimal endometriosis even if there were some bias in this study like the very low pregnancy rate in the control arm, also a meta-analysis tends to give superiority of treatment versus expectant management but other authors do not find any effect of minimal endometriosis on infertility.

If it seems rather evident to treat symptomatic patient suffering from pain. It is more debatable to treat endometriosis in non-symptomatic infertile patients.

Unfortunately at that stage, we are far from being able to give a definitive answer, however, enlighten by new diagnostic approach it seems possible to give some clue.

The management of asymptomatic endometriosis will depend on the circumstances of diagnostic.

Prevalence of Asymptomatic Endometriosis

If there is a consensus to consider that the prevalence of endometriosis in normal patient is around 3-5%.

In case of infertile patients, the prevalence is found in the literature between 20 to 45%.

This important variation depends probably on diagnostic tools used to diagnose endometriosis in infertile patients. For instance in series where endoscopy is performed systematically frequency of endometriosis is higher than in series where only basic tests are practised.

On the contrary in a recent study, it was found that 30% of patients with endometriosis were infertile whereas 67% were nulliparous.

Evolution of Endometriosis in Asymptomatic Patients

It is indeed a crucial question, because if aggravation is obvious, the therapeutic consequences are evident.

In fact, there is very few data available. In baboon it has been demonstrated that the natural history of the disease shows a systematic and continuous evolution, but there is a potential bias in the study since these animals have several laparoscopies to observe the evolution and consequently endoscopies may have an impact on the natural history of endometriosis.

In human Mahmood et al found an aggravation in 43% of cases, stability in 33% and diminution of lesions in 24% but the power of this study is limited since only 45 patients were involved.

Other solder studies suggest that asymptomatic endometriosis is so frequent that it is probably a normal condition which may regress or disappear spontaneously in more than 50% of cases.

Therefore, we have no real arguments coming from the natural evolution of endometriosis to decide to treat or not

Diagnostic of Nonsymptomatic Endometriosis

One of the challenges of endometriosis when non-symptomatic is to establish a diagnostic. It is accepted that the only mean to prove that endometriosis exists is to see it and to have a histological evidence whenever it is possible. Therefore, it is recognized that only Endoscopic evaluation may give the definitive answer.

However, there are other situations where the diagnosis of endometriosis is strongly suspected with only clinical examination or ultra scan examination before any invasive approach.

Therefore, there are three circumstances where non-symptomatic endometriosis may be discovered.

Clinical Diagnosis

There is a situation where it is possible to predict endometriosis when the disease is located either in the recto-vaginal septum or on uterosacral ligaments. In these cases, a careful vaginal examination is sufficient. In fact, this diagnosis is often missed since it appears that quite often the vaginal examination is well done on the cervix, uterine body and adnexae but forget to go deeper in the posterior cul-de-sac.

In case of deep endometriosis, it is possible to feel a nodule in the recto-vaginal septum or sometimes only a fibrous aspect. Sometimes also a typical blue lesion may be seen at the speculum examination.

In all these situations, if laparoscopy is performed, endometriosis will be found.

That situation is rather common: a systematic evaluation of the pouch of Douglas in infertile patients allowed us to detect 5% of patients with deep endometriosis which was not diagnosed before. Confirmation by laparoscopy was done in all cases.

Ultrasound Diagnosis

Diagnosis of endometriosis may also be made by ultrasound in asymptomatic patients when, for any reason, an ultrascan allows to detect an ovarian endometrioma. In fact with ultrasound, endometrioma has the appearance of an hemorrhagic cyst but when this image is persistent at two exams separated by several weeks, endometriosis is strongly suspected **(Figure 15-1)**.

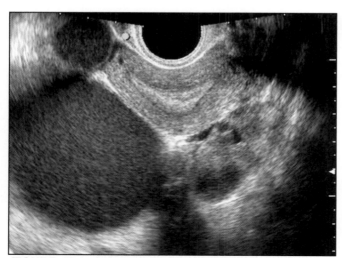

FIGURE 15-1: Appearance of endometrioma in ultrasound.

Endoscopic Diagnosis

It is not rare to discover endometriotic asymptomatic lesions during endoscopy performed for infertile reason.

Nowadays, the classical diagnostic laparoscopy (lap and dye) is rarely performed because it is considered as rather heavy and risky. Therefore, in vitro fertilization (IVF) is often proposed directly to patients with no obvious pathology. In contrary, when endoscopy is practised in patients with no obvious pathology, between 25 to 35% of patients are found with abnormalities such as adhesions or endometriotic lesions.

This is why we have developed a mini invasive technique namely the fertiloscopy in order to have an acceptable systematic endoscopic approach for infertile patients.

We described fertiloscopy **(Figures 15-2 and 15-3)** after the initial works of Gordts in 1997. The technique of this hydrovaginal pelviscopy has been already described several times. Fertiloscopy is feasible under strict anesthesia and have been demonstrated to be as efficient as laparoscopy thanks to the FLY study.

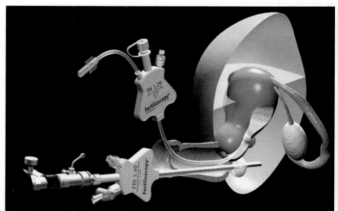

FIGURE 15-2: Principle of fertiloscopy: transvaginal hydropelviscopy.

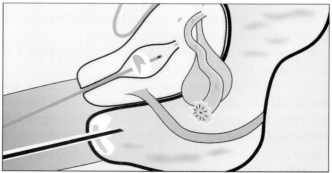

FIGURE 15-3: Principle of fertiloscopy: position of the telescope in the pouch of Douglas.

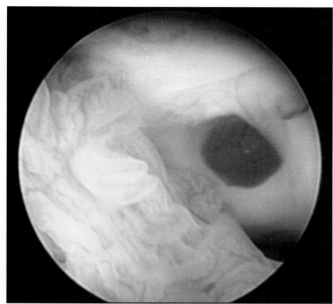

FIGURE 15-4: Endometriotic lesions seen during fertiloscopy.

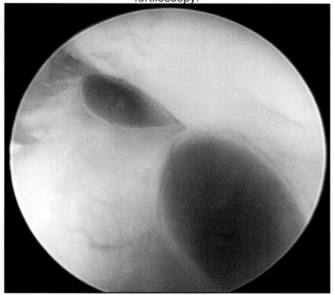

FIGURE 15-5: Endometriotic lesions in the left fossa ovarica.

The results of fertiloscopy performed in all infertile patients with a hysterosalpingogram (HSG) non-conclusive allowed us to detect abnormalities in 556 cases in a series of 1783 patients (31,1%). Among them 15.5% of patients were found to have endometriotic lesions **(Figures 15-4 and 15-5).**

In 8.1% of cases (n=136) endometriosis was considered as minimal according to the AFS classification In 5.3% of cases (n=99) endometriosis was considered as mild and in 2.2% (n=53) endometriosis was considered a severe. To this total we have to add 78 (4.3%) patients where endometriosis

of the recto-vaginal septum was found prior to fertiloscopy and therefore being a contraindication to fertiloscopy were excluded of the series. So in all it is 9, 8 %, of patients who presented endometriotic lesions in this quite extensive series of asymptomatic "unexplained infertility".

What to do in Cases of Asymptomatic Endometriosis?

It mainly depends on the circumstances of diagnostic.

1. In case of endometriosis diagnosed clinically: If endometriotic lesions are clinically evident then it means that the disease is mild or severe. It is in these cases that endometriosis may impaire fertility through mechanical effects, therefore, it seems logical to complete the evaluation with pelvic ultrasound , MRI and then to propose a laparoscopy after clear information of the patient. Laparoscopy in these cases will be able to precise the lesions, and their involvement in the infertility. In some cases, it is possible to treat and restore fertility, when endometriosis is severe indication of extensive surgery is probably not the good answer if the patient has no symptoms since this is a difficult surgery with a complication rate quite high.

2. In case of endometrioma discovered by ultrasound, it is logical to propose a laparoscopy except if the endo-metrioma is less than 3 cm in diameter. In case of laparoscopy, excision of endometrioma has to be preferred to the cystectomy followed by coagulation of the cystic wall, due to the risk of damaging the normal ovarian tissue. When there is recurrence of endomet-rioma, it is not appropriate to operate again since every cystectomy is at risk to reduce the follicles reserve.

   There is one exception which is the ruptured endo-metrioma where surgery is compulsory, but in these cases endometriosis is not any more asymptomatic.

3. In case of endoscopic discovery it is rather evident to treat even the small lesions. That is possible during fertiloscopy since the operative channel of the fertiloscope allows introducing bipolar needle such as Versapoint (Gynecare USA) in order to vaporize the brown or red lesions and divide adhesions frequently associated **(Figure 15-6).**

If lesions are more important during a fertiloscopy practised under general anesthesia then there is a discussion to convert or not fertiloscopy to laparoscopy. This is why a complete information (and consent) of patient is important to decide "on the spot" whereas or not to practice an operative complementary laparoscopy.

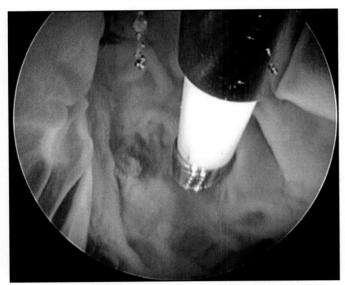

FIGURE 15-6: Use of bipolar Versapoint to vaporize endometriosis during fertiloscopy.

When fertiloscopy is practiced under local anesthesia it has to stay purely diagnostic. So after the operation a decision has to be taken, either to perform an operative laparoscopy or to go directly to IVF which is the preferred option in case of mild or severe asymptomatic endometriosis.

Discussion

At that stage it seems important to try to establish a decision tree for infertile patients with asymptomatic endometriosis **(Figure 15-7).**

In case of endoscopic diagnostic (per fertiloscopy or laparoscopy) surgical treatment has to be done as the first line treatment. In case of recurrence, IVF has to be the preferred option and best results are achieved in the patients is prepared with LHRH agonists for a period of two of three months.

In case of endometrioma, laparoscopic treatment is also necessary if the diameter is bigger than 3 cm. In case of recurrence repeat surgery has to be avoided, because every surgical procedure on the ovary will impair the ovarian reserve. When IVF is practiced, it is better not to puncture the endometrioma even if contamination of follicular fluid by endometriotic liquid has no deleterious effect on the IVF results. In case of IVF practiced in patients with endometriotic lesions, risk of pelvic infection is a real concern which has to be addressed by the adjunction of antibiotics at the time of egg collection.

When diagnosis is purely clinical with no symptoms the best treatment is probably IVF since surgery is difficult and not without risks. In fact, when reviewing these patients after the diagnosis has been done, very often symptoms like dysmenorrhea are found and therefore surgery has to be discussed with very well informed patients after careful exploration and with a multidisciplinary surgical team.

There is no place for medical treatment because this treatment is very effective on pain (which is by definition not the case in asymptomatic patients) but not on fertility. Only preparation of IVF as described above is of real interest.

Lastly it is important to underline not only the interest to treat endometriosis in infertile patients but also to

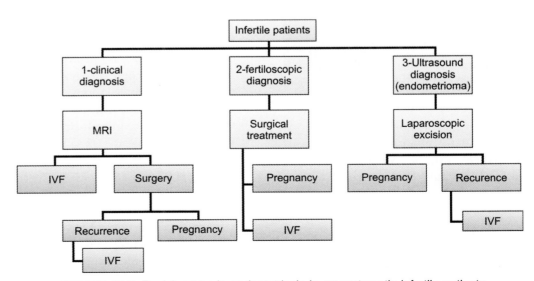

FIGURE 15-7: Decision tree in endometriosis in asymptomatic infertile patients.

preserve fertility in patients with endometriosis. So knowing that the natural evolution of endometriosis is generally to become more and more severe, asymptomatic endometriotic nulliparous patients should be treated taking in account their future wish to conceive.

The decision tree mentioned above has to be the same except indeed the use of IVF. It means that if an endoscopic treatment is performed then medical treatment like progesterone may be useful to try to prevent a recurrence until the patient decides to become pregnant. Also counseling is important to inform patient of the risks of recurrence and the interest, if possible, to become pregnant as soon as possible.

Conclusion

Asymptomatic endometriosis in infertile patient is a frequent situation. Circumstances of diagnostic are multiple even if the definitive diagnostic is endoscopic. The improvement of fertility after treatment is still controversial but recent publications tend to show an interest to treat these patients. It is quite evident when the disease is discovered during a fertiloscopy or a laparoscopy. Nevertheless in case of deep endometriosis in asymptomatic infertile patient the two options which are surgery and IVF has to be discussed with a well informed patient. And quite often it will be the association surgery first then IVF which will be able to allow these patients to conceive.

Bibliography

1. Allaire C. Endometriosis and infertility: A review. Reprod Med 2006;51(3):164-68.
2. Antoine JM. Mémoire académie de cirurgie. 2004;3(1): 14-16.
3. Gordts S, Campo R, Rombauts L, Brosens I. Transvaginal hydrolaparoscopy as an out patient procedure for infertility investigation. Hum Reprod 1998;13:99-103.
4. Gordts S, Watrelot A, Campo R, Brosens I. Risk and outcome of bowel injury during transvaginal pelvic endoscopy. Fertil Steril 2001;76:1238-41.
5. Gruppo Italiano per la Studio dell´Endometriosis Ablation of lesions or not in minimally-mild endometriosis in infertile women: A randomized trial. Hum Reprod 119; 14:1332-34.
6. Konninckx P, Meuleman C, Diemeyere S. Suggestive evidence that pelvic endometriosis is a progressive disease, whereas deeply infiltrating endometriosis is associated with pelvic pain. Fertil Steril 1991;55:759-65.
7. Mahmood TA, Templeton A. The impact of treatment on the natural history of endometriosis. Hum Reprod 1990; 5: 965-70.
8. Marcoux S, Maheux R, Berube S. Laparoscopic surgery in infertile woman with minimal or mild endometriosis. N Engl J Med 1997;24:337, 217-22.
9. Meuleman C, Vandenabeele B, Fleuwes S, Spiessens C, Timmerman D, D´Hooghe T. High prevalence of endometriosisin infertile women with normal ovulation and normospermic partners. Fertil Steril 2008, 4 Epub ahead of print.
10. Ozkan S, Murk W, Arici A. Endometriosis and infertility: epidemiology and evidence based treatments. Ann NY Acad Sci 2008;1127:92-100.
11. Pellicano M, Catena U, Di Zorio P, Simonelli V, Sorrentino F, Stella N, Bonifacio M, Crillo D, Nappi C. Diagnostic and operative fertiloscopy. Minerva Gynecol 2007;59:175-81.
12. Rodgers AK, Falcone T. Treatment strategies of endometriosis. Expert Opin Pharmacother 2008;9(2): 243-55.
13. Tanahatoe S, Lambalk C, McDonnell J, Dekker J, Mijatovic V, Hompes P. Diagnostic laparoscopy is needed after abnormal Hysterosalpingography to prevent over-treatment with IVF. Reprod Biomed Online 2008;16:410-15.
14. Wardle PG, Hull MG. Is endometriosis a disease ? Bailleres Clin Obstet Gynecol 1993;7:673-85.
15. Watrelot A, Dreyfus JM, Andine JP. Evaluation of the performance of Fertiloscopy in 160 consecutive infertile patients with no obvious pathology. Hum Reprod 1999;14: 707-11.
16. Watrelot A, Gordts S, Andine JP, Brosens I. Une nouvelle approche diagnostique: La Fertiloscopie. Endomag 1997; 21: 7-8.
17. Watrelot A, Nisolle M, Hocke C, et al. Is laparoscopy still the gold standard in infertility assessment? A comparison of Fertiloscopy versus laparoscopy in infertility. Hum Reprod 2003;18:834-39.
18. Watrelot A. Place of transvaginale fertiloscopy in the management of tubal factor disease. RBMonline 2007;15(4): 389-95.

Botros RMB Rizk, Christopher B Rizk, Mohamed Aboulghar

Chapter 16

Endometriosis and Infertility: Much Ado about Nothing?

Introduction

Does endometriosis cause infertility? Despite a long history of clinical experience and experimental research, the pathogenesis and management of endometriosis still have a lot of uncertainty.[1-3] Except in the case of obvious anatomical distortion by adhesions or tubal occlusion, the exact mechanism by which endometriosis causes subfertility has yet to be determined, but is likely to be a consequence of local inflammation and an altered immune response in the pelvis mediated by cytokines.[4] The fact that not all women with endometriosis experience

Table 16-1: Pelvic factors and infertility in patients with moderate-to-severe endometriosis*
• Adhesions with distortion of pelvic architecture interfering with the release of the oocytes and the tubal pick-up of these oocytes
• Fimbrial distortion or even occlusion can occur
• Hydrosalpinx can occur if the distal end of the tube is damaged
• Tubal narrowing and constriction
• Proximal tubal obstruction

*Reproduced with permission from: Botros Rizk and Hossam Abdalla (Eds): Endometriosis, 2nd Edition. Oxford, UK: Health Press 2003: p. 38.

infertility and up to 50% of women with infertility are diagnosed with endometriosis underscores the complexity of the mechanisms involved in the development of infertility in women with endometriosis.[5] Endometriosis can present in a variety of anatomical variations **(Figure 16-1)**.[6] Disruption of pelvic anatomy, distortion of the fallopian tubes and destruction of ovarian tissue by endometriomas could simply result in mechanical infertility **(Table 16-1)**.[7] However, there is controversy about whether minimal endometriosis causes infertility **(Table 16-2)**.[2,7]

The relationship between endometriosis and infertility is critically analyzed in this review. The clinical evidence for and against the association between endometriosis and infertility is presented. The mechanisms by which endometriosis could cause infertility will be discussed. Based on basic science research, the indirect evidence that may shed light on the pathophysiology of endometriosis-associated infertility will be reviewed . Data from assisted reproduction and oocyte donation programs may clarify the relative contribution of the follicular environment to the endometrial receptivity in patients with endometriosis.

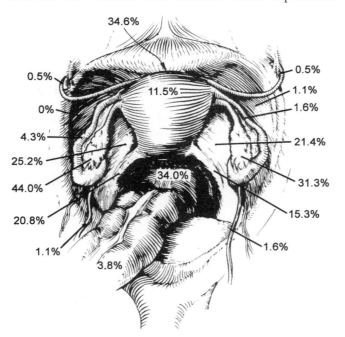

FIGURE 16-1: Distribution of endometriotic implants found at laparoscopy in 182 infertility patients. The numbers represent the proportion of all patients with implants at that site. Reproduced with permission from Jenkins S, Olive DL, Haney AF (1986).

Table 16-2: Possible mechanisms of infertility in patients with mild-to-moderate endometriosis*

Changes in peritoneal fluid
- Increase in volume
- Reduced sperm motility and binding
- Presence of interleukins and tumor necrosis factor
- Increased prostaglandin levels
- Increased number of macrophages

Eutopic endometrium abnormalities
Myometrial and peristalsis abnormalities
Follicular environment and embryo quality
- Increased progesterone and interleukin-6
- Decreased vascular endothelial growth factor

Ovulation disorders
- Anovulation
- Hyperprolactinemia
- Abnormal follicular genesis
- Premature follicular rupture
- Luteinized unruptured follicles
- Luteal phase defect

Pelvic pain
Immunological abnormalities
- T-lymphocytes
- Antigen-specific B-lymphocyte activation
- Non-specific B-lymphocyte activation
- Anti-endometrial antibodies

Spontaneous abortion
Implantation disorders

*Reproduced with permission from: Botros Rizk and Hossam Abdalla (Eds): Endometriosis, 2nd Edition. Oxford, UK: Health Press 2003: p. 34.

Is there an Association Between Endometriosis and Clinical Infertility?

Reproductive researchers differ in their opinion as to whether endometriosis can cause infertility.[7,8]

Yes, There is an Association

Garcia-Velasco and colleagues carefully studied the monthly fecundity rate (MFR) in women with endometriosis and expectant management.[2] A low MFR, 8 percent, has been described in these women.[9,10] In a study from Spain, women with minimal endometriosis had a minimal 6 percent MFR with a cumulative pregnancy rate of 47 percent at twelve month.[11] From the Canadian study, they evaluated the benefit of laparoscopic intervention in women with minimal and mild endometriosis (ENDOCAN) and even lower MFR of 2.5 percent was observed.[12,13] A close correlation can be observed between MFR and severity of the disease as the MFR was 8.7, 3.2 and 0 percent in women with mild, moderate and severe endometriosis, respectively. In the baboon model, the MFR drops from 24% in baboons with normal pelvis to 18% if minimal endometriosis developed and even lower if mild, moderate or severe forms of the disease were present.[14]

Laparoscopic surgeons have always observed that endometriosis is much less frequently documented in patients undergoing laparoscopic sterilization compared to patients with infertility **(Tables 16-3 to 16-7)**.[3] In couples undergoing treatment using artificial insemination by donor, the pregnancy rate was lower if the female partner had pelvic endometriosis **(Tables 16-8 to 16-9)**.[3] Whereas medical therapy does not impact the pregnancy outcome in women with endometriosis, conservative laparoscopic management improves the pregnancy rate.[15,16] Adamson and Pasta (1994) based on a meta analysis of the world literature concluded that surgical treatment by laparoscopy or laparotomy improves the pregnancy rate whereas medical therapy does not **(Figure 16-2)**.[17] Collins elegantly reviewed the literature and concluded from cohort studies

Table 16-3: Prevalence of endometriosis among previously fertile patients undergoing sterilization, 1970-1987

Reference	N	N (%) w/Endo	Min/Mild	Mod/Severe	Histological confirmation
Hasson, 1976	296	4(1.5)	—	—	No
Drake and Grunert, 1980	43	2(5)	—	—	No
Strathy, et al, 1982	200	4(2)	4	0	No
Liu and Hitchcock, 1986	74	32(43)	32	0	No
Moen, 1987	108	19(18)	15	4	No
Subtotal, 1976-1987	721	61(8)	51/54(93%)	4/55(7%)	

Table 16-4: Prevalence of endometriosis, 1988-2000					
Reference	N	N (%) w/Endo	Min/Mild	Mod/Severe	Histological Confirmation
Kirshon et al, 1989	566	42(7.5)	28	4	No
Wheeler 1989	3060	49(1.6)	—	—	No
Trimbos et al, 1990	200	5(2.5)	1	4	No
Moen and Muus, 1991	107	24(22)	23	1	Yes
Mahmood and Templeton, 1991	598	37(6)	30	7	No
Rawson, 1991	8	4(50)	—	—	No
Sangi-Haghpeykar and Poindexter, 1995	3384	126(3.7)	121	5	No
Balasch et al, 1996	30	13(43)	13	—	No
Subtotal 1988-2000	7953	300(4)	216/239 (91%)	21/239 (9%)	
Total	8674	361 (4)	267/292 (91%)	25/292 (9%)	

Table 16-5: Prevalence of endometriosis among infertile patients, 1970-1987		
Reference	Total N	N (%) with endometriosis
Peterson and Behrman, 1970	204	70 (33)
Duignan et al, 1972	675	52 (8)
Liston et al, 1972	312	25 (8)
Pent, 1972	22	1 (5)
Goldenberg and Magendatz, 1976	112	29 (26)
Hasson, 1976	66	15 (23)
Cohen, 1976	1380	320 (23)
Musich and Behrman, 1982	182	63 (35)
Strathy et al, 1982	100	19 (19)
Nordenskjold and Ahlgren, 1983	433	69 (16)
Chang et al, 1987	2053	44 (2)
Subtotal, 1970-1987	5539	707 (13)

Table 16-6: Prevalence of endometriosis among infertile patients, 1988-2000		
Reference	Total N	N (%) with endometriosis
Mahmood and Templeton, 1989	490	101
Koninckx et al, 1991	416	283 (68)
Mahmood and Templeton, 1991	654	133 (21)
Gruppo Italiano, 1996	660	195 (30)
Balasch et al, 1996	52	26 (50)
Corson et al, 2000	100	43 (43)
Subtotal	2372	781 (33)
Total	7911	1068(13.5)

as well as the Canadian endometriosis study (ENDOCAN)[12] that surgical therapy improves the odds of pregnancy in women suffering with endometriosis.[18]

No, There is no Association

Evers and Dunselman , in a thought provoking discussion during the World Congress of Endometriosis, argued that endometriosis is not a disease but an epiphenomenon .[19] Their first argument is that endometriosis is not more frequent in subfertile women. Their second argument is that endometriosis patients do not have a lower fecundity rate and finally, that treatment does not improve pregnancy rate. They carefully analyzed the study demonstrating that

Table 16-7: Prevalence of endometriosis according to stage of disease in infertile and fertile women

Fertility Status	Number	Endometriosis	Minimal-Mild	Mod-Severe
Previously fertile	7953	300 (4%)	216 (91%)	21 (9)
Infertile	2372	781 (33%)	463 (58%)	215 (32%)
P value	P < 0.0001		P < 0.0001	

Table 16-8: Cycle fecundity rate and implantation rate per cycle after intrauterine insemination in women with minimal-mild endometriosis and women with unexplained infertility

Rate	Reference	Minimal-Mild Endometriosis	Unexplained Infertility	P Value
Cycle fecundity rate	Omland et al, 1998	8/49 (16%)	40/119 (34%)	<0.05
	Nuojua-Huttunen et al, 1999	9/138 (6%)	63/413 (15%)	0.05
Implantation rate	Omland et al, 1998	9/49 (18%)	52/119 (44%)	<0.05

Table 16-9: Cycle fecundity rate and cumulative pregnancy rate after donor insemination in women with minimal-mild endometriosis and women with a normal pelvis

Rate	Reference	Minimal-Mild endometriosis	Unexplained Infertility	P Value
Cycle fecundity rate	Hammond et al, 1986 Toma et al, 1992	9/218 (4%) 5/86	38/196 (20%) 29/212 14% (95%CI, 8-20%)	< 0.05
	Jansen et al, 1986	2/56 (4%)	12% (46/380)	< 0.05
Cumulative Pregnancy rate after 6 cycles	Hammond et al, 1986 Toma et al, 1992	20% 38%	55% 80%	

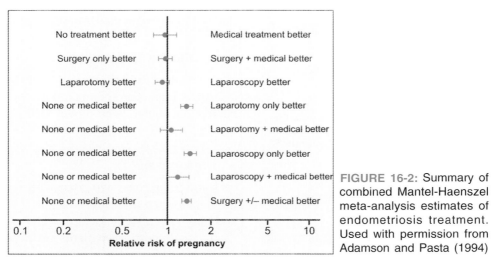

FIGURE 16-2: Summary of combined Mantel-Haenszel meta-analysis estimates of endometriosis treatment. Used with permission from Adamson and Pasta (1994)

6-12% of random biopsies from normal appearing peritoneum in patients without endometriosis show endometriosis histologically. They hypothesized that if several biopsies per patient on all patients were done, then the incidence would increase to almost 100%. On the second issue, they suggested that theoretically, the best way to determine the pregnancy rate in endometriosis without treatment is to compare the pregnancy rate in patients with untreated mild endometriosis with that in fertile normal women. As this is not possible, Evers and Dunselman compared the pregnancy rate in 2026 patients with unexplained infertility to patients with endometriosis in the control group of the randomized controlled studies on endometriosis treatment. They found the pregnancy rates to be very similar (33% versus 28%). The rate in published studies of women with endometriosis undergoing artificial insemination by donor is comparable to that of women without laparoscopic evidence of endometriosis (64% versus 51%). They also argued that the five randomized studies on medical therapy for endometriosis have shown no impact on the pregnancy rate. They admitted that Canadian Endometriosis Study, showed an improvement in pregnancy rate after the surgical treatment of mild and minimal endometriosis; however, the treatment effect was moderate **(Figure 16-3)**.[12] Grunert and Franklin critically appraised the literature and could not establish an undisputed relationship between endometriosis and infertility.[20]

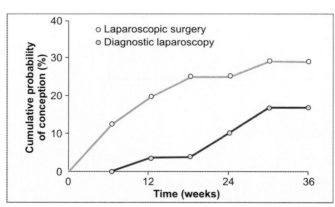

FIGURE 16-3: Cumulative probability of a pregnancy carried beyond 20 weeks in the 36 weeks after laparoscopy in women with endometriosis. Used with permission from Marcoux S, Maheux R, Berube S (1997)

Pathophysiology of Infertility in Patients with Endometriosis

Rizk and Abdalla investigated the pathophysiology of infertility in patients with endometriosis **(Table 16-2)**.[17]

Peritoneal Fluid Abnormalities

Cellular Components of Peritoneal Fluid; Macrophages and Lymphocytes

Badawy and colleagues elegantly investigated the cellular components in peritoneal fluid in 102 infertile women with and without endometriosis.[21] They used Wright's-Giemsa and Papanicolau stains and also evaluated the secretory activity of these cells indirectly by assaying acid phosphatase, prostaglandin $F_{2\alpha}$ and PGE_2 and complement components C_{3c} and C_4. Badawy's results showed that macrophages and lymphocytes were the dominant cells in the peritoneal fluid of patients with endometriosis. These cells were significantly increased in patients with endometriosis compared to control subjects without endometriosis. The peritoneal fluid acid phosphatase, prostaglandin $F_{2\alpha}$ and PGE_2 and complement components C_{3c} and C_4 were significantly increased with endometriosis. These cellular changes and their activation in peritoneal fluid may explain infertility associated with endometriosis.[21]

Embryo Growth

Research from our department has demonstrated that peritoneal fluid from women with endometriosis inhibit two cell mouse embryo growth.[8,22] Prough and colleagues studied the effect of five molecular weight fractions used as media supplement from the peritoneal fluid of patients with endometriosis compared with normal controls. They observed that all fractions observed from patients with endometriosis inhibited mouse embryo growth to a greater extent than normal controls. Interestingly, the MW fractions of more than 100,000 Daltons showed greater inhibition of embryo development than did fractions of less than 100,000 Daltons. The authors suggested the presence of a humoral factor larger than 100,000 Daltons that is inhibitory on mouse embryo growth.[22]

Sperm Motility and Binding

The peritoneal fluid from women with endometriosis has a negative impact on sperm motility. Sperm binding to the zona pellucida has been shown to be reduced *in vitro*.

Vascular Endothelial Growth Factor (VEGF) and Interleukins

Rizk and colleagues have extensively reviewed the role of interleukins in human reproduction.[23] VEGF, interleukins and tumor necrosis factor alpha (TNF-α) in the peritoneal fluid of endometriosis patients are involved in inhibiting sperm motility and function, oocyte fertilization, and embryo growth. Granulosa cells from women with endometriosis express lower levels of VEGF and unchanged levels of IL-6 compared with the cells from unaffected women.[23,24] Vascular endothelial growth factor is important in the development of the oocyte due to increased angiogenesis suggesting that patients with severe endometriosis experience compromised oocyte maturity.[25] This may offer an explanation to the decrease in ovarian reserve in patients with moderate to severe endometriosis.[26]

Prostaglandin Levels

Increased prostaglandin levels in the peritoneal fluid of patients with endometriosis are another possible explanation of infertility.[21]

Prostaglandins alter tubal motility and collection of oocytes, and can lead to luteinized unruptured follicle syndrome and defects in the corpus luteum.

Increase in Fluid Volume

Patients with endometriosis have more free fluid in the pelvis on ultrasound and at laparoscopy.[7,8] While several studies have confirmed an increase in the volume of peritoneal fluid in women with pelvic endometriosis, the correlation between fluid volumes and fertility outcome has not been similarly consistent.[21]

Eutopic Endometrium Abnormalities

The biochemical abnormalities in the eutopic endometrium of women with endometriosis include altered local immune cell population, aberrant expression of proinflammatory chemotactic cytokines, impaired expression of differentiation markers and altered local steroid biosynthesis and metabolism.[7, 8] Aromatase p450 mRNA expression in the endometrium of patients with endometriosis has been extensively investigated in the hope of finding a non-invasive method for diagnosing endometriosis. However, a recent study from Belgium suggested that aromatase p450 mRNA is not a specific marker.[27] Using a global gene expression approach through microarray analysis, Kao et al detected more than 100 aberrantly regulated genes in eutopic endometrium of women with versus without endometriosis during the window of implantation.[28] These aberrant regulated genes may contribute to implantation failure in women with this disorder on the level of embryonic attachment, survival and embryo-decidua signaling.[28] These changes affect cell adhesion molecules, endometrial epithelial secreted proteins, transporters, and immune modulators.[5]

Myometrial Architecture and Peristalsis Abnormalities

The presence of adenomyosis could cause uterine hyperperistalsis and dysperistalsis which may negatively impact the rapid sperm transport and implantation in patients suffering with endometriosis-associated infertility. Garcia-Velasco et al (2009) elegantly demonstrated the utilization of transvaginal ultrasonography and 3D imaging in the visualization of the uterine musculature and the dysfunctional motions of the uterus.[29,30]

Follicular Environment and Embryo Quality

Rizk (2002) reviewed the outcome of ART in patients with pelvic endometriosis.[31] Analyses of IVF and oocyte donation programs have been extremely useful to understand the role of the oocytes and microfollicular environment versus the endometrium in endometriosis associated infertility.[8] Decreased levels of granulosa cell steroidogenesis was demonstrated[32] thereby contributing to decreased oocyte maturation and therefore decreased ovarian reserve.[5,32]

Ovulation Disorders

Rizk and Abdalla reviewed the ovulatory disorders that could possibly be encountered in infertile patients with endometriosis **(Table 16-2)**.[7]

Anovulation

Anovulation may occur in 15-25% of patients with endometriosis. Combining medical treatment of the disease with induction of ovulation appears to increase the pregnancy rate.[33]

Hyperprolactinemia

Hyperprolactinemia has been observed in several studies of patients with different stages of endometriosis. It may simply be that the two conditions coexist and there is insufficient evidence to demonstrate a causal relationship.

Abnormal Follicular Dynamics

Abnormal follicular dynamics in the form of mainly abnormal rates of follicular development and premature follicular rupture are more frequently in patients with endometriosis. The effect of delayed follicular growth leading to asynchrony of oocyte maturation and ovulation was also observed.[34]

Luteinized Unruptured Follicle Syndrome

Luteinized unruptured follicle syndrome has been described in monkeys with surgically induced periovarian endometriotic adhesions. Ultrasound studies have failed to show a consistent increase in incidence of this syndrome in patients with endometriosis.[8]

Luteal Phase Defect

Luteal phase defect (LPD), detected by out-of-phase endometrial development or asynchronous development of endometrial glands and stroma, could be the consequence of abnormal follicular development, inadequate production of progesterone or lack of response of the endometrium to progesterone.[8] Hormonal abnormalities in patients with endometriosis, with a major emphasis on progesterone levels are well documented.

Immunological Abnormalities

Several components of peritoneal fluid (PF), such as growth factors, hormones, and cytokines, are known to be present at different levels in women with endometriosis compared to women without disease.[5] These alterations in the peritoneal environment may affect sperm motility, oocytes maturation, fertilization, embryo survival and tubal function (refer to chapter on immunology of endometriosis by Demowski). Hill (1997) argued whether immunologic abnormalities in patients with endometriosis is a fact, artifact or epiphenomenon.[35]

Cell Mediated Immunological Factors

Changes in T-lymphocyte function have long been suspected as being involved in endometriosis as endometriosis involves transplantation of autologous endometrium, and T-lymphocytes are concerned with the rejection of homographs. Increased numbers of T-cells and B-cells and higher CD4:CD8 ratios in blood and peritoneal fluid have also been reported.

Oosterlynck and colleagues investigated the role of natural killer cells in the decreased cellular immunity of women with endometriosis.[36] They studied prospectively 34 women before laser laparoscopy for infertility or pain at the University of Leuven in Belgium. The NK activity and cytotoxicity against autologous endometrial cells were decreased in women with endometriosis and correlated with the severity of the disease. The Belgian researchers suggested that the decreased cytotoxicity to endometrial cells in women with endometriosis is mainly because of a defect in NK activity and partially because of a resistance of the endometrium.[36]

Humoral Immunological Factors

An autoimmune syndrome characterized by polyclonal B-lymphocyte activation has been suggested as a cause for infertility, though the exact mechanism is unclear.

Antibodies directed towards endometrial cell antigens have been reported in the serum of women with endometriosis, but the reason for their existence is controversial. Anti-endometrial antibodies have also been detected in women with a wide range of pelvic pathologies.

Spontaneous Abortion

Many clinicians have observed that women suffering from endometriosis, spontaneous abortion is more common. Furthermore, treatment of the endometriosis decreases the occurrence of spontaneous abortion.

Implantation

Successful implantation requires a functionally normal embryo at the blastocyst stage and a receptive endometrium. Various genes such as integrins (e.g. $\alpha V\beta3$), matrix metalloproteinases (e.g. MMP-7 and -11), transcription factors (e.g. hepatocyte nuclear factor), endometrial bleeding factor (ebaf), enzymes involved in steroid hormone metabolism (e.g. aromatase, 17β-hydroxysteroid dehydrogenase), leukemia inhibitory factor (LIF), Hox genes, and progesterone receptor isoforms are aberrantly expressed during the window of implantation and at other times of the cycle in women with versus those without endometriosis.[1,37] Integrins are cell adhesion molecules. A deficiency of integrin $\alpha_3\beta_v$, a component of the embryo implantation cascade in the uterus, may reduce the likelihood of embryo implantation in women with early-stage endometriosis.[38] This can apparently be corrected when the disease is treated. Implantation of embryos in patients with endometriosis undergoing ART has been extensively investigated.[31]

Pelvic Pain

Pain can lead to a reduction in the frequency of intercourse and, therefore, reduce the likelihood of pregnancy.

Assisted Reproductive Technology in Patients with Endometriosis

Garcia-Velasco (2008) elegantly reviewed their experience in assisted reproductive technology in patients with endometriosis.[2] Rizk (2002) observed that over the last twenty years, there have been changes in the trends of thought about whether endometriosis influences the success of IVF.[31,39-43] In the early eighties, endometriosis was thought to significantly decrease the pregnancy rate in IVF patients. Tan et al (1989) and Rizk, et al (1989) based on our data from Bourn Hall and Hallam Medical Center found similar pregnancy rates in patients with endometriosis compared to patients with tubal factor infertility.[39-43] The outcome of IVF was similar in cases of endometriosis when compared with other causes of infertility as shown in the 2006 SART data **(Figure 16-4)**.[44] Barnhart and colleagues' meta-analysis,[45] on the outcome of ART in patients with endometriosis suggest a possible role of endometriosis in lower success rates after IVF **(Figure 16-5)**.[45]

Toya and colleagues[46] performed a study at the Yamagata University school of medicine in Japan on 30 women undergoing IVF in order to determine whether folliculogenesis is impaired in women with endometriosis. The patients were divided into 4 groups according to their cause of infertility: tubal factor (n=7), male factor (n=7), idiopathic (n=7), endometriosis (n=9). The rate of apoptosis in the granulosa cells in patients with endometriosis was the highest out of the 4 groups. The authors concluded that endometriosis would impair the cell cycle in granulosa cells. This phenomenon may have a detrimental effect on folliculogenesis.

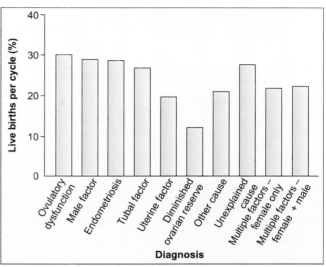

FIGURE 16-4: Live birth rates in women with endometriosis compared with other diagnoses after ART cycles with fresh non-donor eggs or embryos. (SART, 2006)

Simon and colleagues performed a series of interesting studies in an attempt to gain clinical knowledge of the factors involved in the pathogenesis of endometriosis associated infertility.[47] These studies were designed to determine whether the problem lies in the quality of the embryos or the endometrium. In the first study, the authors compared the IVF outcome from 96 cycles in 78 patients

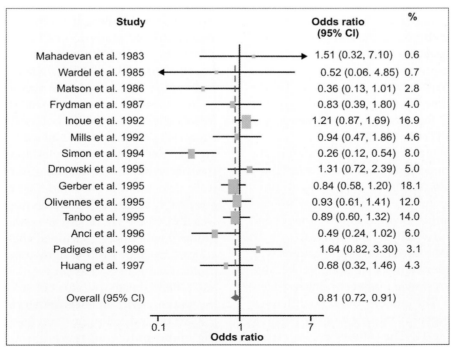

FIGURE 16-5: Unadjusted meta-analysis of the odds of pregnancy in endometriosis patients vs. tubal factor patients as controls. Used with permission from Barnhart, et al (2002)

Table 16-10: Outcome of IVF in endometriosis and tubal factor in infertility				
Diagnosis	*Tubal factor*	*Endometriosis*		
		Total	*I and II*	*III and IV*
No. of cycles	96	96	14	82
No. of patients	78	59	9	50
Age (years)	32.2 ± 0.4*	31.9± 0.3	32.1±0.9	31.9± 0.3
#oocytes fertilized (%)	12.1± 0.7	9.6 ± 0.7	9.6±1.0	9.6± 0.7
Type 1 (%)	61.8	55.7	55.4	57.1
# oocytes fertilized (%)	57.7 ± 2.9	43.5 ± 3.4	55.6±8.9	54.1±3.7
# transfer cycles	91	79	12	67
# embryos transferred/cycle	3.6 ± 0.1	3.5 ±0.2	3.6 ± 0.4	3.4 ± 0.2
# type I transferred	3.0 ± 0.3[a]	2.2 ± 0.2	2.3 ± 0.6	2.2 ± 0.3
# pregnancies/cycle (%)	34/96 (34.4)[b]	12/96 (12.5)	2/14(14.2)	10/82(12.1)
# pregnancies/transfer (%)	34/91 (37.3)[c]	12/79 (15.1)	2/12(16.6)	10/67(14.9)
Implantation rate (%)	44/329 (13.4)[d]	16/275 (5.8)	3/43(6.9)	13/232(5.6)

Simon et al, Hum Reprod 1994;9(4):725-729
* Values are mean ± SEM [a]$p < 0.001$, [b]$p < 0.0004$, [c]$p<0.002$, [d]$p <0.003$

with tubal infertility and from 96 cycles in 59 women with endometriosis **(Table 16-10)**. The endometriosis patients had poor outcome in terms of pregnancy rate/cycle ($p<0.004$) and in reduced pregnancy rate/transfer ($p<0.002$) and a reduced implantation rate ($p<0.003$). The dialogue between the embryo and the endometrium was clearly altered in these patients but the factor responsible for this impairment was initially unknown. At this point the authors felt that the endometrial environment could be blamed since the two clinical parameters regarding oocyte quality (grading and fertilization) were normal in endometriosis patients **(Table 16-10)**.

In an attempt to resolve this dilemma, they studied the results of oocyte donation according to the recipients' cause of infertility. The oocyte recipients were divided into 3 groups. The first group (n=54) were women who were diagnosed with premature ovarian failure; the second group were women who were low responders to ovarian stimulation (n=77) and the third group were women with endometriosis who underwent oocyte donation because of low response (n=11). A similar number of embryos were replaced in each group. The authors found no difference among groups in the pregnancy rate per woman, per cycle or implantation **(Table 16-11)**. The authors' final approach to the analysis of endometriosis was to investigate the implantation potential of embryos derived from women with different types of infertility including endometriosis

(Table 16-12). A trend towards reduced pregnancy rates in women receiving oocytes from endometriotic ovaries and significantly lower implantation rates were observed ($p<0.05$) **(Table 16-12)**.

Diaz and colleagues (2000) performed a matched case-controlled study to evaluate the impact of severe endometriosis on IVF outcome in women receiving oocytes from the same donor.[48] Fifty-eight recipients were included in the study, 25 patients were diagnosed with stage III-IV endometriosis by laparoscopy while the remaining 33 were free of the disease. On the day of oocyte retrieval, the oocytes from a single donor were donated to recipients from both groups. The number of oocytes donated and fertilized as well as the number of available and transferred embryos were similar. Pregnancy and miscarriage rates were not affected by stage III-IV endometriosis. The live birth rate was 28% in the endometriosis and 27.2% in the control group. The authors concluded that implantation is not affected by stage III-IV endometriosis and that given the contemporary methods of preparation of the endometrium, any potential negative effect of severe endometriosis on the uterine environment is undetectable.[48]

Garrido and colleagues[49] reviewed the contribution of the embryonic quality versus the endometrium in endometriosis associated infertility. Having analyzed in detail the investigations over the last decade, the authors found several studies that suggest an altered follicular

Table 16-11: Outcome of oocyte donation according to the recipient's cause of infertility

Diagnosis	Premature ovarian failure	Low response	Endometriosis
# patients	54	77	10
Age (years)	34.7±0.7[b]	37.2±0.5[a]	30.0±0.8[b]
# transfer cycles	71	96	11
# oocytes donated/cycle	7.8±0.3	7.7±0.3	7.6±0.6
# embryos transferred/cycle	3.8±0.2	4.1±0.2	3.6±0.4
# pregnancies	35	51	8
# sacs	51	68	10
PR/transfer (%)	49.3	53.2	72.7
PR/patient (%)	64.8	66.2	80.0
Implantation rate (%)	19.2	17.0	25.0

[a] vs [b] p<0.05
Simon et al, Hum Reprod, 1994;9(4):725-729

Table 16-12: Outcome of oocyte donation according to the donor's cause of infertility

Oocyte donor Characteristics	No. of cycles	Pregnancy rate/transfer	Implantation rate
Fertile	34	15 (44.0)	23/142 (16.2)
Polycystic ovaries	58	35 (6-.3)	55/233 (23.6)
Idiopathic infertility	20	9 (45.0)	9/80 (11.2)
Tubal infertility	27	15 (55.5)	18/96 (18.7)
Male infertility	28	17 (60.7)	21/110 (19.1)
Endometriosis	11	3 (27.3)	3/43 (7.0)[a]

[a] p<0.05
Simon et al, Hum Reprod, 1994;9(4):725-729

microenvironment or an intrinsic ovarian problem. These could be responsible for defective oogenesis and possibly lower quality of oocytes and embryos that have diminished ability to implant. Many molecules that are related to different physiological processes of oocyte maturation and development have been investigated. These include steroidogenesis, angiogenesis and apoptosis. The authors concluded that mixed causes, defects in both the embryo and the endometrium could not be ruled out however, in the ovum donation program, good embryos could possibly bypass an affected endometrium. Rizk et al (2009)[50] suggested that proteomics of the eutopic endometrium could be the future diagnostic modality for endometriosis.

Conclusion

While there is significant controversy as to whether endometriosis causes infertility, the accumulated evidence favors causation. There is also a substantial body of data that explains how endometriosis alters the hormonal, immunologic, and physiology of the reproductive system. These data lead to plausible hypotheses concerning mechanisms of action of decreasing fecundity by endometriosis. However, it is the data from ART and oocyte donation programs that convinced us of the negative impact of endometriosis on human reproduction. Further clinical and basic science research using genomic and proteomic data will elucidate the fundamental mechanisms by which this puzzling disease results in infertility.

References

1. Atabekoglu CS, Arici A. Endometriosis associated infertility. In Rizk B, Garcia-Velasco J A , Sallam H N, Makrigiannakis A (Editors). Infertility and Assisted Reproduction . Cambridge and New York : Cambridge University Press, 2008; Chapter 32:302-08.

2. Garcia-Velasco JA , Guillen A, Quea G , Requena A Endometriosis and assisted reproductive technology In Rizk B, Garcia-Velasco J A , Sallam H N, Makrigiannakis A (Editors). Infertility and Assisted Reproduction . Cambridge and New York : Cambridge University Press, 2008; Chapter 42:381-85.

3. D'Hooghe TM, Debrock S, Hill JA, etal. Endometriosis and subfertility: Is the relationship resolved? Semin Reprod Med 2003;21(2):243-53.

4. Kim AH, Adamson D. Reproductive surgery for endometriosis-associated infertility. In: Rizk B, Garcia-Velasco JA, Sallam HN, Makrigiannakis A (Editors). Infertility and Assisted Reproduction. Cambridge and New York: Cambridge University Press, 2008; Chapter 34:318-26.

5. Germeyer A, Giudice LC. How does endometriosis cause infertility? In: Tulandi T, Redwine D (Eds). Endometriosis: Advanced and Controversies. New York, NY: Marcel Dekker, 2004; Chapter 9:151-66.

6. Jenkins S, Olive DL, Haney AF. Endometriosis. Pathogenetic implications of the anatomic distribution. Obstet Gynecol 1986;67:335.

7. Rizk B, Abdalla H. Endometriosis and infertility. In: Rizk B and Abdalla H (Editors). Endometriosis, 2nd Ed. Oxford, U K: Health Press; 2003;32-41.

8. Rizk B, Nawar MG, Angell NF. Does endometriosis cause infertility? In: Allahabadia G and Merchant R (eds) Gyneco-logical Endoscopy and Infertility. New Delhi, Jaypee Brothers Medical Publishers, 2005; Chapter 4:28-38.

9. Olive D, Stohs F, Metzger D, Franklin R. Expectant management and hydrotubations in the treatment of endo-metriosis-associated infertility. Fertil Steril 1985;44: 35-42.

10. Portuondo JA, Echanojauregui A, Herran C, et al. Early conception in patients with untreated mild endometriosis. Fertil Steril 1983; 39: 22-25.

11. Rodriguez-Escudero F, Negro J, Corcostegui B, etal. Does minimal endometriosis reduce fecundity? Fertil Steril 1988; 50: 522-24.

12. Marcoux S, Maheux R, Berube S. Laparoscopic surgery in infertile women with minimal or mild endometriosis. Canadian Collaborative Group on Endometriosis. N Eng J Med 1997;337:217-22.

13. Berube S, Marcoux S, Langevin M, etal. Fecundity of infertile women with minimal or mild endometriosis and women with unexplained infertility. Fertil Steril 1998; 69: 1034.

14. D'Hooghe T, Bambra C, Koninckx P. Cycle fecundity in baboons of proven fertility with minimal endometriosis. Genecol Obstet Invest 1994; 37:63-65.

15. Rizk B, Abdalla H. Medical treatment of endometriosis. In: Rizk B, Abdalla H (Editors). Endometriosis, 2nd Ed. Oxford, U K: Health Press; 2003;55-70.

16. Rizk B, Abdalla H. Surgical treatment of endometriosis and infertility. In: Rizk B, Abdalla H, editors. Endomet-riosis, 2nd Ed. Oxford, U K: Health Press; 2003;71-80.

17. Adamson GD, Pasta DJ. Surgical treatment of endometriosis-associated infertility: meta-analysis compared with survival analysis. Am J Obstet Gynecol 1994;171:1488-505.

18. Collins J. Endometriosis management: past, present and future. In: Lemay A, Maheux R, editors. Understanding and managing endometriosis: advances in research and practice. New York: Parthenon; 1999;153-58.

19. Evers JL, Dunselman GAJ. Endometriosis is not a disease but an epiphenomenon. In: Lemay A, Maheux R (Editors). Understanding and managing endometriosis: advances in research and practice. New York: Parthenon; 1999;31-40.

20. Grunert GM, Franklin RR. Pathogenesis of infertility in endometriosis. In: Nezhat CR, Berger GS, Nezhat FR, Buttram, VC, Nezhat CH (Editors). Endometriosis: advanced management and surgical techniques. New York: Springer, 1995;45–59.

21. Badawy SZ, Cuenca V, Marshall L, Munchback R, Rinas AC, Coble DA. Cellular components in peritoneal fluid in infertile patients with and without endometriosis. Fertil Steril 1984;42:704–08.

22. Prough SG, Aksel S, Gilmore SM, Yeoman R. Peritoneal fluid fractions from patients with endometriosis do not promote two-cell mouse embryo growth. Fertil Steril 1990; 54:927-30.

23. Rizk B, Aboulghar M, Smitz J, Ron-El R. The role of vascular endothelial growth factor and interleukins in the pathogenesis of severe ovarian hyperstimulation syndrome. Hum Reprod Update 1997;3:255–66.

24. Yamashita Y, Ueda M, Takehera M, et al. Influence of severe endometriosis on gene expression of vascular endothelial growth factor and interleukin-6 in granulosa cells from patients undergoing controlled ovarian hyperstimulation for in vitro fertilization-embryo transfer. Fertil Steril 2002;78(4):865.

25. Geva E, Jaffe RB. Role of vascular endothelial growth factor in ovarian physiology and pathology. Fertil Steril 2000; 74(3):429-38.

26. Hock DL, Sharafi K, Dagostino L, etal. Contribution of diminished ovarian reserve to hypofertility associated with endometriosis. J Reprod Med 2001; 46(1):426-29.

27. Dheenadayalu K, Mak I, Gordts S. Aromatase P450 messenger RNA expression in eutopic endometrium is not a specific marker for pelvic endometriosis. Fertil Steril 2002;78:825–35.

28. Kao LC, Germeyer A, Tulac S, etal. Expression profiling of endometrium from women with endometriosis reveals candidate genes for kisease-based implantation failure and infertility. Endocrinology 2003; 177(7):2870-81.

29. Garcia-Velasco J, Cerillo M, Ornat L. Ultrasonography of pelvic endometriosis. In: Rizk B (ed). Ultrasonography in Reproductive Medicine and Infertility. Cambridge University Press 2009: Chapter 17.

30. Garcia-Velasco J, Puente JM. Ultrasound 3D imaging and infertility. In: Rizk B (Eds). Ultrasonography in Reproduc-tive Medicine and Infertility. Cambridge University Press 2009: Chapter 9.

31. Rizk B. Endometriosis and in vitro fertilization. A clinical step-by-step course for assisted reproductive technologies.

American Society for Reproductive Medicine. 35th Annual Postgraduate Program, 57th Annual Meeting, 2002; 15-23.

32. Harlow CR, Cahill DJ, Maile LA, et al. Refuced preovulatory granulosa cell steroidogenensis in women with endometriosis. J Clin Endocrinol Metab 1996;81:426-29.

33. Haney AF. Endometriosis. In: Lobo RA, Mishell DR, Paulson RJ, Shoupe, D (Editors). Mishell's textbook of infertility, contraception and reproductive endocrinology, 4th ed. Oxford, U K: Blackwell Scientific; 1997; 653–55.

34. Doody MC, Gibbons WE, Buttram VCJ. Linear regression analysis of ultrasound follicular growth series: Evidence for an abnormality of follicular growth in endometriosis patients. Fertil Steril 1988; 49(1):47-51.

35. Hill JA. Immunology and endometriosis: fact, artifact, or epiphenomenon? Endometriosis. Obstet Gynecol Clin N Am 1997;24:291–306.

36. Oosterlynck DJ, Cornillie FJ, Waer M, Vandeputte M, Koninckx PR. Women with endometriosis show a defect in natural killer activity resulting in a decreased cytotoxicity to autologous endometrium. Fertil Steril 1991;56:45-51.

37. Giudice LC, Telles TL, Lobo S, Kao L. The molecular basis for implantation failure in endometriosis: on the road to discovery. Ann NY Acad Sci 2002;955:252-64.

38. Lessey BA, Castelbaum AJ, Sawin SW, Buck CA, Schinnar R, Bilker W, et al. Aberrant integrin expression in the endometrium of women with endometriosis. J Clin Endocrinol Metab 1994;79:643-49.

39. Rizk B, Abdalla H. Assisted reproductive technology and endometriosis. In: Rizk B, Abdalla H (Editors). Endometriosis, 2nd Ed. Oxford, UK: Health Press; 2003;92-102.

40. Buckett WM, Too LL, Tan SL. Treatment of endometriosis associated with infertility – IVF is the best treatment. In: Lemay A, Maheux R (Editors). Understanding and managing endometriosis: advances in research and practice. New York: Parthenon; 1999;165–77.

41. Rizk B, Aksel S, Helvacioglu A. Gamete intrafallopian transfer in patients with pelvic endometriosis. Gynecol Obstet Reprod Med 1995;1:124-26.

42. Tan SL, Mason BA, Rizk B, et al. The relation between age and etiology and success in in-vitro fertilisation. 7th World Congress on Human Reproduction, Helsinki, Finland, 1989.

43. Rizk B, Tan SL, Edwards RG. Cumulative pregnancy rates in IVF. British Fertility Society Annual Meeting, The London Hospital, London, December 1989.

44. Society of Assisted Reproductive Technology and U.S. Department of Health and Human Services, Centers for Disease Control and Prevention. Assisted reproductive technology success rates – national summary and fertility clinic reports, 2006.

45. Barnhart K, Dunsmoor-Su R, Coutifaris C. Effect of endometriosis on in vitro fertilization. Fertil Steril 2002;77:1148–55.

46. Toya M, Saito H, Ohta N, et al. Moderate and severe endometriosis is associated with alterations in the cell cycle of granulosa cells in patients undergoing in vitro fertilization and embryo transfer. Fertil Steril 2000;73(2): 344-50.

47. Simon C, Gutierrez A, Vidal A, de los Santos MJ, Tarin JJ, Remohf J, et al. Outcome of patients with endometriosis in assisted reproduction: results from in-vitro fertilization and oocyte donation. Hum Reprod 1994;9:725–29.

48. Diaz I, Navarro J, Blasco L, et al. Impact of stage III-Iv endometriosis on recipients of sibling oocytes: matched case-control study. Fertil Steril 2000;74(1):31-34.

49. Garrido N, Navarro J, Remohi J, Pellicer A, Simon C. The endometrium versus embryonic quality in endometriosis-related infertility. Hum Reprod Update 2002;8(1):95-103.

50. Rizk B, Rocconi R, Finan M, Pannell L. Proteomics of the eutopic endometrium as a novel non-invasive tool for diagnosis and characterization of endometriosis. 2009, In Press.

Attila Bokor, Thomas M D'Hooghe

Chapter 17

Endometriosis and Miscarriage: Is there any Association?

There is no unequivocal evidence for an association between endometriosis and spontaneous/recurrent pregnancy loss.[1,2] In this chapter, we would like to assess the possible link between endometriosis and spontaneous/recurrent miscarriage or implantation failure and to focus on potential immunological explanations for such an association.

Definitions

Abortion

Clinical Abortion

The diagnosis of clinical spontaneous abortion or miscarriage can be made in the presence of a non-evolutionary gestational sac on ultrasonography with a positive pregnancy test or the presence of chorionic tissue in uterine curettings at a gestational age of less than 20 weeks. Spontaneous abortion occurs in about 15-25% of all clinically recognized pregnancies.[1]

Preclinical Abortion (Biochemical Pregnancy)

A preclinical abortion or biochemical pregnancy is diagnosed only by the detection of HCG in serum or urine and is a sign of embryo implantation/trophoblastic activity that does not develop into a clinical pregnancy. defined by two criteria.

Recurrent Abortion

Recurrent miscarriage is usually defined as the occurrence of two or more clinically recognized pregnancy losses before 20 weeks of gestation. It occurs in nearly 1% of all women. Most of the miscarriages are caused by chromosomal abnormalities (trisomies, especially trisomy 16, monosomy X, and triploidy).[1] Besides genetic factors, anatomical abnormalities (e.g. certain Müllerian malfor-

mations), endocrine problems (e.g. luteal phase deficiency), infections and thrombophilias (e.g. antiphospholipid syndrome) have been linked to recurrent miscarriage.[2]

Implantation Rate per Embryo

The implantation rate per embryo can be defined as the number of gestational sacs observed on ultrasound, divided by the number of embryos transferred.

Association between Endometriosis and Spontaneous/Recurrent Abortion

The data supporting a possible association between endometriosis and (recurrent) miscarriage are not convincing. Most available studies are non-randomized, have reached conflicting conclusions and have only studied spontaneous miscarriage rates, rather than recurrent miscarriage rates.[2]

According to 2 cohort studies,[3,4] there is no association between endometriosis and spontaneous abortion, and no correlation between the extent of endometriosis and the spontaneous abortion rate. Indeed, the spontaneous miscarriage rate has been reported to be similar (OR: 1.05, CI 95% 0.71-1.56) in women with minimal-mild endometriosis (32.4%) and those with moderate-severe endometriosis (33.3%).[4,5]

The effect of laparoscopic surgical treatment of minimal-mild endometriosis on reproductive outcome including spontaneous miscarriage has been compared to the effect of diagnostic laparoscopy in two randomized controlled studies.[6,7] In the Canadian study,[7] early fetal losses occurred with the same prevalence in the laparoscopic surgery group (20.6%) as in the diagnostic laparoscopy group (21.6%). In the multicentric Italian study,[6] the prevalence of spontaneous abortion before laparoscopy was equally observed in the laparoscopic surgical group (5.8%) as in the diagnostic laparoscopy group (6.7%). During the follow-up period after laparoscopy, the abortion rates were also similar in the laparoscopic surgical group (16.7%) and in the diagnostic laparoscopy group (23.1%). The results from both randomized trials,[6,7] do not support the view that laparoscopic treatment of endometriosis reduces the risk of spontaneous abortion in infertile women when compared to diagnostic laparoscopy.

Taken together, these data do not confirm that endometriosis is associated with an increased risk for spontaneous abortion and that this risk is reduced following laparoscopic surgical treatment of endometriosis.

Endometriosis and Implantation Failure after Assisted Reproduction

Recurrent implantation failure is usually defined as three or more failed attempts of IVF with embryo transfer (ET), or failure to conceive after ET of 10 or more embryos, especially in younger patients who fail to conceive despite ET of (multiple) good quality embryos.[8,9]

The etiology of recurrent implantation failure is even less understood than that of recurrent miscarriage. Possible causes include embryonic aneuploidy, abnormalities of the uterine cavity, altered endometrial receptivity and suboptimal embryo transfer techniques.[10]

A negative association between endometriosis and reproductive outcome after IVF has been reported in a meta-analysis[11] using data pooled from 22 non-randomized studies after adjustment for confounding variables, and comparing patients with endometriosis and controls without endometriosis and with tubal infertility. Not only pregnancy rates, but also fertilization rates, implantation rates, peak estradiol concentrations and the number of retrieved oocytes were significantly lower in women with endometriosis than in controls, and these parameters were negatively related to the degree of endometriosis. Indeed, implantation rates, peak estradiol concentrations and the number of retrieved oocytes were significantly lower in women with moderate-severe endometriosis when compared with women with minimal-mild endometriosis. Overall, the authors of this meta-analysis concluded that there was a 54% reduction in pregnancy rate after IVF in patients with endometriosis, and that the success was even poorer when the staging of endometriosis was higher,[5] but no solid data on spontaneous abortion rate following IVF were presented in this meta-analysis.

It has been postulated that IVF with ICSI may improve oocyte and embryo quality in women with endometriosis.

Indeed, there is no evidence that the presence and extent of endometriosis has a negative effect on implantation and pregnancy rates in patients treated with ICSI, but this observation is based on only two retrospective studies.[12] Clearly, randomized trials comparing reproductive outcome in patients with endometriosis after IVF and ICSI are needed before this hypothesis can be accepted.

In patients treated with Assisted Reproductive Technology (ART), some available data suggest a possible association between spontaneous miscarriage and endometriosis. In a recent retrospective cohort study[13] pregnancy outcome after IVF or ICSI was assessed in 1026 patients with unexplained subfertility (n = 274), endometriosis associated subfertility (n = 212), and tubal factor infertility (n = 540). The unexplained infertility group had a higher live birth rate compared with both the endometriosis associated and tubal infertility groups. Both the spontaneous miscarriages rate before 6 weeks of gestation and before 12 weeks of gestation were higher in the endometriosis group than in the unexplained group, respectively. In the total cohort, the probability of first trimester miscarriage was higher if the BMI was >25 kg/m^2 compared with women with a BMI <25 kg/m^2. After adjustment for age and body mass index (BMI, kg/m^2) the probability of first trimester miscarriage remained higher both for the endometriosis group [OR = 1.96 95% CI= 1.25-3.09] compared with the unexplained group. These data were confirmed in another study performed in ART patients reporting that the prevalence of spontaneous abortions was significantly higher in women with endometriosis than in infertile women without endometriosis 126/457 (27.6%) vs. 36/200 (18.0%); OR = 1.7, 95% CI = 1.1 - 2.6; p = 0.01).[8]

Taken together, these studies suggest that IVF is associated with impaired reproductive outcome and an increased spontaneous abortion rate in women with endometriosis when compared to controls.

Possible Mechanisms involved in the Reduction of Implantation Rates after ART in Women with Endometriosis

Immunobiological mechanisms implicated in the physiopathology of endometriosis have been extensively studied. Endometriosis is associated with increased inflammation both in the pelvic cavity and in peripheral blood.[2] However, it has also been postulated that there is a defective immunosurveillance in patients with endometriosis. The appearance of an excess of endometrial proteins in the pelvic cavity during retrograde menstruation may provoke an autoimmune response, either immunological tolerance or rejection of the homograft with alloantigenic potential, resulting in either the development of endometriosis or the maintenance of a normal pelvis respectively.[15] Humoral immunological changes in women with endometriosis include autoimmune phenomena such as autoantibodies against endometrial antigens, and generalized polyclonal B-cell autoimmune activation.[14]

Anti-endometrial Autoantibodies

Concentrations of transferrin, iron and alpha 2-heat shock glycoprotein are elevated in PF of patients with endometriosis when compared to controls.[16,17] High iron concentrations may be detrimental for oocyte quality.[15] Endogenous immunoglobulins (Ig) G derived from serum and peritoneal fluid (PF) has been shown in immunohistochemical studies to bind specifically to transferrin and alpha 2-heat shock glycoprotein in glandular epithelial endometrial cells. These autoantibodies against transferrin and alpha 2-HS glycoprotein adversely affect in-vitro sperm motion and survival and their presence may affect fertility in patients with endometriosis.[15]

Anti-laminin-1 Autoantibodies

Laminin is thought to enhance trophoblast adhesion to the maternal matrix in the peri-implantation period, to be required for initial anchorage and migration of the trophoblast cells into the maternal deciduas during implantation, and to regulate trophoblast proliferation and differentiation during implantation and placentation through an interaction with integrin receptors. Animal studies have shown that immunization of monkeys with laminin-1 can lead to embryotoxicity of their sera, infertility or spontaneous abortion.[18] In humans, anti-laminin-1 IgG has been reported in infertile women with mild-severe endometriosis and laminin-1 mRNA can also be detected in endometriosis lesions.[18] In women with recurrent (two or more consecutive) miscarriages, higher concentrations of anti-laminin-1 IgG were associated with recurrent miscarriage and subsequent pregnancy outcome of recurrent aborters.[19]

Other Autoantibodies

Numerous autoantibodies have in the past been associated with both recurrent pregnancy loss and reproductive failure after assisted reproduction. The first study to draw attention to the effect of circulating autoantibodies on the success of IVF procedures in women with endometriosis was carried out by Dmowski and coworkers. In a retrospective study,[20] they studied the effect of autoantibodies on IVF outcome during 237 consecutive cycles in 193 women (119 cycles in 84 women with and 118 cycles in 109 women without endometriosis). These antibodies were IgG, IgM and IgA isotype antibodies to cardiolipin, phosphatidylserine (PS), phosphatidylethanolamine (PE), phosphatidylglycerol (PG), phosphatidylinositol (PI), phosphatic acid (PA), histone 2A (H2A) and 2B (H2B) fractions, single-stranded DNA (ssDNA) and double-stranded DNA (dsDNA). Autoantibodies were positive (three or more) in 50% of patients with endometriosis. Pregnancy rates were twice as low in the autoantibody-positive group (23%) when compared with the autoantibody-negative group (46%).

Other investigators[21] assessed 591 women with reproductive failure for the presence of several different antinuclear antibodies (ANA), antiphospholipid antibodies (APA), antithyroid antibodies (ATA) and lupus anticoagulant. The patients were subdivided into different groups: recurrent pregnancy loss (n = 302, minimum three miscarriages), unexplained subfertility (n = 97), recurrent implantation failure after IVF/embryo transfer (n = 122), ovarian dysfunction (n = 47) and endometriosis (n = 23). Results are shown in **Table 17-1**. At least one positive test result was observed in 74% of the patients with recurrent pregnancy loss, 70% of the patients with failed IVF/embryo transfer and 52% of those with endometriosis, but in only 10% of normal fertile controls. Lupus anticoagulant was not found to be increased in any subgroup. It was

Table 17-1: Proportion of patients with recurrent pregnancy loss, implantation failure after ART and endometriosis who have positive auto-antibodies for ANA, APA and ATA (based on Kaider et al, 1999)

	Recurrent pregnancy loss (%)	Implantation failure after ART (%)	Endometriosis(%)
Positive ANA	35.1	33.6	21.7
Positive APA	22.5	27.9	21.7
Positive ATA	22.8	15.6	8.7

ANA = antinuclear antibodies; APA = antiphospholipid antibodies; ATA = antithyroid antibodies; ET = embryo transfer.

concluded that the presence of these autoantibodies was significantly more prevalent among women with reproductive failure than in fertile controls. Since both patients with recurrent pregnancy loss and patients with endometriosis were positive for similar tests in this study,[21] it may be tempting to postulate that there is an immunological link between these two conditions. However, this hypothesis is not supported by significant clinical evidence: an association between endometriosis and recurrent pregnancy loss has not been observed so far.

Cell-mediated Immunological Changes in Endometriosis

Endometriosis is a local pelvic inflammatory process with altered concentrations and function of immune-related cells in the peritoneal fluid, including increased concentrations of cytokines, growth factors and activated macrophages, that may have an adverse effect on sperm function and embryo survival.[22] These inflammatory factors may offer new therapeutic opportunities, illustrated by the observation that selective inhibition of tumor necrosis factor α (TNFα), can prevent the development of endometriosis in baboons.[23]

Peritoneal macrophages are the major resident cells in the peritoneal cavity, and their number, concentration and activity is higher in patients with endometriosis than in controls.[24] T-lymphocytes have been demonstrated to have impaired function in endometriosis, especially Th1 cells.[24]

Impaired natural killer (NK) cell function is suggested by the observation that the concentration of interferon-gamma, produced by NK cells, is reduced in PF from patients with endometriosis when compared to controls.[25] Furthermore, reduced NK cytotoxicity in peritoneal fluid[25] may contribute to a decreased cytotoxicity towards ectopic endometriosis lesions.[21] However, it is difficult to reconcile the evidence of subclinical pelvic inflammation in women with endometriosis with the hypothesis that endometriosis is a state of reduced immunosurveillance.

Cytokines

Since both ovaries and fallopian tubes are bathed in PF, increased concentration of relevant cytokines in PF can be related to infertility and reduced success of IVF in women with endometriosis.[24] These PF cytokines are not only produced by peritoneal immune cells, but also by endometriotic lesions.[24] An overview of relevant peritoneal cytokines is presented in **Table 17-2.**

Table 17-2: Overview of specific proteins (mainly cytokines, angiogenic, adhesion and growth factors) with reported increased expression in peritoneal fluid and endometriotic lesions from women with endometriosis when compared to controls (endo= endometriosis)

Proteins	Molecular Weight (kDa)	Peritoneal fluid	Endo-lesion
IL-6	23-30 kDa	↑	
IL-8	8kDa	↑	↑
VEGF	32-42	↑	
TNF alpha	17.5 kDa	↑	
Insulin-like growth factor binding protein-3 (IGF-BP 3)	17.7 kDa		↑
IL-10	39 kDa	↑	
MMP-1	54 kDa		↑
MMP-9	92 kDa		↑
Transgelin	22-23 kDa		↑
TGF-β	dimeric (25 kDa)	↑	
ICAM-1	85-110 kDa		↑
IL-1β	17 kDa	↑	
IL-12	75 kDa	↑	
CA-125	200 kDa	↑	
Aromatase	58 kDa		↑
RANTES	8 kDa	↑	
COX-2	72 kDa		↑
MCP-1	8.7 kDa	↑	↑
HGF	85 kDa	↑	
CD44	85-90 kDa	↑	
cognate chemokine receptor 1(CCR1)	41 kDa	↑	
Bcl-2 (B-cell lymphoma/leukemia-2)	26 kDa		↑
Macrophage colony stimulating factor (M-CSF),	45-100 kDa	↑	

IL = interleukin, VEGF = vascular endothelial growth factor, TNF = tumor necrosis factor, MMP = matrix metalloprotease, TGF = transforming growth factor, ICAM = intercellular adhesion molecule, CA-125= cancer antigen 125, RANTES= regulated upon activation normal T cell expressed and secreted, COX-2= cyclooxygenase-2, HGF= hepatocyte growth factor, MCP = monocyte chemotactic protein, Bcl-2 = mitochondrial protein

In women with endometriosis, an inherent impairment of granulosa cell steroidogenesis, follicular and oocyte function has been recognized as an important contributory cause of the associated subfertility and implantation failure after ART.[1, 26] Granulosa cells from women with endometriosis also have a higher apoptotic incidence, more alterations of the cell cycle and a higher incidence of oxidative stress than those from women with infertility caused by other pathologies.[27] It has been proposed that the increased PF concentration of inflammatory cytokines like IL-1, IL-6, IL-8 and IL-10 in PF from women with endometriosis can activate several cyclin-dependent kinase inhibitors in various cells.[27] Furthermore, the concentration of TNFa has been shown to be increased in the follicular fluid from women with endometriosis when compared with controls and its concentrations are related to poor-quality oocytes.[2] Alterations in the follicular fluid content of women with endometriosis may result in poor quality oocytes and consequently in embryos of lesser quality.[27,28]

Effects on Early Embryonic Development

Several investigators have reported an increased number of aberrant nuclear and cytoplasmic events in embryos, decreased embryo cleavage rates, increased percentage of arrested development, and a significant decrease in the number of blastomeres in women with endometriosis when compared to controls,[2] possibly also associated with the PF alterations mentioned above.[14]

Abortion and Aberrantly Expressed Genes and Gene Products in Endometrium

The endometrium is receptive to embryonic implantation during a well-defined 'window of implantation' in the midsecretory phase, when pinopods appear on the surface of the endometrium. Genes and gene products aberrantly expressed in endometrium from women with endometriosis include aromatase, endometrial bleeding factor, hepatocyte growth factor, 17β-hydroxysteroid dehydrogenase, homeobox genes A-10 and A-11, leukemia inhibitory factor, matrix metalloproteinase-7 and -11 and progesterone receptors.[22]

Aromatase is only expressed in the eutopic and ectopic endometrium of women with endometriosis, but not in the endometrium of healthy women.[29] Endometrial bleeding factor is downregulated during the window of implantation. It is a marker of uterine non-receptivity and is abundantly expressed during the window of implantation in women with endometriosis and infertility.[2]

Matrix metalloproteinases degrade extracellular matrix components, and are normally expressed in the endometrium during menstrual breakdown and subsequent estrogen-mediated endometrial growth, and are suppressed by progesterone during the secretory phase. It has been shown that there is a persistent expression of MMP-7 and -11 during the secretory phase in women with endometriosis when compared to controls, probably caused by complex interactions between progesterone and local cytokines.[30]

The αVβ3 integrin chain is co-expressed with other specific integrins only during the implantation window, and is a biomarker for endometrial receptivity.[31] In women with endometriosis, it appears that αVβ3 integrin expression is reduced.[31] It was suggested that a direct effect is exerted on the endometrium by inflammatory factors contained in the PF from women with endometriosis.

Micro Array studies have shown a marked up-regulation of mRNA for cytokines, growth factors and other gene products in decidualized stromal cells from women with endometriosis when compared to controls, suggesting paracrine interactions between the stroma and other endogenous and transient cell populations within the endometrium and during early pregnancy.[22] Proposed candidate genes involved in implantation failure and infertility in endometriosis include GlcNAc6ST, olfactomedin, C4BP, IL-15, Dickkopf-1, purinenucleoside phosphorylase, neuronal pentraxin II, glycodelin, S100E and BSEP.[32] However, other candidate genes may also promote an inhospitable endometrial milieu for embryonic implantation, due to embryo toxicity, immune dysfunction, inflammatory or apoptotic responses.[32]

Recently, Montgomery et al reviewed gene mapping studies in endometriosis and the prospects of finding gene pathways contributing to disease using the latest genome-wide strategies.[33] Genetic variants in 76 genes have been examined for association, but none shows convincing evidence of replication in multiple studies. Although there is evidence for genetic linkage to chromosomes 7 and 10, the genes (or variants) in these regions contributing to disease risk have yet to be identified.[33]

Although the above mentioned data suggest that the main reason for reproductive failure in women with endometriosis lies can be found in the altered immunobiology of the endometrium during the implantation window, it has been shown[2] that patients with endometriosis receiving donor eggs have the same chances of implantation and pregnancy as oocyte recipients without endometriosis, if the donated oocytes originated from donors without known endometriosis. However, patients who received embryos originating from eggs derived from endometriotic ovaries showed a significantly reduced implantation rate as compared with the remaining groups.[34] These data suggest that dysfunctional endometrial function is not responsible for endometriosis-associated implantation failure in an IVF context. In contrast, endometriosis-related infertility and implantation failure may be more related to alterations within the oocyte, which in turn result in embryos with decreased ability to implant.

Prevention of (Recurrent) Abortion in Women with Endometriosis

As proposed in the ESHRE guidelines for endometriosis, treatment of endometriosis must be individualized, taking into consideration the clinical problem in its entirety, including the impact of the disease and the effect of its treatment on quality of life.[35] It also is important to involve the woman in all decisions, to be flexible in considering diagnostic and therapeutic approaches, and to maintain a good relationship with the patient. It may be appropriate to seek advice from more experienced colleagues or to refer the woman to a center with the necessary expertise to offer all available treatments in a multidisciplinary context.[35]

Specific Interventions

When endometriosis co-exists with other medical conditions that cause recurrent abortion, the treatment strategy should be specific for these medical conditions (e.g. in case of antiphospholipid syndrome, administration of aspirin and low molecular weight heparin).

Non-specific Interventions

Although there appears to be no biological mechanism for supportive care to reduce miscarriages, it has been shown that proper care and support do reduce the miscarriage rate in women suffering from unexplained recurrent miscarriages. For up to half of women suffering from recurrent miscarriages, no known cause can be identified. Studies have been conducted, in which these women received specific antenatal counselling; close weekly supervision by ultrasound scan at a dedicated early pregnancy clinic until the 12th gestational week and formal emotional support.[36] Progesterone can be used for

the prevention of recurrent miscarriage according to a limited number of RCTs carried out in small patient groups.[37] The role of vitamins and uterine relaxing agents is not clear at present. The role of expensive immunotherapy (IVIG) remains highly controversial and should not be used outside a research context.

Summary

In this chapter we reviewed the lack of association between endometriosis (and its treatment), spontaneous abortion and recurrent abortion, and the possible association between endometriosis and reproductive failure after IVF. Although several immunological factors have been identified that could affect/impair embryo implantation and spontaneous fertility in patients with endometriosis, it appears that the impaired reproductive outcome after ART in women with endometriosis when compared to controls is related to alterations within the follicle or oocyte, resulting in embryos with a decreased ability to implant or to lead to a live birth.

References

1. Vercammen EE, D'Hooghe TM. Endometriosis and recurrent pregnancy loss. Semin Reprod Med 2000;18: 363-68.
2. Tomassetti C, Meuleman C, Pexsters A, Mihalyi A, Kyama C, Simsa P, et al. Endometriosis, recurrent miscarriage and implantation failure:is there an immunological link? Reprod Biomed Online 2006;13:58-64.
3. Matorras R, Rodriguez F, Guttierez de Teran G et al. Endometriosis and spontaneous abortion rate: a cohort study in infertile women. Eur J Obstet Gynecol and Reprod Biol 1998; 7: 101-05.
4. Sinaii N, Plumb K, Cotton L, Lambert A, Kennedy S, Zondervan K, Stratton P. Differences in characteristics among 1,000 women with endometriosis based on extent of disease Fertil Steril 2008; 89: 538-45.
5. Revised American Society for reproductive Medicine classification of endometriosis: 1996. Fertil Steril 1997; 67: 817-21.
6. Gruppo Italiano per lo Studio dell' Endometriosi. Hum Reprod 1999; 14: 1332-34.
7. Marcoux S, Maheux R, Bérubé S and the Canadian Collaborative Group on Endometriosis N Engl J Med 1997;337: 217–22.
8. Matalliotakis I, Cakmak H, Dermitzaki D, Zervoudis S, Goumenou A, Fragouli Y Increased rate of endometriosis and spontaneous abortion in an in vitro fertilization program: no correlation with epidemiological factors. Gynecol Endocrinol. 2008; 24:194-98.
9. Taranissi M, El-Thoukhy T, Verlinsky Y Influence of maternal age on the outcome of PGD for aneuploidy

screening in patients with recurrent implantation failure. Reproductive BioMedicine Online 2005; 10:628-32.

10. Urman B, Yakin K, Balaban B Recurrent implantation failure in assisted reproduction: how to counsel and manage. B. Treatment options that have not been proven to benefit the couple. Reproductive BioMedicine Online 2005; 11: 382-91.

11. Barnhart K, Dunsmoor-Su R, Coutifaris C Effect of endometriosis on in vitro fertilisation. Fertil Steril 2002; 77: 1148–55.

12. De Hondt A, Peeraer K, Meuleman C et al. Endometriosis and subfertility treatment: a review. Minerva Ginecol 2005; 57:257-67.

13. Omland AK, Abyholm T, Fedorcsak P, et al. Pregnancy outcome after IVF and ICSI in unexplained, endometriosis-associated and tubal factor infertility. Hum Reprod 2005; 20:722-27.

14. Lebovic DI, Mueller MD, Taylor RN Immunobiology of endometriosis. Fertil Steril 2001;75:1-10.

15. Mathur SP Autoimmunity in endometriosis: relevance to infertility. Am J Reprod Immunol 2000;44:89-95.

16. Mathur SP, Lee JH, Jiang H et al. Levels of transferrin and alpha 2-HS glycoprotein in women with and without endometriosis. Autoimmunity 1999; 29:121-27.

17. Defrère S, Lousse JC, Gonzalez-Ramos R, Colette S, Donnez J, Van Langendonckt A. Potential involvement of iron in the pathogenesis of peritoneal endometriosis. Mol Hum Reprod. 2008 ;14: 377-85.

18. Inagaki J, Sugiura-Ogasawara M, Nomizu M et al. An association of IgG anti-laminin-1 autoantibodies with endometriosis in infertile patients. Hum Reprod 2003;18: 544-49.

19. Inagaki J, Matsuura E, Nomizu M et al. IgG anti-laminin-1 autoantibody and recurrent miscarriage. Am J Reprod Immunol 2001;45:232-38.

20. Dmowski WP, Rana N, Michalowska J, et al. The effect of endometriosis, its stage and activity and of autoantibodies on in vitro fertilisation and embryo transfer success rates. Fertil Steril 1995; 63:555-62.

21. Kaider AS, Kaider BD, Janowicz PB, Roussev RG Immunodiagnostic evaluation in women with reproductive failure. Am J Reprod Immunol 1999; 42: 335-46.

22. Giudice LC, Telles TL, Lobo S, Kao L. The molecular basis for implantation failure in endometriosis. Ann NY Acad Sci 2002; 955: 25-64.

23. D'Hooghe TM, Nugent NP, Cuneo S et al. Recombinant Human TNFRSF1A (r-hTBP1) inhibits the development of endometriosis in baboons: a prospective, randomized, placebo- and drug controlled study. Biol Reprod 2006;74: 131-36.

24. Wu MY, Ho HN The role of cytokines in endometriosis. Am J Reprod Immunol 2003;49:285-96.

25. Oosterlynck DJ, Meuleman C, Waer M, Koninckx PR Transforming growth factor-beta activity is increased in peritoneal fluid from women with endometriosis. Obstet Gynecol 1994; 83: 287-92.

26. Cahill DJ, Hull MGR Pituitary ovarian dysfunction and endometriosis. Hum Reprod Update 2000; 6: 56-66.

27. Pellicer A, Albert C, Garrido N et al. The pathophysiology of endometriosis-associated infertility: follicular environment and embryo quality. J Reprod Fertil 2000; Suppl. 55, 109-19.

28. Saito H, Seino T, Kaneko T et al. Endometriosis and oocyte quality. Gynecol Obstet Invest 2002;53: 46-51.

29. Bulun SE, Mahendroo MS, Simpson ER. Polymerase chain reaction amplification fails to detect aromatase cytochrome P450 transcripts in normal human endometrium or deciduas. J Clin Endocrinol Metab 1993; 76:1458-63.

30. Osteen KG, Keller NR, Feltus FA, Melner NH Paracrine regulation of matrix metalloproteinase expression in the normal human endometrium. Gynecologic and Obstetric Investigation 1999; 48: 2-13.

31. Lessey BA, Damjanovich L, Coutifaris C et al. Integrin adhesion molecules in the human endometrium. Correlation with the normal and abnormal menstrual cycle. J Clin Invest 1992; 90: 188-95.

32. Kao LC, Germeyer A, Tulac S et al. Expression profiling on endometrium from women with endometriosis reveals candidate genes for disease-based implantation failure and infertility. Endocrinology 2003; 144: 2870-81.

33. Montgomery GW, Nyholt DR, Zhao ZZ, Treloar SA, Painter JN, Missmer SA, et al. The search for genes contributing to endometriosis risk. Hum Reprod Update 2008;14: 447-57.

34. Garcia-Velasco JA, Arici A Is the endometrium or oocyte/embryo affected in endometriosis? Hum Reprod 1999;14 (Suppl. 2): 77-89.

35. Kennedy S, Bergqvist A, Chapron C, D'Hooghe T, Dunselman G, Greb R, Hummelshoj L, Prentice A, Saridogan E; ESHRE Special Interest Group for Endometriosis and Endometrium Guideline Development Group. ESHRE guideline for the diagnosis and treatment of endometriosis. Hum Reprod 2005; 20: 2698-704.

36. Clifford K, Rai R, Regan L. Future pregnancy outcome in unexplained recurrent first trimester miscarriage. Hum Reprod 1997;12:387-89.

37. Haas DM, Ramsey PS. Progesterone for preventing miscarriage. Cochrane Database of Systematic Reviews 208, Issue 2. Art. No.: CD003511.

Anabel Salazar, Juan A Garcia-Velasco

Chapter 18

Assisted Reproductive Technology and Endometriosis

What is the Real Chance of Conceiving? Is it Really Worth the Effort?

Endometriosis is a challenging disease characterized by the presence and proliferation of both endometrial glands and stroma outside the uterine cavity. It affects approximately 10-20% of the female population of reproductive age, and occurs in patients from all ethnic and social groups. Only a few cases have been described in adolescents and/or postmenopausal women. Although the relationship between endometriosis and infertility is well documented, because of the higher overall prevalence of disease reported in infertile women, some authors still debate the true occurrence of infertility in endometriosis patients. The exact mechanism remains unclear and a cause and effect relationship has not been established.[1]

This does not mean that all women with endometriosis are infertile or need assisted reproduction techniques (ART). In fact, many women with endometriosis are fertile and successfully reproduce. Nevertheless, their fecundability or chances of achieving pregnancy per month seem to be reduced, as endometriosis may have adverse effects on several aspects of reproductive physiology, including folliculogenesis, ovulation, sperm motility, fertilization, and embryo quality.[1, 2]

Fecundity is defined as the probability of a woman achieving a live birth for any given month.[3] In normal couples, the monthly fecundity rate (MFR) is in the range of 0.15 to 0.20 per month.[4] In untreated women with endometriosis and infertility, MFR is 0.02 to 0.10.[5] The prospective study by Jansen et al demonstrated that endometriosis was a detrimental factor for women undergoing donor insemination, and reported that MFR was 0.12 in women without endometriosis and 0.036 in those with minimal endometriosis.[6] However, other authors have reported that the fecundity of women with minimal or mild endometriosis is similar to healthy women undergoing donor insemination, in terms of cumulative pregnancy rates (CPR), thus these women should not be treated for a trial period of at least 18 months.[7, 8] In contrast, the Canadian Collaborative Group on Endometriosis has compared outcomes following laparoscopic resection or ablation versus expectant management of endometriosis to determine whether laparoscopic surgery enhanced fecundity in infertile women with minimal or mild disease. They followed 341 infertile women with minimal or mild endometriosis for 36 weeks after laparoscopic surgery. The MFR per person was 0.047 and 0.024 in the treated and control groups, respectively. They conclude that surgical resection increases fecundity rates in patients with endometriosis stage I/II.[9]

Conversely, the Gruppo Italiano per lo Studio dell'Endometriosi conducted a randomized, controlled trial[10] in order to define the improvement with resection or ablation in minimal and mild endometriosis. They compared two treatment groups, diagnostic laparoscopy only versus resection or ablation of visible lesions. They found no significant differences between the groups in terms of conceiving: 12 (24%) in the resection/ablation group and 13 (29%) in the no-treatment group. Finally, the 1 year birth rate was 10 out of 51 women (20%) in the resection/ablation group and 10 out of 45 (22%) in the no treatment group. Based on these reports, results do not confirm that resection or ablation of minimal and mild endometriosis increases the short-term likelihood of pregnancy in infertile women when compared to diagnostic laparoscopy alone.

Although fecundity was significantly improved in the Canadian surgical trial, fecundity remained significantly lower than that observed in normal fertile women. Thus, infertile women that have been diagnosed with endometriosis should begin ART, in a reasonable period of time, considering that they will probably have lower chances of conceiving naturally on their own. This period should be established as one year for patients under thirty-five years old with minimal-mild endometriosis, but should be set at six months in patients over thirty-five years old and in those with severe disease. Thus, we can finally conclude that treatment of endometriosis patients with ART is helpful in improving the chance of viable pregnancy.

Where Exactly is the Endometriosis Problem Located?

Many factors have been described as a cause of decreased fertility found in endometriosis patients without tubal involvement. Although it may affect the reproductive process at different levels, ART should make it possible to overcome these obstacles, but this remains to be determined. Some of the potential causes of infertility include defective folliculogenesis, poor oocyte quality, luteinized unruptured follicle, altered tubal permeability and functionality, diminished sperm motility in the uterus, reduced oocyte fertilization, slower embryo cleavage, and reduced embryo implantation.[11]

One of these factors, the altered follicular environment, was studied by Harlow et al,[12] who investigated the production of estradiol (aromatase activity) and progesterone of freshly isolated granulosa cells from women with mild endometriosis and from a control group with tubal or unexplained infertility, undergoing IVF during unstimulated or gonadotropin-stimulated cycles. They found a lower median basal aromatase activity and progesterone production, as well as a reduced fertilization and cleavage rate in mature oocytes from women with endometriosis. Thus, a defect in granulosa cell steroidogenesis associated with endometriosis could adversely affect oocyte function and may partially explain the reduction in fertilizing capacity. We also evaluated the endocrine milieu to determine steroid production of granulosa cells from women with endometriosis.[13] *In vitro* experiments confirmed that, under basal conditions and after hCG stimulation, cells from women with endometriosis showed differential steroid production, which may have an impact on oocyte quality.

The role of oxidative stress in endometriosis associated infertility has been extensively studied in the last few years by Gupta et al. Oxidative stress markers, including production of large amounts of reactive oxygen species,

high levels of nitric oxide and nitric oxide synthase, and others have been found in the endometrium and in the peritoneal and follicular fluid of women with endometriosis. The increased DNA damage in the oocyte induced by oxidative stress may contribute to poorer egg/embryo quality, lower fertilization and implantation rates, and increased miscarriage rates in these patients.[14]

Embryo quality may be altered in women with endometriosis. Clinical observations suggest that implantation rate may be diminished in these patients.[15,16] To address this issue, Pellicer et al[17] evaluated *in vitro* embryo development in women with and without endometriosis undergoing IVF. They showed a significantly reduced number of blastomeres in embryos from endometriosis patients compared with controls ($P < 0.04$), as well as an increased incidence of arrested embryos after 72h of *in vitro* culture ($P < 0.05$). This finding leads us to suggest that the reduced implantation observed in patients with endometriosis may be due to a reduction in embryo quality. Confirmatory evidence comes from oocyte donation programmes, where success rates are unaffected by the presence of endometriosis and are comparable to outcomes following oocyte donation for other indications. Patients with severe endometriosis receive eggs from healthy oocyte donors and show excellent implantation and pregnancy rates.[18]

Proper Selection of Patients and Appropriate Treatment

Intrauterine Insemination (IUI) and Controlled Ovarian Hyperstimulation (COH)

It has been widely described in the literature that empirical treatment with COH and IUI is beneficial in couples with persistent unexplained infertility.[19] Although this treatment also appears to be effective in patients with endometriosis, there seems to be some controversy on this issue amongst authors. Some have reported lower fecundity and pregnancy rates in endometriosis patients, while others find a decreased rate only in mild to severe disease.

The ESHRE guidelines for the diagnosis and treatment of endometriosis recommend that treatment with IUI improves fertility in minimal–mild endometriosis (evidence 1b): COH and IUI is effective but the role of unstimulated IUI is uncertain, based on a systematic review.[20]

Tummon et al[21] reported in a randomized controlled trial the efficacy of COH and IUI versus expectant management in 311 cycles in 103 couples, in whom infertility was associated only with minimal or mild endometriosis (diagnosed laparoscopically 12 months prior). Ovarian stimulation was performed with FSH, and live-birth rate was the main outcome measure. The live birth rate was 11% (14 of 127) in the COH and IUI cycles and 2% (4 of 184) in the no treatment cycles, with an odds ratio of 5.6 (95% confidence interval 1.8 to 17.4) in favor of COH and IUI. Along the same line, Ozkan et al[22] concluded in a recent review that COH with IUI is recommended in early-stage and surgically corrected endometriosis when pelvic anatomy is normal.

A meta-analysis by Hughes[23] showed that both COH and IUI in patients with persistent infertility significantly increased fecundity rates. Twenty-two trials contributed a total of 5214 cycles to this analysis. The evidence showed a 2-fold fecundity increase with FSH, an approximately 3-fold increase with IUI, and a 5-fold increase when both were used compared to untreated cycles (adjusted odds ratios for the likelihood of conception per cycle). The unadjusted data are as follows: 4.6% in all clomiphene citrate and unstimulated cycles versus 11.7% in all FSH cycles; similarly, the ratios are 3.7% with timed intercourse and 9.4% with IUI. Additionally, the authors found that some independent infertility factors, like endometriosis, could reduce treatment effectiveness by approximately half. Omland et al,[24] in a prospective cohort study included 168 patients with unexplained infertility or minimal-mild endometriosis (laparoscopically diagnosed) undergoing COH and IUI, reported a significantly higher pregnancy rate in the unexplained infertility group (33.3% vs 16.3% [p < 0.05]).

As we have seen, COH and IUI are good approaches for the treatment of unexplained infertility, but concerning endometriosis-associated infertility we find different opinions and many inconclusive studies. Taking into acount this problem, we must make a choice regarding which treatment to offer to our patients.

In an effort to identify different prognostic factors associated with treatment outcome, Nuojua et al[25] retrospectively analyzed 811 COH and IUI cycles using clomiphene citrate/human menopausal gonadotrophin (HMG). The study assessed different infertility etiologies, including minimal (stage I) and mild (stage II) endometriosis. The lowest pregnancy rate per cycle (6.5%; 9/138) was found in endometriosis patients. This is slightly lower than that reported previously by Tummon et al (9–16%).[21] These results suggest that there may be other factors affecting fertility in patients with endometriosis, in addition to tubal patency, although this remains unclear. The data from all these studies could suggest that IVF may overcome some of these factors **(Table 18.1).**

Table 18-1: Factors related to infertility in endometriosis disease
• Altered follicular environment
• Impaired oocyte quality
• Reduced implantation rate
• Endometrial receptivity
• Gametotoxic effect induced by endometriosis
• Altered tubal permeability and functionality
• Distorted pelvis anatomy

Conversely, a recent retrospective, controlled, cohort study from Werbrouck et al[26] calls into question the foregoing and suggests another interesting hypothesis, assuming an equal or higher PR per cycle and cumulative live-birth rate after COH and IUI in women with recently surgically treated minimal to mild endometriosis. The study included 107 patients undergoing 259 cycles of COH (23 cycles with clomiphene citrate and 236 with gonadotropins) and IUI. The endometriosis group consisted of 58 patients recently operated (within 7 months before the onset of treatment), 41 for minimal and 17 for mild endometriosis. The main outcome measure was clinical PR per cycle and cumulative live-birth rate within four cycles of treatment. PR per cycle in women with minimal (21%) or mild endometriosis (18.9%) were similar to women with unexplained infertility (20.5%). The cumulative live-birth rate was also comparable in women with minimal endometriosis, mild endometriosis, and unexplained infertility (70.2%, 68.2 %, and 66.5%, respectively).

Although there is still much controversy about this subject, we have to determine the best treatment option for each individual according to additional factors such as age, previous surgery for endometriosis, ovarian reserve, male factor (associated or not), social and emotional issues, and of course previous obstetric history. With all this information and the correct diagnosis of current endometriosis stage, we should make the most appropriate decision to provide the most accurate treatment.

At our institution, if the patient has at least one patent tube and is under 38-40 years of age with normal semen parameters in her partner, we suggest starting with IUI combined with COH for up to 3 attempts. Acknowledging a lower success rate as compared to "good prognosis" patients (20% per cycle), there is still an 8% chance of achieving pregnancy. According to the severity of the disease, the age of the patient, and taking into consideration their anxiety with infertility, we may reduce the number of attempts to 1 or 2, and in some selected cases, start directly with IVF, especially in severe endometriosis with previous surgery, where adhesions may compromise tubal functionality.

In Vitro Fertilization

According to the ESHRE 2005 guidelines for the diagnosis and treatment of endometriosis, IVF is an appropriate treatment, especially if tubal function is compromised, if there is also male factor infertility, and/or when other treatments have failed – (evidence level 2b). IVF pregnancy rates are lower in patients with endometriosis than in those with tubal infertility – (evidence level 1a).[20]

In 2002, a meta-analysis was performed by Barnhart et al,[16] which included twenty-two published studies. The main outcome measures were pregnancy rates, fertilization rate, implantation rates, and numbers of oocytes retrieved in endometriosis patients and in controls. The pregnancy rate was significantly lower for endometriosis patients (odds ratio, 0.56; 95% confidence interval, 0.44-0.70) when compared with tubal factor-associated infertility patients (controls). A decrease in fertilization and implantation rates and a significant decrease in the number of oocytes retrieved for endometriosis patients were also demonstrated, as well as a difference in peak estradiol (E2) concentrations. When they compared women with stage III or IV endometriosis to women with tubal infertility a diminished pregnancy rate was confirmed (OR, 0.46; CI, 0.28–0.74). The same was also demonstrated in women with mild endometriosis compared with tubal factor-associated infertility (OR, 0.60; 95% CI, 0.42-0.87). Although significant differences in all variables except for pregnancy rate were reported, the strength of association was similar to other comparisons, but the results did not achieve statistical significance.

When the stage of endometriosis was taken into account, IVF outcome was quite poor in severe disease (stage III/IV). A 36% decrease in pregnancy rate was observed in women with severe endometriosis compared with mild disease. Also, the number of oocytes retrieved and the peak E2 level were dismished, although fertilization rate was similar between groups. This meta-analysis is in contrast with data generated by large registries such as CDC-ASRM or FIVNAT, where endometriosis patients perform similarly to other diagnostic groups. Probably, the way patients are diagnosed with endometriosis in these registries is not as accurate as in those entering a clinical trial. Barnhart´s meta-analysis pulled together many different trials including some old reports – when IVF results where much poorer than today, with many different heterogeneous protocols of stimulation. However, although bias may exist, a clear conclusion can be drawn that endometriosis reduces IVF success rates, and this reduction correlates with severity of the disease.

Some authors have questioned if GnRH agonists treatment prior to IVF or ICSI would be more effective in terms of pregnancy rate in women with endometriosis. In 2006, Sallam et al[27] performed a review that included three randomized controlled trials (with 165 women) using GnRH agonist 3 to 6 months prior to IVF or ICSI to treat women with any degree of endometriosis diagnosed by laparoscopy or laparotomy. The clinical pregnancy rate per woman was significantly higher (three studies: OR 4.28, 95% CI 2.00 to 9.15). Finally, it was concluded that the administration of GnRH agonists for a period of three to six months prior to IVF or ICSI in women with endometriosis increases the odds of clinical pregnancy by fourfold. The rationale behind these findings might be modulation of the uterine natural killer (NK) cell population or normalization of endometrial aromatase expression, although further trials are needed prior to recommending its routine use.

It seems clear that endometriosis has an impact on IVF outcome, although ART may overcome some of the pathogenic mechanisms implicated, with the except of oocyte quality.

Oocyte Donation

The egg donation program may be a successful alternative for those endometriosis patients with advanced disease, poor response to COH, and previous IVF failure attempts, in order to improve their chances of achieving a pregnancy. The key question here may be if endometrial receptivity in patients with severe endometriosis is diminished.

In vitro experiments to evaluate endometrial receptivity evaluating a morphological marker – pinopods - have been performed. Garcia-Velasco et al[28] studied pinopode expression pattern in two sequential endometrial biopsies obtained in the same cycle of each patient undergoing oocyte donation under hormone replacement therapy. Pinopode expression in women with endometriosis did not differ from that of patients without endometriosis and no differences were found in terms of clinical outcome. Endometrial receptivity in terms of pinopode expression seemed to be unaffected in women with endometriosis undergoing hormonal replacement therapy.

Clinical factors affecting the outcome of oocyte donation have been thoroughly studied, including women suffering from endometriosis. Soares et al[29] recently reviewed different factors affecting the recipient (other than those associated with uterine cavity abnormalities) on the outcome of egg donation. They found that endometriosis has no negative impact when standard endometrial priming protocols were used in oocyte donation.

The best design to confirm whether endometrial receptivity is impaired in women with endometriosis would be to study those recipients sharing eggs from the same donor, with one of the recipients suffering from severe disease while the other undergoes egg donation for a reason unrelated to endometriosis. This study was performed by Diaz et al[30] in a matched, case-control design. They reported no differences between pregnancy, implantation, miscarriage, and live birth rates in endometriosis stage III/IV group when compared with the control group. The study enrolled 25 patients diagnosed by laparoscopy with stage III-IV endometriosis (group I), and 33 disease free women undergoing egg donation (group II). On the day of retrieval, oocytes from a single donor were shared with two recipients: one with severe endometriosis and the other disease free. The number of oocytes donated and fertilized, as well as the number of available and transferred embryos, was comparable between the two groups. Similar PR/ET and LBR was found, suggesting that moderate/severe endometriosis does not affect endometrial receptivity in HRT egg donation cycles.

Oocyte Cryopreservation

Vitrification is indeed a promising method for oocyte cryopreservation, and it offers a good opportunity for young women requiring fertility preservation. It has become an attractive alternative for women with the desire of preserving their fertility for many different reasons, including diseases like cancer but also mutilating surgery such as endometriosis. Among the different techniques available, from slow freezing to ultra rapid freezing, vitrification seems to offer the best outcome.[31] Recently published experience with vitrification, specifically with the cryotop method, showed comparable results in egg donation cycles whether the eggs where fertilized fresh or after vitrification,[32] which is very reassuring when considering postponing fertility by egg banking.

Egg freezing has already been offered to women with severe endometriosis. Shai et al[33] performed three COH cycles with egg retrieval in a young woman with severe endometriosis with the purpose of preserving her fertility, as she had had four complicated endometriosis surgeries, including unilateral oophorectomy due to uncontrolled bleeding. They obtained 21 cryopreserved oocytes after three attempts in a 25-year-old nulliparous woman with severe and symptomatic endometriosis and low antral follicle count.

The hypothetical risk of growth of the endometriotic lesions with the hyperestrogenemic induced by COH has been recently discarded by D´Hooghe et al.[34] In a retrospective cohort study, women who underwent fertility surgery for endometriosis stage III or IV and then either IVF or IUI – which would yield exposure to either high or moderate serum E2 levels due to COH–were evaluated through life table analysis for cumulative endometriosis recurrence rate. Authors concluded that temporary exposure to very high E2 levels in women undergoing ART is not a major risk factor for endometriosis recurrence. Thus, COH and oocyte retrieval for egg banking and fertility preservation could be a good option for those young women who require complicated surgery for endometriosis. Adequate counselling must be given to these patients with extensive surgeries about the risk of damaging their ovarian reserve as well as the limitations of egg banking.

How can Endometriosis Surgery Affect IVF Outcome?

It has been classically admitted that endometriomas in infertile women require surgery to improve their fertility status, as they may negatively influence ovarian function and impose difficulties and risks during oocyte retrieval, although the way in which they can really dismiss the ovarian reserve remains unknown **(Figure 18-1A to C)**. Still today, there are no definitive data clarifying whether the treatment of endometriomas increases (or decreases) the chances of successful IVF.[35, 36]

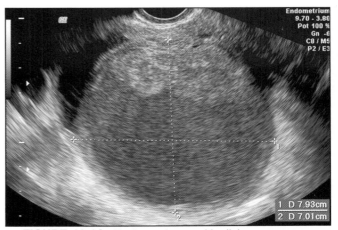

FIGURE 18-1A: Endometrioma with dishomogeneous content

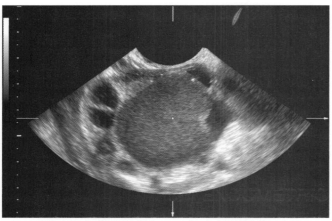

FIGURE 18-1B: Endometrioma with healthy antral follicles surrounding the cyst

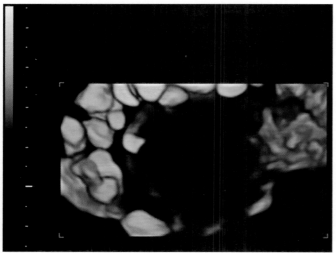

FIGURE 18-1C: Inverse mode 3D image of endometrioma with antral follicles surrounding the endometriotic cyst

But the really decisive question for clinicians is whether surgery would improve outcomes and if the benefits outweigh the risks. We have to balance the benefit of this surgery for the patient versus the potential damage to ovarian reserve, apart from the risks strictly associated with surgery. Most studies suggest that ovarian response to gonadotrophins may be reduced after cystectomy, especially when the endometriotic cyst removal is bilateral.

Some studies have specifically focused on results of IVF cycles in patients with endometriomas. Garcia-Velasco et al,[37] in a retrospective matched case–control study, compared outcomes in patients who underwent laparoscopic ovarian cystectomy with endometriomas >3 cm to patients who had endometriomas and no treatment. Patients who had surgery required more gonadotropins and had lower peak E2 levels compared to controls. There were no

differences between surgery and control groups with regard to implantation rate, clinical pregnancy, and miscarriage rate. Thus, laparoscopic cystectomy does not offer any benefit in terms of fertility outcome. Hence, in asymptomatic patients with endometriomas not larger than 4 cm we should offer direct COH and IVF prior to surgery because of its shorter time to pregnancy, decreased cost, and avoidance of the risk of surgery.

On the other hand, symptomatic women can be counseled that surgery will not decrease their chances of successful IVF outcomes. Risk of surgery are minor, however we have to take into account a 20-30% recurrence rate and less than 3% risk of POF after bilateral cyst removal.[38] Finally, the true question is whether surgery adds anything of value for infertile women with moderate to severe endometriosis.

Somigliana et al[35] concluded in their recent review that results from large randomized trials are needed to solve the issue of endometrioma removal prior to or after IVF cycle. The chances of conceiving are not the main factor to take into account before deciding to operate on endometriosis prior to IVF. Obviously, if there is an endometrioma larger than 4 cm, the oocyte retrieval will be more difficult, with the added risk of puncturing the cyst during the procedure with the subsequent possibility of rupture, infection, and follicular fluid contamination. Clinicians may advise patients individually, taking into account factors such as age, symptomatic disease, previous surgeries, ovarian reserve, and the possibility of occult malignancy. Complete information about the risks and benefits of treatment alternatives must be given to patients in order to allow them to make the most appropriate decision.

Conclusions

According to the best available evidence, endometriosis compromises fertility by several different mechanisms. Advanced stages of the disease compromise the monthly fecundity rate even further. Different ART available are able to bypass most of the endometriosis-related mechanisms of infertility in order to achieve a pregnancy, except for oocyte/embryo quality. Endometrial receptivity does not seem to be affected, as results from egg donation are not diminished in endometriosis patients. When considering surgery prior to ART, it is crucial to consider patient symptoms as well as the potential benefit of this surgical procedure, as ovarian reserve may be compromised after surgery; however, careful technique does not compromise ovarian reserve. In cases where the ovarian function may be seriously compromised, egg banking may be offered.

References

1. D´ Hooghe T, Debrock S, Hill J, Meuleman C. Endometriosis and subfertility: is the relationship resolved? Sem Reprod Med 2003; 21: 243-253.
2. Gianetto-Berrutti A, Feyles V. Endometriosis related to infertility. Minerva Ginecol 2003; 55 :407-16.
3. Chandra A, Mosher WD. The demography of infertility and the use of medical care for infertility. Infertil Reprod Med Clin North Am 1994; 5: 283-96.
4. Schwartz D, Mayaux MJ. Female fecundity as a function of age: results of artificial insemination in 2193 nulliparous women with azoospermic husbands. N Engl J Med 1982;306:404-06.
5. Hughes EG, Fedorkow DM, Collins JA. A quantitative overview of controlled trials in endometriosis-associated infertility. Fertil Steril 1993; 59 : 963-70.
6. Jansen RP. Minimal endometriosis and reduced fecundability: prospective evidence from an artificial insemination by donor program. Fertil Steril 1986; 46: 141-43.
7. Portuondo JA, Echanojauregui AD, Herran C, Alijarte I. Early conception in patients with untreated mild endometriosis. Fertil Steril 1983; 39: 22-25.
8. Rodriguez-Escudero FJ, Neyro JL, Corcostegui B, Benito JA. Does minimal endometriosis reduce fecundity? Fertil Steril 1988; 50: 522- 24.
9. Marcoux S, Maheux R, Bérubé S. Laparoscopic surgery in infertile women with minimal or mild endometriosis. Canadian Collaborative Group on Endometriosis. N Engl J Med 1997; 337:217-22.
10. Gruppo Italiano per lo Studio dell'Endometriosi. Ablation of lesions or no treatment in minimal-mildendometriosis in infertile women: a randomized trial. Hum Reprod 1999; 14 :1332-34.
11. Garrido N, Navarro J, García-Velasco J, Remohí J, Pellicer A, Simón C. The endometrium versus embryonic quality in endometriosis-related infertility. Hum Reprod Update 2002; 8: 95-103.
12. Harlow CR, Cahill DJ, Maile LA. Reduced preovulatory granulosa cell steroidogenesis in women with endometriosis. J Clin Endocrinol Metab 1996;81:426-29.
13. Pellicer A, Valbuena D, Bauset C, Albert C, Bonilla-Musoles F, Remohí J, Simón C. The follicular endocrine environment in stimulated cycles of women with endometriosis: steroid levels and embryo quality. Fertil Steril 1998; 69: 1135-41.
14. Gupta S, Goldberg M, Aziz N, Goldberg E, Krajcir N, Agarwal A. Pathogenic mechanisms in endometriosis-associated infertility. Fertil Steril 2008; 90: 247-57.
15. Simón C, Gutiérrez A, Vidal A, Santos MJ, Tarín JJ, Remohí J, Pellicer A. Outcome of patients with endometriosis in assisted reproduction: results from in-vitro fertilization and oocyte donation. Hum Reprod 1994; 9: 725-29.
16. Barnhart K, Dunsmoor-Su R, Coutifaris C. Effect of endometriosis on in vitro fertilization. Fertil Steril 2002; 77:1148-55.
17. Pellicer A, Oliveira N, Ruiz A, Remohí J, Simón C. Exploring the mechanism(s) of endometriosis-related infertility: an analysis of embryo development and implantation in assisted reproduction. Hum Reprod 1995;10:91-97.
18. Budak E, Garrido N, Reis Soares S, Barreto Melo MA, Meseguer M, Pellicer A, Remohí J. Improvements achieved in an oocyte donation program over a 10-year period: sequential increase in implantation and pregnancy rates and decrease in high-order multiple pregnancies. Fertil Steril 2007; 88: 342-49.
19. Verhulst SM, Cohlen BJ, Hughes E, te Velde E, Heineman MJ. Intra-uterine insemination for unexplained subfertility. Cochrane Database of Systematic Reviews 2006; 4.
20. Kennedy S, Bergqvist A, Chapron C, D'Hooghe T, Dunselman G, Greb R, Hummelshoj L, Prentice A, Saridogan E on behalf of the ESHRE Special Interest Group for Endometriosis and Endometrium Guideline Development Group. ESHRE guideline for the diagnosis and treatment of endometriosis. Hum Reprod 2005; 20: 2698-2704.
21. Tummon IS, Asher LJ, Martin JS and Tulandi T. Randomized controlled trial of superovulation and insemination for infertility associated with minimal or mild endometriosis. Fertil Steril 1997; 68, 8-12.
22. Ozkan S, Murk W, Arici A. Endometriosis and infertility: epidemiology and evidence-based treatments. Ann N Y Acad Sci 2008; 1127:92-100.
23. Hughes EG. The effectiveness of ovulation induction and intrauterine insemination in the treatment of persistent infertility: a meta-analysis. Hum Reprod 1997; 12:1865-72.
24. Omland AK, Tanbo T, Dale PO, Abyholm T. Artificial insemination by husband in unexplained infertility compared with infertility associated with peritoneal endometriosis. Hum Reprod 1999; 13: 2602-05.
25. Nuojua-Huttunen S, Tomas C, Bloigu R, Tuomivaara L, Martikainen H. Intrauterine insemination treatment in subfertility: an analysis of factors affecting outcome. Hum Reprod 1999; 14: 698-703.
26. Werbrouck E, Spiessens C, Meuleman C, D'Hooghe T. No difference in cycle pregnancy rate and in cumulative live-birth rate between women with surgically treated minimal to mild endometriosis and women with unexplained infertility after controlled ovarian hyperstimulation and intrauterine insemination. Fertil Steril 2006; 86: 566-71.
27. Sallam HN, Garcia-Velasco JA, Dias S, Arici A. Long-term pituitary down-regulation before in vitro fertilization (IVF) for women with endometriosis. Cochrane Database of Systematic Reviews 2006.
28. García-Velasco JA, Nikas G, Remohí J, Pellicer A, Simon C. Endometrial receptivity in terms of pinopode expression is not impaired in women with endometriosis in artificially prepared cycles. Fertil Steril 2001; 75: 1231-33.
29. Soares SR, Velasco JA, Fernandez M, Bosch E, Remohí J, Pellicer A, Simón C. Clinical factors affecting endometrial

receptiveness in oocyte donation cycles. Fertil Steril 2008; 89:491-501.

30. Diaz I, Navarro J, Blasco L, Simon C, Pellicer A, Remohi J. Impact of stage III-IV endometriosis on recipients of sibling oocytes: matched case-control study. Fertil Steril 2000;74: 31-34.

31. Cil AP, Oktem O, Oktay K. A meta-analytic comparison of oocyte vitrification to slow freezing: time trends and the current state of the technology. Fertil Steril 2008; 90: 269-70.

32. Cobo A, Kuwayama M, Pérez S, Ruiz A, Pellicer A, Remohí J. Comparison of concomitant outcome achieved with fresh and cryopreserved donor oocytes vitrified by the Cryotop method. Fertil Steril 2008;89: 1657-64.

33. Shai E, Elizur MD, Ri-Cheng Chian PD. Cryopreservation of oocytes in a young woman with severe and sympto-matic endometriosis: A new indication for fertility preservation. Fertil Steril 2009;91:293.e1-293.e3.

34. D'Hooghe T, Denys B, Spiessens C, Meuleman C, Debrock S. Is the endometriosis recurrence rate increased after ovarian hyperstimulation? Fertil Steril 2006; 86: 283-90.

35. Somigliana E, Vercellini P, Vigano P, Ragni G, Crosignani P. Should endometriomas be treated before IVF-ICSI cycles? Hum Reprod Update 2006;12:57-64.

36. Garcia-Velasco JA, Somigliana E. Management of endometriomas in women requiring IVF: to touch or not to touch. Hum Reprod 2009;24:496-501.

37. Garcia-Velasco JA, Mahutte NG, Corona J, Zúñiga V, Gilés J, Arici A, Pellicer A. Removal of endometriomas before in vitro fertilization does not improve fertility outcomes: a matched, case-control study. Fertil Steril 2004; 81: 1194-97.

38. Busacca M, Riparini J, Somigliana E, Oggioni G, Izzo S, Vignali M, Candiani M. Postsurgical ovarian failure after laparoscopic excision of bilateral endometriomas. Am J Obstet Gynecol 2006; 195: 421-25.

Section 5

Surgical Treatment

Charles Chapron, Bruno Borghese, Dominique de Ziegler

Chapter 19

What is Good Surgery for Endometriosis Patients?

Introduction

There are three anatomopathological types of endometriotic lesions: superficial endometriotic lesions (peritoneal and/or ovarian), endometriotic cysts (ovarian endometriomas (OMAs)), and deeply infiltrating lesions (DIE). DIE is a specific entity defined histologically as lesions that penetrate to a depth of 5 mm or more.[1] The pathogenesis of endometriosis is very controversial. Two main theories are proposed: that of regurgitation in which, secondary to reflux menstruation, endometrial cells implant and develop in ectopic locations, mainly in the pelvis;[2] and that of metaplasia,[3] which may involve either the peritoneal serosa[4] or Müllerian remnants[5] resulting in endometrial tissue in ectopic locations. Analysis of the anatomical distribution of endometriotic lesions is in favor of the regurgitation and implantation theory.[6]

Surgical treatment of superficial endometriotic lesions and ovarian endometriomas has been properly classified now: destruction of superficial endometriotic lesions is efficient with respect to pain,[7,8] whatever the technique used (excision or ablation),[9] and increases the chances for pregnancy',[10] intraperitoneal cystectomy via laparoscopy is the technique of reference today to treat OMAs: it reduces the risk of recurrence,[11] is efficient with respect to pain[10] and preserves the chances of fertility.[10] The same is not at all true for DIE treatment. This surgery is far more difficult, non classified, and there are no randomized prospective studies in the literature.

In this chapter we will concentrate on specifying the respective indications for the various treatment possibilities for patients presenting DIE. We will pay particular attention to the methods for surgical treatment, taking the characteristics of this pathology into account. Defining a good surgical treatment for patients presenting DIE requires in fact not only a definition of the pre and peroperative treatment modalities, but also the situations to be described for which there are alternative treatments.

Deeply Infiltrating Endometriosis: Two Major Specificities

DIE presents two essential specificities:

DIE is a Multifocal Pathology

Multifocality is a major characteristic of DIE lesions **(Table 19-1).**[12] Study of the anatomical distribution of DIE lesions pleads in favor of the regurgitation and implantation theory to explain its pathogenesis.[12] This multifocal distribution of DIE lesions is a factor of prime importance to be taken into account for management when surgical treatment is decided.[13]

DIE is Very Often Associated with Other Endometriotic Lesions

DIE lesions are isolated and unique in less than 10% of cases.[14] DIE lesions are associated with superficial lesions, endometriomas and/or adhesions in respectively 61.3%, 50.5% and 74.2% of cases.[14] We have shown that DIE lesions in our experience were associated with OMAs in one out of four cases.[15] When DIE lesions are associated with an OMA, the multifocality of the DIE lesions is greater, and the DIE lesions are more severe, with significantly more associated intestinal and ureteral lesions. In this situation surgical treatment will require more difficult procedures to be carried out, which are not without risk. Ovarian endometrioma must be considered as a marker for severity of DIE.[15]

These two characteristics are crucial when defining the modalities for surgical treatment. Because success of surgery is correlated to the radicality of the exeresis,[16] it is

Table 19-1: Deeply infiltrating endometriosis (n = 500 patients)*: Anatomical distribution of DIE lesions

| Main lesion[a] | N[b] | Associated lesions | | | | | | | Total[c] |
| | | USL | | | Va | Bl | Ur | In | |
		R	L	B					
USL	240	67	115	58					298 (32.2)
Vagina	82	12	12	12	82				132 (14.3)
Bladder	43	2	1	3	3	43			55 (5.9)
Intestine	118	20	17	28	71	10		198	372 (40.2)
Ureter	17	2	4	4	11	3	19	21	68 (7.4)
	500	103	149	106[d]	167	56	19	219	925

( ): values in parentheses are percentages.
[a]According to a previously published surgical classification for deeply infiltrating endometriosis (12)
[b]Number of patients
[c]Number of histologically proven deeply infiltrating endometriosis lesions
[d]Each lesion of bilateral pair counted as part of pair, so total number of individual lesions = 212.
Bl: Bladder; USL: Uterosacral ligament; Va: Vagina; Bl: Bladder; Ur: Ureter; In: Intestine; R: Right; L: Left; B: Bilateral
*: Adapted from Chapron et al[15]

absolutely necessary in this context to make a precise diagnosis of the location and type of endometriotic lesions prior to making the slightest decision.

Deeply Infiltrating Endometriosis: How to make a Correct DIE Diagnosis

Due to the DIE characteristics, there is a specific strategy for diagnosing DIE. The goal of the diagnostic phase, too often neglected, is to establish an accurate map of the location of the DIE lesions prior to any decision. Diagnosis of DIE relies on questioning, clinical examination and imaging investigations.

Questioning

Provided sufficient time is taken for a good quality interview establishing a climate of confidence between the practitioner and his patient, this first phase in the clinical examination is potentially very fruitful. In cases of DIE the main symptom is pelvic pain,[14] sometimes associated with infertility. The clinical symptoms (dysmenorrhea, deep dyspareunia, chronic pelvic pain, bowel and/or urinary functional symptoms, etc) are correlated with DIE lesions location.[15] Detailed questioning will tell the practitioner much about the topography of the DIE lesions, providing considerable help for prescription of the appropriate additional investigations.[17,18]

Clinical Examination

While bluish lesions located in the upper third of the posterior vaginal wall at speculum observation are pathognomonic for DIE, they are not systematically observed.[19] The lesions may present in less typical forms such as an irregular, reddish surface that bleeds easily on contact, or an area that seems "thickened, stiff and less mobile". Inspection via the speculum may also be strictly normal.[17]

During the vaginal touch, although a nodular lesion is the most standard form observed, this is by no means an absolute rule.[17, 18] In certain cases only the most primitive signs will be evident: lateral deviation of the cervix, asymmetry of the utero-sacral ligaments with an irregular, hardened and tense presentation instead of a nodule. The essential semiological point is that firm palpation of these lesions causes pain.

Normal clinical examination can in no way be considered as ruling out a diagnosis of DIE.[17, 18] The accuracy of clinical examination can be increased by carrying out the examination during menstruation.[18-21]

Radiological Work-up

The limits of questioning and clinical examination mean that additional investigations are absolutely essential to establish preoperatively an accurate map of the DIE lesions.[22] Rectal endoscopic ultrasonography (REUS) is a reliable means of diagnosing infiltration of the bowel wall.[20, 21] Magnetic resonance imaging (MRI) presents the great advantage of providing a complete work-up of both the anterior and posterior pelvic compartments at one time.[22, 23] This point is important because of the multifocality of DIE lesions.[12] For this main reason, MRI is, in our opinion, a key means of investigation in the preoperative work-up for patients presenting with DIE. In cases of ureteral involvement, which must be suspected for large, lateralized posterior DIE lesions,[24] MRI offers the possibility of diagnosing ureteral DIE with Uro-MRI shots. Today there is no indication for intravenous pyelography[25] in cases of suspected ureteral endometriosis.

In the preoperative radiological workup, the most recent development concerns the possibilities afforded by transvaginal ultrasonography (TVUS). The preliminary results for transvaginal ultrasonography are very encouraging, both for diagnosing pelvic endometriosis[26] and detecting bowel involvement.[27-29] These excellent results today support the statement that TVUS must be the first line radiological examination to use in cases of clinically suspected DIE. Although TVUS is efficient for the diagnosis of rectal involvement, this technique does give rise to two controversial points. Firstly, TVUS is an operator-dependant procedure. Specific training for the practitioners is essential to learn the DIE TVUS imaging semiology. Secondly, in our experience rectosigmoid lesions are associated with ileo-cecum DIE lesions (cecum and/or terminal ileum) in 28% of cases.[29] These "right bowel lesions" (cecum and/or ileum) will be more difficult to diagnose with TVUS. Studies are needed to find out if multislice computerized tomography is of interest in this context.[30]

The results afforded by properly conducted questioning and clinical investigation carried out under good conditions combined with the efficiency of complementary radiological investigations mean we can state that in 2009 there is no place for purely diagnostic laparoscopy in a context of suspected DIE.

Table 19-2: Deeply infiltrating endometriosis: Principles for surgical treatment

Principles

- Surgery only for symptomatic DIE lesions
- Patient's informed consent
- Multidisciplinary approach for diagnosis and treatment
- Complete surgical exeresis :
  - Of all symptomatic deep endometriotic lesions
  - One-step surgical procedure, each time this is possible
- Referral center for diagnosis, management and research

Deeply Infiltrating Endometriosis: What are the Therapeutic Options?

The treatment modalities for patients presenting with DIE are numerous: expectant management; reproductive endocrinology (ovarian stimulation, intrauterine insemination); surgery; assisted reproductive technologies (IVF, ICSI); association of medical and surgical treatment. The choice depends on the clinical context.

Context of Pelvic Pain

In a context of pelvic pain treatment may be surgical or medical.

Surgical treatment: DIE surgical treatment must comply with the five rules presented in **Table 19-2**. The DIE lesions anatomical distribution provides a basis for proposing a "surgical classification" for DIE, with the aim of establishing the methods for surgery **(Table 19-3)**.[13] In this classification, each location corresponds to a clearly

Table 19-3: Deeply infiltrating endometriosis: Classification according to Chapron.* Proposition for surgical procedure according to the classification

Classification	Operative procedure
A Anterior DIE	
A1: Bladder	**Laparoscopic partial cystectomy**
P: Posterior DIE	
P1: Uterosacral ligament	**Laparoscopic resection of USL**
P2: Vaginal	**Laparoscopically assisted vaginal resection of DIE infiltrating the posterior fornix**
P3: Intestinal	
P3a: Solely intestinal location	
- without vaginal infiltration (V-)	**Intestinal resection by laparoscopy or by laparotomy**
- with vaginal infiltration (V+)	**Laparoscopically assisted vaginal intestinal resection or exeresis by laparotomy.**
P3b: Multiple intestinal location	**Intestinal resection by laparotomy**

DIE: Deeply infiltrating endometriosis; USL: Uterosacral ligament
*: Adapted from Chapron *et al*[13]

Table 19-4: Deeply infiltrating endometriosis : Results of surgical treatment*			
1. *Subjective* evaluation			
	N	%	
* Improvement	148	97.4	
- Excellent	63	41.5	
- Satisfactory	66	43.4	
- Slight	19	12.5	
* No improvement	4	2.6	
2. *Objective* evaluation			
Symptoms	Pre-op	Post-op	Delta
Dysmenorrhea*	8.1 ± 1.8	2.8 ± 3.1	5.2 ± 3.5
Deep dyspareunia*	6.5 ± 2.2	1.9 ± 2.6	4.6 ± 3.0
Painful defecation*	6.6 ± 2.4	2.1 ± 2.8	4.5 ± 3.5
Urinary tract symptoms*	6.1 ± 2.1	1.2 ± 2.6	4.9 ± 3.2
Gastrointestinal symptoms*	6.8 ± 2.2	2.7 ± 3.1	4.1 ± 3.5
NCCPP*	7.5 ± 1.6	2.8 ± 3.6	4.8 ± 3.4

* : $p < 0.001$
Urinary tract symptoms: Hematuria, nonmicrobial cystitis, recurrent urinary tract infections, pain on urinating, pollakiuria, dysuria
Gastrointestinal symptoms: Diarrhea, constipation, rectal bleeding, proctitis, tenesmus, colic rectal pain
NCCPP: Non-cyclic chronic pelvic pain
* : adapted from Chopin *et al*[16]

established operating technique, which is reproducible and of proven efficiency. When there are multiple lesions various surgical procedures need to be associated. The multifocal nature of lesions may prompt the surgeon to favor laparotomy for selected cases in order to achieve complete surgical exeresis in a one-step surgical procedure.

When the principles for DIE surgical treatment, presented in **Table 19-2**, are applied, the results observed for pain are good in terms of both objective and subjective assessments **(Table 19-4)**.[16] These results are observed whatever the location of the main DIE lesion (uterosacral ligament, vagina, bladder or intestine) according to the "surgical classification".[16] Similar satisfactory results have been reported by other teams.[31-36] These good results should not make the risk of complications go overlooked. These are mainly of three types: (i) Gastro-intestinal tract fistulas; (ii) post-operative difficulties with bladder voiding function; (iii) recurrences because of an inadequate preliminary surgical procedure. In our experience the risk of fistulas is 2.5% (data in preparation). In order to keep the risk of bladder voiding dysfunction to a minimum, nerve sparing surgical procedures must be used as far as possible.[37, 38] The success of the operation is correlated with the radicality of surgical exeresis.[39-41]

Medical treatment: The good results obtained with surgical treatment do not mean however that there is no place left for a medical approach. In selected cases, medical treatment (oral contraceptive, progestogens, danazol, LH-RH analogs, etc) is also efficient and represents a reliable alternative to surgery. The various treatments available are of comparable efficiency.[42-45] The choice depends on the contraindications, side effects and cost.[46] The limits for medical treatments are their side effects and the desire for pregnancy.

The main indications for medical treatment are the following:

1. *Doubt about the diagnosis:* It is not appropriate to propose extensive surgery without being certain about the diagnosis of DIE. If the painful functional symptoms disappear with medical treatment, this is a strong semiological argument in favor of endometriosis being responsible for the pain.[47] In certain difficult diagnostic situations, this therapeutic test provides the means for avoiding potentially dangerous surgical procedures being carried out with a very doubtful promise of improvement.

2. *The patient who decides to refuse surgery:* In this context of functional pathology it is impossible to impose an operation with non negligible risks for these patients who are often young.[48] Proposing this type of operation to a patient who is not convinced of the need is neither reasonable nor possible.

3. Recurrence after initial surgical treatment that was carried out correctly. In women with recurrent pelvic

pain after surgical treatment, medical treatment must be the first choice option proposed as alternative to repeat surgery.[49,50]

4. *As a complement to surgery:* Today no studies have established whether or not preoperative medical treatment should be prescribed. After surgery there would appear to be advantages in prescribing postoperative medical treatment.[51] Medical treatments do not reduce the risk of recurrence but they do increase the length of time before recurrence.[45]

Context of Infertility

In a context of infertility there is no place for medical treatments—they do not increase the chances for pregnancy and indeed delay this occurring for as long as they last.[52,53] The only two possibilities are surgery and assisted reproductive technologies (ART). If the infertility is isolated, meaning there is no significant associated pelvic pain, ART can be the first option. If the infertility is associated with pelvic pain, surgery enables 50% of patients to obtain pregnancy whether the procedure is carried out by laparotomy[54, 55] or laparoscopy,[54, 55] with an efficiency of 80 to 85% with respect to the pelvic pain. Just as for pain management, the fertility results are significantly increased when surgical exeresis of the lesions is total.[56] In this context, the risk of ART is that there may be a phase where the disease progresses to the point of needing treatment to be halted, or even requiring emergency surgery.[57] Further studies are essential concerning DIE-associated infertility in order to clarify the respective places for surgery and ART.

Conclusion

A work-up to establish the extent of the disease is indispensable. The goal is to establish a precise map of the lesions preoperatively. DIE treatment may be surgical or medical, each of these approaches having specific indications. In case of surgery, success of the treatment will depend on how radical exeresis is. The methods used for surgery are dictated by the location, extent and multifocal nature of the DIE lesions. Further studies are required in order to specify the place and modalities of pre - and postoperative medical treatments.

DIE lesions multifocality prompts us to cease considering DIE as a pathology affecting organs (vaginal, bowel, ureteral or bladder endometriosis, etc) but instead to see it as an "abdomino-pelvic multifocal pathology". This is the major reason why management of both diagnosis

and treatment must be multidisciplinary. DIE treatment must not focus on a single organ, but should allow management of all the different locations in one-step.

Defining what a good surgical treatment is for endometriotic patients is not limited to specifying the surgical procedures. It requires a global approach to the problem, for which the patient deserves to be managed by a surgeon who is not only technically competent but also open to the other treatment possibilities, after making a comprehensive workup for the situation.

References

1. Cornillie FJ, Oosterlynck D, Lauweryns JM, Koninckx PR. Deeply infiltrating pelvic endometriosis: histology and clinical significance. Fertil Steril 1990;53:978-83.
2. Sampson JA. Peritoneal endometriosis due to premenstrual dissemination of endometrial tissue into the peritoneal cavity. Am J Obstet Gynecol 1927;14:422-69.
3. Meyer R. Ueber den stand der Frage der Adenomyositis und Adenomyome in algemeinen und insbesondere über Adenomyositis serosoepithelialis und Adenomyometritis sarcomatosa. Zentralbl Gynäkol 1919;43:745-50.
4. Gruenwald P. Origin of endometriosis from mesenchyme of the coelomic walls. Am J Obstst Gynecol 1942;44:470-74.
5. Donnez J, Nisolle M, Casanas-Roux F, Bassil S, Anaf V. Rectovaginal septum, endometriosis or adenomyosis: laparoscopic management in a series of 231 patients. Hum Reprod 1995;10:630-35.
6. Bricou A, Batt RE, Chapron C. Peritoneal fluid flow influences anatomical distribution of endometriotic lesions: why Sampson seems to be right. Eur J Obstet Gynecol Reprod Biol 2008;138:127-34.
7. Sutton CJ, Ewen SP, Whitelaw N, Haines P. Prospective, randomized, double-blind, controlled trial of laser laparoscopy in the treatment of pelvic pain associated with minimal, mild, and moderate endometriosis. Fertil Steril 1994;62:696-700.
8. Abbott J, Hawe J, Hunter D, Holmes M, Finn P, Garry R. Laparoscopic excision of endometriosis: a randomized, placebo-controlled trial. Fertil Steril 2004;82:878-84.
9. Wright J, Lotfallah H, Jones K, Lovell D. A randomized trial of excision versus ablation for mild endometriosis. Fertil Steril 2005;83:1830-36.
10. Hart RJ, Hickey M, Maouris P, Buckett W, Garry R. Excisional surgery versus ablative surgery for ovarian endometriomata. Cochrane Database Syst Rev 2005: CD004992.
11. Vercellini P, Chapron C, De Giorgi O, Consonni D, Frontino G, Crosignani PG. Coagulation or excision of ovarian endometriomas? Am J Obstet Gynecol 2003;188:606-10.
12. Chapron C, Chopin N, Borghese B, Foulot H, Dousset B, Vacher-Lavenu MC, et al. Deeply infiltrating endometriosis: pathogenetic implications of the anatomical distribution. Hum Reprod 2006;21:1839-45.
13. Chapron C, Fauconnier A, Vieira M, Barakat H, Dousset B, Pansini V, et al. Anatomical distribution of deeply

infiltrating endometriosis: surgical implications and proposition for a classification. Hum Reprod 2003;18:157-61.

14. Somigliana E, Infantino M, Candiani M, Vignali M, Chiodini A, Busacca M. Association rate between deep peritoneal endometriosis and other forms of the disease: pathogenetic implications. Hum Reprod. 2004;19:168-71.

15. Chapron C, Pietin-Vialle C, Borghese B, Davy C, Foulot H, Chopin N. Associated ovarian endometriomas is a marker for greater severity of deeply infiltrating endometriosis. Fertil Steril (in press).

16. Chopin N, Vieira M, Borghese B, Foulot H, Dousset B, Coste J, et al. Operative management of deeply infiltrating endometriosis: results on pelvic pain symptoms according to a surgical classification. J Minim Invasive Gynecol 2005;12:106-12.

17. Chapron C, Barakat H, Fritel X, Dubuisson JB, Breart G, Fauconnier A. Presurgical diagnosis of posterior deep infiltrating endometriosis based on a standardized questionnaire. Hum Reprod 2005;20:507-13.

18. Fedele L, Bianchi S, Carmignani L, Berlanda N, Fontana E, Frontino G. Evaluation of a new questionnaire for the presurgical diagnosis of bladder endometriosis. Hum Reprod 2007;22:2698-701.

19. Chapron C, Dubuisson JB, Pansini V, Vieira M, Fauconnier A, Dousset B. Routine clinical examination is not sufficient for the diagnosis and establishing the location of deeply infiltrating endometriosis. J Am Assoc Gynecol Laparosc 2002;9:115-19.

20. Chapron C, Dumontier I, Dousset B, Fritel X, Tardif D, Roseau G, et al. Results and role of rectal endoscopic ultrasonography for patients with deep pelvic endometriosis. Hum Reprod 1998;13:2266-70.

21. Fedele L, Bianchi S, Portuese A, Borruto F, Dorta M. Transrectal ultrasonography in the assessment of rectovaginal endometriosis. Obstet Gynecol 1998;91:444-48.

22. Kinkel K, Chapron C, Balleyguier C, Fritel X, Dubuisson JB, Moreau JF. Magnetic resonance imaging characteristics of deep endometriosis. Hum Reprod 1999;14:1080-86.

23. Bazot M, Darai E, Hourani R, Thomassin I, Cortez A, Uzan S, et al. Deep Pelvic Endometriosis: MR Imaging for Diagnosis and Prediction of Extension of Disease. Radiology 2004;232:379-89.

24. Donnez J, Nisolle M, Squifflet J. Ureteral endometriosis: a complication of rectovaginal endometriotic (adenomyotic) nodules. Fertil Steril 2002;77:32-37.

25. Balleyguier C, Roupret M, Nguyen T, Kinkel K, Helenon O, Chapron C. Ureteral endometriosis: the role of magnetic resonance imaging. J Am Assoc Gynecol Laparosc 2004;11:530-36.

26. Bazot M, Thomassin I, Hourani R, Cortez A, Darai E. Diagnostic accuracy of transvaginal sonography for deep pelvic endometriosis. Ultrasound Obstet Gynecol 2004; 24:180-85.

27. Bazot M, Detchev R, Cortez A, Amouyal P, Uzan S, Darai E. Transvaginal sonography and rectal endoscopic sonography for the assessment of pelvic endometriosis: a preliminary comparison. Hum Reprod 2003;18:1686-92.

28. Abrao MS, Goncalves MO, Dias JA, Jr., Podgaec S, Chamie LP, Blasbalg R. Comparison between clinical examination, transvaginal sonography and magnetic resonance imaging for the diagnosis of deep endometriosis. Hum Reprod 2007;22:3092-97.

29. Piketty M, Chopin N, Dousset B, Millischer-Bellaische AE, Roseau G, Leconte M, et al. Preoperative work-up for patients with deeply infiltrating endometriosis: transvaginal ultrasonography must definitely be the first-line imaging examination. Hum Reprod (in press).

30. Biscaldi E, Ferrero S, Fulcheri E, Ragni N, Remorgida V, Rollandi GA. Multislice CT enteroclysis in the diagnosis of bowel endometriosis. Eur Radiol 2007;17:211-19.

31. Redwine DB, Wright JT. Laparoscopic treatment of complete obliteration of the cul-de-sac associated with endometriosis: long-term follow-up of en bloc resection. Fertil Steril 2001;76:358-65.

32. Abbott JA, Hawe J, Clayton RD, Garry R. The effects and effectiveness of laparoscopic excision of endometriosis: a prospective study with 2-5 year follow-up. Hum Reprod 2003;18:1922-27.

33. Ford J, English J, Miles WA, Giannopoulos T. Pain, quality of life and complications following the radical resection of rectovaginal endometriosis. Bjog 2004;111:353-56.

34. Hollett-Caines J, Vilos GA, Penava DA. Laparoscopic mobilization of the rectosigmoid and excision of the obliterated cul-de-sac. J Am Assos Gynecol Laparosc 2003;10:190-94.

35. Anaf V, Simon P, El Nakadi I, Simonart T, Noel J, Buxant F. Impact of surgical resection of rectovaginal pouch of douglas endometriotic nodules on pelvic pain and some elements of patients' sex life. J Am Assoc Gynecol Laparosc 2001;8:55-60.

36. Dubernard G, Piketty M, Rouzier R, Houry S, Bazot M, Darai E. Quality of life after laparoscopic colorectal resection for endometriosis. Hum Reprod 2006;21:1243-47.

37. Landi S, Ceccaroni M, Perutelli A, Allodi C, Barbieri F, Fiaccavento A, et al. Laparoscopic nerve-sparing complete excision of deep endometriosis: is it feasible? Hum Reprod 2006;21:774-81.

38. Possover M, Quakernack J, Chiantera V. The LANN technique to reduce postoperative functional morbidity in laparoscopic radical pelvic surgery. J Am Coll Surg 2005;201:913-17.

39. Garry R. Laparoscopic excision of endometriosis: the treatment of choice? Br J Obstet Gynaecol 1997;104:513-15.

40. Vignali M, Bianchi S, Candiani M, Spadacini G, Oggioni G, Busacca M. Surgical treatment of deep endometriosis and risk of recurrence. J Minim Invasive Gynecol 2005; 12:508-13.

41. Fedele L, Bianchi S, Zanconato G, Berlanda N, Borruto F, Frontino G. Tailoring radicality in demolitive surgery for deeply infiltrating endometriosis. Am J Obstet Gynecol 2005;193:114-17.

42. Kennedy S, Bergqvist A, Chapron C, D'Hooghe T, Dunselman G, Greb R, et al. ESHRE guideline for the diagnosis and treatment of endometriosis. Hum Reprod 2005;20:2698-704.

43. Ozawa Y, Murakami T, Terada Y, Yaegashi N, Okamura K, Kuriyama S, et al. Management of the pain associated with endometriosis: an update of the painful problems. Tohoku J Exp Med 2006;210:175-88.

44. Olive DL, Pritts EA. Treatment of endometriosis. N Engl J Med 2001;345:266-75.

45. Vercellini P, Cortesi I, Crosignani PG. Progestins for symptomatic endometriosis: a critical analysis of the evidence. Fertil Steril 1997;68:393-401.

46. Vercellini P, Cortesi I, Crosignani PG. Progestins for symptomatic endometriosis: a critical analysis of the evidence. Fertil Steril 1997;68:393-401.

47. Hurd WW. Criteria that indicate endometriosis is the cause of chronic pelvic pain [see comments]. Obstet Gynecol 1998;92:1029-32.

48. Koninckx PR, Timmermans B, Meuleman C, Penninckx F. Complications of CO_2-laser endoscopic excision of deep endometriosis. Hum Reprod 1996;11:2263-68.

49. Vercellini P, Pietropaolo G, De Giorgi O, Pasin R, Chiodini A, Crosignani PG. Treatment of symptomatic rectovaginal endometriosis with an estrogen-progestogen combination versus low-dose norethindrone acetate. Fertil Steril 2005; 84:1375-87.

50. Razzi S, Luisi S, Calonaci F, Altomare A, Bocchi C, Petraglia F. Efficacy of vaginal danazol treatment in women with recurrent deeply infiltrating endometriosis. Fertil Steril 2007;88:789-94.

51. Sesti F, Pietropolli A, Capozzolo T, Broccoli P, Pierangeli S, Bollea MR, et al. Hormonal suppression treatment or dietary therapy versus placebo in the control of painful symptoms after conservative surgery for endometriosis stage III-IV. A randomized comparative trial. Fertil Steril 2007;88:1541-47.

52. Adamson GD, Pasta DJ. Surgical treatment of endometriosis-associated infertility: meta-analysis compared with survival analysis. Am J Obstet Gynecol 1994;171:1488-504; discussion 504-05.

53. Olive DL, Lindheim SR, Pritts EA. Endometriosis and infertility: what do we do for each stage? Curr Womens Health Rep 2003;3:389-94.

54. Bailey HR, Ott MT, Hartendorp P. Aggressive surgical management for advanced colorectal endometriosis. Dis Colon Rectum 1994;37:747-53.

55. Coronado C, Franklin RR, Lotze EC, Bailey HR, Valdes CT. Surgical treatment of symptomatic colorectal endometriosis. Fertil Steril 1990;53:411-16.

56. Suginami H, Tokushige M, Taniguchi F, Kitaoka Y. Complete removal of endometriosis improves fecundity. Gynecol Obstet Invest 2002;53 Suppl 1:12-18.

57. Anaf V, El Nakadi I, Simon P, Englert Y, Peny MO, Fayt I, et al. Sigmoid endometriosis and ovarian stimulation. Hum Reprod 2000;15:790-94.

Michelle Nisolle, P Nervo

Chapter 20

Risk of Recurrence after Surgery

Introduction

Endometriosis has been studied for years. It is usually considered as a benign disease and as a recurrent condition which is nearly impossible to cure completely. However, fundamental research has improved our understanding of the disease. Nisolle et al have shown that endometrial cells that were transplanted to ectopic sites had features of neoplastic cells, i.e. the ability to proliferate, to migrate, to induce angiogenesis and to cause reactive fibrosis.[1] This may explain the high rate of recurrence of the disease after surgical treatment and should be kept in mind for the management of patients suffering from infertility or pelvic pain due to endometriosis. The aim of this chapter is to review the rate and risk factors of recurrence of ovarian and deep infiltrating endometriosis after surgery, and to discuss its medical and surgical treatment.

Definition

"Reccurent lesions" after medical or surgical treatment have to be distinguished from "persistent lesions". The former refer to "de novo" formation of endometriotic lesions after complete surgical resection, while the latter result from their incomplete surgical removal and their reactivation once medical therapy is discontinued or once some time has elapsed after surgery. Complete removal of endometriotic lesions may be very difficult to perform, even for experienced surgeons, and requires technical skills, training and adequate knowledge of the pathology. In addition, the rate of recurrence is not accurately known. This is partly due to the lack of clear definitions for recurrent endometriosis. Several criteria have been used.
- The recurrence of symptoms.
- The presence of deep infiltrating endometriosis (DIE) at clinical examination.
- The presence of endometrioma at ultrasonography or magnetic resonance imaging (MRI).
- The presence of DIE at MRI.
- The presence of endometriotic lesions at repeat laparoscopy with histological confirmation.

Rate of Recurrence and Risk Factors

Several studies have investigated the rate of recurrence and the risk factors. Different numbers have been reported with different periods of follow up.

In 1987, Wheeler and Malinak reported a recurrence rate of 19.5% five years after surgery and of 31.6% seven years post-operatively.[2] According to Waller and Shaw, recurrence was found in 53% of patients 5 years after surgery, with 37% in stage I-II and 74% in stage III-IV of the r-AFS (revised American Fertility Society) classification.[3]

In a large study on 458 patients who underwent laparoscopic excision of ovarian endometrioma, Busacca et al reported a cumulative rate of recurrence of 3.0%, 6% and 11.7% diagnosed by ultrasonography after 1, 2 and 4 year(s) respectively.[4] They identified the stage of the disease and a previous surgical treatment as risk factors for recurrence.

In a prospective cohort multicenter study, Parazzini et al investigated clinically detectable endometriosis.[5] The overall clinical recurrence of endometriosis was 4.6% after one year and 9.0% after 2 years. However this could be confirmed at surgery in only 3.3% and 6.3% of cases respectively. For ovarian endometriosis, the recurrence rate was 7.1% after one year and 11.3% after 2 years. In that study, age was a relevant but not statistically significant factor as only 4.6% of women less than 30 years old had recurrent endometriosis in comparison to 13.1% of women over 30. However, a statistically significant difference was observed between stages of endometriosis: after 2 years, the recurrence rate was 5.7% for patients with stage I-II and 14.4% for those with stage III-IV (p< 0.05) endometriosis. The authors concluded that recurrence rate of clinically detectable endometriosis was higher in women in advanced stages of the disease at first surgery.

Kikuchi et al reported a rate of recurrence of ovarian endometrioma (diagnosed by ultrasonography) after laparoscopic cystectomy of 15.9% for a period of follow up of 21.4 ± 16.8 months.[6] The cumulative recurrence rate per patient was 31.7% in 60 months. Young age and severe endometriosis at first laparoscopy were identified as risk factors.

In a series of 224 patients who underwent laparoscopic excision of endometrioma, Koga et al observed a high recurrence rate of 30% when using a cut off value of 2 cm for the size of endometrioma at ultrasonography.[7] Previous medical therapy of endometriosis and the presence of large cystic lesion(s) at first laparoscopy were associated with a higher recurrence rate while post-operative pregnancy seemed to be protective.

Recently, Liu et al, using survival analysis, researched on 20 potential risk factors for recurrence of endometrioma and dysmenorrhea in a sample of 710 patients.[8] For endometrioma, 3 risk factors were identified: a high revised American Fertility Society (r-AFS) score, young age at surgery, and previous medical treatment of endometriosis. For dysmenorrhea, only a high r-AFS score increased the risk.

Very recently, Cheong et al observed retrospectively the rate of repeated surgery in women with endometriosis over a 10-year period.[9] In 486 patients undergoing a second surgery, the reasons for intervention were pelvic pain (49%) and sub-fertility (51%). A second intervention was less likely in older women, or when a pregnancy had been achieved, or when symptoms had improved.

In a prospective observational study of 166 women who underwent complete laparoscopic excision of endometrioma, Porpora et al reported a recurrence of ovarian endometrioma in 9.6% of patients.[10] Risk factors of recurrence were a previous surgery, the presence of adhesions and the use of ovulation drugs.

In summary, according to the above studies, a young age and a high total r-AFS score appear to be the most relevant risk factors for recurrent endometriosis. Pregnancy should be protective. However, the use of the rAFS score to predict the risk has not reached agreement between authors. Vercellini et al concluded that the r-AFS classification was not useful to predict the recurrence of symptoms of endometriosis.[11] On 729 women undergoing conservative laparoscopic surgery, the cumulative probability of moderate or severe dysmenorrhea recurrence was 24% in 425 symptomatic women. While, referring to the r-AFS score, 32% women had a stage I endometriosis, 24% a stage II, 21% a stage III and 19% a stage IV (p =0.094). Recently, the poor prognostic value of the r-AFS scoring system was corroborated by Liu et al.[8] Finally, assessment of risk factors of recurrence after surgical management of DIE is unfortunately lacking in the literature.

Place of Medical Therapy

The administration of medical treatment pre- and post-operatively, or both, to prevent recurrence of symptoms of endometriosis and to delay the need for additional treatment has been investigated.

Preoperative Medical Therapy

Preoperative medical therapy for 3 months aims to decrease the severity of endometriosis and the size of endometrioma, in order to facilitate laparoscopic removal of the lesions. This was reported in two studies by Hemmings et al and by Donnez et al.[12,13] Comparing a group of 40 infertile patients receiving a subcutaneous GnRH analog (goserelin) implant four times a week for 12 weeks, with a group of 40 infertile patients who did not receive any medication, Donnez et al showed a statistically significant effect of treatment in reducing total AFS scores (weighted mean difference (WMD) of – 9.60; 95% CI, –11.42 to –7.78).[13] There was also a statistically significant reduction in implant AFS scores (WMD, –8.70; 95% CI, –10.67 to –6.73). No beneficial effect was observed in the adhesion AFS scores (WMD, –0.90; 95% CI, –3.42 to 1.62). Unfortunately, according to Donnez et al, preoperative medical therapy nor reduced recurrence rates neither increased pregnancy rates. On the contrary, Liu et al concluded to a negative effect of medical therapy before surgery.[8] This was also suggested by Koga et al.[9] An estimated odd ratio of 1.9 was reported by these authors. Under medical treatment, morphologic changes of the endometriotic lesions have been observed such as atrophy, and reduction in size and in vascularization. This may impact negatively the detection of lesions. Undetected lesions are not removed during first laparoscopy and cause future recurrence. In addition, medical therapy induces atrophy of the hormonally dependent ectopic endometrium. After discontinuation of therapy, endometriotic foci regain activity. In consequence, medical treatment is often associated with surgical management.

Postoperative Medical Therapy

A 3 to 6 months postoperative medical therapy aims to treat microscopic endometriosis which was not visible at surgery or macroscopic lesions that could not be completely removed.[14,15] A systematic review of 8 randomized control trials (RCTs) comparing postoperative medical therapy with surgery alone and with surgery plus placebo was published by Yap et al in the Cochrane Library in 2004.[16] Postoperative medical therapy (danazol, GnRHa, oral contraceptive pill), when compared with surgery alone, did not reduce significantly the recurrence of pain after 12 months while significance was reached after 24 months. There was no evidence of decreased recurrence of the disease after medical therapies. On the other hand, postoperative medical therapy with surgery plus placebo had no effect. In their meta-analysis, Yap et al concluded that post-operative medical therapy, when compared with surgery alone or with surgery plus placebo, was not associated with an improvement of pelvic pain, a higher pregnancy rate and a lower rate of recurrence.

This was confirmed recently in another study by Loverro et al.[17] Their RCT showed that GnRHa treatment after laparoscopy in patients with stage III/IV endometriosis was not superior to placebo to prevent recurrence of symptoms and relapse of endometrioma. In a recent retrospective cohort study by Jee et al, a reduction of recurrence was noticed in patients treated with GnRH agonists for 3 to 6 months after conservative laparoscopic surgery of stage III/IV ovarian endometrioma, but it did not reach statistical significance.[18] Recurrence was delayed by 2 and by 5 months when given for 3 months and for 4 to 6 months respectively.

Very recently Vercellini et al suggested that postoperative use of a cyclic, low-dose, monophasic oral contraceptive pill effectively prevents endometrioma recurrence.[19] The recurrence rate was 27%. However, the cumulative proportion of subjects free from endometrioma after 36 months was 94% when contraceptive pills were used and 51% when they were not (p<0.001). The absolute risk reduction of endometrioma recurrence in "always users" compared with "never users" was 47% (95% CI, 37-57). This means that regular postoperative use of an estrogen-progestin combination would prevent endometrioma recurrence in 1 out of 2 patients (95% CI,0.2-7) three years after surgery, with a relative risk reduction of 80%. This observation is in contradiction with Muzzi's study.[20] In a RCT comparing the use of adjuvant oral contraceptive pill for 6 months with no medical treatment after laparoscopic excision of ovarian endometrioma, no significant difference was noticed in the long-term recurrence rate of cysts. Therefore, randomized controlled trials are required to confirm the results of Vercellini et al before post-operative long term ovarian suppression with estrogen-progestin can be recommended after endometrioma surgery.[19]

Comparison between Preoperative or Postoperative Medical Therapy

In a study of 55 women with endometriosis, Audebert et al compared the benefits of medical therapy (intranasal nafarelin for 6 months) administered before or after surgery.[21] In cases with stage III-IV endometriosis, pain was not improved significantly.

Place of Surgery

The complete removal of endometriotic lesions at the first surgical procedure seems to be the key point for successful treatment.

Ovarian Endometrioma

Simple cyst aspiration has been associated with a high rate of recurrence or persistence. This procedure is not an efficient surgical procedure of ovarian endometrioma and is not recommended. Two other procedures have been described for the management of ovarian endometrioma: the "endometrioma excision" which consists to remove the cyst wall from the ovarian cortex by sharp excision, and the "endometrioma ablation" where the cyst wall is destroyed by using several sources of energy (laser vaporization or electrocautery coagulation). Both procedures can be performed by laparotomy or by laparoscopy. In their retrospective study on ovarian endometrioma surgery, Hemmings et al showed that similar recurrence rate could be expected when cystectomy was performed by laparotomy (9% at 1 year) and by laparoscopy (8% at 1 year).[22] The recurrence rate of endometrioma after one year per surgical procedure can be found in **Table 20-1**.

In 2003, Vercellini et al, reviewed four trials[22,24-26] and concluded that endometrioma was more likely to reccur in women treated with electrocautery coagulation or laser vaporization (18.4%) than in women who underwent sharp cystectomy (6.4%).[23] The ORs of endometrioma recurrence for the 4 studies ranged from 1.41 to 9.38. The common OR was 3.09 (95% CI 1.78-5.36), suggesting that coagulation or vaporization without excision of the cyst wall considerably increases the risk of cyst recurrence.

Table 20-1: Recurrence rate of endometrioma after one year per surgical procedure

Author	Type of study	Excision	Ablation
Hemmings et al,[22] 1998	Retrospective	8 %	12 %
Beretta et al,[25] 1998	RCT	6 %	18 %
Saleh and Tulandi,[26] 1999	Retrospective	6.1 %	21.9 %
Alborzi et al,[28] 2004	RCT	5.8 %	22.9 %

A meta-analysis was performed by Hart et al to assess whether laparoscopic surgical excision or ablation of endometriomas was optimal to improve pain and fertility, the primary outcomes of the study.[27] Secondary outcomesd were the recurrence rate of endometriomas. Only 2 prospective RCTs fulfilled the inclusion criteria (randomization at the time of surgery by computer randomization; patient's and surgeon's awareness of the type of procedure that had been performed).[25,28] In both studies, the recurrence rate of ovarian endometrioma was recorded by ultrasound examination every 3 months for the first year, then every 6 months (Alborzi et al) or every 12 months (Beretta et al). The authors assessed also whether a second surgery was required after the initial laparoscopic procedure. In both studies, the 2 laparoscopic procedures of endometriomas management resulted in relief of pelvic pain in all cases. The recurrence of dysmenorrhea and pelvic pain was significantly greater in the drainage and ablation group in both studies. The laparoscopic excision of ovarian endometrioma was associated with a reduction of recurrence of dysmenorrhea (OR 0.15, CI 0.06-0.38), of dyspareunia (OR 0.14, CI 0.05-0.44) and of non-menstrual pelvic pain (OR 0.10, CI 0.02-0.56). Endometrioma was less likely to recur (OR 0.41, CI 0.18-0.93) after sharp excision of endometriomas than after drainage and coagulation. Hart et al concluded there was some evidence that excisional surgery for endometriomas is better than drainage and ablation to reduce recurrence of the endometrioma and symptoms.[27]

Deep Infiltrating Endometriosis

Most publications about DIE involving the rectum referred to the surgical technique, clinical improvements and complications, but little information could be found about the recurrence rate after surgery.

In cases of DIE involving the cul de sac of Douglas and the rectum, different laparoscopic procedures have been recommended: the "shaving technique" without bowel resection, the segmental rectal resection, and the full-thickness rectal disk excision.[29] In the literature, there are no RCTs studying radical excision of DIE involving the rectum, and comparing it with no rectal amputation. It has been reported that complete removal of DIE is associated with improvement of pelvic pain. Validated questionnaires have shown that quality of life can be improved.[30] Excision of posterior vaginal fornix in cases of DIE without rectal involvement was found to be beneficial to reduce postoperative pelvic pain.[31]

Recurrence associated with DIE seems to be higher than that observed after surgical removal of ovarian (12% at 4 years) and peritoneal endometriosis (19% at 5 years). This is clearly related to the technical difficulties encountered during surgery due to severe fibrosis involving several pelvic structures and impeding complete removal of endometriotic lesions. In some cases, incomplete removal of lesions was elected because of the severity of complications that might occur after bowel resection and anastomosis.[32]

In a series of 83 women who underwent surgery for rectovaginal endometriosis, Fedele et al reported that, 36 months after surgery, pain recurred in 28% of patients, and clinical signs or ultrasonographic lesions in 34%. A new treatment was required in 27% of cases.[33] A higher risk of recurrence was observed in younger women and when bowel endometriosis was not removed. As already mentioned for ovarian endometriosis, a distinction between residual and recurrent disease is crucial especially in DIE involving the rectum. In a series of 95 women, undergoing laparoscopic colorectal resection, a recurrence rate of 5.3% was observed.[34] Similar numbers were reported by Panel et al (4.8%) in a series of 21 women after a follow up of 13 months.[35] Daraï et al measured a rate of 16.4% by using a post-operative questionnaire.[32]

The relationship between inadequate surgical procedure (incomplete removal of endometriotic lesions) and the risk of pelvic pain was confirmed by Vignali et al in a retrospective study with a follow-up of at least 12 months.[36] Among 115 symptomatic patients who underwent conservative surgery for DIE, 28 patients had pain recurrence, 15 demonstrated recurrent clinical signs, and 12 required reoperation for DIE. Recurrence rates of pain and clinical signs after 36 months were 20.5% and 9% respectively. By multivariate analysis the authors demonstrated that only the age was a significant predictor of pain recurrence (OR 0.9, 95% CI 0.81-0.99, p<0.5), younger patients being at higher risk. In DIE, obliteration of the pouch of Douglas increased the risk of recurrence of clinical signs (OR 1.46, 95% CI 1.16-16.2, p<0.5), and patients were more likely to be re-operated after an incomplete surgical removal at first operation (OR 21.9, 95% CI 3.2-146.5, p<0.001).

Conservative treatment of recto-vaginal endometriosis necessitates a difficult and challenging surgery with potential complications. The ability to perform complete eradication of endometrioc lesions may have significant influence on the recurrence of the disease. Carmona et al recently demonstrated that an increasing learning curve was associated with a decrease of recurrence rate.[37] In a series of 213 rectal procedures, Brouwer and Woods described a recurrence rate of 22.2% (95% CI (2.5-4.0)) after dissection of the rectal wall.[38] It was significantly lower in cases of anterior wall excision (5.17%; CI 95%; 0.0-10.9) and in cases of segmental rectal resection (2.19%; CI 95%; 0.0-4.6). The overall rectal recurrence was 4.69% (95% CI;1.8-7.5).

Surgeons in favor of the shaving technique justify their choice not to excise the bowel by the likely stability of the remaining lesions ("fibrosis" is not expected to progress with time). However, it is very difficult to prove that lesions do not worsen. The absence of recurrence of pelvic pain could support this hypothesis. Imaging is not suitable to study the evolution of the lesions. On the contrary, histological analysis of bowel endometriosis specimens could assess with precision the degree of infiltration in the different layers of the bowel wall and link the completeness of surgical removal with recurrence. Results of histological studies are shown in **Table 20-2**. Infiltration of the different layers of the bowel wall was considered positive when endometriotic glands surrounded by scanty

stroma were noticed. Fibrosis or smooth muscle hyperplasia are possible findings associated with endometriotic lesions . In the different studies, the serosa and the muscular layer were infiltrated by endometriotic glands in 100% of cases. The infiltration of the submucosal layer was present in 34 to 68% of cases. However mucosal infiltration was less frequently encountered (10 to 38% of cases). In the series of Brouwer and Woods, extension of lesion into the submucosa was present in 36% of cases. In conclusion, by using the shaving technique, complete removal of endometriotic lesions is unlikely as only a part of the muscular layer is amputated. This could explain the higher recurrence with this technique.

Conclusion

Recurrence of endometriosis is a complication that surgeons must be aware of.

So far, no well-designed studies have demonstrated the efficacy of peri-operative medical therapy to reduce recurrence of the symptoms or the disease. Further studies, especially in women suffering from large endometriomas or deep infiltrating endometriosis with or without bowel infiltration, are required to clarify the indications of medical therapy in association with a surgical intervention.

According to the literature, incomplete removal of the lesions seems to be the main cause of recurrence after surgery. Differences in the recurrence rate have been observed between peritoneal, ovarian and DIE with or without bowel infiltration. The age of the patient at first surgery is also determinant and could justify a more radical treatment (bowel resection instead of shaving), taking into account the morbidity related to the surgery.

Surgical techniques for endometriosis are advanced and complex and necessitate a long training. The benefits must balance the risks and complexity of the procedure. Benefits are well-known and include improvement of clinical signs and fertility. Complications vary with anatomical regions. Surgery might induce ovarian lesions that result in an impaired ovarian function, especially if the procedure is

Table 20-2: Colorectal resection: histological analysis of bowel wall infiltration by endometriotic lesions				
Authors	*Serosal layer*	*Muscular layer*	*Submucosal layer*	*Mucosal layer*
Kavallaris et al,[39] 2003	100%	100%	34%	10%
Anaf et al,[40] 2004	100%	100%	68%	26%
Abrao et al,[41] 2006	100%	40%	37.1%	22.9%
Nisolle et al (unpublished data)	100%	100%	61%	38.8%

repeated. If lesions involve resection of the rectum or the sigmoid junction, post-operative leakage and dehiscence may occur at the suture line and necessitates a colostomy.

Therefore, this surgery should be performed only in referral centers where specialists of different disciplines (gynecologists, urologists, surgeons) can collaborate. This will insure an optimal service and limit complications and postoperative recurrence.

References

1. Nisolle M, Alvarez ML, Colombo M, Foidart JM. Pathogenesis of endometriosis. Gynecol obstet Fertil. 2007; 35: 898-903.

2. Wheeler JM, Malinak LR. Recurrent endometriosis: incidence, management and prognosis. Am J Obstet Gynecol 1983; 146: 247-50.

3. Waller KG, Shaw RW. Gonadotropin releasing hormone analogues for the treatment of endometriosis: long term follow-up. Fertil Steril 1993; 59:511-15.

4. Busacca M, Marana R, Caruana P, Candiani M, Muzii L, Calia C et al. Recurrence of ovarian endometrioma after laparoscopic excision. Am J Obstet Gynecol 1999; 180:519-23.

5. Parazzini F, Bertulessi C, Pasini A, Rosati M, Di Stefano F et al. Determinants of short term recurrence rate of endometriosis. Eur J of Obstet Gynecol and Reprod Biol 2005; 121: 216-19.

6. Kikuchi I, Takeuchi H, Kitade M, Shimanuki H, Kumakiri J, Kinoshita K. Recurrence rate of endometriomas following a laparoscopic cystectomy. Acta Obstet Gynecol Scand 2006; 85: 1120-24.

7. Koga K, Takemura Y, Osuga Y, Yoshino O, Hirota Y, Hirata T, Morimoto C, Harada M, Yano T, Taketani Y. Recurrence of ovarian endometrioma after laparoscopic excision. Hum reprod 2006; 21: 2171-74.

8. Liu X, Yuan L, Shen F, Zhu Z, Jiang H, Guo SW. Patterns of and Risk Factors for Reccurrence in Women With Ovarian Endometriomas. Obstetrics and Gynecology 2007; 109: 1411-20.

9. Cheong Y, Tay P, Luk F, Gan HC, Lit C, Cooke I. Laparoscopic surgery for endometriosis: how often do we need to re-operate? J Obstet Gynaecol 2008; 28:82-85.

10. Porpora MG, Pallante D, Ferro A, Crisafi B, Bellati F, Benedetti Panici P. Pain and ovarian endometrioma recurrence after laparoscopic treatment of endometriosis: a long-term prospective study. Fertil Steril, 2008.

11. Vercellini P, Fedele L, Giorgio A, De Giorgi O, Consonni D, Crosignani P G. Reproductive performance, pain recurrence and disease relapse after conservative surgical treatment for endometriosis: the predictive value of the current classification system. Hum Reprod 2006; 21: 2679-85.

12. Hemmings R. Combined treatment of endometriosis, GnRH agonists and laparoscopic surgery. J Reprod Med 1998; 43: 316-20

13. Donnez J, Anaf V, Nisolle M et al. Ovarian endometrial cysts: the role of gonadotropin-releasing hormone agonist and/or drainage. Fertil Steril 1994; 62:63-66.

14. Kettel LM, Murphy AA. Combination medical and surgical therapy for infertile patients with endometriosis. Obstet Gynecol Clin North Am 1989; 16: 167-77.

15. Thomas EJ. Combining medical and surgical treatment for endometriosis: the best of both worlds? Br J Obstet Gynaecol 1992; 99: 5-8.

16. Yap C, Furness S, Farquhar C. Pre and postoperative medical therapy for endometriosis surgery. Cochrane Database Syst Rev 2004; 3: CD003678.

17. Loverro G, Carriero C, Cristina Rossi A, Putignano G, Nicolardi V, Selvaggi L. A randomized study comparing triptorelin or expectant management following conservative laparoscopic surgery for symptomatic stage III-IV endometriosis. EJOG 2008; 136:194-98.

18. Jee BC, Lee JY, Suk Suh C, Kim SH, Choi YM, Moon SH. Impact of GnRH agonist treatment on recurrence of ovarian endometriomas after conservative laparoscopic surgery. Fertil Steril 2008.

19. Vercellini P, Somigliana E, Daguati R, Vigano P, Meroni F, Crosignani P G. Postoperative oral contraceptive exposure and risk of endometrioma recurrence. Am J Obstet Gyn 2008; 198: 504.e1-5.

20. Muzii L, Marana R, Caruana P, Catalano GF, Margutti F, Paniei PB. Postoperative administration of monophasic combined oral contraceptives after laparoscopic treatment of ovarian endometriomas: a prospective, randomised trial. Am J Obstet Gynecol 2000; 183: 588-92.

21. Audebert A, Descamps P, Marret H, et al. Pre or postoperative medical treatment with nafarelin in stage III-IV endometriosis: a French multicenter study. Obstet Gynecol 1998; 79: 145-48.

22. Hemmings R, Bissonnette F, Bouzayen R. Results of laparoscopic treatments of ovarian endometriomas: laparoscopic ovarian fenestration and coagulation. Fertil Steril 1998; 70:527-29.

23. Vercellini P., Chapron Ch, De Giorgi O, Consonni D, Frontino G, Crosignani P G. Coagulation or excision of ovarian endometriomas? Am J Obstet Gynecol, 2003; 188: 606-10.

24. Fayez J, Vogel MF. Comparison of different treatment methods of endometriomas by laparoscopy. Obstet Gynecol 1991; 78:660-65.

25. Beretta P, Franchi M, Ghezzi F, Busacca M, Zupi E, Bolis P. Randomized clinical trial of two laparoscopic treatments of endometriomas: cystectomy versus drainage and coagulation. Fertil Steril 1998; 70: 1176-80.

26. Saleh A, Tulandi T. Reoperation after laparoscopic treatment of ovarian endometriomas by excision and fenestration. Fertil Steril 1999; 72:322-24.

27. Hart R, Hickey M, Maouris P, Buckett W, Garry R. Excisional surgery versus ablative surgery for ovarian endometriomata: a Cochrane Review. Human reprod 2005; 20:3000-07.

28. Alborzi S, Momtahan M, Parsanezhad M E, Dehbashi S, Zolghadri J, Alborzi S. A prostpective, randomized study comparing laparoscopic ovarian cystectomy versus fenestration and coagulation in patients with endometriomas. Fertil Steril 2004; 82: 1633-37.

29. Redwine DB, Wright JT. Laparoscopic treatment of complete obliteration of the cul-de-sac associated with endometriosis: long-term follow-up of en bloc resection. Fertil Steril 2001;76:421-22

30. Dubernard G, Piketti M, Rouzier R et al. Quality of life after laparoscopic colorectal resection for endometriosis. Hum reprod 2006; 21:1243-47.

31. Angioni S, Peiretti M, Zirone M, Palomba M, Mais V, Gomel V, Melis GB. Laparoscopic excision of posterior vaginal fornix in the treatment of patients with deep endometriosis without rectum involvement: surgical treatment and long-term follow-up. Hum Reprod 2006; 21: 1629-34.

32. Daraï E, Bazot M, Rouzier R, Houry S, Dubernard G. Outcome of laparoscopic colorectal resection for endometriosis. Curr Opin Obstet Gynecol 2007; 19:308-13.

33. Fedele L, Bianchi S, Zanconato G, Bettoni G, Gotsch F. Long-term follow-up after conservative surgery for rectovaginal endometriosis. Am J Obstet Gynecol 2004;190:1020-24.

34. Jatan AK, Solomon MJ, Young J, et al. Laparoscopic management of rectal endometriosis. Dis Colon Rectum 2006; 49:169-74.

35. Panel P, Chis C, Gaudin S et al. Laparoscopic surgery of deep endometriosis. About 118 cases. Gynecol Obstet Fertil 2006; 34:583-92.

36. Vignali M, Bianchi S, Candiani M, Spadoccini G, Gagiani G, Busacca M. Surgical treatment of deep endometriosis and risk of recurrence. J Minim Invasive Gynecol 2005; 12: 508-13.

37. Carmona F, Martinez-Zamora A, Gonzales X, Gines A, Bunesch L, Balasch J. Does the learning curve of conservative laparoscopic surgery in women with rectovaginal endometriosis impair the recurrence rate? Fertil Steril 2008.

38. Brouwer R, Woods RJ. Rectal endometriosis: results of radical excision and review of published work. ANZ J Surg 2007; 77:562-71.

39. Kavallaris A, Kohler C, Kuhne-Heid R, Schneider A. Histopathological extent of rectal invasion by rectovaginal endometriosis. Hum Reprod 2003;18:1323-27.

40. Anaf V, El Nakadi I, Simon P, Van de Stadt J, Fayt I, Simonart T, Noel JC. Preferential infiltration of large bowel endometriosis along the nerves of the colon. Hum Reprod 2004;19: 996-1002.

41. Abrao MS, Podgaec S, Dias JA Jr, Averbach M, Garry R, Ferraz Silva LF, Carvalho FM. Deeply infiltrating endometriosis affecting the rectum and lymph nodes. Fertil Steril 2006; 86: 543-47.

Classical Medical Treatments

Juan Balasch

Chapter 21

Oral Contraceptive Pills (OCPs) for Treatment of Endometriosis

Introduction

Endometriosis is a common gynecologic disorder defined by the presence of the endometrial gland and stroma outside the uterus and it is estimated that it occurs in 7-10% for women in the general population and up to 50% of premenopausal women. It is a progressive condition where macroscopically minimal disease may be associated with severe symptomatology and yet extensive disease may be clinically silent.[1] The main manifestations of endometriosis are pelvic pain, adnexal masses and infertility with a prevalence of 38% (range, 20-50%) in infertile women, and in 71-87% of women with chronic pelvic pain.[1] Thus, the goals of treatment for women with endometriosis should ideally be treatment directed at endometriosis itself, alleviation of symptoms, promotion of fertility, and prevention of disease progression. Unfortunately, however, no therapy fulfilling these requirements exists and all conservative treatment regimens, either medical or surgical, are associated with disease recurrence.

Originally the disease was felt to be best treated surgically and with the progressive development of operative laparoscopy the treatment of endometriosis could be instituted at the time of diagnosis, resulting in a more efficient but not necessarily more effective therapy. However, as the complexity and chronicity of endometriosis has been recognized, the pendulum has been swinging relentlessly towards medical options and it is now accepted that medical treatment that can induce a generalized suppression of the disease is necessary.[2,3]

Historically, endometriosis has been seen as an endocrine disease since steroid hormones have been considered as the major regulators of growth and function of endometriotic tissue. Thus, most medical treatments for women with endometriosis have been based on the idea that the condition is a hormonally responsive disease and in fact, their evolution has paralleled the advent and introduction of potent synthetic steroid hormones. Hormonal therapy for endometriosis dates back more than five decades. In the 1940s and 1950s, diethylstilbestrol and methyltestosterone were used. Therapy with progestin alone or estrogen and progestin combinations were used in the 1960s and 1970s. Danazol was introduced in the early 1970s, followed by the gonadotropin-releasing hormone agonists and gestrinone in the late 1980s and early 1990s. Overall, these therapies have focused on the hormonal alteration of the menstrual cycle in an attempt to produce a pseudo-pregnancy, pseudo-menopause, or chronic anovulation. Each of these situations is considered to cause a suboptimal environment for the growth and maintenance of endometrium and, by extension, of endometriotic implants.[2]

Over the past recent years, however, the approach has changed. At present, there is a much better understanding of the pathogenesis, growth and maintenance of ectopic endometrium, specially at the molecular level. This has provided drug developers with precise molecular targets for treatment of endometriosis. Currently under development, these newer agents hold the potential of greater efficacy and flexibility with fewer systemic effects.[3] This notwithstanding, at present, progestogens alone or in the form of oral contraceptive pills (OCP) are gradually regaining popularity as a treatment for endometriosis.

It is in this scenario that this chapter will analyze the rationale and potential indications for the use of OCP in the current therapy of endometriosis. Although most treatments for endometriosis are directed at the implants themselves, the symptoms can be treated directly and thus, these aspects are analyzed separately.

Biological Rationale for the Use of OCP in the Treatment of Endometriosis

In the late 1950s, Kistner reported that combined estrogen-progestagen contraceptives were effective in the treatment of endometriosis. He first noticed by the appearance of endometriosis at the time of cesarean section that pregnancy transforms functioning ectopic endometrial tissue into decidua that ultimately undergoes decidual necrosis and involution and appears to be of benefit with a documented regression of endometriosis after completion of gestation. That author suggested this deciduation of endometriotic tissue resulting from increased blood levels of estrogen and progesterone would explain that signs and symptoms of endometriosis frequently regress during the period of gestation and for varying periods of time thereafter.

The pharmacologic induction of an iatrogenic "pseudopregnancy" with a 6- to 12-month continuous course of estrogen plus progestin attempts to mimic the hormonal profile and thus the endometrial changes seen in pregnancy. Progestogens with or without estrogens induce anovulation and amenorrhea according to their dosage, provoke marked decidualization, acyclicity and atrophy of eutopic and ectopic endometrium, and decrease intraperitoneal inflammation.[4] This has been observed in women but it is in direct disagreement with data from the rhesus monkey demonstrating larger implants with considerable local growth following such a therapeutic approach.[3] In fact, pseudopregnancy regimens produce an acyclic hormone environment, but do expose the endometriotic lesions to significant amounts of estrogen **(Figure 21-1).** Although most synthetic progestins have sufficient androgenic and progestational activity to block the effects of co-administered estrogen, it is conceivable that in some patients the administered estrogen actually stimulates metabolic activity in endometriotic tissue.

In fact, in spite that OCP are the most commonly prescribed drug for endometriosis symptoms, data regarding mechanism of action are scanty. Recently, however, the effect of OCP on regulation of *in vitro* endometrial cell growth has recently been investigated.[5] Apoptosis (or programmed cell death) of the endometrium

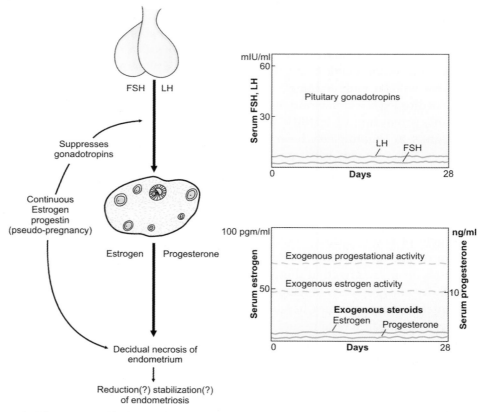

FIGURE 21-1: Effects of continuous estrogen-progestin therapy on the pituitary-ovarian axis. Gonadotropin release and ovarian steroidogenesis are suppressed with the exogenous estrogen and progestin, causing decidual necrosis of the endometrium (Reproduced from Hammond CB, Haney AF, Fertil Steril 1978; 30: 497-509) (Reproduced with Permission)

is regulated by steroid hormones and is controlled by the expression of several regulatory genes. Eutopic epithelial and stromal endometrial cells from patients with endometriosis show an augmented survival capability probably caused by an abnormal high effect of genes blocking apoptosis. Exposure to a monophasic OCP containing desogestrel 0.15 mg + ethinylestradiol 30 mcg per pill for 30 days significantly increases endometrial apoptosis in comparison with pretreatment levels, both in epithelial and stromal cells, producing values similar to those observed in the endometrium from control women without endometriosis. Thus, OCPs enhance cell death and, in addition, endometrial cell proliferation in subjects with the disease is significantly reduced by exposure to an OCP.

Also, dienogest, a synthetic steroid used as a progestogen in OCP is currently being investigated in the treatment of endometriosis.[5] In the rat model, it has been reported that dienogest reduces the volume of autologous transplanted endometrium, inhibits angiogenesis, decreases the number of inflammatory peritoneal fluid cells, increases the natural killer activity of peritoneal fluid cells, decreases interleukin production by peritoneal macrophages, induces prolactin production (a typical marker of decidualization) by human endometrial stromal cells, and causes a dose-dependent inhibition of stromal endometrial cell proliferation. The above recent findings may thus provide a mechanistic clue to the action of OCP in endometriosis.[5]

OCP for Treatment of Endometriosis Itself

As stated above, regression of the endometriotic lesions leading to reduction or elimination of symptoms as well as enhancing fertility should be the goals of medical therapy. All clinical studies conducted on hormonal management of endometriosis were based on the presupposed response of endometriotic implants to an adverse endocrine environment. Also, it was assumed that the more drastic the drug impact, the higher the chance of success in terms of lesion regression and, consequently, pregnancy rate in infertile women and pain relief in symptomatic patients. The field of application of medical approaches has been mostly limited to early stages of the disease, as surgery remains the mainstay of treatment for endometriomas and extensive disease.[6]

The effect of medications on implant number, volume, and extensiveness has been examined for a numer of drugs in different ways. Many are poorly controlled or uncontrolled investigations, and often the observation searching for effect is carried out during administration of the drug itself. Thus, what occurs after drug disconti-nuation is frequently unknown.[3]

A standard 6-month course of hormonal therapy of endometriosis with medroxyprogesterone acetate, danazol or GnRH agonist is usually associated with a total or partial resolution of peritoneal implants in approximately 60% of patients and in an improvement in American Fertility Society (AFS) scores when compared with placebo.[3,7] The OCP commonly prescribed today are most likely to produce a progestogen-dominant picture similar to that of progestagen and thus, results are expected to be similar to those obtained with medroxyprogesterone acetate alone but no specific published data on OCP exist. In fact, it is accepted that medical therapy of endometriosis results, in general, in an improvement of AFS scores and there is no difference in the effectiveness of the different hormonal therapies in this regard.[7]

However, considerations based on the effects of available drugs on the extent of endometriotic implants should no longer be accounted useful, since it has been repeatedly demonstrated that the lesions persist, although in quiescent and microscopic forms, and that a repeated laparoscopy at the end of medical treatment is not predictive of the course of the disease in the short and medium term. In fact, the natural course of endometriosis is a mystery, and it is almost impossible to reach valid conclusions regarding the pathophysiologic development of the disease and its disappearance or recurrence after (or due to) therapy. Approximately one-third of endometriosis patients in a placebo treatment group showed spontaneous improvement in AFS scores, one-third deterioration, and the remainder no change.[8]

Pseudopregnancy regimens have been administered both orally and parenterally and many estrogen-progestin combinations have been used. High-dose OCPs were used initially in an increasing dosage schedule to mimic the pregnancy state. With increased experience, however, it was recognized that the continuous use of low-dose OCP, which were associated with fewer side effects, have similar beneficial results. The choice of the pill matters little, although a monophasic formulation seems more logical than a multiphasic pill for continuous therpay. Almost all estrogen-progestin combinations result in progressive decidualization, and ultimate necrobiosis and resorption of ectopic endometrial tissue. Current technique involves the use of low-dose (20-35 mcg ethinylestradiol) OCP continuously for 6-12 months. The treatment usually is begun with one pill daily and increased to two or more pills per day only if breakthrough bleeding occurs. The administration of doses higher than two pills is not recommended, however, because of increasing undesirable side effects, the lowest dose of hormone that produces amenorrhea then is maintained during the course of therapy. Estrogen (estradiol 2 mg or conjugated estrogens 1.25 mg daily for 1 week) can be added as needed to control episodic breakthrough bleeding, which is more common with continuous than with cyclic therapy. The decidual reaction and necrobiosis produced by low-dose formulations are just as extensive as noted in previously used high-dose regimens.[9]

During the initial 2-3 months of therapy, most patients are beset with worsening symptomatology referable to the endometriosis in addition to those specifically related to OCP. The latter undesirable side effects are frequent and sometimes severe. They may include abdominal swelling, breast pain and tenderness, increased appetite, depression, weight gain, edema, nausea, and breakthrough bleeding. In addition, high dose OCPs increase thromboembolic risk. Ovulation and menstruation usually resume 4 to 8 weeks after therapy has been discontinued.[9]

Pseudopregnancy represented the most effective medical therapy of its time. Because of its side effects, however, many patients were unable or unwilling to continue its use and physicians were hesitant to prescribe it. Today, OCPs are the most commonly prescribed treatment for endometriosis symptoms but interestingly there seems to be a lack of consensus in the literature on a relationship between cyclic OCP use and risk of endometriosis.[10,11] An early study containing the results of the Oxford Family Planning Association concluded that the risk of endometriosis was lower in current users of OCP, but after the pill is stopped the risk is higher than in never users (i.e., current OCP would temporarily suppress endometriosis but the risk is increased thereafter). A similar pattern of risk was also reported in other cohort and case-control studies conducted in Italy and North European and American countries. However, in other epidemiological studies, the risk of developing the disease was reduced by use of the pill whereas in others it was not influenced.

The interpretation of these findings should therefore be cautious. Selection is the major bias in studies on methods of contraception and risk of endometriosis. The elevated risk for ever and ex-users of OCP may be explained by selection bias. Dysmenorrhea is an usual symptom of the disease and also an indication for OCP use. Thus, women with dysmenorrhea related to endometriosis may be excluded selectively from the never users category, with a consequent increased risk for ever use. In addition, patients

with endometriosis may be more frequently infertile, and less fertile women are less frequently users of contraception.[11]

To re-analyze the subject of the association between OCP use and the risk of endometriosis but taking into account the potential differences in selection between cases with the disease and control women, a multicenter study was carried out in women with and without endometriosis who underwent laparoscopy for infertility or pelvic pain in a network of hospitals in Italy, an area characterized by a lower rate of OCP use than that in Northern Europe and North America.[11] This study suggested that the risk of endometriosis is higher in women who have taken OCP. The risk was observed both in current and ex-users, but tended to decrease slightly with time since last use of OCP. These findings are in disagreement with most of previous case-control and cohort studies, but not all. There is not a definite explanation for this fact and it may be due to residual confounding. On the other hand, alternative biological explanations for the actions of OCP in endometriosis have been postulated.[11] OCP causes a regular menstrual pattern, and regular menses tend to increase the risk of endometriosis. Further, studies conducted on castrated monkeys showed that endometrial tissue seeded into the peritoneum did not require steroid supplementation for the initiation of endometriosis, but estradiol and progesterone were indispensable for survival of implants. Also, it has been postulated that estrogens and progestins depress cellular immune response and theoretically could further inhibit the pelvic elimination of the regurgitated endometrial cells.[12] Clearly, further studies on the relationship between OCP use and risk of endometriosis are needed.

OCP for Treatment of Infertility Associated with Endometriosis

Most of the established medical therapies used to treat endometriosis-associated infertility inhibit ovulation and thus are used to treat the disease for a period of time prior to allowing an attempt at conception. Early uncontrolled case-series studies using OCP in women who had infertility in addition to endometriosis reported pregnancy rates ranging from 10% to 60%.[9] However this supposedly beneficial effect on fertility is not supported by data from the evidence-based medicine. A recent Cochrane review[13] reported on 13 randomized clinical trials that included nearly 800 women in order to determine the effectiveness of: a) ovulation suppression with danazol, medroxy-progesterone acetate, gestrinone, combined OCP pills and

GnRH analogs versus placebo or no treatment; and b) any of the above agents versus danazol; and c) GnRH analogs versus OCP for the treatment of endometriosis-associated subfertility. This systematic review and meta-analysis concluded that in the treatment of endometriosis-associated subfertility, the combined data from trials comparing ovulation suppression for up to 6 months with danazol, gestrinone or medroxyprogesterone acetate with placebo or no treatment, showed no evidence of benefit on fertililty. In addition, trials comparing gestrinone, medroxyprogesterone, or OCP with an "active control" (with danazol), demonstrated no statistically significant difference in subsequent fecundity between groups. Finally, the single study comparing GnRH agonist versus OCP indicated no evidence of benefit of one intervention over the other.

Therefore, there appears to be no role for hormone therapy in the treatment of infertility associated with endometriosis. Remarkably, it has been stressed that frequently overlooked is the fact that not only do these hormones fail to enhance fertility, they may also delay fertility in that the patient is unable to conceive while being medicated for several months.[3] If those controlled trials are reanalyzed with follow-up beginning at the time of diagnosis rather than at the conclusion of therapy, medical therapy is significantly worse than no treatment and thus suppressive medical therapy proves significantly detrimental to fertility.[3]

OCP for Treatment of Pain Associated with Endometriosis

Symptomatic endometriosis is a frequent cause of pelvic pain. The pain may occur at the same time as menstrual bleeding (dysmenorrhea), during or after sexual intercourse (dyspareunia or postcoital pain) or be present as other pelvic pain occurring in a cyclical or non-cyclical pattern. Dysmenorrhea is the most common painful symptoms in patients with endometriosis.

OCP are believed by many gynecologists to be the drug of choice in managing women with endometriosis and for many years they have been extensively used in clinical practice for the reduction of painful symptoms associated with this disease. Numerous uncontrolled trials have evaluated pain relief with OC, generally demonstrating improvement in 75 to 90%[3] but only a few formal studies have quantified their effects or compared these with those obtained during administration of other drugs.

In randomized clinical trials comparing hormonal suppressive therapy with danazol, GnRH agonist or medroxyprogesterone versus placebo, medical treatment was found to be more effective than placebo for the treatment of the pain associated with endometriosis, but no one treatment seems to be better than any other.[3,7,14] The only study included in a recent Cochrane review[15] showed no significant difference between GnRH agonist and cyclic low-dose OCP in pain relief at the end of treatment. Six months after treatment, symptoms had recurred in all patients. No comparison of dysmenorrhea during treatment could be made as GnRH agonist induces amenorrhea. However, six months after treatment no women in either group had experienced complete resolution of dysmenorrhea. There was no significant difference between OCP and GnRH agonist in the treatment of dyspareunia, either at the end of treatment or after six months follow-up. In addition, the first placebo-controlled, double-blind, randomized trial investigating low-dose OCP for dysmenorrhea associated with endometriosis showed the efficacy and safety of this therapeutic approach.[16]

OCP used cyclically are the only treatment for endometriosis that permits monthly uterine bleeding. Dysmenorrhea is considered as the most frequent complaint in women with this disease. Therefore, the symptom may not subside completely during administration of OC. Recent studies have demonstrated that women with menstrual-related problems during cyclic use of an OCP may benefit from a shift to continuous administration. Thus, continuous use of a low-dose OCP may be useful in controlling symptomatic endometriosis and menstruation-related pain symptoms in patients who do not respond to a cyclic pill regimen after conservative surgical treatment[5] but no data address the use of cyclic versus noncyclic combined OCP for chronic pelvic pain.[17,18]

No study with appropriate prospective design has evaluated routine post-operative OCP administration following conservative surgery for endometriosis[14] but a recent report suggest that a cyclic, low-dose OCP use after operative laparoscopic treatment of ovarian endometriomas may not only increase the symptom-free period but also prevent endometrioma recurrence.[19] Ovarian endometrioma should not be considered a contraindication to the administration of OCP after surgery if it is necessary, or desirable. A study compared the effectiveness of an OCP (desogestrel 0.15 mg and ethinylestradiol 20 mcg) with that of cyproterone acetate in the treatment of endometriosis-associated recurrent pelvic pain after surgery and both schemes used showed to be an effective, safe and inexpensive treatment for pain recurring after conservative surgery for symptomatic endometriosis.[5] Also, anastrozole plus a low-dose OCP has been proposed for patients with documented endometriosis and chronic pelvic pain refractory to multiple medical and surgical treatments.[20]

Remarkably, OCP has the great advantage over other hormonal treatments in that it can be taken indefinitely and is generally more acceptable to women than alternative hormonal treatments, which improves compliance. Thus, OCP are an appropriate first-line medical therapy for women with endometriosis-related dysmenorrhea and pelvic pain. In fact, no data are available to support the belief that OCP are to be considered as second-line drugs as suggested by a study investigating whether a GnRH agonist administered for 4 months before starting treatment with a cyclic OCP would improve results compared with the immediate use of an OCP (gestodene 0.75 mg and ethinyl estradiol 30 mcg) for 12 months. One year after randomization the two treatment modalities showed similar relief of pelvic pain in women with endometriosis.[5]

OCP in the Empirical Treatment of Chronic Pelvic Pain and Endometriosis

There is no doubt that there are different effective treatments for women with endometriosis, but all have limitations. Given that surgical therapy and medical therapies have similar effectiveness with respect to pain relief, the optimal surgical approach for the pain associated with endometriosis has yet to be defined, and combination treatment with surgery and drugs may offer an advantage in treating pain but the extent of the advantage is unclear, it is not surprising that there are still many unanswered questions regarding the most appropriate treatment for women with this disorder.[2,17]

A comparison of the surgical and medical approach to endometriosis in Europe and the United States reveals similar management strategies for the disease. Laparoscopy is used for diagnosis in 54% and 66% of cases in Europe and the United States, respectively. The most frequently used medical treatments for endometriosis in Europe and the United States are OCP and nonsteroidal antiinflammatory drugs.[21] However, at present, the value of laparoscopy in the diagnosis of endometriosis and chronic pelvic pain is being debated and different shortcomings for this use have been stressed.[21,22] While laparoscopy is the current gold standard for diagnosis, there is wide variation between diagnostic findings between surgeons and between countries. Findings in Belgium show that 70% of women with chronic pelvic pain have visualized endometriosis at laparoscopy. However, in Spain 44% of women undergoing laparoscopy

for chronic pelvic pain were found to have laparoscopic evidence of endometriosis, and of these 11% had the endometriosis confirmed by uterosacral biopsy.[10,21] The positive predictive value for visual versus histological diagnosis of endometriosis has been reported to be 45%. In addition, random biopsy of the peritoneum in patients with pelvic pain showed that approximately 25% of the biopsies reveal endometriosis on pathological evaluation. These findings indicate that diagnosis of endometriosis through laparoscopic visualization is unreliable because negative laparoscopy findings do not imply that the patient has no endometriosis, nor do positive results indicate that the disease is present.[21]

Accordingly with the above evidence, the American College of Obstetricians and Gynecologists,[1,18] the Royal College of Obstetricians and Gynecologists,[23] and the European Society of Human Reproduction and Embriology,[24] have issued clinical guidelines recommending the empirical medical treatment of pain symptoms presumed to be due to endometriosis without a definitive diagnosis. The rationale for this approach is that pelvic pain with a negative work-up is considered to be endometriosis, and that if history, physical examination, laboratory and ultrasound evaluation suggest endometriosis (and in the absence of adnexal masses), empirical treatment is indicated.

Medical treatment of women with chronic pelvic pain suspected to be related to endometriosis should begin with a trial of nonsteroidal anti-inflammatory drugs or OCP or a combination of both. Selection of a first-line medical therapeutic agent should be based on the nature of the pain (cyclic or noncyclic), contraindications to nonsteroidal anti-inflammatory drugs or OCP, desire for contraception, and other factors. If adequate pain relief is obtained from nonsteroidal anti-inflammatory drugs or OCP (individually or in combination), then a maintenance management regimen should be considered. If first-line therapy with OCP and nonsteroidal anti-inflammatory drugs fail to improve symptoms within a reasonable time (3-6 months), a second-line therapy with GnRH agonists and add-back should be tried, for a time. If second-line therapy fails, the clinician should reconsider other causes of pain and laparoscopy. This plan for the management of pain and endometriosis **(Figure 21-2)** was ratified by consensus panels made up of practicing gynecologists from both the United States and Europe.[21,25]

Recently, the American College of Obstetricians and Gynecologists Committee on Adolescent Care wrote a Committee Opinion regarding endometriosis in adolescents which has also changed the diagnosis and treatment

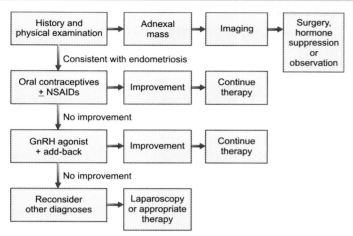

FIGURE 21-2: Recommended strategy for the management of women with endometriosis and pain symptoms. NSAIDs = nonsteroidal antiinflammatory drugs; GnRHa = gonadotropin-releasing hormone agonists. (Reproduced from Winkel CA, Obstet Gynecol 2003; 102:397-408) (Reproduced with Permission)

used for maintenance treatment following GnRH agonist therapy. However, as previously stressed,[12] it is evident that the medical treatments currently available do not cure endometriosis, independently of the hormonal milieu induced and the presence of amenorrhea. Ectopic endometrial implants survive, although in atrophic form, ready for reactivation when suspension of the treatment occurs. A more rationale therapeutic objective might be simple limitation of the growth of eutopic and ectopic endometrium; hypomenorrhea obtained with OCP containing a prevalent progestogen component and low estrogen doses, could reduce the amount of retrograde menstruation and endometrial synthesis of prostaglandins, with decreased myometrial contractility and pelvic pain. This could give patients with endometriosis an acceptable quality of life. However, the relationship between early OCP use and risk of endometriosis as well as specific disease outcomes remains to be determined.

of endometriosis.[26] They recommend that laparoscopic evaluation be offered to adolescents under the age of 18 years only if they have persistent pain while taking OCP and nonsteroidal anti-inflammatory drugs given their safety profiles. In fact, most experts think it is reasonable to begin with this first-line empiric therapy but it has been reported that 50%-70% of adolescents with pelvic pain not responding to combination hormone therapy (such as OCP and nonsteroidal antiinflammatory drugs) have endometriosis at the time of laparoscopy.[26] Therefore, while the need for an early diagnosis and treatment of endometriosis during adolescence has been emphasized,[26] there is often a long delay in the diagnosis and treatment of the condition and it has been suggested that in the long term there may be psychologic and social disadvantages associated with delaying diagnoses.[22] On the other hand, it is not known how the use of OCP masks the diagnosis and no studies have shown that early intervention limits specific disease outcomes. In this regard, it must be emphasized that there are no data available regarding medical therapy for prevention of disease progression or for prevention of future pain and fertility preservation, a fact to be considered mainly in asymptomatic women in whom endometriosis is discovered incidentally.[1]

Summary and Concluding Remarks

OCP are widely used as first-line treatment for painful symptoms associated with endometriosis and they are also

References

1. ACOG. Medical management of endometriosis. ACOG Practice Bulletin No. 11, December 1999; reaffirmed date 2007.
2. Olive DL, Pritss EA. Treatment of endometriosis. N Engl J Med 2001; 345:266-75.
3. Olive DL. Medical therapy of endometriosis. Sem Reprod Med 2003; 21:209-21.
4. The ESHRE Capri Workshop Group. Ovarian and endometrial function during hormonal contraception. Hum Reprod 2001; 16:1527-35.
5. Vercellini P, Fedele L, Pietropaolo G, Frontino G, Somigliana E, Crosignani PG. Progestogens for endometriosis: forward to the past. Hum Reprod Update 2003; 9:387-96.
6. Vercellini P, De Giorgi O, Pesole A, Zaina B, Pisacreta A, Crosignani PG. Endometriosis: drugs and adjuvant therapy. In: Templeton A, Cooke I, Shaughn O'Brien PM, eds. Evidence-based Fertility Treatment. London, RCOG Press, 1999; 225-45.
7. Farquhar C, Sutton C. The evidence for the management of endometriosis. Curr Opin Obstet Gynecol 1998; 10: 321-32.
8. Evers JLH, Dunselman GAJ, Land JA, Bouckaert XJM. Endometriosis: prevention of recurrences. In: Kempers RD, Cohen J, Haney AF, Younger JB (Eds). Fertility and Reproductive Medicine, Amsterdam, Elsevier Science BV, 1998; 387-96.
9. Moghissi KS. Medical treatment of endometriosis. Clin Obstet Gynecol 1999; 42:620-32.
10. Balasch J, Creus M, Fábregues F, Carmona F, Ordi J, Martinez-Romás S et al. Visible and non-visible endometriosis at laparoscopy in fertile and infertile women and in patients with chronic pelvic pain: a prospective study. Hum Reprod 1996; 11:387-91.

11. Italian Endometriosis Study Group. Oral contraceptive use and risk of endometriosis. Br J Obstet Gynaecol 1999; 106:695-99.

12. Vercellini P, Ragni G, Trespidi L, Oldani S, Crosignani PG. Does contraception modify the risk of endometriosis? Hum Reprod 1993; 8:547-51.

13. Hughes E, Brown J, Collins JJ, Farquhar C, Fedorkow DM, Vandekerckhove P. Ovulation suppression for endometriosis. Cochrane Database of Systematic Reviews 2007;3: CD000155.

14. The Practice Committee of the American Society for Reproductive Medicine. Treatment of pelvic pain associated with Endometriosis. Fertil Steril 2006; 86(suppl. 4):S18-S27.

15. Davis L, Kennedy SS, Moore J, Prentice A. Modern combined oral contraceptives for pain associated with endometriosis. Cochrane Database of Systematic Reviews 2007;3: CD001019.

16. Harada T, Momoeda M, Taketani Y, Hoshiai H, Terakawa N. Low-dose oral contraceptive pill for dysmenorrhea associated with endometriosis: A placebo-controlled, double-blind, randomized trial. Fertil Steril 2008;90: 1583-88.

17. Winkel CA. Evaluation and management of women with endometriosis. Obstet Gynecol 2003; 102:397-408.

18. ACOG. Chronic pelvic pain. ACOG Practice Bulletin No. 51. Obstet Gynecol 2004; 103:589-605.

19. Vercellini P, Somigliana E, Daguati R, Vigano P, Meroni F, Crosignani PG. Postoperative oral contraceptive exposure and risk of endometrioma recurrence. Am J Obstet Gynecol 2008; 198:504.e1-504.e5.

20. Amsterdam LL, Gentry W, Jobanputra S, Wolf M, Rubin S, Bulun SE. Anastrazole and oral contraceptives: a novel treatment for endometriosis. Fertil Steril 2005; 84:300-04.

21. Opinion Leaders' Advisory Panel. 2005 Women's Health Global Opinion Leaders'Advisory Panel. Drugs of Today, 2005; vol. 41, Suppl.A.

22. Ballard K, Lowton K, Wright J. Balancing the risks and benefits of different diagnostic interventions for chronic pelvic pain. Fertil Steril 2006; 86:1317.

23. Royal College of Obstetricians and Gynaecologists. The initial management of chronic pelvic pain. Guideline No. 41, April 2005.

24. Kennedy S, Bergqvist A, Chapron C et al. ESHRE guideline for the diagnosis and treatment of endometriosis. Hum Reprod 2005; 20:2698-2704.

25. Gambone JC, Mittman BS, Munro MG et al. Consensus statement for the management of chronic pelvic pain and endometriosis: proceedings of an expert-panel consensus process. Fertil Steril 2002; 78:961-72.

26. ACOG Committee on Adolescent Care. Endometriosis in adolescents. Committee Opinion No. 310, April 2005. Obstet Gynecol 2005; 105:921-27.

Tony G Zreik, Rana Skaf, Chakib M Ayoub

Chapter 22

Nonsteroidal Anti-inflammatory Drugs

Introduction

Endometriosis is a common gynecological condition that affects women in their reproductive years, and can lead to painful symptoms and infertility.[1] The actual prevalence of the disease is unknown and its epidemiology is rather difficult to determine precisely as it requires surgery for diagnosis.[2-4] However, in the year 2005, there were 1.67 billion women aged 15 to 49 years in the world (www.prb.org). Assuming a1% prevalence means that there could be 16 million women with endometriosis worldwide; whereas a 20% prevalence implies there are 334 million women with endometriosis. The actual number probably lies somewhere in between.

According to The National Endometriosis Society (www.endo.org.uk), 65% of women with endometriosis reported that their condition had adversely affected their employment. Ten per cent of women had to reduce their working hours and 30% had not been able to continue in the same employment. As many as 16% of women were unable to continue in any employment and 6% needed to claim state benefits. Thus, in addition to their feelings of loss as contributors to society, they became dependent upon others. This clearly added to the feeling of low esteem some women with endometriosis express due to their incapacitating disease.

Endometriosis is still an enigma and deciding on the optimal treatment for a patient can be very difficult for several reasons. First, there is no complete understanding of the etiology of the disease or its development or recurrence. Second, the pathophysiology leading to the pain and infertility associated with endometriosis is still not completely clear **(Figure 22-1)**. Third, not only the

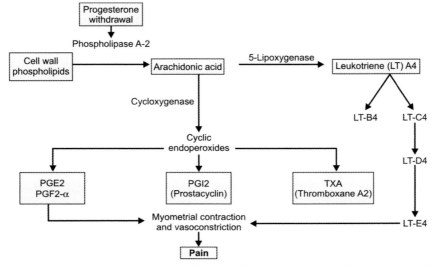

FIGURE 22-1: Pathophysiology of dysmenorrhea. Harel Z. Dysmenorrhea in Adolescents and Young Adults: Etiology and Management. J Pediatr Adolesc Gynecol (2006) 19:363-71 (Reproduced with Permission).

Table 22-1: Medical interventions for the treatment of endometriosis			
The medical interventions within each one of these categories			
Analgesia/anti-inflammatory agents	*Suppression of ovulation/estrogen*	*Direct action in endometriotic deposits*	*Immunomodulation*
NSAIDs*	Contraceptive pill* Danazol* Gestrinone* GnRH agonists* ≠ add back HRT AIs* (+ direct action)	LNG IUS* Progesterone antagonists** SPRMs*** AIs* (+ estrogen suppression) ER ligands*** Angiogenesis inhibitors** Statins**	Inflammatory modulators***

*Currently available and sufficient evidence to recommend usage
** currently available but insufficient evidence to recommend usage
*** product(s) in development (basic science or phase I, II, III trials)
Reference: Panay N. Advances in the medical management of endometriosis. BJOG. 2008 Jun; 115(7):814-7.

mechanism(s) by which pain is caused are not fully understood, the link between the pain experienced and the extent of endometriosis is not well recognized. And even when endometriosis is diagnosed, it may not be the cause of a woman's painful symptoms. Finally, although the severity of symptoms and the probability of diagnosis increase with age, peaking at about age 40 years old,[5,6] the severity of pain experienced does not always directly correlate with the severity of endometriosis.[7,8]

Sampson's theory of retrograde menstruation, which describes endometrial cells that may implant, infiltrate, and grow, seems plausible because peritoneal lesions are most frequently found in the ovaries left more than right, and the posterior cul-de-sac, where regurgitated menstrual material pools.[9] However, despite extensive research efforts, the exact pathogenetic pathways are still in question.[9-11]

Despite lack of evidence confirming the relationship between Nonsteroidal anti-inflammatory Drugs (NSAIDs) and endometriosis, NSAIDs are commonly prescribed treatments for endometriosis-related pain **(Table 22-1)**. This chapter will attempt at elucidating the relationship between endometriosis, prostaglandins and the logic behind treatment with NSAIDs. It will also shed some light on the available evidence-based modalities of treatment using cyclooxygenase (COX) inhibitors.

Endometriosis as an Inflammatory Process

Although retrograde menstruation occurs in about 90% of cycling women, endometriosis is diagnosed in only about 10% of women. This discrepancy raises questions about features of refluxed eutopic endometrium in patients with endometriosis, which may have distinct features for adherence or proliferation at the ectopic sites. Endometriosis is an inflammatory condition.[12,13] PGE_2[14,15] TNF-α and IL-1β[16,17] are all elevated in peritoneal macrophage-conditioned media or in the peritoneal fluid from women with endometriosis when compared with disease-free women. Such an inflammatory stimulus induces an altered biologic response by ectopic endometrial implants in the pelvis and their possible secretion of compounds such as cytokines that can influence the inflammatory response by the host. Host immunologic dysfunctions have been invoked as an important factor in the development of this disorder.[18]

Various studies[10,19-23] have shown that affected women have an increased concentration and activation of endometrial and peritoneal macrophages and polymorphonuclear leukocytes, occurring early in the recruitment sequence of immune cells, which can mediate the release of growth factors, prostaglandins (PGs), complement components, and lymphokines with subsequent effect on monocyte/macrophage activity and natural killer cell cytotoxicity, leading to growth and development of seeded ectopic endometrial implants **(Table 22-2)**.

Garzetti et al reported that the peripheral blood polymorphonuclear leukocyte chemotactic index and cytotoxic activity of natural killer cells were decreased with respect to the stage of endometriosis and were inversely related to plasma PGE_2 and estradiol levels.[24] In addition, PGE_2 (the main prostaglandin product of the COX pathway) has been shown to act post-transcriptionally to stabilize COX-2 transcripts promoting sustained COX-2 enzyme activity in an inflammatory environment.[25,26]

Furthermore, in physiologic conditions, PG production as well as COX-2 increase during the luteal phase and

Table 22-2: Findings suggesting that endometriosis is an inflammatory process
• High PG concentrations of peritoneal fluid in endometriosis (Darke 1981, Badawy 1985)
• High PG concentration in menstrual fluid in dysmenorrheic women (Cham 1978, Lundstrom 1976)
• PGE2 (the main prostaglandin product of the COX pathway) acts post-transcriptionally to stabilize COX-2 transcripts promoting sustained COX-2 enzyme activity in an inflammatory environment.[26]
• The effectiveness of PG synthetase inhibitor in dysmenorrheic women (Pulkkinen 1978)
• Animal studies implicating prostaglandins in uterine implantation of embryos and the decidual cell reaction.
• Elevated TNF-α and IL-1β in the peritoneal fluid from women with endometriosis.[16, 17]
• COX-2 enzyme in not only the eutopic endometrium but also in local lesions of endometriosis, using immunohistochemical techniques.[34]

menstruation.[27, 28] In fact, COX-2 is considered to be involved in cell proliferation, regeneration, and promotion of angiogenesis.[29-32] Higher concentrations of $PGF_{2\alpha}$ due to COX-2 are present in the human endometrium during the luteal phase and menstruation.[33] In addition, increased expression of COX-2 mRNA in the secretory phase was found, with especially pronounced COX-2 staining observed during menstruation.[34] Of Interest, levels of COX-2 mRNA in the endometrium taken from postmenopausal women were decreased when compared with the endometrium of normal menstrual cycles.

At sites of inflammation, hyperalgesic and pro-inflammatory prostaglandins are generated. In addition, transcription and *de novo* synthesis of COX-2 are triggered by exposure of inflammatory cells to endotoxin, interferon and cytokines. In women with endometriosis, peritoneal macrophages have higher levels of COX-2 mRNA and protein than those from women without the disease.[35] Dense staining of COX-2, as well as COX-2 mRNA and protein are present in higher amounts in ectopic endometrial lesions when compared with eutopic endometrium from women with endometriosis.[25,36] Thus suggesting that higher activation of COX-2 in endometriotic tissues may occur in women with dysmenorrhea.

Pathologic angiogenesis occurs in conditions such as malignancy and chronic inflammatory disorders, for example, rheumatoid arthritis, endometriosis, and diabetic retinopathy.[37] Estrogen, a major regulator of endothelial cell growth and angiogenesis in both physiologic and pathologic processes,[38] has been shown to increase the *in vitro* production of PGs by human endometrial fibroblasts. Prostaglandins derived from endothelium, especially PGE_2, are proangiogenic factors that are implicated in altered vascular permeability and angiogenesis. They have also been shown to be involved in the vascular effects of estrogen, the vasculature of the ovary and endometrium being recognized as the most important target of estrogen's action.[39-41]

It has been reported that 17β-estradiol (E_2) could induce COX-2 expression in human umbilical vein endothelial cells, and that E_2 up-regulates COX-2 mRNA and protein levels and PGE_2 production in primary human uterine microvascular endothelial cells (HUMEC) via estrogen receptors.[42, 43] The three key molecules, PGE2, COX-2, and E2, are thus linked together closely with the common thread of angiogenesis.

These observations sparked new insights into the paracrine interactions in the pathophysiology of endometriosis and might well be the basis for new therapeutic strategies capable of interrupting the pathophysiological cascade at key points. Therefore, NSAIDs could have a therapeutic benefit in disrupting the inflammatory processes evident in women with endometriosis.

Prostanoid Biosynthetic and Cyclooxygenase (COX) Signaling Pathways

Prostaglandins

Prostaglandins are ubiquitous bioactive lipids that exert an autocrine or paracrine function by binding to specific G-protein-coupled receptors to activate intracellular signaling and gene transcription. They serve as mediators involved in inflammation and immune response modulation, renal function, vasomotor tone, platelet aggregation and blood clotting, differentiation of immune cells, wound healing, nerve growth, bone metabolism. Prostaglandins are key regulators of reproductive processes, including ovulation, menstruation, implantation and initiation of labor.[44]

Arachidonic acid (AA) is released from plasma membrane phospholipids by phospholipase A2 (PLA2) and used by COX enzymes and specific synthase enzymes, such as prostaglandin D synthase (PGDS), PGES, PGFS, PGIS thromboxane synthase (TXS), to form prostaglandin D_2 (PGD$_2$), PGE$_2$, PGF$_{2\alpha}$, PGI$_2$ and thromboxane A$_2$ (TXA$_2$), respectively. These molecules are actively transported out of the cell by means of a prostaglandin transporter (PGT), where they exert an autocrine or paracrine effect by coupling to their respective heptahelical transmembrane receptors, DP, EP1–EP4, FP, IP and TP, to activate second messengers, such as cyclic AMP (cAMP) and inositol (1,4,5)-trisphosphate (IP$_3$), and intracellular signaling cascades.[45]

At least four isoforms of PGES have been described: two membrane-bound isoforms, mPGES-1 and mPGES-2; a cytosolic isoform, cPGES; and a glutathione *S*-transferase isoform, GST-μ. cPGES preferentially converts COX-1-derived PGH$_2$ to PGE$_2$ and is associated with immediate prostaglandin biosynthesis. The inducible membrane-associated form, mPGES-1, is preferentially associated with COX-2 under conditions of limited AA supply (but can couple to COX-1 under conditions where AA is available) and is associated with delayed biosynthesis of PGE$_2$. mPGES-2 is structurally distinct from mPGES-1 and seems to be expressed in tissues where biosynthesis of mPGES-1 is low. mPGES-2 can couple with both COX-1 and COX-2. The GST-μ isoform of PGES has been described recently; however, its specificity for coupling with either COX isoform remains to be determined.[45]

Prostaglandin Receptors

After biosynthesis, prostanoids are transported out of the cell by means of a prostaglandin transporter (PGT), a protein belonging to a superfamily of 12-transmembrane organic anion-transporting polypeptides.[46] Once released outside the cell, prostaglandins act in an autocrine or paracrine function by binding to specific G-protein-coupled receptors, in the vicinity of their sites of production, to activate intracellular signaling and gene transcription.

PGD$_2$, PGE$_2$, PGF$_{2\alpha}$, PGI$_2$ and TXA$_2$ exert their biological function through interactions with, respectively, the DP, EP, FP, IP and TP prostanoid receptors. There are four subtypes of EP receptor (EP1-EP4), which are encoded by four separate genes. In addition, there are several splice variants of the EP3, FP and TP receptors, which differ only in their carboxy-terminal tails. In general, prostanoid receptor isoforms show similar ligand binding but differ in their signaling pathways, their sensitivity to agonist-induced desensitization, and their tendency towards constitutive activity (**Figure 22-2**).[45]

Among the different receptors, the IP, DP, EP2 and EP4 receptors increase the accumulation of intracellular cyclic (cAMP) via Gα$_s$ and have been termed 'relaxant' receptors because they induce smooth muscle relaxation. The TP, FP and EP1 receptors induce Ca^{2+} mobilization via Gα$_q$ and constitute a 'contractile' receptor group because they cause smooth muscle contraction. The remaining receptor, EP3, is generally associated with a decline in cAMP. This 'inhibitory' receptor usually stimulates smooth muscle contraction; depending on the splice variant and cell type, however, the EP3 receptor can also increase intracellular cAMP and mobilize Ca^{2+}.[47]

Cyclooxygenase Enzymes

Tissue damage activates phospholipase A2, causing arachidonic acid (AA) to be cleaved from cell membrane phospholipids. Upon release, arachidonic acid can proceed down either the lipoxygenase pathway leading to the formation of leukotrienes and lipoxins, or the COX pathway leading to the formation of thromboxanes and prostaglandins.

Currently, the three described isoforms of the COX enzyme (COX-1, COX-2 and COX-3) are responsible in catalyzing the dedicated step in the biosynthesis of prostaglandin and thromboxane (collectively termed 'prostanoids').[48] Following the activation of phospholipase A2 (PLA2), AA is released from plasma membrane phospholipids, and is reduced to the intermediary prostaglandin, prostaglandin H$_2$ (PGH$_2$), by the COX enzymes. PGH$_2$ serves as the substrate for terminal enzymes in the prostanoid biosynthetic pathway, which are designated according to the prostanoid they produce, such that PGD$_2$ synthesized by prostaglandin D synthase (PGDS), PGF$_{2\alpha}$ by PGFS, PGI$_2$ (also known as prostacyclin) by PGIS, thromboxane (TXA$_2$) by thromboxane synthase (TXS), and PGE$_2$ by PGES (**Figure 22-2**).[47]

A role for a functional COX-3 isoform in human physiology and pathophysiology remains to be established.

COX-1 and COX-2 are products of two genes residing on different chromosomes. Both attach to different sites on AA, but convert it to prostaglandins equally efficiently.

COX-1 is ubiquitous to most tissues, and maintains normal gastric mucosa and influences kidney and platelet function. It has long been implicated in normal physiological functions, but more recently it has been shown to be upregulated in various carcinomas and to have a central role in tumorigenesis.[45]

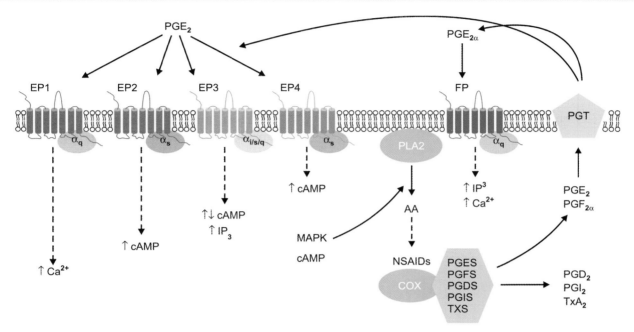

FIGURE 22-2: Schematic representation of the cyclooxygenase–prostanoid biosynthetic and signaling pathway. Arachidonic acid (AA) is released from plasma membrane phospholipids by phospholipase A2 (PLA2) and utilized by cyclooxygenases (COX) and specific synthase enzymes to form prostaglandin (PG), PGD2, PGE2, PGF2, PGI2 and thromboxane (TX) A. These products are actively transported out of the cell by a prostanoid transporter (PGT), on which they exert an autocrine–paracrine effect by coupling to heptahelical transmembrane receptors to activate intracellular signaling. Inhibitors of COX enzyme function such as nonsteroidal anti-inflammatory drugs (NSAIDs) can block PG biosynthesis and subsequent downstream events. IP32: inositol trisphosphate; MAPK: mitogen-associated protein kinase; PGDS: prostaglandin-D-synthase; PGES: prostaglandin-E-synthase; PGFS: prostaglandin-F-synthase; PGIS: prostaglandin-I-synthase; TXS: thromboxane synthase. Reference: Sales KJ, Jabbour HN. Cyclooxygenase enzymes and prostaglandins in pathology of the endometrium. Reproduction 2003;126:559–67.

On the other hand, COX-2 is present in the central nervous system, the gastrointestinal tract, kidneys, bones, ovaries and uterus. The immediate early response gene COX-2 can be induced by proinflammatory or mitogenic stimuli, which include various cytokines, growth factors, and oncogenes.[45] The contributions of COX-2 to angiogenesis include: (1) increased expression of vascular endothelial growth factor (VEGF); (2) the production of the eicosanoid products PGE$_2$, thromboxane A$_2$, and PGI$_2$, which can directly stimulate endothelial cell migration and growth factor-induced angiogenesis; and, potentially, (3) the inhibition of endothelial cell apoptosis. Thus, COX-2 is inducible by pro-inflammatory cytokines and produces prostaglandins that mediate the inflammatory and pain responses. Its inhibition is a therapeutic goal.[49,50]

Ablation of the gene encoding COX-2 in mice results in multiple reproductive failures, including ovulation, fertilization, implantation and decidualization, confirming that the prostaglandins produced by COX-2 have a crucial role in these processes.[51,52]

Chishima and coworkers quantitatively evaluated the expressions of COX-2 mRNA in endometrium, ectopic endometriosis tissue, and peritoneum by competitive reverse transcription–polymerase chain reaction (RT–PCR). They noted that in the uterus, COX-2 was localized in the endometrial epithelium. Eutopic endometrial surface epithelium contained more COX-2 than did glandular epithelium. They also observed more frequent and denser COX-2 staining in the ectopic endometriosis implants when compared with eutopic endometrium **(Figure 22-3)**. Furthermore, the levels of COX-2 mRNA in endometriosis were five times those of eutopic endometria. Hence, the authors concluded that enhanced synthesis of PGs, as a consequence of up-regulated COX-2, possibly contributed to the pathogenesis of endometriosis and disease progression.[25]

Nonsteroidal Anti-inflammatory Drugs

NSAIDs have been in use long before anything was known about their mechanism of action **(Table 22-3)**. They are analgesics which inhibit the cyclooxygenase (COX) enzymes thereby inhibiting the production of prostaglandins and alleviating cramps. The first of the

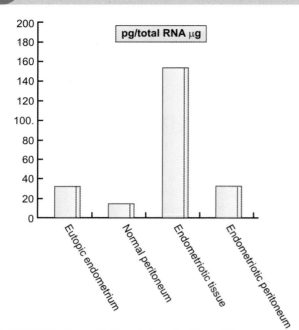

FIGURE 22-3: Quantitative determination of the amounts of COX-2 mRNA in eutopic endometrium, normal peritoneum, endometriotic tissue (ovarian endometriosis), and endometriotic peritoneum. Reference: Chishima F, Hayakawa S, Sugita K, Kinukawa N, Aleemuzzaman S, Nemoto N, Yamamoto T, Honda M. Increased Expression of Cyclooxygenase-2 in Local Lesions of Endometriosis Patients. AJRI 2002; 48:50-6.

drugs with this mode of action was aspirin (acetylsalicylic acid), which was introduced in 1899. However, the term NSAID was not used until the 1950s when phenylbutazone was developed. Since then NSAIDs have become more widely used **(Table 22-3)**.[53]

Traditional NSAIDs inhibit both COX-1 and COX-2 **(Table 22-4)**, and in so doing not only decrease inflammation and pain, but also promote gastrointestinal tract damage and bleeding. Inhibitory potency and selectivity of conventional first-generation NSAIDs for COX-1 and COX-2 vary greatly. However, at therapeutic concentrations none of the currently marketed NSAIDs spare gastric COX-1 activity. It is estimated that 25% of patients using NSAIDs experience some kind of side effect, with 5% developing serious health consequences (massive GI bleeds, acute renal failure, etc.). The occurrence of side effects varies with the traditional NSAIDs.

In the course of the search for a specific inhibitor of the negative effects of prostaglandins which spared the positive effects, it was discovered that prostaglandins could indeed be separated into two general classes which could loosely be regarded as "good prostaglandins" and "bad prostaglandins", according to the structure of a particular enzyme involved in their synthesis, namely cyclooxygenase.

Table 22-3: History of the prostaglandin E pharmacotherapy	
Date	*Breakthrough*
Ancient times	Parts of the willow tree used to relieve pain and inflammation
1897	Acetylsalicylic acid isolated, identified and synthesized
1899	Bayer Company first marketed aspirin
1963	Indomethacin synthesized, followed by several other synthetic and semisynthetic NSAIDs
Mid-1970s	Investigations into development of aromatase inhibitors begins
1971	NSAIDs such as aspirin exert their actions primarily by inhibiting the production of prostaglandins
1976	COX enzyme purified
1984	COX enzyme shown to increase in inflamed tissue
1988	COX enzyme shown to be stimulated by interleukin -1
1988	COX enzyme cloned
1990	COX shown to be induced by endotoxin and prevented by glucocorticoids, but dexamethasone does not affect baseline prostaglandin formation, so postulated a second COX enzyme
1991	Second COX gene discovered and isoform cloned: COX-2
1999	Launch of COX-2 selective inhibitors: rofecoxib and celecoxib
2002	Second-generation COX-2 selective inhibitors: valdecoxib, parecoxib and etoricoxib

COX—cyclooxygenase, NSAIDs—nonsteroidal anti-inflammatory drugs
Reference: Thomas P. Connolly, DO. Cyclooxygenase-2 Inhibitors in Gynecologic Practice. Clinical Medicine & Research 2003; 1(2):105-10.

Table 22-4: Cyclooxygenase modulating medications

NSAIDs

I. Acidic
  A. Carboxylic acids
    1. Fenamic Acids
      a) Meclofenamate
    2. Acetic Acids
      a) Sulindac
      b) Indomethacin
      c) Tolmetin
      d) Diclofenac
      e) ketorolac
    3. Pyranocarboxylic acids
      a) Etodolac
    4. Propionic acids
      a) Naproxen
      b) Flubiprofen
      c) Ibuprofen
      d) Ketoprofen
    5. Salicylic acids
      a) Aspirin
      b) Salsalate
      c) Diflunisal
  B. Enolic acids
    1. Oxicams
      a) Piroxicam
II. Nonacidic
  A. Nephthylalkanones
    1. Nabumetone

Cyclooxygenase-2 inhibitors

I. First generation
  A. Celocoxib
  B. Refocoxib
II. Second generation
  A. Valdecoxib
  B. Etoricoxib
  C. parecoxib

Reference: Thomas P. Connolly, DO. Cyclooxygenase-2 inhibitors in Gynecologic Practice. Clinical Medicine & Research 2003; 1(2):105-10.

Prostaglandins whose synthesis involves the cyclooxygenase-I enzyme, or COX-1, are responsible for maintenance and protection of the gastrointestinal tract, while prostaglandins whose synthesis involves the cyclooxygenase-II enzyme, or COX-2, are responsible for inflammation and pain. The COX-2 enzyme was discovered in 1988 by Daniel Simmons, a Brigham Young University researcher formerly of Harvard University. The same day the enzyme was sequenced, he had his notebook notarized as proof of his discovery. Subsequently, the research firm with whom Dr. Simmons had contracted refused to give him any royalties and profits from his discovery. A lawsuit by Dr. Simmons against the drug developers ensued.

First-generation COX-2 Inhibitors[54]

Rofecoxib was approved as safe and effective by the Food and Drug Administration (FDA) on May 20, 1999 and was subsequently marketed under the brand name Vioxx ®. However, on September 30, 2004, Merck voluntarily withdrew rofecoxib from the market because of concerns about increased risk of heart attack and stroke associated with long-term, high-dosage use. Rofecoxib was one of the most widely used drugs ever to be withdrawn from the market (www.pdr.net).

Celecoxib (Celebrex®) is 375 times more selective for COX-2 than COX-1, and does not inhibit COX-1 at therapeutic doses. It is rapidly and completely absorbed following oral ingestion, even in the presence of food. Steady blood levels are achieved after 10 days. Celecoxib is metabolized by the liver to inactive metabolites that are excreted in the gut and urine. In clinical trials, gastrointestinal toxicity, including mucosal damage, perforation, ulcers and bleeding, occurred significantly less often with rofecoxib than ibuprofen, naproxen or diclofenac. It did not affect bleeding time and platelet aggregation, but had no advantage in terms of renal toxicity (www.pdr.net).

Second-generation COX-2 Inhibitors

Valdecoxib was manufactured and marketed under the brand name Bextra® by G. D. Searle & Company. It has improved potency and a broader therapeutic range than other COX-2 inhibitors. It was approved by the United States Food and Drug Administration on November 20, 2001, and was available by prescription in tablet form until 2005, when it was removed from the market due to concerns about possible increased risk of heart attack and stroke.

In Europe, another second-generation COX-2 specific inhibitor, etoricoxib, is available. Etoricoxib (brand name Arcoxia worldwide; also Algix and Tauxib in Italy) is a new COX-2 selective inhibitor (approximately 106.0 times more selective for COX-2 inhibition over COX-1) from Merck & Co. Doses are 60, 90 mg/day for chronic pain and 120 mg/day for acute pain. Currently it is approved in more than 60 countries worldwide but not in the US, where the Food and Drug Administration (FDA) required additional safety and efficacy data for etoricoxib before it will issue approval. Current therapeutic indications are: treatment of rheumatoid arthritis, osteoarthritis, chronic low back pain, acute pain and gout (www.pdr.net).

Due to the poor water solubility of valdecoxib, the prodrug, parecoxib, is being developed as an injectable form. Parecoxib is a water soluble and injectable prodrug of valdecoxib. It is marketed as Dynastat in the European Union. Parecoxib is a COX-2 selective inhibitor in the same category as celecoxib (Celebrex) and rofecoxib (Vioxx). It is approved through much of Europe for short term perioperative pain control much in the same way ketorolac (Toradol) is used in the United States. However, unlike ketorolac, parecoxib has no effect on platelet function and therefore does not promote bleeding during or after surgery. However, in the United States ketorolac is the only injectable NSAID, although it is banned in many European countries due to concerns about surgical bleeding and stomach ulcers after surgery (www.pdr.net).

In 2005, the FDA issued a letter of non-approval for parecoxib in the United States. One study noted increased occurrences of heart attacks following cardiac bypass surgery compared to placebo when high doses of parecoxib were used to control pain after surgery. The drug is not approved for use after cardiac surgery in Europe. (www.pdr.net)

Nimesulide is a relatively COX-2 selective, non-steroidal anti-inflammatory drug (NSAID) with analgesic and antipyretic properties. Its approved indications are the treatment of acute pain, the symptomatic treatment of osteoarthritis and primary dysmenorrhea in adolescents and adults above 12 years old. Due to concerns about the risk of hepatotoxicity, nimesulide has been withdrawn from market in many countries. (www.pdr.net)

In general, COX-2 inhibitors exhibit improved gastrointestinal safety, are longer lasting, and are more effective at pain and inflammation control.

NSAIDs and Endometriosis

Classically, the main indications for the medical therapy of endometriosis have been dysmenorrhea, pelvic pain, and dyspareunia. However, based on available current data directed at preventing the implantation of endometrium to ectopic sites,[34] controlling growth of the endometriotic lesion, and inducing the regression of endometrial explants in rats[55] and mice,[56] one can speculate that inhibition of COX-2 would be a promising therapy toward treating the disease itself.

Management of Pain Related to Endometriosis

The three most commonly suggested mechanisms for pain production in endometriosis are: (1) production of substances such as growth factors and cytokines by activated macrophages and other cells associated with functioning endometriotic implants; (2) the direct and indirect effects of active bleeding from endometriotic implants; and (3) irritation or direct invasion of pelvic floor nerves or direct invasion of those nerves by infiltrating endometriotic implants, especially in the cul-de-sac. It remains plausible, of course, that in any individual more than one or all of these mechanisms may be in operation.

In addition, the peritoneal fluid of infertile women with endometriosis also exhibits an increased prostaglandin level. This suggests that aberrant endometriotic cells can synthesize and release prostaglandins into the peritoneal fluid and possibly be a cause of various consequences such as: pain and tubal dysfunction.[57]

Simple analgesics (e.g. paracetamol, aspirin) can be used to relieve mild to moderate pain in endometriosis, there being no consistent evidence of significant differences in effectiveness between these first line alternatives.

Dysmenorrhea secondary to endometriosis is, however, frequently treated by NSAIDs as the first option, despite the paucity of randomized controlled trials.

Kauppila et al conducted two prospective studies evaluating the effect of different NSAIDs on overall pain relief in patients with endometriosis. The first trial[58] was a placebo controlled, double-blind, four-treatment crossover trial comparing indomethacin inhibiting PG-synthetase (25 mg, three times per day), acetylsalicylic acid (500 mg, three times per day) exerting a weak PG-synthetase inhibition, tolfenamic acid which both inhibits PG-synthetase and antagonizes PGs at the target level (200 mg, three times per day), and placebo (three times per day) in 18 symptomatic women diagnosed with endometriosis by laparoscopy or by pelvic examination. Each woman received one of the four drugs for two menstrual cycles each, but it was not clear how the women were randomized. Prostaglandin biosynthesis inhibitors did not alleviate premenstrual complaints better than placebo. During menstruation tolfenamic acid relieved endometriotic symptoms more effectively than placebo while indomethacin and acetylsalicylic acid did not differ from placebo.

In his second trial,[8] twenty patients with moderate to very severe painful menstrual periods secondary to endometriosis were treated in a double-blind, four-period, crossover clinical trial with naproxen sodium and placebo. Endometriosis was diagnosed by pelvic examination, history of menstrual distress, or by direct visualization of pelvic regions at laparoscopy or laparotomy. Each woman received either naproxen sodium (275 mg, four times per day) for two menstrual cycles followed by placebo (four times per day) for two menstrual cycles, or placebo for two menstrual cycles followed by naproxen sodium for two menstrual cycles. Complete or substantial pain relief was obtained in 83% of the cases of painful menstruation with naproxen sodium and in 41% with placebo (P = .008); indicating that naproxen sodium is efficacious and safe for the treatment of dysmenorrhea in patients with endometriosis.

There have been a number of studies linking COX-2 expression to endometriosis-related pain. Using immunohistochemical studies, Ota et al (2001), have shown that COX-2 protein is up-regulated in endometriotic lesions.[36] Moreover, Matsuzaki et al (2004), showed that patients with deep endometriosis exhibiting severe dysmenorrhea (pain score for dysmenorrhea >7) had significantly higher levels of COX-2 expression in the eutopic endometrial stromal cells in the secretory phase.[34]

Cobellis et al assessed the use of the COX-2 specic inhibitor (rofecoxib) in the management of pain related to endometriosis. Twenty eight women with stage I-II endometriosis were included in a placebo-controlled double blind study. The diagnosis of endometriosis was based on clinical symptoms, and was confirmed by laparoscopy and histopathological examination. Rofecoxib was given at a dose of 25 mg per day for six months. Folic acid was used as the placebo drug at 4 mg daily for six months. Patents were asked to fill out a questionnaire for assessment of pain before laparoscopy and then after 6 months of treatment. Pain symptoms were divided according to dysmenorrhea, dyspareunia and chronic pelvic pain. The rofecoxib group had a significant decrease in all painful symptoms as compared to the placebo group (p<0.0001) (Cobellis). Despite the small size of the study, rofecoxib group (n = 16) vs. placebo group (n = 12), the results appeared promising in considering COX-2 specific inhibitors as a first line medical treatment for endometriosis.

In their 2003 Cochrane review of 31 studies, Marjoribanks et al[53] compared NSAIDs versus placebo for primary dysmenorrhea. Twenty one different types of NSAIDs were evaluated in the included studies: aspirin, ketoprofen, naproxen, piroxicam, ketoprofen, dexketoprofen, diclofenac, etodolac, fenoprofen, flufenamic acid, flurbiprofen, glucamethacin, ibuprofen, indomethacin, ketoprofen, lysine cloxinate, mefenamic acid, naproxen, niflumic acid, nimesulide and piroxicam. The trials included in this review provided overwhelming evidence of the effectiveness of NSAIDs in providing pain relief from dysmenorrhea. All measures of effectiveness confirmed the overall superiority of NSAIDs to placebo, despite a statistically significant increased risk of adverse effects to the gastrointestinal (for example, nausea and diarrhea) and nervous (for example, headache, drowsiness, dizziness, and dryness of the mouth) systems.[53]

Despite rigorous searches, the authors identified only two randomized controlled trials comparing NSAIDs with placebo in the treatment of women with dysmenorrheal secondary to endometriosis. This is surprising given that NSAIDs are widely prescribed and are available over the counter for the treatment of pain caused by endometriosis. In comparison, there is much literature suggesting the use of NSAIDs as a treatment for primary dysmenorrhea. It is likely, however, that prostaglandins are involved in pain causation in both groups of patients.[53]

The Cochrane Database of Systematic Reviews 2005 showed that there is no conclusive evidence whether NSAIDs, namely naproxen, are effective in managing pain caused by endometriosis (OR 3.27 [0.61–17.69] for active treatment naproxen versus placebo). Moreover, there was no evidence that any individual NSAID is more effective than the rest.[59]

Despite adequate evidence of NSAIDs being effective in treating primary dysmenorrhea, still the evidence is inconclusive when evaluating dysmenorrhea secondary to endometriosis.

More recently, Sinaii et al. in their cross-sectional survey evaluated the usual pattern of medical treatments for pain from endometriosis. In their study of patients lifetime experience in treatment utilization for endometriosis symptoms, they described the sequence of treatments used, based on the calculated probabilities of one treatment to be followed by another from all quantifiable treatment orders provided by the study respondents.[60] Oral Contraceptives (OCs) or analgesics were taken first 83% of the time (47% and 36%, respectively) by surveyed patients. Women taking OCs most often took analgesics next (41%). Similarly, those taking analgesics went on to take OCs (40%), while very few (6%) took OCs again. Surprisingly, 17% started with a second-line hormone as their initial treatment. Of those taking GnRH-a, most then took analgesics (34%), or either danazol or progestins (34%).

NSAIDs Inhibition of Endometriosis

COX-2 over expression was detected in eutopic and ectopic endometrium from patients with endometriosis.[34, 36] Furthermore, the large amounts of PGs found in peritoneal fluid from endometriosis patients and endometriotic lesions may lead to excessive estradiol formation. In turn, estradiol and cytokines (interleukin-1b and tumor necrosis factor-a), which are increased in endometriosis, induce COX-2.[61] The COX-2 vascular endothelial growth factor (VEGF) association has been shown in human samples of non-small cell lung cancer.[62] PGE increases VEGF production[62] and then VEGF stimulates COX-2 expression in endothelial cells.[26] This pathway establishes a positive feedback loop in favor of high concentrations of estrogen, PGE and VEGF in endometriosis.[43]

Based on these data, one can speculate that inhibition of COX-2 would be a promising therapy toward controlling the growth of the endometriotic lesion. In fact, Inhibition of COX-2 has been shown to reduce inflammation, angiogenesis and cellular proliferation. It may also downregulate aromatase activity in ectopic endometrial lesions. Accordingly, ectopic endometrial establishment and growth are therefore potentially suppressed in the presence of COX-2 inhibitors.

Hull et al hypothesized that COX-2 inhibition would reduce the size and number of ectopic human endometrial lesions in a nude mouse model of endometriosis (Hull 2005). The selective COX-2 inhibitor, nimesulide, was administered to estrogen-supplemented nude mice implanted with human endometrial tissue. Ten days after implantation, the number and size of ectopic endometrial lesions were evaluated and compared with lesions from a control group. There was no difference in the number or size of ectopic endometrial lesions in control and nimesulide-treated nude mice. Furthermore, nimesulide did not induce a visually identiable difference in blood vessel development or macrophage or myofibroblast infiltration in the nude mouse explants. The authors concluded that treatment with COX-2 inhibitors such as nimesulide is unlikely to reduce the size or number of endometriotic lesions in women, if administered in a constant estrogenic environment. Possible explanations for this negative effect might be that 1- Prostaglandin production by COX-1- mediated pathways in macrophages and fibroblasts may have masked nimesulide's therapeutic influence. In fact, elevated levels of COX-1 mRNA have been detected in peritoneal macrophages harvested from women with severe endometriosis when compared with normal controls;[35] and macrophages and myofibroblasts were identified in both treated and untreated nude mouse lesions. Thus, prostaglandin production in these cells may have been minimally affected by COX-2 inhibition due to high constitutive COX-1 activity.[63]

Vascular disruption has been shown to influence lesion number and size in the nude mouse model of endometriosis,[64] however, nimesulide treatment did not alter these parameters, suggesting that products of COX-2 do not alter vessel formation. It is possible that the outcome measure of lesion size would not detect subtle changes in vessel development after nimesulide exposure. However, immunohistochemical identification of endothelial cells indicated that there were no differences in vascularity between treatment groups. It is therefore unlikely that COX-2 significantly influences ectopic endometrial vascular supply in the nude mouse model.

In a study of histological samples obtained from 130 women,[65] COX-2 immunostaining was more common in ovarian endometrioma (78.5%) than in peritoneal implants (11%) and rectovaginal nodules (13.3%). It may be that COX-2 inhibitors tend to influence ovarian endometriosis more than disease at other sites.

Intraperitoneal lesions may also have a greater response to COX-2 inhibitors than nude mouse lesions that are supplied by peritoneal blood vessels[64] but lie outside the peritoneal cavity.

It would have been helpful to measure COX-2 enzymatic activity in ectopic human endometrial tissues both in COX-2 inhibitor-treated mice and controls in order to confirm that the dose administered to the nude mice was adequate to inhibit the COX-2 enzyme in human endometrial tissues.

In contradistinction, in a prospective randomized study, Matsuzaki et al evaluated the effect of COX-2 inhibition on surgically induced endometriosis in seventy adult female Sprague-Dawley rats.[34] The aim of their study was to investigate the effects of COX-2 inhibitors on the growth of surgically established implants in protocol 1; the development of ectopic implants in protocol 2; and the preventive effects of COX-2 inhibitor pretreatment on implantation of the ectopic implants in protocol-3.

In the first group of rats, celecoxib (5 mg/kg/day, twice/day by oral gavage) started before auto-transplanting uterine tissues. The size of ectopic implants post-treatment was significantly reduced compared with pretreatment size in the same rat (P <0 .03).

The second group of rats received celecoxib for 2 or 4 weeks starting day 1 after surgical implantation, evaluating the effects on the development of ectopic implants, showed the absence of implants in 50% of the treated rats, while the remaining 50% had smaller implants as compared to controls.

In the third group of rats, evaluating the effect of pretreatment with the COX-2 inhibitor on implantation to ectopic sites, no significant difference was detected in implant size at 2 or 4 weeks of pre-treatment or between treated and control groups.

The authors concluded that celecoxib prevented the establishment of new endometriotic lesions and the growth of already established ones, in addition to a marked reduction in the expression of COX-2 in ectopic implants in treated rats compared with that seen in controls.[34]

This was the rst *in vitro* study suggesting a direct effect of celecoxib COX-2 inhibitor on the reduction of endometrial growth. In humans, only one report has been published and suggested that the use of COX-2-specific inhibitors was effective in the management of pelvic pain associated with endometriosis.[66]

More recently, Olivares et al investigated the effects of this drug on cell proliferation and apoptosis of cultured human endometrial epithelial cells (EECs).[32] The reduction of PGE_2 production induced by 25 mm celecoxib in EECs without the induction of growth inhibition supports the proposal that the growth arrest induced by higher concentrations (50–100 mm) of celecoxib is not simply due to reduced PGE_2 secretion. Similar results were obtained by[67] who speculated that the mechanisms involved in the inhibition of cell proliferation due to celecoxib treatment are independent of COX-2 activity and expression, since the concentrations needed to induce cell cycle arrest and inhibit proliferation are higher than those needed to inhibit COX-2 activity.

In conclusion, chronic administration of NSAIDs limits the progression of endometriosis. Available data suggest that NSAID selection in the treatment of endometriosis should be extended beyond pain management to maximize the inhibitory effect on disease burden. In addition, the NSAID-mediated mechanisms suppressing endometriosis are likely to be multifactorial. These factors include effects on angiogenesis, inflammation, apoptosis, vascular permeability, COX inhibition, and PPAR-activation. Differences in any one of these parameters as well as differences in pharmacokinetics could contribute to differential efficacy.

NSAIDs and Recurrent Lesions of Endometriosis

Recurrence rates of up to 47% after five years of medical or surgical therapy have been reported based on the number of patients who experience recurrent symptoms.[68, 69]

To determine whether the inhibitory effects of celecoxib persisted after the drug was discontinued, Efesthatiou et al conrmed the statistically significant lower incidence of lesion establishment (61.9 ± 21.8%) and smaller lesion size (3.8 + 0.7 mm²) compared with controls (100 ± no establishment; lesion size 6.6 + 2.4 mm²) in mice examined immediately after completing a 4-week course of celecoxib.[70]

Cobellis et al assessed the use of the COX-2 specific inhibitor (rofecoxib) in the management of pain related to endometriosis. The rofecoxib group had a significant decrease in all painful symptoms as compared to the placebo group (p<0.0001).[66] In addition, at the six months follow-up the rofecoxib group did not show any recurrence of endometriosis, while 16% of the placebo group had relapses confirmed by a rise in CA125 and by transvaginal ultrasonography showing an echogenic focus on the ovarian surface.

Conclusion

Because the clinical profile of endometriosis is typical of an inflammatory disease, therapy with anti-inflammatory or anti-cytokine drugs has been proposed. Clinical evidence supports the use of NSAIDs to treat pain and dysmenorrhea associated with endometriosis, but beneficial effects of these agents on pregnancy rate or disease expression have not been demonstrated or well documented.

Endometriotic spread and implants in peritoneal cavity needs angiogenetic factors to permit the ectopic endometrial cells survival. The hypothesis that COX-2 specic inhibitors might block angiogenesis in endometriotic implants seems a favorable effect in the natural history of disease, mainly in the relapse control. NSAIDs are often given to relieve the pain associated with endometriosis. These drugs reduce the release of prostaglandins in endometriotic implants and probably also in the peritoneal fluid. Nevertheless, limitations to NSAIDs use include over-the-counter doses that may be insufficient to relieve pain and the potential for gastrointestinal toxicity when given chronically at high doses.

COX-2 is induced in the proliferative stage of the endometrium, and COX-2, rather than COX-1, is the primary isoenzyme involved in the endometrial productions of prostaglandins. Peritoneal PGE-2 in endometriotic stromal cells may also induce steroidogenic acute regulatory protein, further contributing to the development of endometriosis. Aromatase inhibitors have successfully treated unusually aggressive postmenopausal endometriosis, and future treatment of endometriosis will likely combine both COX-2 and aromatase inhibitors.[71]

Web Resources

The URLs for data presented herein are as follows:
Women of our world 2005, population reference Bureau: www.prb.org
National Endometriosis Society: www.endo.org.uk
Physicians Desk Reference web site: www.pdr.net

References

1. Olive DL, Schwartz LB. Endometriosis. N Engl J Med, 1993; 328:1759-69.
2. Eskenazi B, Warner ML. Epidemiology of endometriosis. Obstet Gynecol Clin North Am, 1997;24:235-58.
3. Mahmood TA, Templeton A. Prevalence and genesis of endometriosis. Hum Reprod, 1991;6:544-49.

4. Berube S, Marcoux S, Maheux R. Characteristics related to the prevalence of minimal or mild endometriosis in infertile women. Canadian Collaborative Group on Endometriosis. Epidemiology 1998;9:504-10.

5. Fedele L, et al. Stage and localization of pelvic endometriosis and pain. Fertil Steril 1990;53:155-58.

6. Redwine DB. Age-related evolution in color appearance of endometriosis. Fertil Steril 1987;48:1062-63.

7. Vincent K, Kennedy S, Stratton P. Pain scoring in endometriosis: entry criteria and outcome measures for clinical trials. Report from the Art and Science of Endometriosis meeting. Fertil Steril 2008.

8. Kauppila A, Ronnberg L. Naproxen sodium in dysmenorrhea secondary to endometriosis. Obstet Gynecol 1985;65:379-83.

9. Zreik TG, Olive DL. Pathophysiology. The biologic principles of disease. Obstet Gynecol Clin North Am 1997; 24:259-68.

10. Gazvani R, Templeton A. Peritoneal environment, cytokines and angiogenesis in the pathophysiology of endometriosis. Reproduction 2002;123:217-26.

11. Pellicer A, et al. The pathophysiology of endometriosis-associated infertility: follicular environment and embryo quality. J Reprod Fertil Suppl 2000;55:109-19.

12. Haney AF, Weinberg JB. Reduction of the intraperitoneal inflammation associated with endometriosis by treatment with medroxyprogesterone acetate. Am J Obstet Gynecol 1988;159:450-54.

13. Hull ML, et al. Nimesulide, a COX-2 inhibitor, does not reduce lesion size or number in a nude mouse model of endometriosis. Hum Reprod 2005;20:350-58.

14. Karck U, et al. PGE2 and PGF2 alpha release by human peritoneal macrophages in endometriosis. Prostaglandins, 1996;51:49-60.

15. Raiter-Tenenbaum A, et al. Functional and phenotypic alterations in peritoneal macrophages from patients with early and advanced endometriosis. Arch Gynecol Obstet 1998;261:147-57.

16. Mori H, et al. Peritoneal fluid interleukin-1 beta and tumor necrosis factor in patients with benign gynecologic disease. Am J Reprod Immunol 1991;26:62-67.

17. Keenan JA, et al. IL-1 beta, TNF-alpha, and IL-2 in peritoneal fluid and macrophage-conditioned media of women with endometriosis. Am J Reprod Immunol 1995;34:381-85.

18. Hill JA. Immunology and endometriosis. Fertil Steril 1992; 58:262-64.

19. Senturk LM, Arici A. Immunology of endometriosis. J Reprod Immunol 1999;43:67-83.

20. Koninckx PR, Kennedy SH, Barlow DH. Endometriotic disease: the role of peritoneal fluid. Hum Reprod Update 1998;4:741-51.

21. Ramey JW, Archer DF. Peritoneal fluid: its relevance to the development of endometriosis. Fertil Steril 1993;60:1-14.

22. D'Hooghe TM, Debrock S. Endometriosis, retrograde menstruation and peritoneal inflammation in women and in baboons. Hum Reprod Update 2002;8:84-88.

23. Garcia-Velasco JA, et al. Macrophage derived growth factors modulate Fas ligand expression in cultured endometrial stromal cells: a role in endometriosis. Mol Hum Reprod 1999;5:642-50.

24. Garzetti GG, et al. Decrease in peripheral blood polymorphonuclear leukocyte chemotactic index in endometriosis: role of prostaglandin E2 release. Obstet Gynecol 1998;91:25-29.

25. Chishima F, et al. Increased expression of cyclooxygenase-2 in local lesions of endometriosis patients. Am J Reprod Immunol 2002;48:50-6.

26. Tamura M, et al. Up-regulation of cyclooxygenase-2 expression and prostaglandin synthesis in endometrial stromal cells by malignant endometrial epithelial cells. A paracrine effect mediated by prostaglandin E2 and nuclear factor-kappa. BJ Biol Chem 2002;277:26208-16.

27. Van Voorhis BJ, et al. Immunohistochemical localization of prostaglandin H synthase in the female reproductive tract and endometriosis. Am J Obstet Gynecol 1990;163:57-62.

28. Kim JJ, et al. Expression of cyclooxygenase-1 and -2 in the baboon endometrium during the menstrual cycle and pregnancy. Endocrinology 1999;140:2672-78.

29. Tsujii M, DuBois RN. Alterations in cellular adhesion and apoptosis in epithelial cells overexpressing prostaglandin endoperoxide synthase 2. Cell 1995;83:493-501.

30. Tsujii M, et al. Cyclooxygenase regulates angiogenesis induced by colon cancer cells. Cell 1998;93:705-16.

31. Basu GD, et al. Mechanisms underlying the growth inhibitory effects of the cyclo-oxygenase-2 inhibitor celecoxib in human breast cancer cells. Breast Cancer Res 2005;7:R422-35.

32. Olivares C, et al. Effects of a selective cyclooxygenase-2 inhibitor on endometrial epithelial cells from patients with endometriosis. Hum Reprod 2008;23:2701-08.

33. Lumsden MA, Brown A, Baird DT. Prostaglandin production from homogenates of separated glandular epithelium and stroma from human endometrium. Prostaglandins 1984;28:485-96.

34. Matsuzaki S, et al. Cyclooxygenase-2 expression in deep endometriosis and matched eutopic endometrium. Fertil Steril 2004;82:1309-15.

35. Wu MH, et al. Distinct mechanisms regulate cyclooxygenase-1 and -2 in peritoneal macrophages of women with and without endometriosis. Mol Hum Reprod 2002; 8:1103-10.

36. Ota H, et al. Distribution of cyclooxygenase-2 in eutopic and ectopic endometrium in endometriosis and adenomyosis. Hum Reprod 2001;16:561-66.

37. Tamura M, et al. Estrogen up-regulates cyclooxygenase-2 via estrogen receptor in human uterine microvascular endothelial cells. Fertil Steril 2004;81:1351-56.

38. Healy DL, et al. Angiogenesis: a new theory for endometriosis. Hum Reprod Update, 1998;4:736-40.

39. Bulun SE, et al. Molecular basis for treating endometriosis with aromatase inhibitors. Hum Reprod Update 2000;6: 413-8.

40. Oosterlynck DJ, et al. Angiogenic activity of peritoneal fluid from women with endometriosis. Fertil Steril 1993;59:778-82.

41. Donnez J, et al. Vascular endothelial growth factor (VEGF) in endometriosis. Hum Reprod 1998;13:1686-90.

42. Bulun SE, et al. Estrogen biosynthesis in endometriosis: molecular basis and clinical relevance. J Mol Endocrinol 2000; 25:35-42.

43. Bulun SE, et al. Mechanisms of excessive estrogen formation in endometriosis. J Reprod Immunol 2002;55:21-33.

44. Sales KJ, Jabbour HN. Cyclooxygenase enzymes and prostaglandins in pathology of the endometrium. Reproduction 2003;126:559-67.

45. Jabbour HN, Sales KJ. Prostaglandin receptor signalling and function in human endometrial pathology. Trends Endocrinol Metab 2004;15:398-404.

46. Schuster VL. Molecular mechanisms of prostaglandin transport. Annu Rev Physiol 1998;60:221-42.

47. Narumiya S, Sugimoto Y, Ushikubi F. Prostanoid receptors: structures, properties, and functions. Physiol Rev 1999; 79:1193-1226.

48. Morita I. Distinct functions of COX-1 and COX-2. Prostaglandins Other Lipid Mediat 2002;68-69:165-75.

49. Laschke MW, Menger MD. In vitro and in vivo approaches to study angiogenesis in the pathophysiology and therapy of endometriosis. Hum Reprod Update 2007;13:331-42.

50. Wu G, et al. Involvement of COX-2 in VEGF-induced angiogenesis via P38 and JNK pathways in vascular endothelial cells. Cardiovasc Res 2006;69:512-19.

51. Langenbach R, et al. Cyclooxygenase-deficient mice. A summary of their characteristics and susceptibilities to inflammation and carcinogenesis. Ann N Y Acad Sci 1999; 889:52-61.

52. Lim H, et al. Multiple female reproductive failures in cyclooxygenase 2-deficient mice. Cell 1997;91:197-208.

53. Marjoribanks J, Proctor ML, Farquhar C. Nonsteroidal anti-inflammatory drugs for primary dysmenorrhoea. Cochrane Database Syst Rev 2003:CD001751.

54. FitzGerald GA, Patrono C. The coxibs, selective inhibitors of cyclooxygenase-2. N Engl J Med 2001;345:433-42.

55. Dogan E, et al. Regression of endometrial explants in rats treated with the cyclooxygenase-2 inhibitor rofecoxib. Fertil Steril 2004;82 Suppl 3:1115-20.

56. Ozawa Y, et al. A selective cyclooxygenase-2 inhibitor suppresses the growth of endometriosis xenografts via antiangiogenic activity in severe combined immuno-deficiency mice. Fertil Steril 2006;86:1146-51.

57. Haney AF. Endometriosis, macrophages, and adhesions. Prog Clin Biol Res 1993;381:19-44.

58. Kauppila A, Puolakka J, Ylikorkala O. Prostaglandin biosynthesis inhibitors and endometriosis. Prostaglandins 1979;18:655-61.

59. Allen C, Hopewell S, Prentice A. Non-steroidal anti-inflammatory drugs for pain in women with endometriosis. Cochrane Database Syst Rev 2005;CD004753.

60. Sinaii N, et al. Treatment utilization for endometriosis symptoms: a cross-sectional survey study of lifetime experience. Fertil Steril 2007;87:1277-86.

61. Attar E, Bulun SE. Aromatase inhibitors: the next generation of therapeutics for endometriosis? Fertil Steril 2006;85: 1307-18.

62. Gately S, Li WW. Multiple roles of COX-2 in tumor angiogenesis: a target for antiangiogenic therapy. Semin Oncol 2004;31:2-11.

63. Evett GE, et al. Prostaglandin G/H synthase isoenzyme 2 expression in fibroblasts: regulation by dexamethasone, mitogens, and oncogenes. Arch Biochem Biophys 1993; 306:169-77.

64. Hull ML, et al. Antiangiogenic agents are effective inhibitors of endometriosis. J Clin Endocrinol Metab 2003;88:2889-99.

65. Fagotti A, et al. Analysis of cyclooxygenase-2 (COX-2) expression in different sites of endometriosis and correlation with clinico-pathological parameters. Hum Reprod 2004; 19:393-97.

66. Cobellis L, et al. The treatment with a COX-2 specific inhibitor is effective in the management of pain related to endometriosis. Eur J Obstet Gynecol Reprod Biol 2004; 116:100-02.

67. Grosch S, et al. COX-2 independent induction of cell cycle arrest and apoptosis in colon cancer cells by the selective COX-2 inhibitor celecoxib. Faseb J 2001;15:2742-44.

68. Revelli A, et al. Recurre nt endometriosis: a review of biological and clinical aspects. Obstet Gynecol Surv 1995; 50:747-54.

69. Wheeler JM, Malinak LR. Recurrent endometriosis: incidence, management, and prognosis. Am J Obstet Gynecol 1983;146:247-53.

70. Efstathiou JA, et al. Nonsteroidal antiinflammatory drugs differentially suppress endometriosis in a murine model. Fertil Steril 2005;83:171-81.

71. Ebert AD, Bartley J, David M. Aromatase inhibitors and cyclooxygenase-2 (COX-2) inhibitors in endometriosis: new questions—old answers? Eur J Obstet Gynecol Reprod Biol 2005;122:144-50.

Edgardo Somigliana

Chapter 23

Progestins in Endometriosis Treatment

Introduction

It has been definitely shown that hormones used in the medical therapy of endometriosis do not eradicate the disease.[1] At restoration of ovulation and of physiologic levels of estrogens, the endometrium, both eutopic and ectopic, resumes its metabolic activity. Since pharmacological treatment is symptomatic and pain relapse at treatment suspension is the rule, drugs that could be administered for long periods of time should be identified.[1] Medical therapy for endometriosis should often be conceived in terms of years, and the use of agents that must be withdrawn after a few months due to poor tolerability, severe metabolic side effects or high cost do not greatly benefit women with symptomatic endometriosis. The characteristics of progestins as well as combined oral contraceptives render these agents the ideal pharmacological choice. Data on the latter has been discussed earlier. In this chapter, the main progestins used for endometriosis and currently available on the market will be reviewed. Data will be presented according to the route of administration **(Table 23-1)**.

Oral Route

Norethisterone Acetate

Norethisterone acetate (or norethindrone acetate, NETA) is a strong progestin derivative of 19-nortestosterone. Its efficacy was initially studied in 52 women with symptomatic and laparoscopically confirmed endometriosis.[2] NETA was started at the beginning of the menstrual cycle at a daily dose of 5 mg, which was increased by 2.5 mg up to 20 mg/day until amenorrhea was achieved. Treatment was continued for 6 months to over 1 year. Dysmenorrhea regressed in 48/52 (92%) subjects and chronic pelvic pain in 25/28 (89%). At the end of treatment 49/52 (94%) women

Table 23-1: Different progestins used for medical treatment of endometriosis
Oral route
Norethisterone acetate
Cyproterone acetate
Dienogest
Intramuscular route
Medroxiprogesterone acetate
Intrauterine route
Levonorgestrel-releasing IUD

had few or no symptoms. Breakthrough bleeding was, however, experienced by 30 (58%) patients. This complaint was the cause of discontinuation in 4 of them (8%). One other patient suspended therapy for severe breast tenderness, and three patients for inefficacy. Overall, treatment was successful in 44/52 (84%) recruited subjects.

Moore et al compared the effect of a 6-month oral treatment with dienogest 2 mg/day (n = 119) versus NETA 10 mg/day (n = 48).[3] Pain relief at the end of therapy was similar, being obtained in 88/97 (91%) of the former group and 46/48 (96%) of the latter.

NETA offers various advantages for the long-term treatment of endometriosis. This progestin allows good control of uterine bleeding as compared with other compounds, has a positive effect on calcium metabolism by producing greater increases in bone mineral density than alendronate, and at low dosages has no negative effects on the lipoprotein profile.[4] NETA administered continuously to treat endometriosis is approved by the United States Food and Drug Administration.

Cyproterone Acetate

A role for cyproterone acetate (CPA), a derivative of 17-hydroxyprogesterone with anti-androgenic and antigonadotropinic properties, in the treatment of endometriosis has been firstly proposed by Fedele et al at the dosage of 27 mg/day.[5]

Subsequently Moran et al evaluated the efficacy of a 6-month treatment with CPA at a reduced dosage (10 mg/day for 20 days followed by 10 days with no treatment) in seven women affected by mild to severe symptomatic endometriosis.[6] Dysmenorrhea was considerably relieved in all the subjects, with oligomenorrhea reported by six and spotting by one. A repeated laparoscopy at the end of treatment demonstrated minimal residual lesions in five women and absence of disease in two.

A similar dosage (12.5 mg/day) but administered continuously was tested in a randomized study that compared its effects to those of an oral contraceptive (desogestrel 0.15 mg and ethynilestradiol 0.02 mg) given continuously for 6 months.[7] Ninety women were recruited with moderate to severe pelvic pain that recurred after conservative surgery for symptomatic endometriosis. The main outcome of the study was patients' degree of satisfaction, which was deemed important in order to be able to consider their point of view in the evaluation of drug efficacy, as well as the impact of side effects. At 6 months, dysmenorrhea, deep dyspareunia and non-menstrual pelvic pain were considerably reduced. In addition the health-related quality of life, psychological profile and sexual satisfaction improved significantly, with no major differences between groups. Metabolic and subjective side effects were limited. According to an intention-to-treat analysis, 33/45 (73%) women in the CPA group and 30/45 (67%) in the oral contraceptive group were satisfied with the treatment received.

CPA may be used when subjective and metabolic effects of estrogens need to be avoided, or in women unwilling to use contraception because of cultural or religious objections. On the other hand, the continuous use of a low-dose monophasic oral contraceptive is most probably the preferred option to prevent the effects of estrogen deprivation in women for whom a long period of therapy is envisaged.

Dienogest

Dienogest is a progestin derived from 19-nortestosterone, has good oral bioavailability and is highly selective for progesterone receptors. Due to its good efficacy and tolerability of dienogest in patients with endometriosis, it has been claimed to represent a valid option in women with the disease. This possibility has been recently confirmed in a large multicenter non-inferiority randomized

clinical trial in symptomatic women with the disease comparing a daily oral dose of 2 mg of dienogest (n=128) to intranasal buserelin 900 μg/day (n=125) for 24 weeks.[8] Dienogest reduced the scores of all symptoms and findings at the end of treatment, and the mean changes in the scores of all pain symptoms were comparable to those obtained with buserelin. Compared with buserelin, Dienogest was associated with irregular genital bleeding more frequently but also with fewer hot flushes. Finally, the reduction in bone mineral density during dienogest treatment was significantly lower than that during buserelin treatment. Overall, these results support the view that dienogest represent a valid option for the long-term treatment of women with endometriosis not aiming to conceive.

Oral Progestins and Rectovaginal Endometriosis

In current practice it is erroneously assumed that medical treatments are not efficacious for rectovaginal endometriosis. This uncritical belief, based on a reportedly different receptor pattern from eutopic endometrium,[9] leads to the obvious conclusion that surgery is the only reasonable therapeutic choice, and thus exposes women to potentially severe morbidity, especially if procedures are performed by gynecologists not specifically trained in this difficult and technically demanding field. This clinical approach should be challenged as in these patients good results are obtainable with safe, tolerable, and inexpensive drugs that can be used for prolonged periods of time.[1]

A RCT was recently conducted on 90 women with recurrent moderate or severe pelvic pain after unsuccessful conservative surgery for symptomatic rectovaginal endometriosis, who were allocated to 12-month continuous treatment with oral ethinyl estradiol 0.01 mg plus cyproterone acetate 3 mg/day, or norethindrone acetate 2.5 mg/day.[10] Seven subjects in the ethinyl oestradiol plus cyproterone acetate arm and five in the norethindrone acetate arm withdrew because of side effects ($n = 5$), treatment inefficacy ($n = 6$), or loss to follow-up ($n = 1$). At 12 months, dysmenorrhea, deep dispareunia, non-menstrual pelvic pain, and dyschezia scores were substantially reduced, without major between-group differences. In particular, moderate to severe deep dispareunia was reported at baseline by 12 women in the ethinyl estradiol and cyproterone acetate group and by 13 in the norethindrone acetate group. The symptom was not relieved in two subjects in each group. Moderate to severe dyschezia was present before treatment in, respectively, 10 and 15 patients and regressed under therapy in all cases. Among the women who completed the study,

17/38 (45%) who took the ethinyl estradiol plus cyproterone acetate combination achieved amenorrhea compared with 29/40 (72%) given norethindrone acetate. Twenty-one women in the former group and 11 in the latter experienced erratic bleeding episodes (spotting in 14 and nine subjects, respectively; breakthrough bleeding in seven and two). These patients were advised to interrupt treatment for 1 week. Side effects were reported by 16/41 (39%) subjects allocated to ethinyl estradiol plus cyproterone acetate, and by 21/42 (50%) of those taking norethindrone acetate. The mean gain in the patients reporting a weight increase was 2.3 ± 1.0 kg (+4%) in seven subjects in the former group, and 3.6 ± 2.3 kg (+7%) in 12 subjects in the latter. Both regimens induced minor unfavorable variations in serum lipid profile. At transrectal ultrasonography, the mean ± SD volume of rectovaginal plaques dropped from a baseline value of 3.1 ± 1.4 mL in the ethinyl estradiol plus cyproterone acetate group and of 3.0 ± 1.3 mL in the norethindrone acetate group to, respectively, 2.2 ± 1.0 mL and 1.9 ± 1.1 mL at the end of treatment. According to an intention-to-treat analysis, 28/45 (62%) patients in the ethinyl estradiol plus cyproterone acetate group and 33/45 (73%) in the norethindrone acetate group were satisfied with the treatment received. In Italy, the monthly cost of treatment with norethindrone acetate 2.5 mg daily is about € 1.5. Consequently, low-dose norethindrone acetate should be considered as the treatment of choice for patients who do not want to conceive and who were diagnosed recurrent or persistent deeply infiltrating lesions after failure of conservative surgery. The ethinyl estradiol plus cyproterone acetate combination was slightly less effective but well tolerated, and could be suggested for women with acne or hypertrichosis and those who experience androgenic side effects with norethindrone acetate.

In our opinion, if other studies confirm the efficacy of progestins in women with symptomatic rectovaginal endometriosis, patients' consent to surgery should no longer be sought based solely on the purported uselessness of medical therapies.

Intramuscular and Subcutaneous Routes: The Depot Medroxyprogesterone (DMPA) Option

The depot formulation of medroxyprogesterone acetate (DMPA) has been widely evaluated for contraceptive purposes and is currently being widely used in women worldwide.[1] The administration modality is extremely convenient and consists of a single 150 mg intramuscular injection every 3 months. The risk of breast cancer in users of DMPA is not superior to that of oral contraceptives while there is evidence showing bone demineralization secondary to hypoestrogenism in chronic users.[1]

Results from the first formal study on the use of DMPA in patients with endometriosis have been published in 1996.[11] The progestin was compared to an association of a monophasic oral contraceptive with low-dose danazol (50 mg/day). After a 1-year treatment, 29/40 women (72%) allocated to DMPA were satisfied versus 23/40 (57%) of those allocated to oral contraceptive plus danazol. A significant reduction in pain symptoms evaluated with a visual analogue and multidimensional scale has been observed in both groups. However, patients in the combined oral contraceptive plus danazol group complained of a greater frequency and severity of dysmenorrhea, which is a logical consequence of cyclic administration. Both treatments induced a similar, significant reduction in serum HDL cholesterol levels, whereas an increase in LDL cholesterol levels was only observed in subjects allocated to the oral contraceptive plus danazol treatment. The incidence of side effects was greater in DMPA users. Moreover, in these women, the mean delay in appearance of a regular menstrual cycle after suspension was 7 months to a maximum of 1 year.

The efficacy of DMPA as a therapy for endometriosis was recently confirmed in two randomized controlled trials conducted in order to investigate a new, subcutaneous formulation of DMPA 104 mg and to assess its equivalence (non-inferiority) to leuprolide acetate 11.25 mg chosen as the standard comparator.[12,13] Both drugs were injected during a menstrual cycle and then after three months, for an overall study period of six months. In one trial, 300 women with surgically diagnosed endometriosis were recruited in Europe, Asia, Latin America and New Zealand,[12] and in the other trial 274 subjects with similar characteristics were recruited in Canada and USA.[13] The DMPA subcutaneous preparation proved statistically equivalent to leuprolide in reducing pain symptoms both at the end of treatment and at 12-months follow-up. Patients in the DMPA group showed significantly less bone mineral density loss than did leuprolide patients. Bone mineral density returned to pre-treatment levels 12 months post-treatment in the progestin but not in the GnRH analogue group. Compared with leuprolide, DMPA was associated with fewer hypo-estrogenic symptoms but more irregular bleeding. In the first study continuation rate was 90% in the DMPA group and 93% in the leuprolide group, whereas in the second study the percentages were 65%

and 74%, respectively. Total productivity and health-related quality of life improved in both groups.

DMPA is an effective, safe, and extremely economic alternative for the treatment of symptomatic endometriosis. However, because of some of its characteristics, candidates for treatment need to be selected carefully. In fact, prolonged delay in resumption of ovulation is a contraindication to the use of DMPA in women wanting children in the near future. Additionally, uterine breakthrough bleeding may be prolonged, repeated and troublesome to correct. More in general, treatment cannot be interrupted in the event of side effects, rendering clinical management complicated when these are severe or scarcely tolerable. Its indication of choice is residual symptomatic endometriosis following definitive surgery in women not wanting children in the near future. In such circumstances, future conception or irregular uterine bleeding do not represent a problem, and use of DMPA allows a simple and well-tolerated suppression of persistent foci after non-radical operations with no need to opt for daily administration of drugs or further surgery.

Intrauterine Route

Levonorgestrel is a potent progestin with androgenic and antiestrogenic activity on the endometrium.[14] An intrauterine device releasing 20 µg/day of levonorgestrel (Lng-IUD), a progestin derived from 19-nortestosterone, may induce amenorrhea in different ways compared to standard treatments and may relieve menstrual pain. In fact, the local administration of levonorgestrel has a profound effect on the endometrium, which becomes atrophic and inactive, although ovulation is generally not suppressed. The identification of safe and effective alternatives to prolong treatment constitutes an essential element in the current clinical research on symptomatic endometriosis. In this regard, the possibility of aiming the therapeutic action of drugs at specific organs, thus reducing the general metabolic impact, is a subject of great interest. Not surprisingly, the Lng-IUD has been tested in patients with several forms of endometriosis including rectovaginal lesions, in those with recurrent endometriotic lesions and also as a postoperative measure.

Symptomatic Peritoneal and Superficial Ovarian Lesions

Lockhat et al studied 37 women of reproductive age who underwent laparoscopy for pelvic pain to investigate the effectiveness of the Lng-IUD for the relief of symptoms associated with minimal to moderate endometriosis.[15] In 34 subjects stage I to III endometriosis was diagnosed but not treated, and a Lng-IUD was inserted intraoperatively. The Lng-IUD was removed soon after surgery in five women because of side effects or pain worsening, and another subject was withdrawn due to protocol violation. At 6-month evaluation, dysmenorrhea was significantly relieved in the remaining 28 women, as the proportion of patients experiencing moderate or severe menstrual pain fell from 96 to 50%. Of the 20 cases experiencing dispareunia at the start of the study, 13 felt this had improved after 6 months therapy, two felt it had worsened, two reported no change and three were no more sexually active. Non-cyclical pelvic pain was not significantly reduced. The mean ± SD number of days of pain experienced per month was 15.0 ± 6.9 at baseline and 10.7 ± 8.7 after 6 months therapy. At the end of treatment, 14 patients were very satisfied, 5 satisfied, 7 uncertain, and 2 dissatisfied. Including dropouts as failures in an intention to treat analysis, slightly more than half of the recruited subjects (19/34, 56%) were satisfied or very satisfied with the treatment received. Six patients requested device removal at the end of the study period.

The same authors recently published the 3-year follow-up data on the subjects enrolled in the 6-month trial that requested continuation of therapy with the Lng-IUD.[16] The device was retained by 23/34 (68%) women at 12 months, 21 (62%) at 24 months, and 19 (56%) at 36 months. Out of a total of 15 discontinuations, five (33%) were for unacceptable irregular bleeding, most of which were within the first 6 months. Pelvic pain (21%) and weight gain (9%) were respectively the second and third most common reasons for requesting removal. There were no expulsions over the 3-year period. Overall, results from this study suggested that the most dramatic improvement in symptoms occurred during the first 12 months of therapy. Thereafter, there were no significant changes over the remaining 24 months.

Recently Petta et al conducted a multicenter randomized controlled trial on 82 subjects to compare the efficacy of the Lng-IUD ($n = 39$) and of leuprolide depot, 3.75 mg/28 days ($n = 43$), in the control of endometriosis-related pain over a period of six months.[17] Pelvic pain decreased substantially from the first month of treatment throughout the study period without significant between-group differences. Lng-IUD users had a higher bleeding score than GnRH analogue users. Quality of life improved similarly in both treatment groups. On these bases, the authors conclude that the Lng-IUD could become the treatment of choice for symptomatic endometriosis, as it does not provoke hypoestrogenism and it requires only one medical intervention for its introduction every 5 years.

Rectovaginal Endometriosis

To evaluate the effectiveness of the Lng-IUD as a therapy for rectovaginal endometriosis, Fedele et al recruited 11 symptomatic women who previously underwent conservative surgery without excision of deep lesions and assessed variations in pain symptoms and size of plaques.[18] At 1-year follow-up nine women were oligomenorrheic and two experienced amenorrhea; dysmenorrhea, which had been moderate or severe in all cases, and nonmenstrual pelvic pain were absent. Of notable interest was the reduction of deep disparcunia, which had been moderate or severe in 8 cases prior to IUD insertion, to absent or mild in all subjects throughout treatment. Dyschezia was relieved in 4 out of 5 women by the sixth month of treatment. Transrectal ultrasonography showed a slight but significant reduction of rectovaginal lesions after six months of therapy. The use of the Lng-IUD was associated with headache in four patients; breast tenderness in four; seborrhea, oily hair, or acne in three; and weight increase in four. In the Authors' opinion, the mechanism of action of the Lng-IUD is a receptor-mediated effect of levonorgestrel that can reach endometriotic foci through blood circulation or direct diffusion from the uterus. Another mechanism of action could be secondary oligoamenorrhea and the consequent reduction in cyclic bleeding at ectopic endometrial site. Relief of organic symptoms such as deep disparcunia and rectal tenesmus is probably due not only to size reduction of the fibronodular rectovaginal plaques, but also to decrease of the intra- and perilesional inflammatory condition.

Recurrent Endometriosis

Vercellini et al studied 20 parous patients previously operated for endometriosis who experienced recurrent moderate to severe menstrual pain.[19] Variations of dysmenorrhea severity as well as patients' satisfaction were assessed after 1 year of therapy with the Lng-IUD. Two women withdrew from the study (1 requested IUD removal because of weight gain and abdominal bloating; in another the medicated IUD was expelled 3 months after insertion) and 1 was lost to follow up. The menstrual pattern in the remaining 17 women after 12 months of treatment was characterized by amenorrhea in 4 (24%), hypomenorrhea or spotting in 8 (47%), and normal flows in 5 (29%). A five-fold reduction in blood loss was documented. During the study period the mean ± SD 100-mm visual analogue score and 0 to 3 verbal rating scale scores dropped, respectively, from 76 ±12 to 34 ± 23 points and from 2.5 ± 0.5 to 1.2 ± 0.5 points. Only 5 (29%) women were considered still symptomatic at final evaluation. Side effects were reported by 9 patients (bloating in 7, weight gain in 5, headache in 4, breast tension in 3, and pelvic pain and decreased libido in 1). Fifteen women (75%) were very satisfied or satisfied with treatment at 12-month follow-up.

Postoperative Adjuvant Treatment

Vercellini et al designed a pilot study to verify if the frequency and severity of dysmenorrhea recurrence is reduced at 1-year follow-up in women in whom a Lng-IUD is inserted immediately after laparoscopic surgery for endometriosis compared with women treated with laparoscopic surgery only.[20] After complete excision or coagulation of all endometriotic lesions, 20 subjects were randomized to Lng-IUD insertion and 20 to postoperative expectant management. Displacement of the Lng-IUD was observed in one woman 5 months after insertion. One subject in each group was lost to follow-up. At the 12-months evaluation, amenorrhea was reported by 5 (28%) of the remaining 18 women in the Lng-IUD arm, hypomenorrhea or spotting by 9 (50%), and normal flows by 4 (22%). Median (interquartile range) dysmenorrhea visual analogue and multidimensional categorical rating scale scores fell by 50 mm (35 to 65) and 1 point (1 to 2) in the postoperative Lng-IUD group and by 30 (25 to 40) and 1 (0 to 2) in the surgery only group (P = .012 and .021). According to an intention-to-treat analysis, postoperative moderate or severe dysmenorrhea recurrence was less frequent in the former group (2/20 subjects, 10%) than in the latter (9/20, 45%; P = 0.03; relative risk = 0.22; 95% CI, 0.05 to 0.90). A Lng-IUD should be inserted postoperatively in three patients to avoid moderate or severe dysmenorrhea recurrence in one of them 1 year after surgery. In addition, dispareunia and nonmenstrual pain scores were reduced to a greater extent with the postoperative use of Lng-IUD. Side effects were reported by 8 of the 20 patients allocated to Lng-IUD insertion (bloating in 6, weight gain in 6, headache in 3, seborrhea and acne in 2, breast tenderness in 1, decreased libido in 1, and pelvic pain in 1), but were deemed tolerable and removal of the IUD was not necessary except in the case of the displaced device. At 12 months, 75% of subjects in the surgery plus Lng-IUD group were satisfied or very satisfied after 1 year of treatment compared with 50% in the surgery-only group.

Insertion of the medicated device after conservative surgery for endometriosis may constitute an innovative, effective, safe and convenient adjuvant treatment for the reduction of risk of dysmenorrhea recurrence.

Advantages and Drawbacks of the Lng-IUD for Endometriosis

The use of a Lng-IUD in women with endometriosis confers several advantages over other conventional systemic therapies (avoidance of the need for repeated administration, effective contraception and, possibly, fewer side effects) and may increase patients' compliance during long-term treatments. Although it may be expensive at the outset, the cumulative final costs could be less than those of other medications.

Women should be informed that during the first 3-4 months of use major menstrual disorders are expected, including spotting, prolonged or continuous bleeding, and even menorrhagia. After the first year of use, few women report intermenstrual bleeding and about 20% to 30% are amenorrheic. This is relevant as dysmenorrhea is the most frequent symptom in patients with endometriosis.

Intrauterine administration of levonorgestrel with a possible direct distribution to pelvic tissues would imply a local concentration greater than its plasma levels. This could translate into a superior effectiveness with limited adverse effects, also due to absence of the hepatic first-pass following oral administration of the drug. Based on the dosage of drug administered, the metabolic consequences of the Lng-IUD should be less pronounced than those of other contraceptive methods. However, a general effect secondary to uterine absorption of levonorgestrel cannot be excluded, as most reported side effects are typical of progestins.

The expulsion rate of the device is over 5% and the risk of pelvic infection about 1.5%.[21] Accordingly, the recommended patient profile is parous women with no history of pelvic inflammatory disease. Nulliparity is not a contraindication, but the use of IUDs in smaller uteri may be associated with increased uterine cramping. This could be particularly worrisome in patients with endometriosis-associated severe dysmenorrhea.

Finally, limited information is available on the risk of endometrioma formation during long periods of therapy. In fact, cumulative evidence suggests that development of endometriotic ovarian cysts is associated with ovulation.[22] Since the Lng-IUD generally does not inhibit ovulation except for the first few months after insertion, one may argue that, in theory, this may constitute a specific drawback of the Lng-IUD in comparison with other forms of progestin treatment. Clinical data are required to disentangle this point. Comparative trials are needed also to confirm the effect on organic pain symptoms, such as dispareunia and dyschezia and to verify whether the good results observed are maintained during the entire 5-year period of efficacy.

Conclusions

Management of endometriosis with oral contraceptive or progestins is safe, effective, well tolerated, and should constitute the first-line medical treatment modality in symptomatic women not wanting children. These pharmacologic options are inexpensive, suitable for prolonged periods of therapy, with the additional advantage of being available all over the world with reproducible results. After attending updating courses, even general practitioners could prescribe and monitor treatments, thus limiting the medical costs of the disease.

About one patient out of four will still need an intervention because of lack of response or intolerance to side effects, but the overall impact of surgery would be limited greatly, with reduction in morbidity and, possibly, long-term complications. In fact, the outcomes of surgery are strictly operator-dependent, and optimal results can be assured only in tertiary-care and referral centres. In the majority of women not seeking pregnancy endometriosis could be controlled, although not cured, in a non-invasive manner.

References

1. Vercellini P, Somigliana E, Viganò P et al. Endometriosis: current and future medical therapies. Best Pract Res Clin Obstet Gynaecol 2008;22:275-306.
2. Muneyyirci-Delale O, Karacan M. Effect of norethindrone acetate in the treatment of symptomatic endometriosis. Int J Fertil Womens Med 1998;43:24-27.
3. Moore C, Kohler G, Muller A. The treatment of endometriosis with dienogest. Drugs Today 1999;35(Suppl C):41-52.
4. Riis BJ, Lehmann HJ, Christiansen C. Norethisterone acetate in combination with estrogen: effects on the skeleton and other organs: a review. Am J Obstet Gynecol 2002;187:1101-06.
5. Fedele L, Arcaini L, Bianchi S, et al. Comparison of cyproterone acetate and danazol in the treatment of pelvic pain associated with endometriosis. Obstet Gynecol 1989;73:1000-04.
6. Moran C, Alcivia JC, Garcia-Hernandez E, et al. Treatment of endometriosis with cyproterone acetate. Preliminary report. Arch Med Res 1996;27:535-38.

7. Vercellini P, De Giorgi O, Mosconi P, et al. Cyproterone acetate versus a continuous monophasic oral contraceptive in the treatment of recurrent pelvic pain after conservative surgery for symptomatic endometriosis. Fertil Steril 2002;77:52-61.

8. Harada T, Momoeda M, Taketani Y, et al. Dienogest is as effective as intranasal buserelin acetate for the relief of pain symptoms associated with endometriosis-a randomized, double-blind, multicenter, controlled trial. Fertil Steril 2008. [Epub ahead of print]

9. Ford J, English J, Miles WA, et al. Pain, quality of life and complications following the radical resection of rectovaginal endometriosis. BJOG 2004; 111: 353-56.

10. Vercellini P, Pietropaolo G, De Giorgi O, et al. Treatment of symptomatic rectovaginal endometriosis with an estrogen-progestogen combination versus low-dose norethindrone acetate. Fertil Steril 2005;84:1375-87.

11. Vercellini P, De Giorgi O, Oldani S, et al. Depot medroxy-progesterone acetate versus an oral contraceptive combined with very-low-dose danazol for long-term treatment of pelvic pain associated with endometriosis. Am J Obstet Gynecol 1996;175:396-401.

12. Crosignani PG, Luciano A, Ray A, et al. Subcutaneous depot medroxyprogesterone acetate versus leuprolide acetate in the treatment of endometriosis-associated pain. Hum Reprod 2006;21:248-56.

13. Schlaff WD, Carson SA, Luciano A, Ross D, et al. Subcutaneous injection of depot medroxyprogesterone acetate compared with leuprolide acetate in the treatment of endometriosis-associated pain. Fertil Steril 2006;85: 314-25.

14. Vercellini P, Viganò P, Somigliana E. The role of the levonorgestrel-releasing intrauterine device in the management of symptomatic endometriosis. Curr Opin Obstet Gynecol 2005;17:359-65.

15. Lockhat FB, Emembolu JO, Konje JC. The evaluation of the effectiveness of an intrauterine-administered progestogen (levonorgestrel) in the symptomatic treatment of endometriosis and in the staging of the disease. Hum Reprod 2004;19:179-84.

16. Lockhat FB, Emembolu JO, Konje JC. The efficacy, side-effects and continuation rates in women with symptomatic endometriosis undergoing treatment with an intrauterine administered progestogen (levonorgestrel): a 3 year follow-up. Hum Reprod 2005;20:789-93.

17. Petta CA, Ferriani RA, Abrao MS, et al. Randomized clinical trial of a levonorgestrel-releasing intrauterine system and a depot GnRH analogue for the treatment of chronic pelvic pain in women with endometriosis. Hum Reprod 2005;20:1993-98.

18. Fedele L, Bianchi S, Zanconato G, et al. Use of a levonorgestrel-releasing intrauterine device in the treatment of rectovaginal endometriosis. Fertil Steril 2001; 75:485-88.

19. Vercellini P, Aimi G, Panazza S, et al. A levonorgestrel-releasing intrauterine system for the treatment of dysmenorrhea associated with endometriosis: a pilot study. Fertil Steril 1999;72:505-08.

20. Vercellini P, Frontino G, De Giorgi O, et al. Comparison of a levonorgestrel-releasing intrauterine device versus expectant management after conservative surgery for symptomatic endometriosis: a pilot study. Fertil Steril 2003;80:305-09.

21. Shulman LP, Nelson AL, Darney PD. Recent developments in hormone delivery system. Am J Obstet Gynecol 2004; 190: S39-48.

22. Vercellini P, Somigliana E, Daguati R, et al. Postoperative oral contraceptive exposure and risk of endometrioma recurrence. Am J Obstet Gynecol 2008;198:504.e1-5.

Richard P Dickey

Chapter 24

Danazol in the Medical Treatment of Endometriosis

Introduction to Danazole

Danazol was the first drug approved for the treatment of endometriosis in the United States. Medical treatment of endometriosis before danazol consisted of 'off label' use of a number of androgenic and progestational drugs, those most often described were methyl testosterone, medroxyprogesterone acetate, and high doses of oral contraceptives. Numerous side effects of other hormonal treatments of endometriosis created a ready market for danazole when it became available. Use of danazol for medical treatment of endometriosis has decreased since the introduction of gonadotropin releasing hormone (GnRH) agonists. The rational for use of progestational drugs and oral contraceptives was that they suppressed ovulation and induced a pseudopregnancy state. It was believed or observed that endometriosis improved during pregnancy.[1] The rational for use of methyl testosterone and similar androgens was that they acted as antagonists of estrogen at the tissue level. Danazol, which is a modified androgen, combined both actions by suppressing ovulation and antagonizing estrogen effects on endometriotic tissue. Modern medical treatment of endometriosis is based on the suppression of ovarian estrogen production necessary for the development and maintenance of the normal endometrium and of ectopic endometrial implants, rather than on the creation of pseudopregnancy.[2] Although both danazol and GnRH agonists can suppress estrogen, their mechanism of action, method of administration, time until onset of action and return to ovulation after treatment are different. Danazol alone has a direct antiestrogen effect on endometriotic lesions. An immunosuppressive effect of danazol on endometriosis has also been suggested.

Chemical Structure and Activity

Danazol (17 α Pregna-2, 4-dien-20-ynol [2, 3-d]-isoxazol-17-0l) is a derivative of 17-α-ethinyl ethisterone. The 17-α-ethinyl group reduces androgenic activity and increases oral activity. The 2,3 isoxazol group blocks the progestational activity present in ethisterone. The relative androgenic activity is 2.5-3.5% that of methyl testosterone. The biological activity of danazol has been compared to that of norethindrone (norethisterone) and lynestrenol, 19-norandrogens used in oral contraceptives (Table 24-1).[3] Danazol is midway in androgenic and metabolic activity between norethindrone and lynestrenol. Unlike the two 19-norprogestins, danazol has no estrogenic or progestational activity. Danazol is metabolized to approximately 70 different compounds, but the principal metabolites are 2-hydroxy methyl ethisterone and 2-ketoethisterone.[4]

Danazol alters pulsatile GnRH patterns thereby diminishing the midcycle LH/FSH surge.[5] Danazol also suppresses serum estradiol (E_2) levels by acting directly on the ovary to inhibit steriodogenesis of androgen

Table 24-1: Comparative biological activity of danazol and some 19-norprogestins				
Drug	Androgenic	Anabolic	Estrogenic	Progestational
Norethindrone	2.0%	10.0%	0.25%	0.38%
Danazol	—	6.0-10.0%	-0-	-0-
Lynestrenol	6.0%	12.5%	2.60%	0.33%

Adapted from Dickey 1985[3]

precursors of estrogen.[6] Specifically, danazol blocks receptor sites in the ovary of 17-α-hydroxylase, 17-ß-hydroxy dehydrogenase, 17-20 lyase, and 3-ß- hydroxy dehydrogenase enzymes necessary for the conversion of progesterone and pregnenalone to androstenedione and dehydroepiandrosterone. Danazol does not alter the conversion of testosterone and dehydroepiandrosterone to estrogen (aromatization). In addition, danazol may directly act on endometriotic implants by binding to and blocking estrogen receptor sites.[7]

At doses of danazol necessary for treatment of endometriosis (600-800 mg daily) androgenic and hypoestrogenic side effects are common **(Table 24-2)**. The androgenic side effects are due more to the increased amount of free testosterone originating from ovarian and adrenal androgens, due to displacement from and reduction in SHBG, than from the androgenic activity of danazol *per se*.[3] By comparison, hypoestrogenic side effects are 2 to 3 times more common in patients using GnRH agonists due to their more profound suppression of estrogen and SHBG, while androgenic side effects are about half as frequent. Additionally loss of bone mass during 6 months of treatment is more pronounced with use of GnRH agonists. Danazol decreases high-density lipoproteins (HDLs) and slightly increases low-density lipoproteins (LDLs), however lipoprotein changes are usually reversed within 5 months after cessation of treatment. Danazol is known to cause insulin resistance and an impeded glucose

Table 24-2: Frequency of symptoms

Symptom	Frequency I	Frequency II
Weight gain, 5 pounds	2.8 – 60%	3.5%
Edema	5.0 – 55%	6.4%
Muscle cramps	4.0 – 52%	4.0%
Flushes and sweats	5.0 – 42%	9.3%
Rash	2.0 – 8%	3.0%
Acne	13 – 27%	17.0%
Voice change	3.0 – 8%	2.6%
Sebum increase, skin and scalp	2.0 – 37%	2.3%
Hirsutism	5.0 – 21%	5.5%
Nervous symptoms	3.0 – 38%	0.6%

*Average gain 9 pounds
I. A Compilation of Six Studies Comprising 1376 Patients Using 800 mg/day
II. Manufacturers data on file with the US FDA
Adapted from Dickey 1985[3]

tolerance curve similar to that seen with oral contraceptive progestins.[8] Danazole has been associated with development of female pseudohermaphroditism *in utero* and should not be given when there is a possibility of pregnancy.[9]

Importance of Measuring Estradiol Levels during Danazol Treatment

In order to optimize effectiveness and minimize side effects during danazol treatment estradiol (E_2) levels must be monitored.[2] This is also true for GnRH treatment of endometriosis. Danazol, similar to oral micronized progesterone, must be taken every 6 hours to achieve maximum suppression of E_2. The serum half-life of danazol is as short as 4.5 hours, and serum levels are markedly decreased or undetectable in plasma after 8 hours.[4, 5, 10] When danazol is given as 400 mg every 12 hours, the dose and interval originally recommended by the manufacturer, E_2 levels are unchanged.[11-13] When danazol is administered at lesser doses but more frequent intervals, E_2 levels are decreased.[14-17] Dmowski who conducted the initial clinical studies emphasized that danazol should be administered every 6 hours because of its short serum half-life.[18] Importantly, in the clinical studies cited by the manufacture as evidence of effectiveness in treating endometriosis, danazol was given as 200 mg every 6 hours, not as 400 mg every 12 hours as stated in the package insert prescribing information for physician. Failure of subsequent post marketing studies to achieve equally good results or suppression of E_2, in all cases, may be attributable to administration of danazol at 12 hour rather than 6 hour intervals.

In a two phase clinical study Dickey et al[2] evaluated the relationship of E_2 levels to objective (laparoscopy or laparotomy visualization) improvement in endometriotic lesions, side effects during danazol treatment, and the relationship of dose and treatment timing to serum E_2 levels. On average, E_2 levels were significantly suppressed by the second week of danazol treatment, but maximum suppression did not occur until after the end of the third week. Improvement in endometriosis was evaluated in 42 women diagnosed with moderate, severe, or extensive disease by laparoscopy who were given danazol 400 mg twice daily for 75-90 days before re-evaluation at the time of microsurgery laparotomy 24 hours following the last dose. Patients with minimal and mild endometriosis did not have additional surgery. Serum for E_2 determine was drawn weekly and the day before surgery. Endometriosis was staged according to the classification of the American

Table 24-3: Relationship between serum E_2 levels and improvement of endometriosis after danazol therapy								
Pretreatment AFS classification	No. of patients	Observed improvement	Serum E_2		Kruskal-Wallis statistic	P value	Spearman correlation	P Value
			Average pg/ml	Range pg/ml				
Moderate	3	Partial	56.7	53-63	5.40	0.0201	-0.822	< 0.005
	6	Complete	20.1	4-40				
Severe	7	None	72.8	56-101	18.70	0.001	-0.944	< 0.001
	8	Partial	40.2	27-49				
	7	Complete	13.7	5-21				
Extensive	5	None	85.2	41-201	8.59	0.0136	-0.927	< 0.001
	2	Partial	29.5	25-34				
	4	Complete	8.8	2-14				
All	42				32.81	0.0001	-0.894	< 0.001

Adapted from Dickey et al 1984[2]

Table 24-4: Relationship between initial weight and serum E_2 levels during danazol treatment							
Weight lbs/kg	No. of patients	Mean E_2[a] pg/ml	% of patients treated with E_2 (pg/ml)				
			<5	5-20	21-50	51-100	>100
Less than 100/45	6	24.8 ± 8.2	33.3	16.7	33.3	16.7	0
101-150/46-68	86	48.8 ± 4.7	3.5	19.7	36.0	33.7	7.0
Over 150/68	12	77.2 ± 11.0	0	0	16.7	66.7	16.7
Total	104	48.0 ± 4.1	4.8	18.3	31.7	37.5	7.7

[a]Mean + SEM, Adapted from Dickey et al 1984[2]

Fertility Society (AFS).[19] Improvement was rated as: "complete" if no endometriosis remained; "almost complete" if there was some hemosiderin reaction and neovascularization remaining; "partial" if there was improvement but still considerable endometriosis remaining; "none" if there was no, or almost no, objective improvement. For analysis, women with complete and almost complete improvement were combined because it was thought that additional days of treatment would have resulted in further improvement.

Relationship of E_2 Levels at the End of Danazol Treatment, Initial Stage of Endometriosis, and Extent of Improvement

The extent of improvement was related to both the E_2 level after 75-90 days of treatment and to the stage of endometriosis observed at the time of pretreatment laparoscopy (Table 24-3). Complete or almost complete improvement occurred when E_2 levels were 15 pg/ml or less in extensive, 21 pg/ml or less in severe, and 40 pg/ml or less in patients with moderate endometriosis. Partial improvement occurred when E_2 levels were < 40 pg/ml in extensive, < 50 pg/ml in severe, and < 65 pg/ml in moderate endometriosis. No improvement was observed when E_2 levels were > 40 pg/ml in extensive or > 50 pg/ml in severe endometriosis.

Relation of E_2 Suppression to Weight

Pretreatment weight strongly influenced E_2 levels in patients treated with 400 mg danazol every 12 hours for 75-90 days (Table 24-4). E_2 levels < 20 pg/ml occurred in 23.1% of patients. There were no women with initial weights over 150 pounds (68 kg) whose E_2 levels were suppressed to < 20 pg/ml, and only 16% in this weight group were suppressed to <50 pg/ml. E_2 levels >100 pg/ml occurred in 7.7% of all patients and in 16.7% of patients who weighed more than 150 pounds (68 kg). The average initial weight was 131 pounds (60 kg). The average weight gain during treatment was 2.2 pounds (1 kg). No relationship was found between RIA E_2 levels during treatment and the patient's age, midluteal phase E_2 level, or P midluteal phase level.

Table 24-5: Relationship of E_2 levels during danazol treatment to side effects					
Symptom	No. of patients	Percentage with symptoms	Serum E_2[a] pg/ml	%E_2	
				< 20 pg/ml	> 100 pg/ml
All patients	104	100	48.0 ± 4.1	23.1	7.7
Amenorrhea	47	45.2	57.1 ± 7.4	23.4	14.9
Spotting	30	28.8	44.4 ± 6.8	30.0	3.3
Bleeding	27	26.0	47.6 ± 4.5	11.1	0
Edema	16	15.4	40.8 ± 5.7	12.5	0
Weight gain over 5 lbs (2.2 kg)	15	14.4	63.7 ± 13.8	20.0	26.7
Hot flashes	12	11.5	49.9 ± 10.5	33.3	8.3
Seburn/hair	12	11.5	42.7 ± 7.1	25.0	0
Muscle cramps	10	9.6	49.5 ± 5.7	10.0	0
Nervousness	6	5.8	39.5 ± 6.3	16.7	0
Nausea	4	3.8	46.8 ± 10.4	0	0
Pelvic Pain	3	2.9	48.0 ± 12.9	0	0

[a]Mean + SEM; Adapted from Dickey et al 1984[2]

Relationship of E_2 Levels to Side Effects

Side effects experienced by patients during treatment with 400 mg danazol every 12 hours were inconsistently related to E_2 levels (Table 24-5). This is especially important because intuitively patients with hot flashes or amenorrhea are assumed to have very low E_2 levels. E_2 levels were suppressed to < 20 pg/ml in only 33% of patients with hot flashes and in only 23% of patients with amenorrhea. E_2 levels were > 100 pg/ml indicating little or no suppression in 8% of patients with hot flashes and 15% of patients with amenorrhea receiving 400 mg danazol twice daily. Patients with amenorrhea and those with weight gain over 5 pounds (2.2 kg) tended to have higher than average E_2 levels. None of the patients with spotting, edema, excess sebum, muscle cramps or nervousness had E_2 levels greater than 100 pg/ml indicating that a lower dose of danazol, which would have reduced these side effects, might have been effective.

Effect of Increasing the Frequency of Danazol Administration

The short serum half-life of danazol and the finding that serum levels are markedly decreased or undetectable after 8 hours,[4, 5, 9] are reasons to suspect that danazol must be given more frequently than 2 times a day to achieve maximum suppression of E_2 levels. This was confirmed when after 4 weeks of danazol 400 mg every 12 hours E_2 levels were measured and patients were assigned to three groups; Group I continued to take danazol 400 mg every 12 hours, Group II began taking danazol 200 mg every 8 hours, and Group III began taking danazol 200 mg every 6 hours (Table 24-6). At the end of 4 weeks E_2 levels were remeasured. There was no change in serum E_2 levels for patients who continued to take 400 mg every 12 hours. There also was no change in E_2 levels when patients took 200 mg every 8 hours even though the total daily dose was 25% lower than when 400 mg danazol was taken every 12 hours. For patients who took danazol 200 mg every 6 hours, serum E_2 levels were reduced 40% compared to when danazol was taken 400 mg every 12 hours.

Effect of Concurrent Administration of Dexamethasone or Spironolactone to Decrease Androgenic Side Effects

Androgenic side effects of danazol treatment may occur because SHBG binding sites for androgens (A) are blocked or SHBG is reduced by danazol thereby increasing the proportion of endogenous A that is free and unbound or because of the androgenic activity of danazol itself. The primary forms of circulating androgen when ovarian steroidogenesis is suppressed are dehydroandrosterone (DHEA) and dehydroandrosterone sulfate (DHEAS) of adrenal origin although some DHEA is produced in the ovaries. Adrenal production of adrenal DHEA and DHEAS is suppressed by dexamethasone at doses as little as 0.5 mg per day and also by prednisone 5 mg per day. Skin and scalp sebum and hirsutism due to dihydro-

Table 24-6: Effect of change in dose and frequency of Danazol on serum E_2 levels

Dose and frequency of administration (first dose and Second dose)	No. of patients	Serum E_2[a] pg/ml	Significance % E_2 change	% E_2 < 20 pg/ml
I. 400 mg/12 hr	18	50.3 ± 5.3	NS[b]	6.2
400 mg/12 hr		50.3 ± 4.9	0	6.2
II. 400 mg/12 hr	18	25.0 ± 3.1	NS[b]	33.3
200 mg/8 hr		24.4 ± 4.1	-2	50
III. 400 mg/12 hr	28	61.1 ± 6.0	0.001	7.1
200 mg/6hr		36.6 ± 6.0	-40	32.1

[a]Mean ± SEM, [b] Not significant, Adapted from Dickey et al 1984[2]

testosterone and other androgens are blocked at the skin receptor level by spironolactone. The effect of concurrent administration of danazole and dexamethasone or spironolactone was evaluated **(Table 24-7)**. Concurrent administration of dexamethasone in patients inadequately suppressed by danazole alone resulted in a 61% decrease in mean E_2 levels. Concurrent administration of dexamethasone resulted in a decrease in androgenic skin effects in 35% of patients, but increased symptoms of fluid retention, edema, and muscle pain in 75% of patients. Concurrent administration of 100 mg spironolactone every 12 hours resulted in marked improvement in sebum and hair growth in 75% of patients and by complete remission of androgenic effects in 67% of patients, but was accompanied by a 49% increase in serum E_2 levels.

Clinical Management of Endometriosis with Danazol

Indication

Medical treatment of endometriosis is indicated when the predominant manifestation of endometriosis is adenomyosis for both patients seeking pain relief and patients desiring fertility. Medical treatment is also indicated when pain returns after surgical treatment. When medical treatment is used for the purpose of pain relief a six month course of either danazol or GnRH will provide continued relief of pain for approximately 18 months after the cessation of treatment, providing E_2 levels are adequately suppressed. The time until return of pain symptoms is approximately the same after laparoscopic laser or electrocautery of endometriosis implants. If pain is not relieved after the first month of medical treatment surgery should be considered instead. In the author's experience and that of his gynecological teachers forty plus years earlier, surgical treatment of endometriosis for relief of pain should include uterosacral ligament transection, uterosacral ligament reattachment to the posterior lower uterine segment, uterosacral ligament plication with non-resorbable suture to elevate the uterus out of the cul de sac, and if the surgeon has been trained in the procedure, presacral neurectomy. The advantages of danazol over GnRH for pain relief are less severe hypoestrogen side effects; less lose, if any, of bone density, and a more rapid onset of estrogen suppression. The onset of E_2 suppression and endometriotic lesion regression is immediate for danazol compared to a delay of 10 to 21 days for GnRH because of an initial flare up of serum E_2 levels. The disadvantages of danazol for pain relief are the need to

Table 24-7: Effect on estradiol levels of concurrent administration of dexamethasone or spironolactone

Drug	No. of patients	Serum E_2[a] pg/ml	Significance % E_2 change	% E_2 < 20 pg/ml
I (A) Danazol	20	65.7 ± 9.0	0.001	15.7
(B) Danazol plus Dexamethasone		25.8 ± 3.6	-61	42.0
II (A) Danazol	20	28.7 ± 4.2	0.01	50.0
(B) Danazol plus Spironolactone		42.7 ± 6.2	+49	25.0

[a] Mean ± SEM, Adapted from Dickey et al 1984[2]

take a pill 3 or 4 times a day, a tendency to weight gain although this averaged only 2.2 pounds in 3 months, and usually mild androgenic effects.

When corneal tubal obstruction is found at laparoscopy or hysterosalpingogram in association with endometriosis a presumptive diagnosis of adenomyosis can be made after ruling out past chlamydia infection with serum IgG assay and tuberculosis in countries where pelvic tuberculosis is endemic. The first line of treatment for proximal tubal obstruction associated with endometriosis and infertility is to use either danazol or GnRH in a short 3 month course followed by repeat hysterosalpingogram. Providing E_2 levels are suppressed to < 20-30 pg/ml, fallopian tubes obstructed because of adenomyosis are nearly always opened. The second situation in which a short course of medical treatment is indicated is preoperatively before surgery. It is imperative to remind readers that post-operative medical treatment reduces pregnancy rates in patients desiring pregnancy. The only exception to the prescription of medical suppression after surgery is when tubal obstruction was not previously known and is discovered during surgery. The advantage of danazol for short-term treatment of infertility patients over depo GnRH are a more rapid return to ovulatory cycles after cessation of treatment; 4 to 5 weeks for danazol compared to 8 to 14 weeks for depo GnRH. A situation where danazol instead of GnRH is absolutely indicated for preoperative medical treatment exists when an endometrioma is present. In these cases the increase in E_2 when GnRH treatment is initiated could potentially cause the endometrioma to rupture.

Initiating and Monitoring Danazol

Danazol treatment should be initiated during menses. Treatment must be started no later than the fifth menstrual cycle day to insure ovarian suppression and preferably earlier as is true for hormonal contraception.[20] Patients who could become pregnant should use non-hormonal methods of contraception until ovulation suppression is assured. Suppression of ovulation can be assumed of the E_2 level is < 50 pg/ml. Amenorrhea is no guarantee that ovulation is suppressed since 15% of patients who were amenorrhic after 75-90 days of danazol had E_2 levels of 100 pg/ml or higher and could possibly have become pregnant. The author knew a physician, now retired, that treated young women with laparoscopy diagnosed endometriosis who were also overweight with the manufactures recommended dose of 400 mg twice daily dose, and who had the experience of several of his patients becoming pregnant while on treatment.

I start with an initial dose of 200 mg danazol every 8 hours for women with mild or moderate endometriosis who weigh less than 150 pounds (68 kg). Patients with severe or extensive endometriosis and those with lesser stages, who weigh more than 150 pounds (68 kg), should be given 200 mg every 6 hours initially. I evaluate serum E_2 levels initially and 3 weeks after the initial dose and after any change in dose. My therapeutic goal is for E_2 levels to be < 20 pg/ml in patient with severe and extensive endometriosis, and < 40 pg/ml in patients with moderate endometriosis. I ordinarily do not treat patients with mild and minimal endometriosis other than by laparoscopy. The exception is when there is cornual tubal obstruction in which case I use a dose and interval that will result in E_2 levels < 20 pg/ml. When it is necessary to increase the danazol to achieve adequate suppression of E_2 levels, the first step up is to 400 mg every 8 hours and then if necessary to 400 mg every 6 hours. Before increasing the daily dose to this extent I first try adrenal suppression with dexamethasone 0.5 mg daily at bedtime. Adrenal androgen levels that are the presumed source of the E_2 levels take a minimum of 4 days to be suppressed so that remeasuring E_2 levels after one week allows adequate time to determine of dexamethasone should be continued. If patients develop increased sebum or hair growth, the dose of danazol may be reduced if E_2 levels are lower than needed to achieve remission of endometriosis. Alternatively, they may be given 100 mg spironolactone twice daily. However, E_2 levels need to be remeasured to ensure they remain adequately suppressed if spironolactone is used.

The determination of serum E_2 levels is essential when either danazol or GNRH agonist are used to treat endometriosis. I measure serum E_2 levels the day treatment is initiated and again 3-4 weeks latter to determine if levels are suppressed. I sometimes measure E_2 levels earlier if a patient has symptoms of excess androgen or hypoestrogenism so that I can decrease the frequency of danazol administration if E_2 levels are adequately or more than adequately suppressed. When decreasing the total daily dose of danazol it can be given as 200 mg 3 instead of 4 times daily or 2 instead of 3 times daily. A 100 mg danazol pill is also available that can be given 2 to 4 times daily. In no case should danazol be given less than twice daily if treatment is to be effective. E_2 assay results much more than other hormones assays give varying results according to the assay technique. The values in **Tables 24-3 to 24-7** were determined by coated tube Radioimmunoassay (RIA) (DPC Cost-A-Count: Diagnostic Products, Los Angeles., CA). Compared to RIA, E_2 levels determined by monoclonal antibody (Tosoh: AIA-600, San

Francisco, CA) average 52% higher, and E_2 levels determined by chemiluminescence (ASC: 180 plus; Chiron/Bayer, Norwood MA) average 18% higher. Clinicians should be aware of the normal menopause E_2 levels in their own or their reference laboratory. A few older E_2 assay methods still in use are not accurate when E_2 levels are < 50 pg/ml.

References

1. Kistner RW. Management of endometriosis in the infertile patient. Fertil Steril 1975; 26:1151-66.
2. Dickey RP, Taylor SN, Curole DN. Serum estradiol and danazol: 1, Endometriosis response, side effects, administration interval, concurrent spironolactone and dexamethasone. Fertil Steril 1984; 42:709-16.
3. Dickey RP. Managing Danazol Patients. Creative Infomatics, Durant OK USA, 1985.
4. Davidson C, Banks W, Fritz A. The absorption, distribution, and metabolic fate of danazol in rats, monkeys and human volunteers. Arch Int Pharmacodyn Ther 1976; 221:294-310.
5. Dmowski WP, Headley S, Radwanska E. Effects of danazol on pulsatile gonadotropin patterns and on serum estradiol levels in normally cycling women. Fertil Steril 1983; 39:49-55.
6. Barbieri RL, Canick JA, Makris A, Todd RB, Davies IJ, Ryan KJ. Danazol inhibits steroidogenesis. Fertil Steril 1977; 28:809-13.
7. Barbieri R, Lee H, Ryan KJ. Danazol binding to rat androgen, glucocorticoid, progesterone, and estrogen receptors: correlation with biologic activity. Fertil Steril 1979; 91:182-6.
8. Wynn V. Metabolic effects of danazol. J Int Med Res 1977; 5 (Suppl 3): 25-35.
9. Quagliarello J, Alba-Greco M. Danazol and urogenital sinus formation in pregnancy. Fertil Steril 1985; 43:939-42.
10. Lloyd-Jones JO. Danazol plasma concentrations in man. J Int Med Res 1977; 5 (Suppl 3):18-24 .
11. Andrews MC, Wentz AC. The effects of danazol on gonadotropins and steroid blood levels in normal and anovulatory women. Am J Obstet Gynecol 1975; 121: 817-28.
12. Luciano AA, Hauser KS, Chapler FK, Sherman BM. Danazol: endocrine consequences in healthy women. Am J Obstet Gynecol 1981; 141:723-7.
13. Hirschowitz JS, Soler NJ, Wortsman J. Sex steroid levels during treatment of endometriosis. Obstet Gynecol 1979; 54:448-50.
14. Rannevik G. Hormonal, metabolic and clinical effects of danazol in the treatment of endometriosis. Postgrad Med J 1979; 55 (Suppl 5):14-20.
15. Ronnberg L, Ylostalo P, Jarvinen PA. Effects of danazol in the treatment of severe endometriosis. Postgrad Med J 1979; 55(Suppl 5):21-26.
16. Wood GP, Wu CH, Flickinger GL, Mikhail G. Hormonal changes associated with danazol therapy. Obstet Gynecol 1975; 45:302-04.
17. Floyd WS. Danazol: endocrine and endometrial effects. Int J Fertil 1980; 25:75-80.
18. Dmowski WP. Endocrine properties and clinical application of danazol. Fertil Steril 1979; 31:237-51.
19. American Fertility Society: Classification of endometriosis. Fertil Steril 1979; 32:633-34.
20. Dickey RP, Dickey RP. Managing Contraceptive Pill Patients. Creative Infomatics, Durant OK USA, 2007.

Engel JB, A Schally

Chapter 25

Agonists and Antagonists of Luteinizing Hormone-releasing Hormone (LHRH) in the Treatment of Endometriosis

Summary

Agonists of LHRH induce a reversible hypoestrogenic state by down-regulation of LHRH receptors and desensitation of the pituitary. Since endometriotic implants are estrogen sensitive, LHRH agonists are frequently used for medical treatment of endometriosis. There are various delivery systems and depot preparations of LHRH agonists with similar therapeutic efficacy. LHRH agonists are used prior to surgery in order to facilitate the operation, as an adjuvant after the surgery to prevent the recurrence or prolong the disease-free interval and in patients scheduled for IVF procedures in order to increase pregnancy rates. Adverse effects are due to hypoestrogenism and include hot flashes, vaginal dryness, loss of libido, sleep disturbances and a decrease of bone density, and limit the duration of administration to 6 months. If a long-term treatment is desired, add-back of estrogen/progestin, or progestin only with or without bisphosphonates has to be applied, but existing studies only cover a 12 months period of treatment.

LHRH antagonists block competitively pituitary receptors for LHRH. Consequently a partial pharmacological hypophysectomy reducing the estrogen levels to a desired level is possible if LHRH antagonists are adequately dosed. As endometriotic implants require relatively high amounts of estrogen, while lower plasma levels are sufficient to prevent the loss of bone density, a long-term treatment without add-back therapy is possible. So far, two trials demonstrated, that 8 weeks of treatment can abolish endometriosis–related symptoms without hypoestrogenic side effects with sustained symptomatic for up to sixteen weeks after therapy in one trial.

Introduction

More than 30 years ago our laboratory first achieved the isolation, elucidation of structure and synthesis of hypothalamic luteinizing hormone-releasing hormone (LHRH).[1-5] Subsequent studies demonstrated that the structure of hypothalamic LHRH is conserved in all mammalian species, including humans.

LHRH is the primary link between the brain and the pituitary in the regulations of the gonadal function and plays a key role in vertebrate reproduction. We showed that both natural LHRH and the synthetic decapeptide possessed major follicle stimulatin hormone (FSH)-releasing as well as luteinizing hormone (LH)-releasing activity.[4] Thus, one of us (A.V.S.) put forward a concept that one hypothalamic hormone, LHRH, which is also known as gonadotrophin hormone-releasing hormone (GnRH), controls the secretion of both gonadotrophins from the pituitary gland. This hypothesis is now well established and upheld by abundant experimental and clinical evidence.[5-11] Because GnRH can be easily confused with GHRH (growth hormone-releasing hormone), we prefer to use the original name LHRH.[8] The endocrine actions of LHRH and its analogs are mediated by high-affinity membrane receptors for LHRH on the pituitary gonadotrophs.[11]

Recently, another isoform of the decapeptide, LHRH-II, has been discovered, which is expressed in the human brain, peripheral organs some and tumors such as breast carcinomas.[12, 13] LHRH type II receptors have been detected in some mammals, but the presence of functional LHRH-II receptors in humans remains controversial.[13-15]

LHRH-analogs: Agonists and Antagonists

In the past 30 years, more than 3000 analogs of LHRH have been synthesized.[8-10] Agonistic analogs, such as triptorelin, leuprolide, goserelin and buserelin, which are

50-100 times more potent than LHRH and available as depot preparations have become well-established therapeutic tools for the treatment of sex steroid dependent diseases such as endometriosis.[8, 9, 16] Potent antagonistic analogs of LHRH, such as cetrorelix, ganirelix, degarelix have also been synthesized.[17, 18]

Acute administration of an agonistic analog of LHRH produces a marked increase of FSH, LH and subsequently of estradiol, the so-called flare-up effect. However, a continuous stimulation of the pituitary with LHRH agonists induces a suppression of the pituitary-gonadal axis. This effect is due to down-regulation of receptors and desensitation to LHRH and leads to a decrease of the circulating levels of LH and sex steroids.[9, 16, 19] Down-regulation of LHRH receptors produced by sustained administration of LHRH agonists is the primary basis for the endocrine treatment of sex-steroid sensitive diseases such as endometriosis.[9, 16, 19] LHRH antagonists exhibit no intrinsic activity, but compete with native LHRH for the same binding sites.[8, 9, 16] By producing a competitive blockade of LHRH receptors, LHRH antagonists cause an immediate suppression of the release of gonadotrophins and sex steroids.[9, 16] As LHRH antagonists compete for their receptors with native LHRH, a dose dependent suppression of the gonadotrophins and subsequently of the sex steroids occurs. Thus, sex steroids can be lowered to a desired level using an adequate dose of an LHRH antagonist.

LHRH Agonists in the Treatment of Endometriosis

Endometriosis is a common gynecological disease affecting approximately 10% of women during premenopause.[20] In selected groups of patients such as sterility patients the incidence is 30-60%.[21] The symptoms, which arise due to aberrant endometrial tissue located in the pelvis, the ovary or the rectouterine cavity, include pelvic pain, dysmenorrhea and infertility.[20] Although endometriosis can be diagnosed quite accurately based on patient history and pelvic exam, if severe dysmenorrhea and nodularity in the cul de sac are present,[22] surgery still remains the most accurate diagnostic measure, which normally is combined with primary treatment by ablation of the endometriotic tissue. However, after a successful surgery, the recurrence rates are as high as 50% 12 months after the operation.[20,23] Other reports indicate that 7–30% of patients experience recurrence of pain symptoms within 3 years of laparoscopic surgery, an estimate that increases to 40-50% at 5 years after surgery.[24] These findings underline the importance of additional medical therapy in order to decrease the recurrence rates and avoid additional surgery.

Dosage and Timing of Administration

The dose of LHRH agonist used for the treatment of endometriosis varies with the specific compound and mode of delivery. For patient convenience depot preparations should be used **(Table 25-1)**. If dosed adequately, no difference with respect to efficacy was noted between the different compounds.[25]

Since LHRH agonists initially induce an increase of the levels of gonadotrophins and estradiol, endometriosis related symptoms may become worse at the initial phases of therapy. However, there are three ways to avoid this unwanted effect. One way is to start with the LHRH agonist in the midluteal phase instead of the follicular phase of the cycle.[26, 27] Thus, due to high progesterone levels at that time of the cycle, the flare–up effect of the gonadotrophins and subsequently of estradiol is prevented. One shortcoming of this approach is the fact that administration of the LHRH agonist may coincide with an inadvertent pregnancy. A second approach may consist of the pretreatment with progesterone or oral contraceptives for several weeks prior to the administration of the LHRH agonist.[27] A third way to avoid the flare-up effect is the cotreatment with an LHRH antagonist for the first week after the administration of the LHRH agonist.

Treatment of Endometriosis-related Symptoms

LHRH analogues are currently one of the most widely used medical therapies for endometriosis.[24] As the endometrial implants are estrogen-sensitive, chronic administration of LHRH-agonists inducing medical

Table 25-1: LHRH agonists and antagonists		
Analog type	*drug*	*dose*
Agonist	Goserelin	3.6 mg/month; 10.8 mg/3 months
Agonist	Triptorelin	3.75 mg/month
Agonist	Leuprolide	3.57 mg/month
Agonist	Buserelin	6.6 mg/2 months; 9.45 mg/3 months
Antagonist	Cetrorelix	0.25 mg/day; 3 mg
Antagonist	Cetrorelix-pamoate	52 mg
Antagonist	Ganirelix	0.25 mg/day

LHRH-agonists are available as depot preparations, which have to be applied at 1-3 monthly intervals to achieve pituitary suppression. LHRH-antagonists are so far given as daily injections. Cetrorelix is available as a 3 mg preparation, which induces pituitary suppression for some days.

menopause can be successfully used for the management of endometriosis. LHRH analogs used for the treatment of endometriosis include nafarelin, buserelin, histrelin, goserelin, triptorelin and leuprolide, which are about equally effective.[25, 28] Recent findings suggest additional direct effects of LHRH analogs at the endometriotic lesions which will be reviewed below. Most patients achieve symptomatic relief within a month of starting therapy. Treatment of women with endometriosis leads to relief of abdominal pain, and reduction in endometrial implants. One study testing leuprolide depot vs placebo demonstrated the effectiveness of the LHRH agonist after 3 months of application.[29] Dysmenorrhea, pelvic pain, and pelvic tenderness were relieved significantly to LHRH agonist treatment in comparison with placebo. About 33% of patients with dysmenorrhea and 75% with dyspareunia had maintained relief at 12 months and 37 % of the group of patients with non-cyclic pain experienced relief at 1 year post-therapy. In numerous comparative trials LHRH agonists, some of which were placebo controlled, have shown similar therapeutic efficacy as compared to other established medical therapies, such as danazol, progestins and oral contraceptives **(Table 25-2)**.[29-39] A special review group performed a meta-analysis of the existing comparative trials.[40] Twenty-six studies were found to be adequately performed and included in the review, of which 15 compared LHRH analogs with danazol, 5 compared LHRH analogs with and without add-back therapy, 3 different doses of LHRH analogs, one LHRH analog with gestrinone and one with an oral contraceptive. No difference between the different treatment modalities was detected with respect to pain relief and reduction in endometriotic deposits. The profiles of side effects, however, varied between the different treatment regimens. The most common adverse events occurring during a therapy with LHRH agonists are hypoestrogenic symptoms such as hot flushes, sleep disturbances, vaginal dryness and decrease of libido.[40] Other non-specific side effects such as joint pain, headache and mood changes may also occur. However, the decrease in bone-density that occurs as a side effect of hypoestrogenism after 3-6 months is a major source of concern and limits the duration of therapy with LHRH-analogs. Although, the recurrence rates after a therapy with LHRH agonists are similar to surgery and endometriosis can be diagnosed clinically with a positive predictive value of more than 90% if patient history and pelvic exam are suggestive, LHRH-agonists are used commonly prior to surgery, in order to reduce the size and activity of the endometriotic lesions, after surgery to prevent or delay the recurrence and prior to IVF/ET to improve the pregnancy rate.[21] Because of a high recurrence rate after surgery, a medical long-term treatment for endometriosis would be desirable.

Surgical Adjunctive Therapy

It has been hypothesized that treatment with LHRH agonists prior to surgery will improve the outcome, due to a decrease of the chronic inflammation and also of endometriotic lesions. Thus, the surgery would be easier to perform and a more complete and less destructive operative approach would be possible. Others, however, are worried that lesions might become less apparent due to shrinkage, and therefore could be missed, leading to incomplete surgery with residual disease. So far, only one randomized study has evaluated the role of preoperative treatment with LHRH agonists.[41] In this study, patients with advanced endometriosis were subjected to 3 months of therapy with LHRH agonists prior to surgery or to surgery alone. Surgery was noted to be easier, though not statistically significant, but surgical outcome in terms of symptomatic relief was not assessed.

Postoperative therapy with LHRH agonists is recommended by its advocates with the aim to decrease residual disease as surgery is thought to be frequently incomplete. Therefore, follow-up medical treatment should result in a therapeutic benefit. Three randomized, controlled trials investigated the use of LHRH agonists after surgery and 3 months duration of treatment proved to be ineffective with regard to enhancing pain relief.[42] However, 6 months of postoperative therapy led to significantly improved pain scores and significantly delayed recurrence of symptoms.[23, 43]

Add-back Therapy

The concept of add-back therapy with LHRH agonist treatment was put forward in order to create a medical long-term treatment for symptomatic endometriosis. This concept was triggered by the "estrogen threshold theory" of Barbieri, who suggested that there was a specific estrogen threshold below which endometriotic tissue was not stimulated, but hot flashes and in particular bone loss were controlled. Various steroidal and non-steroidal agents have been investigated for this purpose, including estrogen alone, progestins alone, estrogens plus progestins and progestins plus bisphosphonates. Each of these regimens

Table 25-2: Prospective controlled studies on the comparative efficacy of LHRH agonist therapy in the treatment of endometriosis

Author	Patient number	Compounds	Design	Duration	Result
Henzl et al 1988[30]	213	Nafarelin vs danazol vs	Randomized, placebo controlled, double blind	6 months	Improvement in all treatment groups
Fedele et al 1989[32]	62	Buserelin vs danazol vs	Randomized, placebo controlled	6 months	Marked pain improvement in both groups
Kennedy et al 1990[32]	85	Nafarelin vs danazol	Randomized, double-blind	6 months	Pain scores improved in both groups
Shaw 1990[33]	73	Nafarelin vs danazol	Randomized, placebo-controlled	6 months	Pain scores improved in both groups
Rolland and van der Heijden 1990[34]	170	Nafarelin vs danazol	Randomized, double-blind, double-dummy	6 months	Pain scores: no difference in both groups
Dlugi et al 1990[29]	63	Leuprolide depot vs placebo	Randomized, placebo-controlled, double blind	6 months	Improvement in treatment group
Nafarelin European Endometriosis Trial Group 1992[35]	263	Nafarelin vs danazol	Randomized, double-blind, double dummy	6 months	No significant difference between two groups
Wheeler et al 1992[36]	253	Leuprolide depot vs danazol	Randomized, double-blind, placebo-controlled	6 months	No difference, improvement in both groups
Fedele et al 1993[37]	35	Buserelin vs expectant management	Randomized	6 months	
Rock et al 1993[38]	315	Zoladex vs danazol	Randomized, open	6 months	Similar efficacy
Bergquist 1998[39]	49	Triptorelin vs placebo	Placebo-controlled, double-blind	6 months	Agonist effective by 2-3 months of treatment

was demonstrated to substantially decrease or abrogate the adverse effects of a LHRH agonist therapy **(Table 25-3).**[44-52] However, some of these regimens resulted in a decreased therapeutic benefit. Estrogen alone, in particular at higher doses (conjugated equine estrogens 1.25 mg daily) induced recurrence of endometriosis-related symptoms and therefore should not be administered as add-back therapy.[48] The other add-back regimens have shown to be equally effective to reduce pain symptoms with LHRH agonist monotreatment. All regimens have shown adequate safety profiles with regard to protection of bone loss for up to 12 months. Calcium supplementation should be an essential part of a bone maintenance program. As the add-back regimens investigated within clinical studies only lasted for up to 12 months, yearly measurement of bone-density should be performed if LHRH therapy with add-back is administered as medical treatment for a long period.

Endometriomas

While LHRH agonists effectively control endometriosis-related symptoms, they failed to show a significant amount of resolution of endometriomas. While volume decrease by > 50% of smaller endometriomas was observed about 50% of the cases, Batioglu and coworkers found resolution of only 18% of endometriomas larger than 3 cm after therapy with LHRH agonists.[53] Furthermore, so far there is also no evidence for preoperative LHRH agonist treatment of endometriomas.[54]

Infertility

Recent available data definitely show that a mere hormonal suppression of ovarian function to improve fertility at any stage of endometriosis is not effective and should not be offered for this indication if it is not combined with an IVF treatment.[55]

Table 25-3: LHRH agonist with add-back regimens for treatment of endometriosis: Comparative studies

Author	Patient number	Design	Agonist	Add-back	Duration	Result
Surrey and Judd 1992[44]	20	Prospective, randomized, masked	Leuprolide	Norethindrone 5 mg/10 mg	24 weeks	Less change in BMD less menopausal symptoms in nortehindrone group, pain efficacy similar
Surrey et al 1995[45]	37	Prospective, randomized, open-label	Leuprolide	Norethindrone 2.5 or 10 mg Etidronate 400 mg 14 d/moVs no treatment	48 weeks	Pain efficacy similar, BMD preserved in treated patients
Mukherjee et al 1996[46]	26	Prospective, randomized, blinded	Leuprolide	Etidronate 400 mg/14 days every other month	6 months	BMD preserved only in treatment group
Moghissi et al 1998[47]	306	Prospective, placebo-controlled, open label for agonist, blinded for HRT	Goserelin	CEE 0.3 or 0.625 mg MPA 5 mg	24 weeks	Similar pain efficacy, decreased bone loss, decreased menopausal symptoms in HRT groups
Hornstein et al 1998[48]	201	Prospective, randomized, double-blind	Leuprolide	Norethindrone 5 mg +Placebo or CEE 0.625 or1.25 mg	1 year	Recurrence of pain in CEE 1.25 mg, BMD preserved in all add-back groups
Franke et al 2000[49]	41	Prospective, randomized, double-blind, placebo-controlled	Goserelin	Placebo or estradiol 2 mg/norethistereone acetate 1 mg	24 weeks	Similar efficacy, BMD and menopausal symptoms attenuated in add-back group
Pierce et al 2000[50]	45	Prospective, randomized, long-term follow-up	Goserelin	Placebo or estradiol 2 mg,/norethisterone acetate 1 mg	2 years active treatment, 6 years follow up	Similar efficacy, BMD less in both groups not fully recovered in 5 years
Surrey and Hornstein 2002[51]	123	Prospective, randomized, double-blind, placebo-controlled	Leuprolide	Placebo or norethindrone 5 mg + CEE 0.625 or 1.25 mg	12 months therapy, 2 years follow-up	Similar efficacy, BMD maintained in add-back groups
Fernandez et al 2004[52]	78	Randomized, double-blind, placebo-controlled	Leuprolide	Promegestone 0.5 mg + placebo/ or estradiol 2 mg + promegestone 0.5 mg	1 year	Similar efficacy, BMD maintained in add-back groups

In a meta-analysis of 22 nonrandomized trials, it has been shown that patients with endometriosis are less likely to get pregnant in IVF cycles than patients with tubal factor sterility,[56] a phenomenon most likely due to a not fully clarified effect on oocyte quality. Thus, the majority of studies indicate that poor oocyte quality, due to the alterations in the follicular environment, may play a major role in reducing the fertilization and implantation rates and in turn, lower pregnancy rates in women with endometriosis suffering from infertility.[57-61] These findings were confirmed by results from oocyte donor cycles, which demonstrated that pregnancy rates were comparable to controls for recipients with endometriosis. However, implantation rates and pregnancy rates were reduced when the donor oocytes were derived from women with endometriosis.[62-64]

Consequently it was investigated, whether the use of long-term LHRH agonists prior to ART can improve pregnancy and implantation rates in women with endometriosis subjected to IVF. To date, several studies have been carried out on the effect of prolonged treatment with LHRH agonist in the management of infertile women with endometriosis.[65,66-71] Salam et al[72] combined the results of the three existing prospective randomized studies in a meta-analysis. According to the combined results of these studies, clinical pregnancy rates in women who received LHRH agonist compared with those who did not were 53 of 88 and 25 of 77, respectively. The pooled odds ratio showed that there was a statistically significant benefit for women who were treated with LHRH agonist as compared to the control group (4.28; 95% CI 2.00–9.15). Thus, the meta-analysis confirmed that in women with endometriosis, treatment with a LHRH agonist for three to six months prior to ART, increases the odds of clinical pregnancy by at least four-fold. The number of oocytes retrieved was significantly higher after long-term treatment with LHRH agonist, while the dose of gonadotrophin required for stimulation did not differ.[71] Thus, evidence is strong that prior to an IVF procedure, endometriosis patients should be treated with an LHRH agonist for 3 to 6 months.

Direct Effects on Endometriotic Tissue

There is growing evidence that LHRH agonists may have direct effects on ovarian steroidogenesis and on the growth of endometriotic implants depending on their endocrine effect. Recent studies *in vitro* showed that an LHRH agonist induced apoptosis and decreased promitogenic cytokines such as interleukin 1 beta and vascular endothelial growth factor (VEGF) in specimens of ectopic endometrium of women with untreated endometriosis.[73,74] Other data suggest that VEGF may be involved in the maintenance of endometriosis and that immunologic mechanisms mediated through IL-1 may act as growth factors and also may prevent apoptosis of ectopic endometrium.[74,75] In addition, receptors for LHRH have been detected on ectopic endometrial cells,[76] Accordingly, cell growth could be inhibited by administration *in vitro* of a LHRH agonist,[76] suggesting that LHRH may be a growth factor in endometriotic tissue, a phenomenon which has already been described for other tumors.[77] Iwabe et al showed that LHRH agonists can reduce serum concentrations of interleukin-6 in patients with ovarian endometriomas.[78] Furthermore, it has been demonstrated that estrogen receptor alpha, but not beta is down-regulated in endometriomas secondary to LHRH agonist therapy.[79] Thus, direct effects of LHRH agonists appear to growth inhibiting effects at the endometriotic tissue in addition to the induction of a hypoestrogenic state by uncoupling the endocrine gonadal axis.

Antagonists of LHRH in the Treatment of Endometriosis

A long-term medical treatment for endometriosis would be desirable because of a high recurrence rate after surgery. As mentioned above, it has been hypothesized that endometriotic lesions need relatively high levels of estrogen for their growth (>40 pg/ml).[9,66]

LHRH antagonists act through a dose-dependent receptor blockade. A fine tuning of the suppression of estradiol should therefore, be possible with LHRH anta-

gonists, and it has been speculated that in this approach hormonal replacement therapy could be avoided. Most available administration forms of LHRH antagonists provide short term (daily or every third-day) dosing as infertility treatment. To date, only two studies on the use of LHRH antagonists for the treatment of endometriosis have been published. Küpker et al administered 3 mg cetrorelix weekly for 8 weeks to 15 patients with pain related to endometriosis. Serum estradiol levels ranged about 50 pg/ml throughout the therapy and no symptoms of estrogen deprivation occurred.[80] All patients were symptoms free during the treatment period.[80] Subsequent laparoscopy indicated a significant regression of the endometriotic implants in 60% of the cases. On the basis of these data, a dose-finding study with cetrorelix was carried out in 60 patients with endometriosis proven by laparoscopy with moderate to severe symptoms.[81] These women were treated for 8 weeks with either weekly or bi-weekly doses of 5 and 10 mg of cetrorelix. All patients had a rapid decrease of endometriosis-related symptoms by the fourth week of treatment, and the effect lasted for 16 weeks, as shown on the basis of pain and dysmenorrheal scores. In the trial women did not suffer from hypoestrogenic symptoms and the medication was well tolerated. Because of the absence of an initial flare-up effect, a long-term intermittent therapy with LHRH antagonists seems to be a new option for the treatment of endometriosis. The antagonist could thus be given at doses that do not lead to suppression of estrogen to castration levels and another treatment cycle could be initiated if symptoms reappear. Development of LHRH antagonists as depot preparations or orally active non-peptidic LHRH antagonists may be of use for such treatment.

One recent study showed, that direct proapoptotic effects on endometriotic tissue may also contribute to the therapeutic effect of LHRH antagonists, as both LHRH agonist leuprolide and the antagonist antide induced apoptosis in endometrial epithelial cell cultures from patients with endometriosis. This effect was accompanied by an increase in the expression of the pro-apoptotic proteins Bax and FasL and a decrease in the anti-apoptotic protein Bcl-2.[82]

Antagonists of Growth Hormone-releasing Hormone (GHRH) in the Treatment of Endometriosis

One recent publication showed that growth hormone and its splice variant SV-1 receptor may play a role in endo-metriosis or development of endometriosis. Consequently it is possible that antagonistic analogs of GHRH could find an application in the treatment of endometriosis alone or in combination with LHRH analogs.[83]

Conclusion

The treatment with LHRH agonists provides proven pain relief in 80 to 90% of women with documented endometriosis. However, after the end of the therapy symptoms recur. The administration of LHRH agonists for 6 months as an adjuvant measure after surgery has been shown to extend the pain-free interval. The addition of immediate add-back therapy does not reduce the efficacy of LHRH agonists, while preventing loss of bone substance and alleviating the symptoms of hypoestrogenism. Thus, in combination with add-back therapy LHRH agonists should be considered a first-line treatment for relief of endometriosis related pain. If IVF is planned in patients with endometriosis, they should receive 3-6 months of therapy with LHRH agonists prior to starting the stimulation, as pregnancy rates are significantly increased by this treatment modality.

LHRH antagonists deserve further consideration because of their immediate onset of action which avoids the flare up effect in the therapy of endometriosis. Still more important is the possibility of titrating estrogen levels with appropriate doses of antagonist, long-term treatment without add-back therapy might be possible with the antagonists of LHRH.

References

1. Matsuo H, Baba Y, Nair RM, Arimura A, Schally AV. Structure of the porcine LH- and FSH-releasing hormone. I. The proposed amino acid sequence. Biochem Biophys Res Commun 1971; 43:1334-39.
2. Matsuo H, Arimura A, Nair RM, Schally AV. Synthesis of the porcine LH- and FSH-releasing hormone by the solid-phase method. Biochem Biophys Res Commun 1971; 45:822-27.
3. Schally AV, Arimura A, Baba Y, Nair RM, Matsuo H, Redding TW, Debeljuk L. Isolation and properties of the FSH and LH-releasing hormone. Biochem Biophys Res Commun 1971; 43:393-99.
4. Schally AV, Arimura A, Kastin AJ, Matsuo H, Baba Y, Redding TW, Nair RM, Debeljuk L, White WF. Gonadotropin-releasing hormone: one polypeptide regulates secretion of luteinizing and follicle-stimulating hormones. Science 1971; 173:1036-38.
5. Schally AV, Kastin AJ, Arimura A. Hypothalamic follicle-stimulating hormone (FSH) and luteinizing hormone (LH)-regulating hormone: structure, physiology, and clinical studies. Fertil Steril 1971; 22:703-21.
6. Schally AV. Aspects of hypothalamic regulation of the pituitary gland. Science 1978; 202:18-28.
7. Reissmann T, Diedrich K, Comaru-Schally AM, Schally AV. Introduction of LHRH-antagonists into the treatment of gynaecological disorders. Hum Reprod 1994; 9:769.
8. Schally AV. LH-RH analogues: I. Their impact on reproductive medicine. Gynecol Endocrinol 1999; 13:401-09.
9. Reissmann T, Schally AV, Bouchard P, Riethmiiller H, Engel J. The LHRH antagonist cetrorelix: a review. Hum Reprod Update 2000; 6:322-31.
10. Kastin AJ, Schally AV, Gual C, Midgley AR, Jr., Bowers CY, Gomez-Perez F. Administration of LH-releasing hormone to selected subjects. Am J Obstet Gynecol 1970; 108:177-82.
11. Clayton RN, Catt KJ. Gonadotropin-releasing hormone receptors: characterization, physiological regulation, and relationship to reproductive function. Endocr Rev 1981; 2:186-209.
12. White RB, Eisen JA, Kasten TL, Fernald RD. Second gene for gonadotropin-releasing hormone in humans. Proc Natl Acad Sci U S A 1998; 95:305-09.
13. Millar R. GnRH II and type II GnRH receptors. Trends Endocrinol Metab 2003; 14:35-43.
14. Enamoto M ED, Kawashima S, Park MK. Human type II receptor mediates effects of GnRH on cell proliferation. Zoological Science 2004; 21:763-70.
15. Maudsley S, Davidson L, Pawson AJ, Chan R, de Maturana RL, Millar RP. Gonadotropin-releasing hormone (GnRH) antagonists promote proapoptotic signaling in peripheral reproductive tumor cells by activating a Galphai-coupling state of the type I GnRH receptor. Cancer Res 2004; 64: 7533-44.
16. Schally AV, Comaru-Schally AM, Nagy A, Kovacs M, Szepeshazi K, Plonowski A, Varga JL, Halmos G. Hypothalamic hormones and cancer. Front Neuroendocrinol 2001; 22:248-91.
17. Bradbeer JN, Lindsay PC, Reeve J. Fluctuation of mineral apposition rate at individual bone-remodeling sites in human iliac cancellous bone: independent correlations with osteoid width and osteoblastic alkaline phosphatase activity. J Bone Miner Res 1994; 9:1679-86.
18. Trachtenberg J, Gittleman M, Steidle C, Barzell W, Friedel W, Pessis D, Fotheringham N, Campion M, Garnick MB. A phase 3, multicenter, open label, randomized study of abarelix versus leuprolide plus daily antiandrogen in men with prostate cancer. J Urol 2002; 167:1670-74.
19. Emons G, Schally AV. The use of luteinizing hormone releasing hormone agonists and antagonists in gynaecological cancers. Hum Reprod 1994; 9:1364-79.
20. Crosignani P, Olive D, Bergqvist A, Luciano A. Advances in the management of endometriosis: an update for clinicians. Hum Reprod Update 2006; 12:179-89.
21. Tavmergen E, Ulukus M, Goker EN. Long-term use of gonadotropin-releasing hormone analogues before IVF in women with endometriosis. Curr Opin Obstet Gynecol 2007; 19:284-88.
22. Cheewadhanaraks S, Peeyananjarassri K, Dhanaworavibul K, Liabsuetrakul T. Positive predictive value of clinical diagnosis of endometriosis. J Med Assoc Thai 2004; 87: 740-44.

23. Hornstein MD, Hemmings R, Yuzpe AA, Heinrichs WL. Use of nafarelin versus placebo after reductive laparoscopic surgery for endometriosis. Fertil Steril 1997;68: 860-64.

24. Valle RF, Sciarra JJ. Endometriosis: treatment strategies. Ann N Y Acad Sci 2003; 997:229-39.

25. Filicori M. Gonadotrophin-releasing hormone agonists. A guide to use and selection. Drugs 1994; 48:41-58.

26. Meldrum DR, Wisot A, Hamilton F, Gutlay AL, Huynh D, Kempton W. Timing of initiation and dose schedule of leuprolide influence the time course of ovarian suppression. Fertil Steril 1988; 50:400-02.

27. Olive DL. Optimizing gonadotropin-releasing hormone agonist therapy in women with endometriosis. Treat Endocrinol 2004; 3:83-89.

28. Child TJ, Tan SL. Endometriosis: aetiology, pathogenesis and treatment. Drugs 2001; 61:1735-50.

29. Dlugi AM, Miller JD, Knittle J. Lupron depot (leuprolide acetate for depot suspension) in the treatment of endometriosis: a randomized, placebo-controlled, double-blind study. Lupron Study Group. Fertil Steril 1990; 54: 419-27.

30. Henzl MR, Corson SL, Moghissi K, Buttram VC, Berqvist C, Jacobson J. Administration of nasal nafarelin as compared with oral danazol for endometriosis. A multicenter double-blind comparative clinical trial. N Engl J Med 1988; 318:485-89.

31. Fedele L, Bianchi S, Arcaini L, Vercellini P, Candiani GB. Buserelin versus danazol in the treatment of endometriosis-associated infertility. Am J Obstet Gynecol 1989; 161:871-76.

32. Kennedy SH, Williams IA, Brodribb J, Barlow DH, Shaw RW. A comparison of nafarelin acetate and danazol in the treatment of endometriosis. Fertil Steril 1990; 53: 998-1003.

33. Shaw RW. Nafarelin in the treatment of pelvic pain caused by endometriosis. Am J Obstet Gynecol 1990; 162:574-76.

34. Rolland R, van der Heijden PF. Nafarelin versus danazol in the treatment of endometriosis. Am J Obstet Gynecol 1990; 162:586-88.

35. Nafarelin for endometriosis: a large-scale, danazol-controlled trial of efficacy and safety, with 1-year follow-up. The Nafarelin European Endometriosis Trial Group (NEET). Fertil Steril 1992; 57:514-22.

36. Wheeler JM, Knittle JD, Miller JD. Depot leuprolide versus danazol in treatment of women with symptomatic endometriosis. I. Efficacy results. Am J Obstet Gynecol 1992; 167:1367-71.

37. Fedele L, Bianchi S, Bocciolone L, Di Nola G, Franchi D. Buserelin acetate in the treatment of pelvic pain associated with minimal and mild endometriosis: a controlled study. Fertil Steril 1993; 59:516-21.

38. Rock JA, Truglia JA, Caplan RJ. Zoladex (goserelin acetate implant) in the treatment of endometriosis: a randomized comparison with danazol. The Zoladex Endometriosis Study Group. Obstet Gynecol 1993; 82:198-205.

39. Bergqvist A, Bergh T, Hogstrom L, Mattsson S, Nordenskjold F, Rasmussen C. Effects of triptorelin versus placebo on the symptoms of endometriosis. Fertil Steril 1998; 69:702-08.

40. Prentice A, Deary AJ, Goldbeck-Wood S, Farquhar C, Smith SK. Gonadotrophin-releasing hormone analogues for pain associated with endometriosis. Cochrane Database Syst Rev 2000:CD000346.

41. Audebert A, Descamps P, Marret H, Ory-Lavollee L, Bailleul F, Hamamah S. Pre- or post-operative medical treatment with nafarelin in stage III-IV endometriosis: a French multicenter study. Eur J Obstet Gynecol Reprod Biol 1998; 79:145-48.

42. Parazzini F, Fedele L, Busacca M, Falsetti L, Pellegrini S, Venturini PL, Stella M. Postsurgical medical treatment of advanced endometriosis: results of a randomized clinical trial. Am J Obstet Gynecol 1994; 171:1205-07.

43. Vercellini P, Crosignani PG, Fadini R, Radici E, Belloni C, Sismondi P. A gonadotrophin-releasing hormone agonist compared with expectant management after conservative surgery for symptomatic endometriosis. Br J Obstet Gynaecol 1999; 106:672-77.

44. Surrey ES, Judd HL. Reduction of vasomotor symptoms and bone mineral density loss with combined norethindrone and long-acting gonadotropin-releasing hormone agonist therapy of symptomatic endometriosis: a prospective randomized trial. J Clin Endocrinol Metab 1992; 75:558-63.

45. Surrey ES, Voigt B, Fournet N, Judd HL. Prolonged gonadotropin-releasing hormone agonist treatment of symptomatic endometriosis: the role of cyclic sodium etidronate and low-dose norethindrone "add-back" therapy. Fertil Steril 1995; 63:747-55.

46. Mukherjee T, Barad D, Turk R, Freeman R. A randomized, placebo-controlled study on the effect of cyclic intermittent etidronate therapy on the bone mineral density changes associated with six months of gonadotropin-releasing hormone agonist treatment. Am J Obstet Gynecol 1996; 175:105-109.

47. Moghissi KS, Schlaff WD, Olive DL, Skinner MA, Yin H. Goserelin acetate (Zoladex) with or without hormone replacement therapy for the treatment of endometriosis. Fertil Steril 1998; 69:1056-62.

48. Hornstein MD, Surrey ES, Weisberg GW, Casino LA. Leuprolide acetate depot and hormonal add-back in endometriosis: a 12-month study. Lupron Add-Back Study Group. Obstet Gynecol 1998; 91:16-24.

49. Franke HR, van de Weijer PH, Pennings TM, van der Mooren MJ. Gonadotropin-releasing hormone agonist plus "add-back" hormone replacement therapy for treatment of endometriosis: a prospective, randomized, placebo-controlled, double-blind trial. Fertil Steril 2000; 74:534-39.

50. Pierce SJ, Gazvani MR, Farquharson RG. Long-term use of gonadotropin-releasing hormone analogs and hormone replacement therapy in the management of endometriosis: a randomized trial with a 6-year follow-up. Fertil Steril 2000; 74:964-68.

51. Surrey ES, Hornstein MD. Prolonged GnRH agonist and add-back therapy for symptomatic endometriosis: long-term follow-up. Obstet Gynecol 2002; 99:709-19.

52. Fernandez H, Lucas C, Hedon B, Meyer JL, Mayenga JM, Roux C. One year comparison between two add-back therapies in patients treated with a GnRH agonist for

symptomatic endometriosis: a randomized double-blind trial. Hum Reprod 2004; 19:1465-71.

53. Batioglu S, Celikkanat H, Ugur M, Mollamahmutoglu L, Yesilyurt H, Kundakci M. The use of GnRH agonists in the treatment of endometriomas with or without drainage. J Pak Med Assoc 1996; 46:30-32.

54. Muzii L, Marana R, Caruana P, Mancuso S. The impact of preoperative gonadotropin-releasing hormone agonist treatment on laparoscopic excision of ovarian endometriotic cysts. Fertil Steril 1996; 65:1235-37.

55. Olive DL, Pritts EA. Treatment of endometriosis. N Engl J Med 2001;345:266-75.

56. Barnhart K, Dunsmoor-Su R, Coutifaris C. Effect of endometriosis on in vitro fertilization. Fertil Steril 2002; 77:1148-55.

57. Akande AV, Asselin J, Keay SD, Cahill DJ, Muttukrishna S, Groome NP, Wardle PG. Inhibin A, inhibin B and activin A in follicular fluid of infertile women with tubal damage, unexplained infertility and emdometriosis. Am J Reprod Immunol 2000; 43:61-69.

58. Pellicer A, Albert C, Mercader A, Bonilla-Musoles F, Remohi J, Simon C. The follicular and endocrine environment in women with endometriosis: local and systemic cytokine production. Fertil Steril 1998; 70: 425-31.

59. Harlow CR, Cahill DJ, Maile LA, Talbot WM, Mears J, Wardle PG, Hull MG. Reduced preovulatory granulosa cell steroidogenesis in women with endometriosis. J Clin Endocrinol Metab 1996; 81:426-29.

60. Carlberg M, Nejaty J, Froysa B, Guan Y, Soder O, Bergqvist A. Elevated expression of tumour necrosis factor alpha in cultured granulosa cells from women with endometriosis. Hum Reprod 2000; 15:1250-55.

61. Morita Y, Kojima T, Takeda S, Kinoshita K, Sakamoto S, Baba K, Itoyama S. Effects of buserelin presurgical treatment on vascularity in the sub-serosal interstitial tissue of the uterus and operative blood loss at hysterectomy in women with uterine leiomyoma and adenomyosis. Nippon Sanka Fujinka Gakkai Zasshi 1991; 43: 197-204.

62. Simon C, Gutierrez A, Vidal A, de los Santos MJ, Tarin JJ, Remohi J, Pellicer A. Outcome of patients with endometriosis in assisted reproduction: results from in-vitro fertilization and oocyte donation. Hum Reprod 1994; 9:725-29.

63. Sung L, Mukherjee T, Takeshige T, Bustillo M, Copperman AB. Endometriosis is not detrimental to embryo implantation in oocyte recipients. J Assist Reprod Genet 1997; 14:152-56.

64. Pellicer A, Navarro J, Bosch E, Garrido N, Garcia-Velasco JA, Remohi J, Simon C. Endometrial quality in infertile women with endometriosis. Ann N Y Acad Sci 2001; 943:122-30.

65. Marcus SF, Edwards RG. High rates of pregnancy after long-term down-regulation of women with severe endometriosis. Am J Obstet Gynecol 1994; 171:812-17.

66. Nakamura K, Oosawa M, Kondou I, Inagaki S, Shibata H, Narita O, Suganuma N, Tomoda Y. Menotropin stimulation after prolonged gonadotropin releasing hormone agonist pretreatment for in vitro fertilization in

patients with endometriosis. J Assist Reprod Genet 1992; 9:113-17.

67. Dicker D, Goldman GA, Ashkenazi J, Feldberg D, Voliovitz I, Goldman JA. The value of pre-treatment with gonadotrophin releasing hormone (GnRH) analogue in IVF-ET therapy of severe endometriosis. Hum Reprod 1990; 5:418-20.

68. Dicker D, Goldman JA, Levy T, Feldberg D, Ashkenazi J. The impact of long-term gonadotropin-releasing hormone analogue treatment on preclinical abortions in patients with severe endometriosis undergoing in vitro fertilization-embryo transfer. Fertil Steril 1992; 57:597-600.

69. Parmar H, Nicoll J, Stockdale A, Cassoni A, Phillips RH, Lightman SL, Schally AV. Advanced ovarian carcinoma: response to the agonist D-Trp-6-LHRH. Cancer Treat Rep 1985; 69:1341-42.

70. Ruiz-Velasco V, Allende S. Goserelin followed by assisted reproduction: results in infertile women with endometriosis. Int J Fertil Womens Med 1998; 43:18-23.

71. Surrey ES, Silverberg KM, Surrey MW, Schoolcraft WB. Effect of prolonged gonadotropin-releasing hormone agonist therapy on the outcome of in vitro fertilization-embryo transfer in patients with endometriosis. Fertil Steril 2002; 78:699-704.

72. Sallam HN, Garcia-Velasco JA, Dias S, Arici A. Long-term pituitary down-regulation before in vitro fertilization (IVF) for women with endometriosis. Cochrane Database Syst Rev 2006:CD004635.

73. Meresman GF, Bilotas M, Buquet RA, Baranao RI, Sueldo C, Tesone M. Gonadotropin-releasing hormone agonist induces apoptosis and reduces cell proliferation in eutopic endometrial cultures from women with endometriosis. Fertil Steril 80 Suppl 2003; 2:702-07.

74. Meresman GF, Bilotas MA, Lombardi E, Tesone M, Sueldo C, Baranao RI. Effect of GnRH analogues on apoptosis and release of interleukin-1beta and vascular endothelial growth factor in endometrial cell cultures from patients with endometriosis. Hum Reprod 2003; 18:1767-71.

75. Donnez J, Smoes P, Gillerot S, Casanas-Roux F, Nisolle M. Vascular endothelial growth factor (VEGF) in endometriosis. Hum Reprod 1998; 13:1686-90.

76. Borroni R, Di Blasio AM, Gaffuri B, Santorsola R, Busacca M, Vigano P, Vignali M. Expression of GnRH receptor gene in human ectopic endometrial cells and inhibition of their proliferation by leuprolide acetate. Mol Cell Endocrinol 2000; 159:37-43.

77. Engel JB, Schally AV. Drug Insight: clinical use of agonists and antagonists of luteinizing-hormone-releasing hormone. Nat Clin Pract Endocrinol Metab 2007; 3:157-67.

78. Iwabe T, Harada T, Sakamoto Y, Iba Y, Horie S, Mitsunari M, Terakawa N. Gonadotropin-releasing hormone agonist treatment reduced serum interleukin-6 concentrations in patients with ovarian endometriomas. Fertil Steril 2003; 80:300-304.

79. Matsuzaki S, Uehara S, Murakami T, Fujiwara J, Funato T, Okamura K. Quantitative analysis of estrogen receptor alpha and beta messenger ribonucleic acid levels in normal endometrium and ovarian endometriotic cysts using a real-time reverse transcription-polymerase chain reaction assay. Fertil Steril 2000; 74:753-59.

80. Kupker W, Felberbaum RE, Krapp M, Schill T, Malik E, Diedrich K. Use of GnRH antagonists in the treatment of endometriosis. Reprod Biomed Online 2002; 5:12-16.

81. Donnez JP, O. Barukov A. Dose-finding study of the LHRH antagonist cetrorelix, given over a period of 8 weeks, in the treatment of endometriosis. Evidence Based Obstet Gynecol 2004; 6.

82. Bilotas M, Baranao RI, Buquet R, Sueldo C, Tesone M, Meresman G. Effect of GnRH analogues on apoptosis and expression of Bcl-2, Bax, Fas and FasL proteins in endometrial epithelial cell cultures from patients with endometriosis and controls. Hum Reprod 2007; 22: 644-53.

83. Fu L, Osuga Y, Yano T, Takemura Y, Morimoto C, Hirota Y, Schally AV, Taketani Y. Expression and possible implication of growth hormone-releasing hormone receptor splice variant 1 in endometriosis. Fertil Steril 2009.

Eric S Surrey

Chapter 26

Controlled Ovarian Hyperstimulation in Endometriosis Patients

Introduction

A detailed discussion of the relationship between endometriosis and infertility is beyond the scope of this chapter and has been discussed extensively elsewhere in this text. However, a variety of mechanisms including alterations in the peritoneal environment, distorted pelvic anatomy, altered immune function, suppressed endometrial receptivity, aberrant folliculogenesis and elevated oxidative stress have been impugned as causative factors.[1-3] It is thought that these factors may all combine to inhibit ovum pick-up, ovulation, oocyte quality, fertilization and/or implantation.

This chapter will discuss the relative outcomes achieved with controlled ovarian hyperstimulation (COH), whether in conjunction with timed intercourse, intrauterine insemination (IUI), or *in vitro* fertilization in infertile patients afflicted with this disorder **(Table 26-1)**.

No therapeutic plan should be formulated until a thorough evaluation of other causes of infertility including ovarian reserve, tubal occlusion and sperm function abnormalities has been completed. Before addressing therapeutic options, it is also important to evaluate the likelihood that a patient will conceive without therapy. This is clearly a function of the degree of mechanical distortion associated with the disease. As would be expected, the likelihood of pregnancy in women with anatomic distortion and severe disease is limited at best.[4] The outcomes are more encouraging in patients with less severe disease. Bérubé[5] and coworkers assessed 168 endometriosis patients in a multicenter prospective cohort study who were managed expectantly.[5] The 36-week cumulative probability of pregnancy after diagnostic laparoscopy was 18.2% in infertile women with endometriosis as opposed to 23.7% in infertile women without endometriosis (RR 0.77; 95% CI: 0.52–1.15). In evaluating 226 women undergoing donor IUI, Hammond et al noted that patients with endometriosis experienced significantly lower monthly fecundity rates (MFR) in comparison to women without infertility factors (0.04 vs. 0.2; P<0.05).[6] Byrd and coworkers reported no differences in overall pregnancy rates in women undergoing IUI in unstimulated cycles than those with cervical or male factor infertility.[7] After following 192 infertile couples for up to 3 years after laparoscopy, Akande et al noted, in contrast, that women with minimal/mild endometriosis experienced a significantly lower probability of pregnancy than women with otherwise unexplained infertility (35% vs. 55%; P<0.05).[8] In another trial of women with a similar extent of endometriosis diagnosed laparoscopically, the 24-month cumulative pregnancy rate in 43 patients managed expectantly was 20.9% with a 16.2% probability of carrying a pregnancy beyond 20 weeks.[9] Thus, a case could certainly be made for expectant management in a subset of younger patients without anatomic distortion and an otherwise normal evaluation.

COH: Clomiphene and Aromatase Inhibitors

The use of clomiphene citrate either with or without IUI has been successfully employed as therapy for patients

Table 26-1: Controlled ovarian hyperstimulation and endometriosis related infertility: therapeutic options

1. Expectant management
2. Clomiphene citrate ± IUI
3. Aromatase inhibitors ± gonadotropins ± IUI
4. Gonadotropins ± IUI
5. Surgical intervention prior to COH
6. ART
7. Medical suppression followed by ART

with unexplained infertility.[10–14] There are a limited number of studies that address the use of clomiphene specifically in endometriosis patients whose disease has not been surgically treated. Simpson et al reported upon the results of the use of clomiphene with intercourse timing in a group of endometriosis patients and described a significantly enhanced likelihood for pregnancy in comparison to untreated controls (OR 2.9; 95% CI: 1.2–7).[15] Dickey and coworkers noted that the presence of endometriosis either with or without tubal adhesions significantly reduced the likelihood of pregnancy in comparison to controls (P=0.013 and P<0.0005, respectively) in a prospective study of 1,974 clomiphene citrate-IUI (CCIUI) cycles performed in 849 patients.[11] In a subsequent report with an enlarged sample size of 3,381 CCIUI cycles, these investigators reported a 34% cumulative pregnancy rate after 4 cycles in comparison to 46% for patients with ovulatory dysfunction.[13]

Aromatase inhibitors have been proposed as an alternative to clomiphene citrate. These agents act to stimulate follicular development without exerting any apparent deleterious effect on the endometrium as has been reported with clomiphene. Bedaiwy and coworkers reported on the outcomes of 31 cycles in endometriosis patients in a larger retrospective series of 872 cycles in women undergoing IUI with FSH alone or in conjunction with the aromatase inhibitor letrozole.[16] Significantly lower cost with similar pregnancy rates was noted with the use of the aromatase inhibitor. It is important to note that these agents have not yet received approval for this indication from the U.S. Food and Drug Administration.

COH: Gonadotropins

Various gonadotropin preparations have also been successfully used in conjunction with IUI to achieve pregnancy in patients with unexplained infertility.[17] Two prospective randomized trials have specifically addressed the use of gonadotropins in the treatment of infertility in women with minimal or mild endometriosis. Fedele and colleagues randomly assigned 49 such women to either 3 superovulation cycles with human menopausal gonadotropins (hMG) after a GnRH agonist had been administered to achieve adequate pituitary gonadotropin down-regulation or to 6 cycles of expectant management.[18] The MFR was significantly higher in those treated with gonadotropins (0.15% vs. 0.045%, P<0.05).

Previously, Tummon and coworkers evaluated a similar patient population of 103 couples who underwent 311

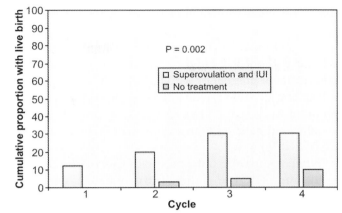

FIGURE 26-1: Cumulative proportion of endometriosis patients with a live birth after either undergoing gonadotropin COH and IUI or expectant management (from Tummon et al, ref. 19. Reprinted with permission from Elsevier Publishers, Inc.)

cycles and were randomized to treatment with 4 cycles of superovulation employing urinary FSH and IUI vs. expectant management.[19] The overall live birth rate was significantly higher after superovulation (11% vs. 7%, or: 5.6; 95% CI: 1.8–17.4) **(Figure 26-1)**. Others have reported that the presence of endometriosis did not affect the likelihood of conception as a result of gonadotropin/ IUI in comparison to patients with unexplained infertility, ovulatory disorders, or cervical factor.[20] Interestingly, Cahill et al reported that the granulosa cells of women with endometriosis may be less sensitive to exogenous luteinizing hormone than those with tubal damage.[21]

Several retrospective studies have further evaluated this approach. Chaffkin et al performed a comparative analysis of MFR in patients with various forms of infertility treated with hMG with or without IUI.[22] MFR in endometriosis patients were 12.85% and 6.6%, respectively, suggesting a beneficial effect of IUI in conjunction with COH. Isaksson et al reported a pregnancy rate of 18.4% with gonadotropin therapy in endometriosis patients, which was not significantly lower than in patients with otherwise unexplained infertility (27.7%).[23] Another investigative team reported an MFR of 0.17 in endometriosis patients who underwent hMG-stimulated IUI cycles in comparison 0.19 for those with idiopathic infertility.[24]

In contrast, others have shown no difference in pregnancy or monthly fecundity rates in patients with minimal endometriosis undergoing IUI after being administered COH with either clomiphene citrate or gonadotropins for 3 cycles (0.13) in comparison to those ovulatory women who underwent IUI in unmedicated cycles (0.14).[25] The results of this study would suggest that IUI in and of itself might be of benefit regardless of the administration of medications.

In a large meta-analysis of the role of gonadotropins with or without IUI, Hughes reported that the common odds ratio for pregnancy with IUI was 2.37 (95% CI: 1.43–3.9) among all patients with infertility based on 5,214 cycles reported in 22 trials.[26] However, this approach was not beneficial in patients with endometriosis (OR: 0.45, 95% CI: 0.27–0.76).

When comparing outcomes with COH-IUI to *in vitro* fertilization (IVF) in endometriosis patients, Dmowski et al evaluated 648 COH-IUI cycles, 139 IVF-cycles and 68 IVF cycles after failed COH-IUI.[27] The life table estimate of first-cycle fecundity with IVF was significantly higher than the cumulative fecundity after six cycles of COH-IUI. The authors noted that failure of prior COH-IUI did not impact the outcomes of IVF in these patients. Thus, although gonadotropin therapy may be a reasonable second line approach in this patient population, it is less successful than IVF, is much more costly than clomiphene citrate, and does pose a significant risk of high order multiple pregnancy.

COH: Assisted Reproductive Technologies (ART)

A detailed analysis of the impact of ART and, more specifically, *in vitro* fertilization (IVF) on the management of endometriosis will be addressed elsewhere in this text. In this section, we shall specifically discuss the issue of ovarian stimulation in preparation for ART in this patient population.

One of the problems with studies evaluating the response of endometriosis patients to COH in preparation for IVF is the lack control for ovarian reserve which would reflect the potential for response prior to determination of dosing regimens. In current practice, an assessment of ovarian reserve, which typically would include measurement of early follicular phase serum FSH and estradiol levels, antral follicle count, and possible serum anti-mullerian hormone (AMH) or inhibin B levels would be performed along with an assessment of prior responses before initiation of treatment. This information plays a critical role in determining both prognosis and the appropriate COH protocol.

In a meta-analysis involving 22 published studies, Barnhart and colleagues noted that the mean number of oocytes obtained was significantly lower in endometriosis patients than in tubal factor controls (adjusted OR: 0.92;

95% CI: 0.85–0.99).[28] Although this would suggest a decrease in ovarian responsiveness in endometriosis patients, the study does not control for ovarian reserve or dosing regimes, however. In contrast, Geber et al reported upon 140 patients with endometriosis undergoing 182 IVF cycles employing GnRH agonists as part of the stimulation regime and compared results to three control groups with male factor, tubal factor, and unexplained infertility.[29] There were no differences among the groups with regards to gonadotropin dose or days of administration, peak estradiol levels or number of oocytes retrieved. These findings have been confirmed by others.[30, 31]

The effect of stage of endometriosis on ovarian response to gonadotropin stimulation prior to IVF has also been evaluated. In the aforementioned meta-analysis, the mean number of oocytes obtained and peak serum estradiol levels achieved during stimulation were significantly lower in those with stages III-IV as opposed to stages I-II disease.[28] This finding was confirmed in a more recent trial.[32] However, others have demonstrated no difference in COH response for patients with more severe disease in comparison to either controls with other forms of infertility or less severe forms of endometriosis.[29,30] Azem and coworkers, in an earlier study, reported that although peak serum estradiol levels and number of oocytes obtained were similar, significantly higher gonadotropin doses were required in age-matched patients with more severe disease than those with less advanced endometriosis.[34]

The effect of ovarian endometriotic cysts (endometrioma) on COH prior to IVF also has been addressed. Al-Azemi et al described a decrease in ovarian response that required the use of higher gonadotropin doses in patients with such lesions.[34] Cumulative pregnancy and live birth rates were unaffected, however. Yanushpolsky et al reported a higher incidence of pregnancy loss and an adverse effect on number of oocytes retrieved with transvaginal ultrasound-guided techniques in patients with endometriosis.[35] Others have demonstrated no effect of persistent endometriomas on any outcome parameter of either controlled ovarian hyperstimulation or IVF.[30] One interesting study compared COH response in ovaries with endometriosis to unaffected contralateral ovaries and noted a significantly lower number of dominant follicles >15 mm in mean diameter in the affected ovaries.[36] This effect was more pronounced in women with larger as well as with multiple endometriomas. Unfortunately, none of these investigators has correlated endometrioma size with outcome. Similarly, it is difficult to differentiate the effect of an isolated endometrioma *per se* on cycle outcome because patients with these lesions may have varying extents of concomitant peritoneal disease that may represent a confounding variable.

Does Adjuvant Therapy Improve COH Outcomes?

The question of whether medical or surgical intervention for endometriosis will improve COH outcomes for those patients who are planning IUI or timed intercourse is somewhat controversial.

The impact of prior surgical ablation or excision of endometriosis has been addressed in several studies of varying design and will be discussed elsewhere in this text. Deaton et al published a prospective randomized crossover trial of clomiphene and IUI versus no treatment, which, unfortunately, combined couples with unexplained explained infertility (48%) and those with endometriosis (52%), of which 24/27 had minimal or mild disease.[37] Based on life-table analysis, the MFR in the treated group was significantly higher than that of the untreated group (0.095 vs. 0.033; p<0.05). Another restrospective series confirmed these findings and demonstrated that COH outcome with gonadotropins or clomiphene and IUI in women who had undergone surgical treatment of stage I or II endometriosis were similar to those with unexplained infertility.[38] The clinical pregnancy rates per cycle were 21% (stage I endometriosis), 18.9% (stage II endometriosis) and 20.5% (unexplained infertility).

In an effort to further address this issue, Karabacak et al followed patients for a mean of 11 months who had undergone laparoscopic cauterization of endometriosis, adhesiolysis and resection of endometriomas when appropriate.[39] The author compared outcomes in patients managed expectantly to those treated with ovulation induction and noted that ovulation induction only had a beneficial effect if performed with gonadotropins (in comparison to clomiphene citrate) and only if the duration of infertility was less than 5 years. However, by failing to include a group of endometriosis patients undergoing COH-IUI who had not undergone surgical management of their disease, any potential benefit of surgical correction cannot be truly ascertained from these studies.

The effect of surgical resection of endometriomas before IVF has also been evaluated. Canis et al reported the outcome of a series of 41 patients who underwent precycle laparoscopic resection of large (>3 cm in diameter) ovarian endometriotic cysts (unilateral in 30 patients and bilateral in 11 patients) in comparison to 139 controls with endometriosis but without endometriomata and 59 additional controls with tubal infertility.[40] Despite extensive ovarian surgery, no differences regarding the resulting number of oocytes or embryos obtained were described. A more recent study reported on 85 patients (187 cycles) who underwent laparoscopic ovarian endometrioma cyst wall vaporization before IVF and compared responses to 289 patients (633 cycles) with tubal factor infertility.[41] Response to stimulation and clinical pregnancy rates were similar between the groups. These findings have been confirmed by others.[42, 43]

In contrast, a series of investigations have demonstrated that regardless of ultimate cycle outcomes, higher gonadotropin doses are required, lower peak estradiol levels are achieved, and lower numbers of mature oocytes are obtained after laparoscopic resection of endometriomas prior to IVF.[44–49] In a case-control study of 189 women with endometriomas of whom 56 proceeded directly to IVF and 133 first underwent resection, Garcia-Velasco and coworkers noted similar outcomes between the groups in general but again peak estradiol levels were lower and gonadotropin dose requirements were higher in those who underwent pre-cycle surgery.[50] It is not clear whether endometrioma size was similar among the groups. Nevertheless, this study suggests that although surgical resection of endometriomas does not adversely impact IVF outcome, it does not appear to be beneficial.

Resection of large lesions clearly enhances access to follicles within underlying normal ovarian tissue and eliminates the potential for rupture during oocyte aspiration. Meticulous surgical technique with an eye toward carefully avoiding compromise of ovarian blood supply and destroying healthy ovarian tissue is mandatory, however.

The question of whether surgical management of endometriosis in the absence of ovarian endometriomata would enhance IVF cycle outcome has been addressed in two retrospective series. Surrey et al reported that COH and IVF cycle outcomes were similar between groups of patients with endometriosis who underwent surgical resection either within 6 months or from longer than 6 months to 5 years prior to oocyte aspiration (ongoing pregnancy rates 63.6% vs. 60.53%, respectively).[51] Bedaiwy and colleagues also demonstrated no association between time of endometriosis surgery and IVF cycle outcome after logistic regression analysis.[52] It seems that the well-described benefit derived from such surgery in enhancing spontaneous conception may be masked by the greater impact on implantation and pregnancy achieved with the assisted reproductive technologies.

The efficacy of hormonal suppression with the use of progestins, danazol and GnRH agonists in the management of symptomatic endometriosis has been well established. However, the benefit of these agents in enhancing fertility has not been demonstrated. Hughes et al evaluated data from nine trials that compared ovulation suppression with either danazol, gestrinone, or medroxyprogesterone acetate to no treatment or placebo, which all failed to show any beneficial effect on enhancing pregnancy rates (OR 0.85; 95% CI: 0.95–1.22).[53] In the same study, an additional six randomized trials that compared a gonadotropin-releasing hormone (GnRH) agonist, gestrinone, or an oral contraceptive to danazol also failed to demonstrated any differences (OR 1.07; 95% CI: 0.71–1.61). More recently, this group performed an expanded meta-analysis and calculated that the odds ratio for pregnancy following ovulation suppression versus either placebo or no treatment was 0.74 (95% CI: 0.48–1.15).[54] These authors suggested that medical suppressive therapy for treatment of endometriosis-associated infertility could not be justified.

Only one trial conflicts with these conclusions. Rickes and colleagues randomized 63 women with stage II–IV endometriosis who had undergone surgery to a 6-month treatment course with a GnRH agonist followed by a maximum of 3 cycles of gonadotropin COH in conjunction with IUI.[55] Pregnancy rates per patient were significantly higher in the GnRH agonist treated group (89% vs. 61%; P<0.03), although both groups underwent the same mean number of treatment cycles.

There are several possible explanations for these findings. One could propose that minimal-to-mild endometriosis has no impact on fertility given the proven efficacy of these agents in treating the underlying disease but lack of efficacy in improving conception. A second explanation is that the mechanism of infertility associated with endometriosis is different from that associated with pelvic pain and is unaffected by these medications. Neither of these explanations can be supported by data. Several investigators have demonstrated that danazol and GnRH agonists may have a positive impact on peritoneal cytokine levels, natural killer cell activity, metalloproteinase-1 tissue inhibitor concentrations, nitric oxide synthase expression, and endometrial cell apoptosis.[56–60]

A third—and perhaps more plausible—explanation may be that by the time a patient resumes normal ovulatory patterns, which may be months after completion of therapy, the deleterious effects of the disease process on fertility that were suppressed initially by medications recur even if the patient remains asymptomatic. If a patient could attempt conception when the disease process is maximally suppressed, pregnancy rates would be heightened. The successful use of prolonged GnRH agonist therapy immediately before IVF would lend support to this hypothesis.

In a prospective multi-center randomized trial, Surrey and coworkers recently evaluated the effect of a 3-month course of a GnRH agonist administered immediately before IVF in patients with surgically confirmed endometriosis.[61] Significantly higher ongoing pregnancy rates with a trend toward higher implantation rates were appreciated in this group of 25 patients in comparison to 26 controls with endometriosis treated with standard COH techniques in the absence of prolonged GnRH agonist before oocyte aspiration **(Table 26-2)**. There were no differences in gonadotropin doses, duration of therapy, or number of oocytes obtained between the groups.

These findings have been confirmed by other researchers as demonstrated by a recent meta-analysis which noted that the live birth rate per woman was significantly higher in those endometriosis patients receiving prolonged GnRH agonist therapy prior to IVF (OR 9.19, 95% CI 1.08–78.22).[62] This analysis did not specifically address COH response. Although these studies would suggest a benefit of therapy, they do not determine whether this approach should be applied to all endometriosis patients undergoing IVF, or rather, to a specific subset.

Summary

Prior to initiation of therapy in patients with infertility and endometriosis, it is critical to complete a thorough evaluation to rule out other or contributory causes.

Table 26-2: Outcome of COH and IVF cycles in endometriosis patients receiving a 3-month course of GnRH agonist prior to IVF (Gr.I) vs. controls (Gr.II). Modified from Surrey et al[61]					
Group	Patient number	Prolonged GnRH agonist	Gonadotropin dose (75 IU Ampoules) (Mean ± SEM)	COH duration (Days) (Mean ± SEM)	Ongoing pregnancy rate	Group implantation rate
I	25	Yes	42.4 ± 3.21	10.12 ± 0.43	80%	42.68%
II	26	No	43.2 ± 2.5	10.08 ± 0.21	53.85%	30.38%

It is important to remember that women with infertility and endometriosis with tubal patency can conceive spontaneously, albeit at lower rates than in the fertile population. Surgical ablation or resection seems to provide benefit if pelvic anatomy can be restored to normal. After reconstruction or in patients with less extensive disease, controlled ovarian hyperstimulation techniques potentially in conjunction with intrauterine inseminations can be effective. Clomiphene citrate is generally considered to be a first-line agent and, if unsuccessful, gonadotropins may then be considered. The question of whether exposure to high estrogen levels associated with COH, particularly in conjunction with preparation for IVF, may have a dele-terious effect on endometriosis has not been extensively evaluated. One retrospective cohort study would suggest that cumulative endometriosis recurrence rates were not affected by short-term exposure to the very high estradiol levels achieved in this patient population.[63] It is important to monitor patients carefully given the risk of high order multiple gestation reported with these agents.

IVF represents an effective means of bypassing the hostile peritoneal environment and anatomic distortion associated with this disease state. Patients with severe endometriosis and ovarian endometriomas which have been resected may have impaired responses. Although medical suppression of endometriosis alone provides virtually no benefit in enhancing fertility, there seems to be significant benefit of pretreatment with GnRH agonists immediately before IVF cycle initiation. Whether only a specific subset or all patients with endometriosis would benefit from this approach has not yet been determined. The use of endometrial implantation markers may be helpful in this regard.

The selection of the most appropriate approach and dose regimen designed to overcome infertility in the endometriosis patient should be individualized and based on an understanding of the extent of the disease, evaluation of ovarian reserve and other fertility factors, as well as a thorough discussion with the patient of risks and likelihood of a successful outcome.

References

1. Gupta S, Goldberg J, Aziz N, Goldberg E, Krajacir N, Agarwal A. Pathogenic mechanisms in endometriosis-associated infertility. Fertil Steril 2008;90:247-57.
2. The Practice Committee of the American Society for Reproductive Medicine. Endometriosis and infertility. Fertil Steril 2004;81:1441-46.
3. Ryan I, Taylor R. Endometriosis and infertility: new concepts. Obstet Gynecol Surv 1997;52:365-71.
4. Olive D, Stohs G, Metzger D, et al. Expectant management and hydrotubations in the treatment of endometriosis associated infertility. Fertil Steril 1985;44:35-40.
5. Bérubé S, Marcoux S, Langevin M, Maheux R, Canadian Collaborative Group on Endometriosis. Fecundity of infertile women with minimal or mild endometriosis and women with unexplained infertility. Fertil Steril 1998;69:1034-41.
6. Hammon M, Jordan S, Sloan C. Factors affecting pregnancy rates in a donor insemination program using frozen semen. Am J Obstet Gynecol 1986;155:480-85.
7. Byrd W, Ackerman G, Carr B, Edman C, Guzick D, McConnell J. Treatment of refractory infertility by transcervical intrauterine insemination of washed spermatozoa. Fertil Steril 1987;48:921-27.
8. Akande U, Hunt L, Cahill D, Jenkins J. Differences in time to natural conception between women with unexplained infertility and infertile women with minor endometriosis. Hum Reprod 2004;19:96-103.
9. Milingos S, Mavromatis C, Elsheikh A, Kallipolitis G, Coutradis D, Diakomanolis E, Michalas S. Fecundity of infertile women with minimal or mild endometriosis. Arch Gynecol Obstet 2002; 267:37-46.
10. Costello M. Systematic review of the treatment of ovulatory infertility with clomiphene citrate and intrauterine insemination. Aust NZ J Obstet Gynecol 2004;44:93-102.
11. Dickey R, Olar T, Taylor S, Curole D, Rye P. Relationship of follicle number and other factors to fecundability and multiple pregnancy in clomiphene citrate-induced intrauterine insemination cycles. Fertil Steril 1992;57:613-19.
12. Guzick D, Sullivan M, Adamson G, Cedars M, Falk R, Peterson E, et al. Efficacy of treatment for unexplained infertility. Fertil Steril 1998;70:207-13.
13. Dickey R, Taylor S, Lu P, Sartor B, Rye P, Pyrzak R. Effect of diagnosis, age, sperm quality, and number of preovulatory follicles on the outcome of multiple cycles of clomiphene citrate-intrauterine insemination. Fertil Steril 2002;78:1088-93.
14. Hammond M, Halme J, Talbert L. Factors affecting the pregnancy rate in clomiphene citrate induction ovulation. Obstet Gynecol 1983;62:196-202.
15. Simpson C, Taylor P, Collins J. A comparison of ovulation suppression and ovulation stimulation in the treatment of endometriosis-associated infertility. Int J Gynaecol Obstet 1993;59:1239-44.
16. Bedaiwy M, Forman R, Mousa N, Al Inany H, Casper R. Cost-effectiveness of aromatase inhibitor cotreatment for controlled ovarian stimulation. Hum Reprod 2006;21:2838-44.
17. Guzick D, Carson S, Coutifaris C, Overstreet J, Factor-Litvak P, Steinkampf M, et al. Efficacy of superovulation and intrauterine insemination in the treatment of infertility. N Engl J Med 1999;340:177-83.
18. Fedele L, Bianchi S, Marchini M, Villa L, Brioschi D, Parazzini F. Superovulation with human menopausal gonadotropins in the treatment of infertility associated with minimal or mild endometriosis: a controlled randomized study. Fertil Steril 1992;58:28-31.

19. Tummon I, Asher L, Martin J, Tulandi T. Randomized controlled trial of superovulation and insemination for infertility associated with minimal or mild endometriosis. Fertil Steril 1997;68:8-12.

20. Göker E, Ozçakir H, Terek M, Levi R, Adakan S, Tavmergen E. Controlled ovarian hyperstimulation and intrauterine insemination for infertility associated with endometriosis: a retrospective analysis. Arch Gynecol Obstet 2002;266:21-24.

21. Cahill D, Harlow C, Wardle P. Pre-ovulatory granulosa cells of infertile women with endometriosis are less sensitive to luteinizing hormone. Am J Reprod Immunol 2003;49:66-69.

22. Chaffkin L, Nulsen J, Luciano A, Metzger D. A comparative analysis of the cycle fecundity rates associated with combined human menopausal gonadotropin (hMG) and intrauterine insemination (IUI) versus either hMG or IUI alone. Fertil Steril 1991;55:252-57.

23. Isaksson R, Tiitinen A. Superovulation combined with insemination or timed intercourse in the treatment of couples with unexplained infertility and minimal endometriosis. Acta Obstet Gynecol Scand 1998;76:550-54.

24. Dodson W, Whitesides D, Hughes C, Easley H III, Haney A. Superovulation with intrauterine insemination in the treatment of infertility: a possible alternative to gamete intrafallopian transfer and in vitro fertilization. Fertil Steril 1987;48:441-45.

25. Serta R, Rufo S, Seibel M. Minimal endometriosis and intrauterine insemination: does controlled ovarian hyperstimulation improve pregnancy rates? Obstet Gynecol 1992;80:37-40.

26. Hughes E. The effectiveness of ovulation induction and intrauterine insemination in the treatment of persistent infertility: a meta-analysis. Hum Reprod 1997;12:1865-72.

27. Dmowski W, Pry M, Ding J, Rana N. Cycle-specific and cumulative fecundity in patients with endometriosis who are undergoing controlled ovarian hyperstimulation-intrauterine insemination or in vitro fertilization-embryo transfer. Fertil Steril 2002;78:750-56.

28. Barnhart K, Dunsmoor-Su R, Coutifaris C. Effect of endometriosis on in vitro fertilization. Fertil Steril 2002;77:1148-55.

29. Geber S, Paraschos T, Atkinson G, Margara R, Winston R. Results of IVF in patients with endometriosis: the severity of the disease does not affect outcome, or the incidence of miscarriage. Hum Reprod 1995;10:1507-11.

30. Olivennes F, Feldberg D, Liu H, Cohen J, Moy F, Rosenwaks Z. Endometriosis: a stage by stage analysis in the role of in vitro fertilization. Fertil Steril 1995;64:392-98.

31. Omland A, Abyholm T, Fedorcsak P, Ertzeid G, Oldereid N, Bjercke S, Tanbo T. Pregnancy outcome after IVF and ICSI in unexplained, endometriosis-associated and tubal factor infertility. Hum Reprod 2005;20:722-27.

32. Kuivasaari P, Hippelainen M, Anttila M, Heinonen S. Effect of endometriosis on IVF/ICSI outcome: stage III/IV endometriosis worsens cumulative pregnancy and live-born rates. Hum Reprod 2005;20:3130-35.

33. Azem F, Lessing J, Geva E, Shahar A, Lerner-Geva L, Yovel I, et al. Patients with stages III and IV endometriosis have a poorer outcome in in vitro fertilization-embryo transfer than patients with tubal infertility. Fertil Steril 1999;72:1107-09.

34. Al-Azemi M, Lopez Bernal A, Steele J, Gramsbergen I, Barlow D, Kennedy S. Ovarian response to repeated controlled stimulation in in vitro fertilization cycles in patients with ovarian endometriosis. Hum Reprod 2000;15:72-75.

35. Yahushpolski E, Best C, Jackson K, Clarke R, Barbieri R, Hornstein M. Effects of endometriomas on oocyte quality and pregnancy rates in in vitro fertilization cycles: a prospective case-controlled study. J Assist Reprod Genet 1998;15:193-97.

36. Somigliana E, Infantino M, Benedetti F, Arnoldi M, Calanna G, Ragni G. The presence of ovarian endometriomas is associated with a reduced responsiveness to gonadotropins. Fertil Steril 2006;86:192-96.

37. Deaton J, Gibson M, Blackmer K, Nakajima S, Badger G, Brumsted J. A randomized controlled trial of clomiphene citrate and intrauterine insemination in couples with unexplained infertility or surgically corrected endometriosis. Fertil Steril 1990;54:1083-88.

38. Werbronck E, Spiessens C, Meuleman C, D'Hooghe T. No differences in cycle pregnancy rate and in cumulative live-birth rate between women with surgically treated minimal to mild endometriosis and women with unexplained infertility after controlled ovarian hyperstimulation and intrauterine insemination. Fertil Steril 2006;86:566-71.

39. Karabacak O, Kambic R, Gursoy R, Ozeren S. Does ovulation induction affect the pregnancy rate after laparoscopic treatment of endometriosis? Int J Fertil Women's Med 1999;44:38-42.

40. Canis M, Pouly J, Tamburro S, Mage G, Wattiez A, Bruhat M. Ovarian response during IVF-embryo transfer cycles after laparoscopic ovarian cystectomy for endometriotic cysts of >3 cm in diameter. Hum Reprod 2001;12:2583-86.

41. Donnez J, Wyns C, Nisolle M. Does ovarian surgery for endometriomas impair the ovarian response to gonadotropin? Fertil Steril 2001;76:662-65.

42. Alborzi S, Ravanbakhsh R, Parsanezhad M, Alborzi M, Alborzi S, Dehbashi S. A comparison of follicular response of ovaries to ovulation induction after laparoscopic ovarian cystectomy or fenestration and coagulation versus normal ovaries in patients with endometrioma. Fertil Steril 2007;88:507-09.

43. Marconi G, Vilela M, Quintana R, Sueldo C. Laparoscopic ovarian cystectomy of endometriomas does not affect the ovarian response to gonadotropin stimulation. Fertil Steril 2002;78:876-78.

44. Cirpan T, Akercan F, Tavmergen Goker E, Ozyurek E, Levi R, Tavmergen E. Laparoscopic resection or sonography-guided vaginal aspiration of endometriomas prior to ICSI-ET does not worsen treatment outcomes. Clin Exp Obstet Gynecol 2007;34:215-18.

45. Loo T, Lin M, Chen S, Chung M, Tang H, Lin L, Tsai Y. Endometrioma undergoing laparoscopic ovarian cystectomy: its influence on the outcome of in vitro fertilization and embryo transfer (IVF-ET). J Assist Reprod Genet 2005;22:329-33.

46. Suzuki T, Izumi S, Matsubayashi H, Awaji H, Yoshikata K, Mukimo T. Impact of ovarian endometrioma on oocytes and pregnancy outcome in in vitro fertilization. Fertil Steril 2005;83:908-13.

47. Somigliana E, Ragni G, Benedetti F, Borroni R, Vegetti W, Crosignani P. Does laparoscopic excision of endometriotic ovarian cysts significantly affect ovarian reserve? Insights from IVF cycles. Hum Reprod 2003;18:2450-53.

48. Ho H, Lee R, Hwu Y, Lin M, Su S, Tsai Y. Poor response of ovaries with endometrioma previously treated with cystectomy to controlled ovarian hyperstimulation. J Assist Reprod Genet 2002;19:507-11.

49. Duru N, Dede M, Acikel C, Keskin U, Fidan U, Baser I. Outcome of in vitro fertilization and ovarian response after endometrioma stripping at laparoscopy and laparotomy. J Reprod Med 2007;52:805-09.

50. Garcia-Velasco J, Mahutt N, Corona J, Zuniga V, Giles J, Arici A, Pellicer A. Removal of endometriomas before in vitro fertilization does not improve fertility outcomes: a matched case-control study. Fertil Steril 2004;81:1194-97.

51. Surrey E, Schoolcraft W. Does surgical management of endometriosis within 6 months of an in vitro fertilization-embryo transfer cycle improve outcome? J Assist Reprod Genet 2003;20:365-70.

52. Bedaiwy M, Falcone T, Katz E, Goldberg J, Assad R, Thornton J. Association between time from endometriosis surgery and outcome of in vitro fertilization cycles. J Reprod Med 2008;53:161-65.

53. Hughes E, Fedorokow D, Collins J. A quantitative overview of controlled trials in endometriosis-associated infertility. Fertil Steril 1993;59:963-70.

54. Hughes E, Fedorkow D, Collins J, Vanderkerckhove P. Ovulation suppression for endometriosis (Cochrane Review). In: The Cochrane Library, 2003 Issue 3, Oxford update software.

55. Rickes D, Nickel J, Kropf S, Kleinstein J. Increased pregnancy rates after ultralong postoperative therapy with gonadotropin-releasing hormone analogs in patients with endometriosis. Fertil Steril 2002;78:757-62.

56. Sharpe-Timms K, Keisler L, McIntush E, Keisler D. Tissue inhibitors of metalloproteinase-I concentrations are attenuated in peritoneal fluid and sera of women with endometriosis and restored in sera by gonadotropin-releasing hormone agonist therapy. Fertil Steril 1998; 69:1128-34.

57. Imai A, Takagi A, Tamay T. Gonadotropin-releasing hormone analog repairs reduced endometrial cell apoptosis in endometrial in vitro. Am J Obstet Gynecol 2000;182:1142-46.

58. Garzetti G, Ciavattini A, Provinciali M, Muzzioli M, di Stefano G, Fabris N. Natural cytotoxicity and GnRH agonist administration in advanced endometriosis: positive modulation on natural killer cell activity. Obstet Gynecol 1996;88:234-40.

59. Taketani Y, Kuo T, Mizuno M. Comparison of cytokine levels and embryo toxicity in peritoneal fluid in infertile women with untreated or treated endometriosis. Am J Obstet Gynecol 1992;167:265-70.

60. Wang J, Zhou F, Dong M, Wu R, Qian Y. Prolonged gonadotropin-releasing hormone agonist therapy reduced expression of nitric oxide synthase in the endometrium of women with endometriosis and infertility. Fertil Steril 2006;80:1037-44.

61. Surrey E, Silverberg K, Surrey M, Schoolcraft W. The effect of prolonged GnRH agonist therapy on in vitro fertilization-embryo transfer cycle outcome in endometriosis patients: a multicenter randomized trial. Fertil Steril 2002;78:699-704.

62. Sallam H, Garcia-Velasco J, Dias S, Arici A. Long-term pituitary down-regulation before in vitro fertilization (IVF) for women with endometriosis. The Cochrane Database of Systemic Reviews 2006, Issue 1. Art. No: CD004635. pub 2.

63. D'Hooghe T, Denys B, Spiessens C, Meuleman C, Debrock S. Is the endometriosis recurrence rate increased after ovarian hyperstimulation? Fertil Steril 2006;86:283-90.

Section 7

New Medical Treatments

Irving M Spitz, Ronald D Wiehle, Andre van As

Chapter 27

Progesterone Receptor Modulators in Endometriosis: A New Therapeutic Option

Introduction

Endometriosis is defined as the presence of functional endometrium outside the uterine cavity. The clinical presentation is variable, with some women having no symptoms and others experiencing dysmenorrhea, dyspareunia, noncyclic pelvic pain, and subfertility. The incidence of endometriosis is 40-60% in women with dysmenorrhea and 20-30% in those with subfertility.[1] This disease affects 5 million American women.[2] Assuming a 10% prevalence rate among women in the reproductive age, it has been estimated that the overall cost of treating endometriosis in the US in 2002 was in the range of $22 billion.[2, 3]

The precise etiology of endometriosis is unclear. The most widely accepted hypothesis for its development is retrograde menstruation, in which fragments of menstrual endometrium are refluxed through the fallopian tubes into the peritoneal cavity. This was first suggested by Sampson more than 80 years ago.[2] Retrograde menstruation occurs in up to 90% of normal women but not all of them develop endometriosis.[2] Thus, this cannot be the sole explanation for this disease and other mechanisms postulated include immunological, inflammatory, genetic and environmental factors as well as an increase in angiogenesis.[2]

Well established, time honored medical therapies for endometriosis include oral contraceptives, danazol (an isoxazol derivative of 17α-ethinyltestosterone), gonadotropin releasing hormone agonists (GnRHa) and antagonists as well as progestogens. The latter include medroxyprogesterone acetate (MPA), the levonorgestrel intrauterine system, norethindrone acetate and lynestrenol. Gestrinone, (a synthetic 19 nortestosterone derivative) is available in Europe but not in the US. All treatments suppress ovarian activity and menses and induce atrophy of endometriotic implants, although the extent to which they achieve this varies.[2]

Since all medical managements are effective in relieving pain during treatment, side effect profiles and costs are important in deciding therapeutic choices.[1] Oral contraceptives are contraindicated in women with a history of thromboembolic disease and in smokers over 35 years of age. The side effects associated with danazol include skin changes, weight gain, and androgenic symptoms and it is contraindicated for women with hepatic, renal, or cardiac problems. GnRHa's suppress gonadotropins, estradiol and progesterone, leading to anovulation, and climacteric symptoms ranging from hot flushes to losses in bone mass.[1] Administration of GnRH antagonists requires careful dose titration since antagonists produce marked gonadotropin and estradiol suppression.[4] Progestins are associated with irregular menstrual bleeding, weight gain, mood swings, decreased libido, nausea, breast tenderness, fluid retention and decrements in HDL. Both androgenic and antiestrogenic side effects have been described with gestrinone.

In view of the side effects associated with established medical methods for the treatment of endometriosis, new approaches are being evaluated. These include inhibitors of aromatase and angiogenesis, matrix metalloproteases modulators, estrogen receptor-β agonists, as well as progesterone receptor modulators (PRMs). This chapter will focus on the role of PRMs in the treatment of endometriosis.

Rationale for the use of Progesterone Receptor Modulators

Mifepristone (RU 486), was the first progesterone antagonist to be described.[5] Numerous related compounds were subsequently synthesized. Because of structural variations and variable binding characteristics to the progesterone receptor (PR), these progesterone receptor ligands may function as progesterone agonists, progesterone antagonists (PAs), or mixed agonists-antagonists. The latter are known as Selective Progesterone Receptor Modulators (SPRMs), a term which is in keeping with the terminology adopted for SERMs.[6] In this manuscript, the term PRM refers to both PAs and SPRMs.

PR Receptor

This exists as two separate isoforms, PR-A and PR-B, which are expressed from a single gene by alternate promoter usage (See (6) for a review). The structural configurations of the PR-A and PR-B isoform are similar although the latter contains an N-terminal fragment of 164 amino acids which is absent from the PR-A isoform. The two forms of the PR have similar steroid hormone and DNA binding activities but they have distinct functional activities which depend on the cell type and context of the target gene promoter. In general, PR-B is a much stronger activator than PR-A. Under certain conditions, PR-A is inactive as a transcription factor but can function as a ligand-dependent transdominant repressor of other steroid receptors including the estrogen receptor.[7]

Estrogen receptor (ER) and PR receptor content in endometriotic implants are heterogeneous and they do not undergo the predictable changes in response to endogenous hormones as does the eutopic endometrium.[8] In endometriotic implants, only the PR-A but not the PR-B is expressed.[9] Hypermethylation occurs in the promoter region of PR-B, but not PR-A in epithelial cells in endometriotic implants.[10] Promoter hypermethylation is associated with transcriptional silencing.[11] This may explain the mechanism responsible for the down-regulation of PR-B in endometriotic implants.

Estrogen and Progesterone Dependency

Endometriosis is an estrogen dependent condition and the beneficial effects of treatment with PRMs reported are probably related to their antiproliferative effects which have been well described in the primate endometrium[6] and in rodent mammary tumors.[12] In the latter model, progesterone was strongly proliferative. The PRMs mifepristone and CDB-4124 differed in their antiproliferative activity with CDB-4124 showing strong reduction in the number of tumor cells positive for the proliferation marker Ki-67 but mifepristone demonstrated no such activity.[12]

PAs and SPRMs are associated with an increase in ER, PR and androgen receptor (AR).[13] Androgens suppress estrogen-induced endometrial proliferation. The increase in AR consequent to PRMs could thus produce these unexpected antiproliferative effects. Further evidence of the role played by androgens in this antiproliferative effect is the observation that the pure antiandrogen, flutamide, blocks the antiproliferative effects of the PRMs ZK137316 and ZK230211 in the endometrium.[13] The effect on the AR appears to be a likely mechanism explaining the antiproliferative effect although it may also be related to the fact that the PR-A isoform inhibits estrogen receptor gene transcription induced by progestins and PAs.[7]

Aromatase expression in endometriosis implants is markedly increased compared to eutopic endometrium and this leads to an increase in estradiol.[2] Mifepristone blocks medroxyprogesterone acetate-induced aromatase activity in endometrial stromal cells.[14]

The enzyme, 17β hydroxysteroid dehydrogenase (17β-HSD) type 2, catalyses the conversion of E_2 to the biologically inactive E_1. Progesterone is the most potent stimulator of this enzyme in the eutopic endometrium during the secretory phase of the cycle but is unable to induce this enzyme in endometriosis[2] and this suggests the presence of progesterone resistance. This is most likely a consequence of over-expression of the repressive PR-A and down-regulation of the stimulatory PR-B.[9]

Matrix Metalloprotease Inhibitors (MMPs)

Several of the MMPs are dysregulated in endometriosis and it has been suggested that inhibition of MMP activity may be used to treat this disease. Cell specific mRNA expression of MMP3 and MMP7 is elevated in the eutopic endometrium of women with endometriosis during the secretory phase whereas they are absent in normal women.[2] Together with the absence of 17β-HSD type 2 in endometriosis, this increase in MMP3 and MMP7 is further evidence of the presence of progesterone resistance.

Apoptosis

The susceptibility of endometrial tissue to spontaneous apoptosis is lower in women with endometriosis than in healthy controls.[2] One of the apoptopic pathways involves the *bcl-2/bax* family of proteins.[15] Increased expression of *bcl-2* protein has been observed in the proliferative eutopic endometrium from patients with endometriosis compared with controls.[15] This balances the pro/anti-apoptotic pathways toward a protective effect on the endometriotic cell, facilitating its survival. Other workers have denied any correlation between apoptosis and expression of *bcl-2* in endometriosis.[16]

Mifepristone has been shown to promote apoptosis by overexpressing *bax* and down-regulating *bcl-2* in cultured Ishikawa endometrial adenocarcinoma cells[17] as well as in the endometrial EM42 cell line.[18] In the latter model, mifepristone stimulated the cellular binding activity of the nuclear transcription factor, nuclear factor-kappa B (NF-kappa B), which has been identified in the promoters of both *bcl-2* and *bax*. Thus growth inhibition and apoptosis in endometrial cells by mifepristone, involves stimulation of NF-kappa B binding with modulation of the apoptosis regulatory genes, *bax* and *bcl-2*.[18]

In the rat DMBA model of breast cancer, both CDB-4124 and mifepristone induced apoptosis.[12] An unpublished study in cynomolgous monkeys also showed that CDB-4124 and mifepristone were pro-apoptotic. Caspase 3, which is associated with the early onset of apoptosis, was enhanced in both endometrial epithelium and stroma with CDB-4124 but only in the epithelium with mifepristone (Wiehle, personal communication).

Angiogenesis

This is involved in the pathogenesis of endometriosis[2] and inhibition of angiogenesis is regarded as a novel therapeutic approach to the disease. Estradiol is a potent stimulus of angiogenesis through the direct increase of Vascular Endothelial Growth Factor (VEGF) expression.[19] VEGF is elevated in the peritoneal fluid of women with endometriosis and is expressed in endometriotic lesions.[2] VGEF is one of the main stimuli for angiogenesis in this disease and PRMs have been shown to suppress VGEF in human and cynomolgus endometrial tissue samples.[20, 21]

Case Studies

Studies in Animals

PAs have been shown to reduce endometriotic lesions in animal models with surgically induced endometriosis. In rats, the PAs, onapristone and ZK 136 799, both induced a reduction in endometriotic lesions and an antiproliferative effect in ectopic but not eutopic endometrium.[22] In monkeys, mifepristone appeared to be as efficient in reducing endometriotic lesions as a GnRH analog.[23] In the macaque endometriosis model, the PA, ZK 223211, was associated with reduction in size of the endometriotic implants.[24]

Studies in Women

Three small clinical trials comprising a total of 22 patients have been reported[25-27] using three dose schedules of mifepristone (5 mg or 50 mg per day for 6 months or 100 mg per day for 3 months). There was an improvement in symptoms with all three dosages. With the highest mifepristone dose, an antiglucocorticoid effect was demonstrated; this was not apparent with the two lower doses. With the 50 mg dose, there was a 55% mean regression of visible endometriosis after 6 months of treatment and all women had amenorrhea. Treatment with the lowest dose for 6 months, revealed no change in surgical staging in 5 of the 7 women and 5 complained of irregular bleeding.[25-27] Thus, the most appropriate dose appeared to be 50 mg daily.

A multi-center, placebo controlled double blind, parallel group study was conducted with asoprisnil in a total of 130 women with laparoscopic evidence of endometriosis. To date, the study has only been reported in abstract form.[28] Doses of asoprisnil used were 5, 10 and 25 mg administered daily for 12 weeks. All 3 doses significantly reduced the dysmenorrhea as well as non-menstrual pain as compared to the placebo and also dose-dependently induced amenorrhea.[28]

CDB-4124 in the Treatment of Endometriosis

The PRM, CDB-4124 (also known as Proellex® or Progenta), is a 21-substituted analog of 19-norprogesterone. Its structure is 17α-acetoxy-11β-(N,N-di-methylamino-phenyl)-21-methoxy-19-norpregna-1,9-diene-3,20-dione. The National Institute of Child Health and Human Development (NICHD) has performed receptor binding and *in vivo* bioassays which showed that CDB-4124 is a more effective progesterone antagonist in the rabbit uterus than mifepristone.[29] CDB-4124 lacks androgenic activity, binds the A and B isoforms of the human PR, and *in vivo* studies show that it has a lower affinity for glucocorticoid receptors than mifepristone.[30] It is being developed by Repros Therapeutics Inc. CDB-4124 administered over three months is effective in uterine fibroids.[31] In view of this, it was decided to determine the efficacy and safety of CDB-4124 in the treatment of endometriosis.

Study Design

This was a randomized, double-blind, multiple-dose study evaluating the effect of CDB-4124 compared to open label leuprolide acetate depot suspension and was conducted in three study centers in Bulgaria. The women underwent screening procedures and assessments for up to four weeks prior to enrollment. At the baseline visit (Day 0), eligible women were randomized in a 1:1:1:1 ratio to one of four treatment groups: CDB-4124 (12.5 mg, 25 mg and 50 mg) or leuprolide acetate. CDB-4124 was administered orally once daily for 6 months and leuprolide acetate in a dose of 3.75 mg by monthly intramuscular treatment. A total of 6 injections were given. Women were seen at monthly intervals and the duration of treatment was 6 months. Following cessation of treatment, the women attended follow-up visits at Month 7 and Month 9.

Women Studied

Regularly menstruating premenopausal women, aged 18-45 years, with symptomatic endometriosis were enrolled. They all had endometriosis documented by historical and laparoscopic assessment, were of child bearing potential and willing to use effective non-hormonal double barrier contraception and be available for all treatment and follow-up visits.

Women who were post-menopausal, pregnant or lactating, using contraceptives or other hormonal treatments within 60 days prior to start of study, had a past or present history of any significant medical disorder, a history of alcoholism or drug abuse, were infected with HIV, Hepatitis B or C and had a body mass index lower than 18 or greater than 37 were excluded from the study.

Results

Demographic Characteristics

A total of 39 women were enrolled and randomized to the study drugs. Details are shown in **Table 27-1**. Treatment compliance was defined as taking 90% of required doses over the course of the study. Based on this criterion, only two women were considered noncompliant to study drug; one in the CDB-4124 (25 mg) and one in the CDB-4124 (50 mg) group.

The median age range of the study population in the four dose groups was 32-36 years. All women in this study were Caucasian. There were no differences between the treatment groups with regard to age, height, weight and body mass index, and vital signs (mean blood pressure, pulse, respiratory rate and temperature).

Table 27-1: Number of women enrolled in the study		
Proellex dose	Enrolled	Completed
12.5 mg	9	7
25 mg	10	8
50 mg	10	8
Leuprolide depot	10	6

Effects on pain: Pain was assessed by the Short Form McGill Pain Questionnaire which is a well accepted method to assess pain.[32] This questionnaire was completed by each woman at every visit. The highest 50 mg dose of CDB-4124 was associated with fewer days of pain, less severe pain and accompanying distress and appeared to be more effective than the lower doses of CDB-4124 and was at least as effective as leuprolide acetate. A representative example demonstrating the sensory pain rating index in the four treatment groups is shown in **Figure 27-1**. The best response occurred with the 50 mg CDB-4124 dose and reduction in the pain rating index was apparent within one month. Reduction in the pain rating index also occurred with leuprolide acetate but appeared to be greater with 50 mg CDB-4124. Improvement in the sensory pain rating index was less dramatic and occurred later with the two lower doses of CDB-4124.

Bleeding: Heavy menstrual bleeding is not a major symptom in endometriosis. Moderate to heavy bleeding was reported at baseline in 50-60% of women assigned to CDB-4124 and in 25% of women who were to receive leuprolide acetate. A rapid reduction in bleeding occurred soon after commencement of treatment in women treated with all three doses of CDB-4124. This was somewhat delayed with leuprolide acetate but after 6 weeks, no bleeding was reported by women in the leuprolide acetate group **(Figure 27-2)**. Some bleeding became apparent four and a half months after commencing treatment with all three CDB-4124 groups but regular menstrual bleeding only occurred 2 to 8 weeks after cessation of treatment. This was delayed to 10 weeks following cessation of leuprolide acetate treatment.

Four women in the CDB-4124 groups had severe bleeding during the study and underwent dilatation and curettage (D&C). In two of these women, bleeding commenced 3 and 4 weeks after the end of the 6 months treatment course and in the remaining 2 women, bleeding commenced after 5 months of treatment **(Table 27-2)**. A further woman also had moderate bleeding after four and a half months of treatment, but did not require D&C.

LH, FSH, estradiol and progesterone responses: During pretreatment, there was a wide scatter of basal LH, FSH, estradiol and progesterone levels. Full suppression of LH was evident during leuprolide acetate treatment. There was no dramatic effect on FSH. With CDB-4124 there were no consistent changes in either LH or FSH **(Figure 27-3)**.

As expected, full suppression of estradiol and progesterone occurred during leuprolide acetate treatment **(Figure 27-4)**. With all 3 doses of CDB-4124, estradiol levels

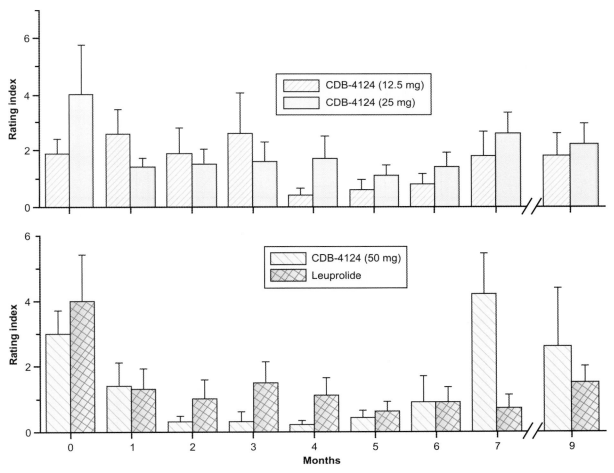

FIGURE 27-1: Sensory pain rating index from the McGill pain questionnaire. The response to CDB-4124 (12.5 and 25 mg) is shown in the upper panel and to CDB-4124 (50 mg) and leuprolide acetate in the lower panel. Values shown are mean ± SEM.

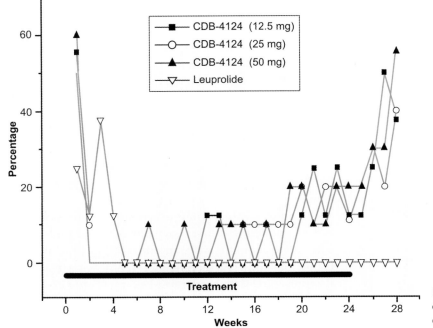

FIGURE 27-2: Percentage of women with moderate or severe bleeding in the four groups. See text for details.

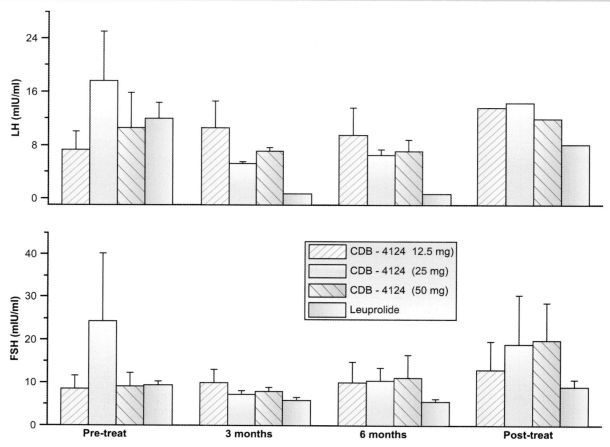

FIGURE 27-3: Mean (±SEM) serum LH (upper panel) and serum FSH responses (lower panel) pretreatment, at 3 and 6 months of treatment and following cessation of treatment in the four groups.

decreased during treatment but mean levels remained above 50 pg/ml. There was still evidence of luteal activity as shown by non-suppressed progesterone levels with the 2 lower doses of CDB-4124 at 3 months although not with the highest 50 mg dose. At 6 months, progesterone levels were suppressed with all three CDB-4124 doses. Following cessation of treatment, LH, FSH, estradiol and progesterone increased in all four groups.

ACTH-cortisol axis: Although the urinary cortisol measurements were not normalized for urinary creatinine, there did not appear to be any increase in urinary cortisol levels. When compared to baseline during the 6 months of therapy **(Figure 27-5)**. Neither were there changes in serum ACTH. The increase in mean ACTH with the highest CDB-4124 dose which occurred at 6 months was due to a single outlier with marked elevation of serum ACTH of 127 pg/ml (normal range 8-66) in the presence of a urinary cortisol of 394.8 nmol/24 hours (normal range 100-1400).

Endometrial thickness: Baseline mean endometrial thicknesses were 10.0, 8.9, 11.1 and 6.4 mm for the 12.5, 25,

50 mg CDB-4124 and the leuprolide acetate treatment groups respectively. After months 3 and 6, these measurements were 13.2, 12.9, 9.3 and 3.5 mm and 21.0, 18.4, 15.0 and 3.5 mm for the four groups respectively. After 3 months of follow-up, all of these CDB-4124 treated patients had endometrial thicknesses of less than 10 mm **(Figure 27-6)**. In all, seven women had mean endometrial thickness greater than 20 mm at any time on treatment. Two women (one each with the 12.5 and 25 mg dose) had thickness which exceeded 20 mm at 3 months. At 6 months, 4 of 8 women receiving 12.5 mg CDB-4124, 1 out of 7 receiving 25 mg CDB-4124 and 2 of 9 women who received the 50 mg dose had endometrial thicknesses greater than 20 mm.

Endometrial thickening exceeding 20 mm occurred in the 4 women who had heavy bleeding and underwent D&C. One woman, with an endometrial thickness of 19 mm four and a half months after commencing treatment, also presented with moderate bleeding **(Table 27-2)**. The remaining 3 women with endometrial thickness above 20 mm did not experience any bleeding of significance.

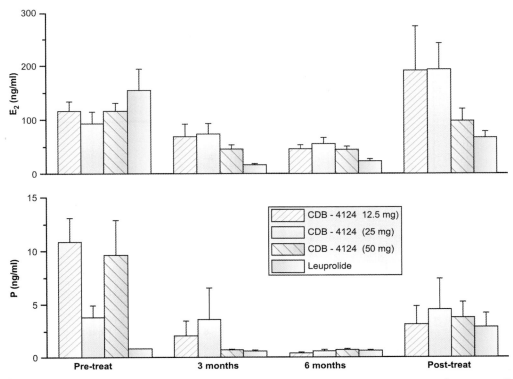

FIGURE 27-4: Mean (± SEM) serum estradiol (upper panel) and serum progesterone responses (lower panel) pretreatment, at 3 and 6 months of treatment and following cessation of treatment in the four groups.

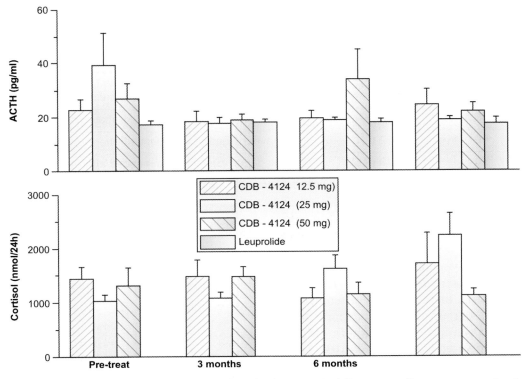

FIGURE 27-5: Mean (± SEM) serum ACTH (upper panel) and urinary cortisol (lower panel) responses pretreatment, at 3 and 6 months of treatment and following cessation of treatment in the four groups. Urinary cortisol levels were not determined during treatment with leuprolide acetate.

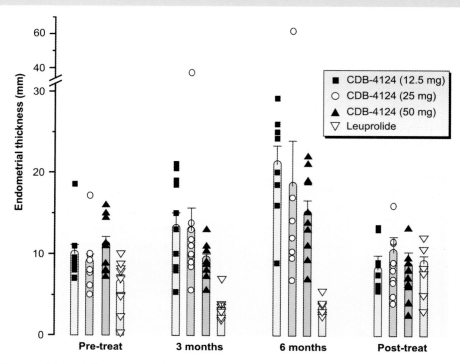

FIGURE 27-6: Mean (±SEM) and individual measurements of endometrial thickening pretreatment, at 3 and 6 months of treatment and following cessation of treatment in the 4 groups.

Table 27-2: Relationship between endometrial thickness and heavy bleeding			
Patient number	CDB-4124 dose	Endometrial thickness (mm)	Bleeding
02 201	12.5	25 (6)*	Completed 6 months of treatment. Severe bleeding commenced 3 weeks after conclusion of treatment**
03-216	50	21 (6)	Completed 6 months of treatment. Severe bleeding commenced one month after conclusion of treatment**
02-202	25	62 (5)	Severe bleeding commenced after 5 months of treatment**
03-209	50	22 (5)	Severe bleeding commenced after 5 months of treatment **
03-219	50	19 (4.5)	Moderate bleeding commenced after 4.5 months treatment

* number in brackets refers to the month following commencement of treatment when endometrial thickness was determined
** patient underwent D&C

Bone mineral density (BMD): BMD of the lumbar spine (L2-L4) and femoral neck was measured by dual-energy X-ray absorptiometry at baseline and at 6 months in the four treatment groups. When compared to their respective baseline determinations, there were no differences in BMD in the 3 CDB-4124 groups; on the other hand, there was an expected and significant reduction in BMD of L2-L4 in the leuprolide acetate group (p < 0.03). There were no differences in femoral neck BMD.

Adverse events: The majority of adverse events were mild to moderate in intensity across all treatment groups. One woman in the leuprolide acetate group developed breast cancer. No clinically relevant changes in median blood chemistry, hematology, vital signs, or ECG intervals were observed with CDB-4124 and it was well tolerated.

Discussion

This small proof of concept study evaluated the safety and efficacy of CDB-4124 (12.5, 25 and 50 mg) compared to open label leuprolide acetate for up to 6 months in the treatment of premenopausal women with symptomatic endometriosis. The doses of CDB-4124 selected were based on previous studies conducted in uterine fibroids.[31] The long acting GnRHa, leuprolide acetate, rather than a placebo, was selected as the active comparator since it is an established and recognized medical treatment for endometriosis.

The principal efficacy endpoint, pain, was reduced by all treatment groups. No differences were observed between the three CDB-4124 doses due to the small sample size. However, the highest dose used (50 mg) appeared to have an advantage over the two lower doses in that the onset of pain relief occurred earlier, and the reduction in pain intensity was the greatest with this dose. This dose was also associated with fewer days of pain and distress and appeared to be more effective than the lower CDB-4124 doses of 12.5 and 25 mg, and at least as effective as leuprolide acetate.

The variable LH, FSH, estradiol and progesterone levels observed during pretreatment sampling presumably reflect the fact that blood samples were taken randomly and not at any specific time in the menstrual cycle. LH suppression is an expected effect of GnRH agonists. With CDB-4124, serum estradiol levels decreased but remained above 50 pg/ml which are levels representative of those seen in the early follicular phase of the menstrual cycle. Similar observations have been observed previously with mifepristone.[33] In contrast there was marked suppression of estradiol with leuprolide acetate. In this six month study, there was a decrease in bone mineral density with leuprolide acetate but no changes with CDB-4124. The profound estrogen deficiency with all its consequences such as a decrease in bone mineral density seen with GnRH agonists is not observed with CDB-4124.

Although the urinary cortisol measurements were not normalized for urinary creatinine, there did not appear to be any increase in urinary cortisol levels and this implies that there is no glucocorticoid receptor blockade. The one patient in this study with an elevated ACTH level had urinary cortisol in the low normal range. This is not the picture seen with glucocorticoid antagonism where urinary cortisol levels would be expected to be elevated. In contrast to these observations, mifepristone administered in a dose of 100 mg daily was associated with glucocorticoid receptor blockade.[25]

Serial ultrasound measurements demonstrated that the endometrium thickens with time of exposure. This has also been observed with other PRMs.[6] With CDB-4124 there was an impression that the higher the dose the less likely the endometrium would thicken excessively in the first 4 months of exposure. Further studies need to be conducted to confirm this. This observation has led to the treatment concept of using a higher CDB-4124 dose (50 mg) for a period of 4 months.

Administration of all three doses of CDB-4124 was associated with a reduction in menstrual bleeding which was more rapid than that observed with leuprolide acetate. Bleeding with CDB-4124 recommenced after four and a half months of continuous treatment. In five women, this bleeding was moderate to heavy and occurred after four and a half months of treatment in one woman, after 5 months in a further two women and 3 and 4 weeks after concluding 6 months of treatment in the remaining two women. D&C was required in four of these women. This type of bleeding occurred only in those women with thickening of the endometrium greater that 19 mm. There was no bleeding of significance in the three additional women with endometrial thickness exceeding 20 mm. This observation has resulted in the employment of a cyclical treatment stratagem of four months of treatment followed by an off drug interval until menstruation occurs. Further four month treatment cycles can then recommence and be repeated as long as required. This proposed regimen will maximize safety by reducing the incidence of breakthrough bleeding and obviate the necessity to monitor the endometrial thickness with regular ultrasound measurements. Continuous long-term administration of CDB-4124, or any other PRM, will lead to endometrial thickening and bleeding and will pose an unnecessary risk that can be avoided by intermittent therapy without diminishing the efficacy of the treatment.

In conclusion, efficacy has been demonstrated in premenopausal women with symptomatic endometriosis treated for 6 months with 12.5, 25 or 50 mg of CDB-4124. The most favorable response in this small study occurred with the highest dose (50 mg). This small proof of concept and safety study is very important in furthering the understanding of the effect of PRMs in general and CDB-4124 in particular in the treatment of endometriosis as well as the effect on bleeding patterns and the endometrium. At the present time, this intermittent regimen appears to be the most appropriate for long-term treatment. Future development of PRMs for the treatment of endometriosis may be the advent of compounds which are selective to the A or B subunit of the PR.

Acknowledgments

The authors would like to thank Dr Regine Sitruk Ware for her helpful comments.

References

1. Farquhar C. Endometriosis. British Medical Journal 2007;334(7587):249-53.
2. Arici A. Endometriosis. Semin Reprod Med 2003;21(2).
3. Simoens S, Hummelshoj L, D'Hooghe T. Endometriosis: cost estimates and methodological perspective. Hum Reprod Update 2007;13(4):395-404.
4. Griesinger G, Felberbaum R, Diedrich K. GnRH-antagonists in reproductive medicine. Arch Gynecol Obstet 2005;273(2):71-8.
5. Philibert D. RU38486: An original multifaceted antihormone in vivo. In: Agarwal M (Ed): Adrenal Steroid Antagonism. Berlin, Germany: Walter de Gruyter and Co.; 1984:77-101.
6. Spitz IM. Progesterone receptor antagonists. Curr Opin Investig Drugs 2006;7(10):882-90.
7. McDonnell DP, Goldman ME. RU486 exerts antiestrogenic activities through a novel progesterone receptor A form-mediated mechanism. J Biol Chem 1994;269(16):11945-9.
8. Fujishita A, Nakane PK, Koji T, et al. Expression of estrogen and progesterone receptors in endometrium and peritoneal endometriosis: an immunohistochemical and in situ hybridization study. Fertil Steril 1997;67(5):856-64.
9. Attia GR, Zeitoun K, Edwards D, Johns A, Carr BR, Bulun SE. Progesterone receptor isoform A but not B is expressed in endometriosis. J Clin Endocrinol Metab 2000;85(8): 2897-2902.
10. Wu Y, Strawn E, Basir Z, Halverson G, Guo SW. Promoter hypermethylation of progesterone receptor isoform B (PR-B) in endometriosis. Epigenetics 2006;1(2):106-11.
11. Bird AP. The relationship of DNA methylation to cancer. Cancer Surv 1996;28:87-101.
12. Wiehle RD, Christov K, Mehta R. Anti-progestins suppress the growth of established tumors induced by 7,12-dimethylbenz(a) anthracene: comparison between RU486 and a new 21-substituted-19-nor-progestin. Oncol Rep 2007;18(1):167-74.
13. Slayden OD, Brenner RM. Flutamide counteracts the antiproliferative effects of antiprogestins in the primate endometrium. J Clin Endocrinol Metab 2003;88(2):946-9.
14. Tseng L, Mazella J, Sun B. Modulation of aromatase activity in human endometrial stromal cells by steroids, tamoxifen and RU 486. Endocrinology 1986;118(4):1312-8.
15. Garcia-Velasco JA, Arici A. Apoptosis and the pathogenesis of endometriosis. Semin Reprod Med 2003;21(2):165-72.
16. Watanabe H, Kanzaki H, Narukawa S, et al. Bcl-2 and Fas expression in eutopic and ectopic human endometrium during the menstrual cycle in relation to endometrial cell apoptosis. Am J Obstet Gynecol 1997;176(2):360-8.
17. Li A, Felix JC, Minoo P, Amezcua CA, Jain JK. Effect of mifepristone on proliferation and apoptosis of Ishikawa endometrial adenocarcinoma cells. Fertil Steril 2005;84(1):202-11.
18. Han S, Sidell N. RU486-induced growth inhibition of human endometrial cells involves the nuclear factor-kappa B signaling pathway. J Clin Endocrinol Metab 2003;88(2):713-9.
19. Hyder SM, Nawaz Z, Chiappetta C, Stancel GM. Identification of functional estrogen response elements in the gene coding for the potent angiogenic factor vascular endothelial growth factor. Cancer Res 2000;60(12):3183-90.

20. Classen-Linke I, Alfer J, Krusche CA, Chwalisz K, Rath W, Beier HM. Progestins, progesterone receptor modulators, and progesterone antagonists change VEGF release of endometrial cells in culture. Steroids 2000;65(10-11): 763-71.
21. Greb RR, Heikinheimo O, Williams RF, Hodgen GD, Goodman AL. Vascular endothelial growth factor in primate endometrium is regulated by oestrogen-receptor and progesterone-receptor ligands in vivo. Hum Reprod 1997;12(6):1280-92.
22. Stoeckemann K, Hegele-Hartung C, Chwalisz K. Effects of the progesterone antagonists onapristone (ZK 98 299) and ZK 136 799 on surgically induced endometriosis in intact rats. Hum Reprod 1995;10(12):3264-71.
23. Grow DR, Williams RF, Hsiu JG, Hodgen GD. Antiprogestin and/or gonadotropin-releasing hormone agonist for endometriosis treatment and bone maintenance: a 1-year primate study. J Clin Endocrinol Metab 1996;81(5):1933-9.
24. Nayak NR, Slayden OD, Mah K, Chwalisz K, Brenner RM. Antiprogestin-releasing intrauterine devices: a novel approach to endometrial contraception. Contraception 2007;75(6 Suppl):S104-11.
25. Kettel LM, Murphy AA, Mortola JF, Liu JH, Ulmann A, Yen SS. Endocrine responses to long-term administration of the antiprogesterone RU486 in patients with pelvic endometriosis. Fertil Steril 1991;56(3):402-7.
26. Kettel LM, Murphy AA, Morales AJ, Ulmann A, Baulieu EE, Yen SS. Treatment of endometriosis with the antiprogesterone mifepristone (RU486) [see comments]. Fertil Steril 1996;65(1):23-8.
27. Kettel LM, Murphy AA, Morales AJ, Yen SS. Preliminary report on the treatment of endometriosis with low-dose mifepristone (RU 486). Am J Obstet Gynecol 1998; 178(6): 1151-6.
28. Chwalisz K, Mattia-Goldberg K, Lee M, Elger W, Edmonds A. Treatment of endometriosis with the novel selective progesterone receptor modulator (SPRM) asoprisnil. Fertil Steril 2004;82(Suppl 2):S83.
29. Kim HK, Blye RP, Rao PN, Cessac JW, Acosta CK. 21-substituted progesterone derivatives as new antipro-gestational agents. US Patent No 6,861,415 B2, March 1, 2005.
30. Attardi BJ, Burgenson J, Hild SA, Reel JR. In vitro anti-progestational/antiglucocorticoid activity and progestin and glucocorticoid receptor binding of the putative metabolites and synthetic derivatives of CDB-2914, CDB-4124, and mifepristone. J Steroid Biochem Mol Biol 2004;88(3):277-88.
31. Wiehle RD, Goldberg J, Brodniewicz T, Jarus-Dziedzic K, Jabiry-Zienieiwicz Z. Effects of a new progesterone receptor modulator, CDB-4124, on fibroid size and uterine bleeding. US Obstetrics and Gynaecology 2008;3(1):17-20.
32. Melzack R. The short-form McGill Pain Questionnaire. Pain 1987;30(2):191-7.
33. Yen SSC. Use of antiprogestins in the management of endometriosis and leiomyoma. MS Donaldson, L Dorflinger, SS Brown and LZ Benet (Eds): In Clinical Applications of Mifepristone (RU496) and other Antiprogestins 1993; National Academy Press, Washington DC:189-209.

Anna Sokalska, Antoni J Duleba

Chapter 28

Statins as Potential Novel Medical Treatment of Endometriosis

Introduction

Scope of Problem

Endometriosis is one of the most common and yet still poorly understood gynecologic disorders affecting approximately 6-10% of women.[1,2] It is defined as the presence of ectopic endometrial tissue, usually in the peritoneal cavity. The most frequent clinical presentations of endometriosis include dysmenorrhea, intermenstrual pelvic pain, dyspareunia, infertility and/or pelvic mass. Less commonly, bowel and bladder function may be also affected. The relationship between the extent of endometrial implants and clinical presentation is often poor. In the presence of advanced endometriosis, pelvic anatomy is grossly distorted by adhesions, inflammatory induration and fibrosis. However, even minimal or mild endometriosis may be associated with infertility and/or significant pain.

Various theories on the pathogenesis of endometriosis have been advanced. Dominant concepts are: (i) retrograde menstruation-induced implantation of endometrium and (ii) coelomic metaplasia. Postulated predisposing factors include immune dysfunction, genetic predisposition and environmental pollutants.[3]

Available treatments of endometriosis are associated with significant side effects and hence their long-term use is often problematic. GnRH analogs induce a hypoestrogenic state associated with a broad range of menopausal-like symptoms and their long-term use may be associated with serious health issues such as osteoporosis. Danazol use leads to profound hyperandrogenic symptomatology and is usually poorly tolerated. Progestagens often cause weight gain, depressed mood and breakthrough bleeding. The above therapies are often effective, but upon discontinuation of these medications, symptoms of endometriosis frequently return.

An ideal treatment of endometriosis would induce regression of the disease with minimal or no side effects and with proven long-term safety. This chapter will explore the concept that statins may hold promise as a potentially effective and well-tolerated therapy addressing a broad range of pathophysiologic features of endometriosis.

Hypothesis

Statins may be effective in the treatment of endometriosis, targeting growth and invasiveness of ectopic endometrial tissues as well as inflammation and oxidative stress associated with this condition.

Formation of endometriotic implants requires ectopic attachment and proliferation of endometrial stroma and glands. Prominent features of endometriosis include inflammatory reaction, increased oxidative stress and intense angiogenesis surrounding the implants.[4]

The rationale for considering statins as a promising treatment of endometriosis is based on several considerations. First, statins are competitive inhibitors of 3-hydroxy-3-methylglutaryl-coenzyme A (HMG-CoA) reductase, a rate-limiting step of the mevalonate pathway. The inhibition of HMG-CoA reductase depletes downstream products of the mevalonate pathway, especially isoprenyls.[5] Depletion of isoprenyls decreases activity of small GTPases such as Ras and Rho resulting in decreased signaling of important growth-regulating pathways.[6] Second, inhibition of HMG-CoA reductase may reduce another downstream product, dolichol, which is required for maturation of type I IGF-I receptor, and hence may decrease the mitogenic effect of IGF-I on endometrial stromal cells. Third, statins can interfere with angio-genesis, which is necessary for the development of endometriotic implants. In addition, statins possess anti-inflammatory and immuno-modulatory properties, which may reduce the inflammatory reaction associated with endometriosis.

Another and related aspect of the actions of statins pertains to their anti-oxidant properties. Proliferation of endometrial stroma is stimulated by moderate oxidative stress, but inhibited by a broad range of antioxidants.[7] Statins may reduce oxidative stress by decreasing activity of a small GTPase, Rac, which is essential for generation of reactive oxygen species (ROS) by NADPH oxidase.[8] In addition, statins possess intrinsic antioxidant activity.[9]

The hypothesis that statins may be used in the treatment of endometriosis is also supported by the evidence that in several tissues, such as vascular smooth muscle, products of the mevalonate pathway have been shown to facilitate isoprenylation of small GPTases and thus activate signal transduction pathways promoting growth while inhibition of the mevalonate pathway by statins decreases growth and exerts antioxidant effects **(Figure 28-1)**.[5, 10]

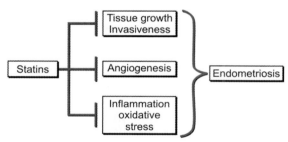

FIGURE 28-1: Proposed role of statins in treatment of endometriosis.

Endometriosis: Relevant Pathophysiology

Growth of Endometrial Stroma and Invasiveness

Endometriosis is characterized by inappropriate invasiveness and excessive growth of tissues. Excessive proliferation may be induced by a broad range of cytokines and growth factors.

Monocyte chemotactic protein 1 (MCP-1) has been shown to stimulate endometrial cell proliferation both directly and by stimulation of macrophages to secrete various growth factors (e.g. VEGF, TGF-β, EGF) and cytokines (e.g. IL-1, IL-6, IL-8, IL-12, RANTES, TNF-α).[11] Another potentially relevant contributor to development of endometriosis is insulin-like growth factor type I (IGF-I). Both endometrial stroma and glands express type I and type II IGF receptors[12] and the expression of these receptors may be stimulated by estrogens. IGF-I and IGF-II are mitogenic factors for endometrial stromal cells in culture and antibodies blocking IGF-I receptor induce partial inhibition of endometrial stromal cell proliferation.[13]

Formation of endometriotic implants requires attachment and proliferation of endometrial stroma and glands. The attachment may be enhanced by excessive expression of adhesion molecules and matrix metalloproteinases (MMPs) leading to local destruction of extracellular matrix and hence invasion and establishment of the disease.[14] Several MMPs are inappropriately expressed in the endometrium of women with endometriosis and are upregulated by tumor necrosis factor alpha (TNF-α) and interleukin 1 (IL-1). While the role of autoantibodies in endometriosis is still not well understood, it has been shown that a hemopexin domain expressed by MMPs, except MMP-7, can be recognized and bound by T-like autoantibodies in women with endometriosis leading to dysregulation of MMPs and tissue inhibitors of MMP (TIMP) in ectopic lesions.[15] All the mechanisms listed above, in association with a reduced sensitivity of MMPs to progesterone in the endometrium of women with this disease, lead to invasive potential of refluxed endometrium.[14] Furthermore, a continuous expression of several MMPs, and especially MMP-3 and MMP-7 in endometriotic lesions plays a role in the establishment of endometriosis.[16]

Endometriosis and Angiogenesis

Angiogenesis is an important component of the pathogenesis of endometriosis. Establishment of blood supply through angiogenesis seems to be a second basic step in the development of the disease after implantation of endometrial fragments in the peritoneal cavity. Several studies have reported that endometriosis is associated with an increased level of angiogenesis inducers: vascular endothelial growth factor (VEGF) and transforming growth factor β (TGF-β).

VEGF promotes endothelial cell proliferation, migration, differentiation and capillary formation and it may play an important role in the progression of the disease.[17] Activated peritoneal macrophages, endometrium and endometriotic implants have the capacity to secrete VEGF, while TGF-β is mainly produced by platelets, activated lymphocytes and macrophages.[15]

Endometriosis: Inflammation and Oxidative Stress

Although the precise etiology of endometriosis is still not known, there is substantial evidence that the pathogenesis of this condition involves increased concentrations of activated macrophages and changes in the cytokine network including interleukin-8 (IL-8), tumor necrosis factor-α (TNF-α), monocyte chemoattractant protein-1

(MCP-1), transforming growth factor β (TGF-β) and several other proinflammatory chemoattractant cytokines (e.g. IL-1, IL-4, IL-5, IL-6, IL-10, IL-13, IL-15, INF-γ, MCSF, RANTES).[15, 18]

Systemic inflammation may be induced by oxidative stress, another important component of endometriosis.[4] Leukocytes attracted to and activated by the above mentioned chemokines are a major source of oxidative stress. Furthermore, it appears that endometriosis is associated with depletion of antioxidant capacity. Intraperitoneal levels of vitamin E are decreased, likely due to consumption by oxidation reactions.[19] These observations are also in accord with the findings of Ota et al, who has demonstrated elevated levels of several enzymes involved in the generation and metabolism of reactive oxygen species in endometrial tissues and endometrial implants of women with endometriosis.[20-23] Also Foyouzi et al found that proliferation of endometrial stroma is stimulated by moderate oxidative stress and inhibited by antioxidants.[7]

Another important consideration relates to the association of endometriosis with impaired immune recognition and clearance of ectopic endometrial cells, suppressed cytotoxicity of natural killer (NK) cells, as well as activation of B-cells accompanied by increased production of the antinuclear autoantibodies (ANA).[15,24,25]

Statins: Pleiotropic Activities

Overview

Statins exert a broad range of effects on tissues and the organism. Many actions of statins may address the major features of endometriosis outlined above. This section will present evidence supporting the concept that statins may reduce excessive tissue growth, angiogenesis, oxidative stress and inflammation.

The major mode of action of statins is related to their competitive inhibition of the key enzyme regulating the mevalonate pathway: HMG-CoA reductase. The mevalonate pathway is comprised of the reactions starting from acetyl-coenzyme A (acetyl-CoA) and leading to the formation of farnesyl pyrophosphate (FPP): the substrate for several biologically important agents including cholesterol, isoprenylated proteins, coenzyme Q, and dolichol.[26] The most crucial seem to be components of the pathway leading to isoprenylation of proteins: farnesyl-pyrophosphate (FPP) and geranylgeranyl-pyrophosphate (GGPP) **(Figure 28-2)**.

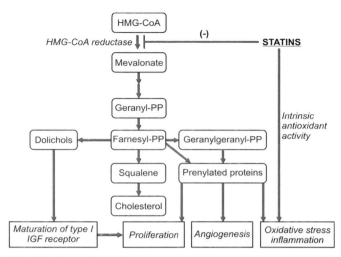

FIGURE 28-2: The outline of mevalonate pathway and the site of action of statins. (HMG-CoA, 3-hydroxy-3-methyl-glutaryl-coenzyme A; PP, pyrophosphate; IGF, insulin-like growth factor)

Isoprenylation is the process of attachment of FPP (farnesylation) or GGPP (geranylgeranylation) to the carboxyl terminus of the proteins.[27] This posttranslational modification is important to membrane attachment and the function of several families of proteins including Ras and Ras-related GTP binding proteins (small GTPases), subunits of trimeric G proteins and protein kinases.[27] The functions of these proteins depend on association with the cytoplasmic leaflet of the cellular membrane: farnesylation of Ras and geranylgeranylation of Rho, Rac and Cdc42. Since these small GTPases modulate proliferation, apoptosis and function of cells, any interference with isoprenylation may have profound effects. Statins can impair both geranylgeranylation and farnesylation by depletion of GGPP and FPP.

Effects on Growth of Mesenchymal Tissues

As noted above, the mevalonate pathway can affect several key signal transduction steps relevant to regulation of tissue growth by modulation of isoprenylation of several small GTPases. The most important pathways regulating proliferation include mitogen-activated protein kinase (MAPK) pathways, which may be stimulated by growth factors such as IGF-I, as well as by other stimuli including oxidative stress. Another aspect of tissue growth regulation involves modulation of apoptosis; this process is largely controlled via the phosphatidylinositol 3'-kinase/ protein kinase B (PI3 kinase/PKB) pathway. Key steps required for activation of the above pathways include isoprenylation of several small GTPases.

Consistent with the above concepts, inhibition of HMG-CoA reductase by statins blocks proliferation of several cell types including vascular smooth muscle, hepatocytes, mesangial cells, ovarian theca-interstitial cells and several cancer cells.[5, 28-31] In these tissues, statin-induced inhibition of proliferation is partly abrogated by the addition of agents such as mevalonic acid and FPP but not squalene, suggesting an important role of isoprenylation.

However, the above mechanisms are not ubiquitous and appear to depend on the cell type. Thus, for example, in endothelial progenitor cells, a statin-induced increase of proliferation has been observed.[32] The variable responses to statins underscore the complexity of the interactions between pathways regulating proliferation and apoptosis. Variability of responses to statins may be related to different effects of individual small GTPases.[33]

Statins and Endometrium: Inhibition of Endometrial Stromal Growth

Endometriosis may be associated with abnormal activation of MAPK and/or PI3K/PKB pathways, leading to excessive growth of endometriotic implants.[34] The inhibitory effect of statins on endometrial stromal cell proliferation was confirmed by *in vitro* studies. Piotrowski et al has shown that statins induce a potent, concentration-dependent, inhibition of proliferation of endometrial stromal cells; this inhibition was noted irrespective of the supply of cholesterol. The effect of statins was, at least in part, due to decreased production of mevalonate and was associated with decreased activity of the MAPK pathway, possibly due to decreased isoprenylation of Ras. In addition, statins induced apoptosis.[35] These observations were consistent with results published by Esfandiari et al[36] who found a concentration-dependent inhibitory effect of lovastatin on tissue growth in an *in vitro* model of endometriosis.

Effects on MMPs

Many studies on the pathogenesis and treatment of cardiovascular diseases have demonstrated that statins inhibit MMPs. Thus, for example, statins reduced MMP secretion and activity and increased TIMP-1, consistent with their plaque-stabilizing effect in humans.[37] Furthermore, Porter et al found that statins inhibit MMPs and block migration through a matrix barrier of cultured human saphenous vein smooth muscle cells, preventing vein graft stenosis.[38] Statins were also studied as a new therapeutic strategy for human immunodeficiency virus (HIV). An imbalance between MMPs and tissue inhibitors of MMPs

(TIMPs) might contribute to HIV-associated pathology by inducing extracellular matrix remodeling; this process may be inhibited by statins.[39] The effects of statins on MMPs are likely mediated by protein prenylation.[40]

Statins and Endometrium: Inhibition of MMPs

As discussed above, development of endometriosis requires ectopic attachment of endometrial tissue by a process involving MMPs. Statins may interfere with this process in several ways. First, MMP9 production may be affected by modulation of prenylation.[40] Second, statins may decrease MMP9 production by monocytes via activation of the nuclear receptor transcription factor peroxisome-proliferator-activated receptor-γ (PPARγ).[41]

More recently, Bruner-Tran et al have shown that simvastatin inhibits expression of MMP-3 in human endometrial stroma.[42] The cells were cultured in the presence of estradiol (E; 1 nM). In addition, the cells were treated either with medroxyprogesterone acetate (MPA; 50 pM) and/or simvastatin (1 and 10 μM). Some cultures were also exposed to interleukin-1α (IL-1α; 200 ng/ml). Collected media were tested by Western analysis for expression of MMP-3. Endometrial stromal cells expressed abundant levels of MMP-3 following treatment with E, but minimal levels in cultures also containing MPA or simvastatin. While IL-1α induced a profound increase in MMP-3 secretion from cells pretreated with E alone, treatment with either MPA or simvastatin abrogated this effect. Cultures containing MPA and simvastatin were the most resistant to MMP-3 induction by IL-1α.

Effects on Angiogenesis

The effects of statins on angiogenesis are complex. They appear to be tissue-specific and dependent on the dose of statin. Skaletz-Rorowski et al demonstrated that low doses of statins have a pro-angiogenic effect through increased nitric oxide production and serine/threonine protein kinase Akt activation, whereas high doses promote decreased protein prenylation, inhibit capillary tube formation and decrease VEGF production, having an overall angiostatic effect.[43, 44] Furthermore, inhibitory or stimulatory actions of statins on blood vessel formation in primary invasive tumors or metastases depend on statin doses and also on tumor cell type.[44]

Studies of Park et al, confirmed the role of protein prenylation in angiogenesis and demonstrated that statins also inhibit VEGF-stimulated phosphorylation of the VEGF receptor and prevent the progression of atherosclerosis by the inhibition of plaque angiogenesis.[45]

Statins and Endometrium: Inhibition of Angiogenesis

To date little is known regarding the effects of statins on angiogenesis in endometriosis. Initial studies using an *in vitro* model of endometriosis are encouraging and have indicated an inhibitory effect of statin on angiogenesis.[36] Growth of human endometrial biopsy tissues in a three-dimensional culture in fibrin matrix was observed for several weeks. Lovastatin induced a concentration-dependent inhibitory effect on cell growth and angiogenesis. The authors proposed that the probable mechanism of diminished blood-vessel formation was related to the inhibition of expression of VEGF by statins.[36]

Effects on Inflammation and Oxidative Stress

Statins exert anti-inflammatory effects manifested by lowering C-reactive protein levels and suppressing pro-inflammatory agents such as TNF-α and interleukins.[46] As immunomodulators, statins may also have a beneficial action in autoimmune diseases.[47] Inhibition of protein prenylation appears to be a key mechanism by which statins alter immune function.[40] Furthermore, it was also suggested that statins can directly bind the beta 2 integrin leukocyte function antigen-1 (LFA-1), resulting in reduced adhesion and stimulation of leukocytes.[48]

Increased major histocompatibility complex (MHC) class II molecule expression occurs in several autoimmune diseases. Statins have been shown to alter the function of antigen-presenting cells (APCs) by inhibiting interferon-γ (INF-γ)-inducible expression of the MHC class II transactivator (CIITA) and by preventing cytokine-induced maturation of APCs.[49, 50] MHC class II molecule expression could also be affected by statins via reduced cholesterol level and altered integrity of cell-membrane lipid rafts, however this concept still needs to be verified.[51, 52]

Statin-induced reduction in activity of small GTPases may alter the formation of the immunological synapses between T-cells and APCs and decrease T-cell proliferation. Moreover, statins can modulate disease progression through alteration of T-cell phenotype. Results of studies differ regarding a shift in T-cell phenotype, from Th1 to Th2, causing a strong attenuation of the Th1-type immune response (IL-2, IL-12, INF-γ, TNF-α) and increased secretion of anti-inflammatory Th2-type cytokines (IL-4, I-5, IL-10). However, the most consistent finding is a beneficial suppression of the Th1-cell response by statins.[40]

Statins may also modulate immune response by changing the expression of leukocyte and endothelial-cell adhesion molecules (i.e. ICAM, VCAM) as well as reducing leukocyte extravasation and infiltration of the target tissue. In addition, leukocyte motility and migration are affected.[40]

Statins may also have a significant effect on the level of oxidative stress. A broad range of nonphagocytic cells produce superoxide anions and other reactive oxygen species (ROS) in response to extracellular stimuli such as platelet-derived growth factor (PDGF) or epidermal growth factor (EGF).[53, 54] The mevalonate pathway may profoundly affect oxidative stress in several ways including: (i) modulation of the synthesis of an antioxidant, coenzyme Q and (ii) isoprenylation-related changes in the activity of NADPH oxidase, an important source of reactive oxygen species (ROS).

Studies in vascular smooth muscle, cardiac muscle and ovarian theca-interstitial cells confirmed the role of statins in reducing oxidative stress level in association with inhibition of isoprenylation.[8, 55, 56] Thus, for example, Wassmann et al reported that atorvastatin decreased oxidative stress, and that this effect was reversed by the addition of mevalonate but not 25-hydroxycholesterol indicating the importance of isoprenylation rather than cholesterol synthesis in the regulation of oxidative stress.[8] In other experiments in vascular smooth muscle, inhibition of geranylgeranylation reduced angiotensin II-mediated oxidative stress.[56] Statins also decreased oxidative stress in coronary smooth muscle via mechanisms involving suppression of phospholipase D (PLD) and protein kinase C-α (PKC-α).[57] Overall, it is apparent that the net effect of inhibition of the mevalonate pathway is the reduction of oxidative stress.

In vitro, statins have pronounced intrinsic antioxidant activity: simvastatin was the most effective as an anti-hydroxyl radical antioxidant while fluvastatin was the most effective as an anti-peroxyl radical antioxidant.[9] *In vivo*, statins have been shown to exert potent antioxidant effects including reduction of plasma levels of nitrotyrosine and chlorotyrosine.[58]

It is likely that the above listed actions of statins may decrease inflammation and oxidative stress associated with endometriosis. Furthermore, in view of the auto-immune aspects of endometriosis, the immunomodulatory properties of statins may also have beneficial effects **(Figure 28-3)**.

Statins: Effects *in vivo* (Rodent Models of Endometriosis)

To the best of our knowledge, to date, only two reports addressed *in vivo* effects of statins on endometriosis. The first study was published by Oktem el al[59] who presented

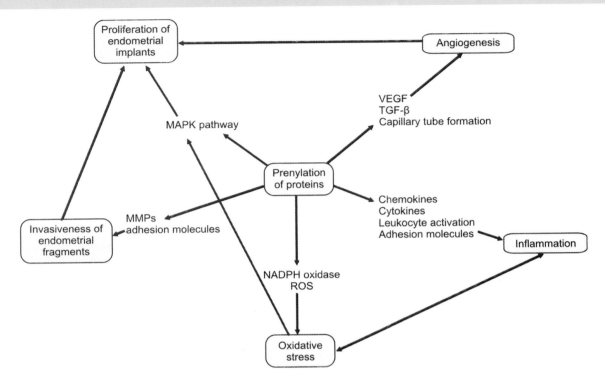

FIGURE 28-3: Proposed mechanisms of actions of statins in relation to modification of isoprenylation. (NADPH oxidase, nicotinamide adenine dinucleotide phosphate oxidase; ROS, reactive oxygen species; MAPK, mitogen-activated protein kinase; MMPs, metrix metaloproteinases; VEGF, vascular endothelial growth factor; TGF-β, tumor transforming growth factor-β)

the anti-angiogenic effects of atorvastatin on experimentally induced endometriosis in the rat model. Wistar-Albino rats received endometrial implants into the peritoneal cavity and were randomly divided into four groups three weeks later. Animals in group I were given 0.5 mg/kg/day oral atorvastatin (low-dose atorvastatin group), group II received 2.5 mg/kg/day oral atorvastatin (high-dose atorvastatin group), group III was given a single dose of 1 mg/kg s.c. leuprolide acetate (GnRH agonist group), and group IV received no medication (control group). After 21 days of treatment the rats were euthanized and implant size, vascular endothelial growth factor (VEGF) level in peritoneal fluid and histological score were assessed. The mean areas of implants were smaller and VEGF levels in peritoneal fluid were lower in groups II and III than those in group I and the control group (P<0.05). The mean areas of implants decreased from 41.2±13.9 to 22.7±13.9 mm² in group II (P<0,05) and from 41.2±18.1 to 13.1± 13.8 mm² in group III (P<0.05). In group I the mean area increased from 43.0±12.7 to 50.5±13.9 mm². The authors concluded that high-dose atorvastatin caused a significant regression of endometriotic implants.

The second study evaluated the effects of simvastatin on a nude mouse model of endometriosis and the role of simvastatin in modulation of MMP-3.[42] Proliferative phase human endometrial biopsies were obtained and established as organ cultures. To establish endometriosis in the nude mouse, endometrial tissues were maintained in 1 nM estradiol (E) for 24 hrs and subsequently injected intraperitoneally into ovariectomized nude mice. Mice were treated with E (8 µg, silastic capsule implants) and placebo or simvastatin (5 and 25 mg/kg/day) by gavage for 10 days beginning 1 day after tissue injection. The animals were then sacrificed and endometrial implants were evaluated. In mice treated with simvastatin, a dose-dependent inhibition of the number and the volume of endometrial implants was observed.

The presented findings are encouraging and indicate that statins may hold promise as a possible novel treatment of endometriosis. However, one has to bear in mind that rodent models of endometriosis are only distantly related to endometriosis in humans, because of significant differences in reproductive anatomy and physiology. Rodents do not undergo menstruation and do not develop spontaneous endometriosis. Moreover, these models use endometrial tissues without potentially important blood components present in retrograde menstruation in humans.

Overview

Summary

Inhibition of the mevalonate pathway by statins may exert several beneficial effects on endometriosis including decreased endometrial stromal proliferation, angiogenesis, inflammation and oxidative stress. These experimental data suggest that statins alone or in combination with other therapeutic options may improve clinical outcomes and may inhibit the initiation and progression of the disease.

Future Directions

While interesting and promising effects of statins were observed *in vitro* and in rodent studies, further research is needed to determine whether statins would be useful in clinical practice as a treatment of endometriosis. Such studies may first require work on a primate model, such as baboon, and ultimately a completion of clinical trials in women with endometriosis. These trials would need not only to determine whether statins are effective but also to identify optimal regimens including duration of treatment, minimal effective doses and long-term safety.

References

1. Propst AM, Laufer MR. Endometriosis in adolescents. Incidence, diagnosis and treatment. J Reprod Med 1999; 44:751-58

2. Mahmood TA, Templeton A. Prevalence and genesis of endometriosis. Hum Reprod. 1991;6:544-49.

3. Giudice LC, Kao LC. Endometriosis. Lancet 2004 ;364:1789-99.

4. Santanam N, Murphy AA, Parthasarathy S. Macrophages, oxidation, and endometriosis. Ann N Y Acad Sci. 2002;955:183-98; discussion 19-200, 396-406.

5. Danesh FR, Sadeghi MM, Amro N, Philips C, Zeng L, Lin S, et al. 3-Hydroxy-3-methylglutaryl CoA reductase inhibitors prevent high glucose-induced proliferation of mesangial cells via modulation of Rho GTPase/ p21 signaling pathway: Implications for diabetic nephropathy. Proc Natl Acad Sci U S A. 2002 ;11;99:8301-05.

6. Mattingly RR, Gibbs RA, Menard RE, Reiners JJ, Jr. Potent suppression of proliferation of a10 vascular smooth muscle cells by combined treatment with lovastatin and 3-allylfarnesol, an inhibitor of protein farnesyltransferase. J Pharmacol Exp Ther. 2002 ;303:74-81.

7. Foyouzi N, Berkkanoglu M, Arici A, Kwintkiewicz J, Izquierdo D, Duleba AJ. Effects of oxidants and antioxidants on proliferation of endometrial stromal cells. Fertil Steril 2004;82 :1019-22.

8. Wassmann S, Laufs U, Muller K, Konkol C, Ahlbory K, Baumer AT, et al. Cellular antioxidant effects of atorvastatin *in vitro* and *in vivo*. Arterioscler Thromb Vasc Biol 2002;22:300-05.

9. Franzoni F, Quinones-Galvan A, Regoli F, Ferrannini E, Galetta F. A comparative study of the in vitro antioxidant activity of statins. Int J Cardiol 2003 ;90:317-21.

10. Porter KE, Naik J, Turner NA, Dickinson T, Thompson MM, London NJ. Simvastatin inhibits human saphenous vein neointima formation via inhibition of smooth muscle cell proliferation and migration. J Vasc Surg 2002; 36:150-57.

11. Arici A, Oral E, Attar E, Tazuke SI, Olive DL. Monocyte chemotactic protein-1 concentration in peritoneal fluid of women with endometriosis and its modulation of expression in mesothelial cells. Fertil Steril 1997;67: 1065-72.

12. Giudice LC, Dsupin BA, Jin IH, Vu TH, Hoffman AR. Differential expression of messenger ribonucleic acids encoding insulin-like growth factors and their receptors in human uterine endometrium and decidua. J Clin Endocrinol Metab 1993 ;76:1115-22.

13. Giudice LC, Dsupin BA, Gargosky SE, Rosenfeld RG, Irwin JC. The insulin-like growth factor system in human peritoneal fluid: its effects on endometrial stromal cells and its potential relevance to endometriosis. J Clin Endocrinol Metab 1994 ;79:1284-93.

14. Osteen KG, Yeaman GR, Bruner-Tran KL. Matrix metalloproteinases and endometriosis. Semin Reprod Med 2003; 21:155-64.

15. Siristatidis C, Nissotakis C, Chrelias C, Iacovidou H, Salamalekis E. Immunological factors and their role in the genesis and development of endometriosis. J Obstet Gynaecol Res 2006 ;32:162-70.

16. Bruner-Tran KL, Eisenberg E, Yeaman GR, Anderson TA, McBean J, Osteen KG. Steroid and cytokine regulation of matrix metalloproteinase expression in endometriosis and the establishment of experimental endometriosis in nude mice. J Clin Endocrinol Metab 2002; 87:4782-91.

17. Donnez J, Smoes P, Gillerot S, Casanas-Roux F, Nisolle M. Vascular endothelial growth factor (VEGF) in endometriosis. Hum Reprod 1998;13:1686-90.

18. Arici A. Local cytokines in endometrial tissue: the role of interleukin-8 in the pathogenesis of endometriosis. Ann NY Acad Sci 2002 ;955:101-9; discussion 18, 396-406.

19. Murphy AA, Santanam N, Morales AJ, Parthasarathy S. Lysophosphatidyl choline, a chemotactic factor for monocytes/T-lymphocytes is elevated in endometriosis. J Clin Endocrinol Metab 1998 ;83:2110-13.

20. Ota H, Igarashi S, Hatazawa J, Tanaka T. Immunohistochemical assessment of superoxide dismutase expression in the endometrium in endometriosis and adenomyosis. Fertil Steril 1999 ;72:129-34.

21. Ota H, Igarashi S, Kato N, Tanaka T. Aberrant expression of glutathione peroxidase in eutopic and ectopic endometrium in endometriosis and adenomyosis. Fertil Steril 2000;74:313-18.

22. Ota H, Igarashi S, Tanaka T. Xanthine oxidase in eutopic and ectopic endometrium in endometriosis and adenomyosis. Fertil Steril 2001; 75:785-90.

23. Ota H, Igarashi S, Sato N, Tanaka H, Tanaka T. Involvement of catalase in the endometrium of patients with endometriosis and adenomyosis. Fertil Steril 2002; 78:804-09.

24. Chishima F, Hayakawa S, Hirata Y, Nagai N, Kanaeda T, Tsubata K, et al. Peritoneal and peripheral B-1-cell populations in patients with endometriosis. J Obstet Gynaecol Res 2000 ;26:141-49.

25. Gupta S, Goldberg JM, Aziz N, Goldberg E, Krajcir N, Agarwal A. Pathogenic mechanisms in endometriosis-associated infertility. Fertil Steril 2008;90:247-57.

26. Goldstein JL, Brown MS. Regulation of the mevalonate pathway. Nature 1990;343:425-30.

27. Zhang FL, Casey PJ. Protein prenylation: molecular mechanisms and functional consequences. Annu Rev Biochem 1996;65:241-69.

28. Corsini A, Raiteri M, Soma MR, Bernini F, Fumagalli R, Paoletti R. Pathogenesis of atherosclerosis and the role of 3-hydroxy-3-methylglutaryl coenzyme A reductase inhibitors. Am J Cardiol. 1995 ;76:21A-28A.

29. Rombouts K, Kisanga E, Hellemans K, Wielant A, Schuppan D, Geerts A. Effect of HMG-CoA reductase inhibitors on proliferation and protein synthesis by rat hepatic stellate cells. J Hepatol 2003;38:564-72.

30. Seeger H, Wallwiener D, Mueck AO. Statins can inhibit proliferation of human breast cancer cells in vitro. Exp Clin Endocrinol Diabetes 2003;111:47-48.

31. Izquierdo D, Foyouzi N, Kwintkiewicz J, Duleba AJ. Mevastatin inhibits ovarian theca-interstitial cell proliferation and steroidogenesis. Fertil Steril 2004;82:1193-97.

32. Assmus B, Urbich C, Aicher A, Hofmann WK, Haendeler J, Rossig L, et al. HMG-CoA reductase inhibitors reduce senescence and increase proliferation of endothelial progenitor cells via regulation of cell cycle regulatory genes. Circ Res 2003;92:1049-55.

33. Choi JA, Park MT, Kang CM, Um HD, Bae S, Lee KH, et al. Opposite effects of Ha-Ras and Ki-Ras on radiation-induced apoptosis via differential activation of PI3K/Akt and Rac/p38 mitogen-activated protein kinase signaling pathways. Oncogene 2004;23:9-20.

34. Yoshino O, Osuga Y, Hirota Y, Koga K, Hirata T, Harada M, et al. Possible pathophysiological roles of mitogen-activated protein kinases (MAPKs) in endometriosis. Am J Reprod Immunol 2004;52:306-11.

35. Piotrowski PC, Kwintkiewicz J, Rzepczynska IJ, Seval Y, Cakmak H, Arici A, et al. Statins inhibit growth of human endometrial stromal cells independently of cholesterol availability. Biol Reprod 2006;75:107-11.

36. Esfandiari N, Khazaei M, Ai J, Bielecki R, Gotlieb L, Ryan E, et al. Effect of a statin on an in vitro model of endometriosis. Fertil Steril 2007;87:257-62.

37. Sluijter JP, de Kleijn DP, Pasterkamp G. Vascular remodeling and protease inhibition—bench to bedside. Cardiovasc Res 2006;69:595-603.

38. Porter KE, Turner NA. Statins for the prevention of vein graft stenosis: a role for inhibition of matrix metalloproteinase-9. Biochem Soc Trans 2002;30:120-26.

39. Mastroianni CM, Liuzzi GM. Matrix metalloproteinase dysregulation in HIV infection: implications for therapeutic strategies. Trends Mol Med 2007;13:449-59.

40. Greenwood J, Steinman L, Zamvil SS. Statin therapy and autoimmune disease: from protein prenylation to immuno-modulation. Nat Rev Immunol 2006;6:358-70.

41. Grip O, Janciauskiene S, Lindgren S. Atorvastatin activates PPAR-gamma and attenuates the inflammatory response in human monocytes. Inflamm Res 2002;51:58-62.

42. Bruner-Tran KL, Osteen KG, Duleba AJ. Simvastatin inhibits development of experimental endometriosis; role of inhibition of MMP-3. . In: Taylor HS (Editors). SGI 55th Annual Meeting; March 26-29, 2008; San Diego: SAGE Publications; 26-29, 2008. p. 313A.

43. Skaletz-Rorowski A, Walsh K. Statin therapy and angiogenesis. Curr Opin Lipidol 2003;14:599-603.

44. Hindler K, Cleeland CS, Rivera E, Collard CD. The role of statins in cancer therapy. Oncologist 2006;11:306-15.

45. Park HJ, Zhang Y, Georgescu SP, Johnson KL, Kong D, Galper JB. Human umbilical vein endothelial cells and human dermal microvascular endothelial cells offer new insights into the relationship between lipid metabolism and angiogenesis. Stem Cell Rev 2006;2:93-102.

46. Ando H, Takamura T, Ota T, Nagai Y, Kobayashi K. Cerivastatin improves survival of mice with lipopoly-saccharide-induced sepsis. J Pharmacol Exp Ther 2000; 294:1043-46.

47. Weber MS, Stuve O, Neuhaus O, Hartung HP, Zamvil SS. Spotlight on statins. Int MS J 2007;14:93-97.

48. Weitz-Schmidt G, Welzenbach K, Brinkmann V, Kamata T, Kallen J, Bruns C, et al. Statins selectively inhibit leukocyte function antigen-1 by binding to a novel regulatory integrin site. Nat Med 2001;7:687-92.

49. Kwak B, Mulhaupt F, Myit S, Mach F. Statins as a newly recognized type of immunomodulator. Nat Med 2000;6:1399-402.

50. Yilmaz A, Reiss C, Tantawi O, Weng A, Stumpf C, Raaz D, et al. HMG-CoA reductase inhibitors suppress maturation of human dendritic cells: new implications for athero-sclerosis. Atherosclerosis 2004;172:85-93.

51. Kuipers HF, Biesta PJ, Groothuis TA, Neefjes JJ, Mommaas AM, van den Elsen PJ. Statins affect cell-surface expression of major histocompatibility complex class II molecules by disrupting cholesterol-containing microdomains. Hum Immunol 2005;66:653-65.

52. Dunn SE, Youssef S, Goldstein MJ, Prod'homme T, Weber MS, Zamvil SS, et al. Isoprenoids determine Th1/Th2 fate in pathogenic T cells, providing a mechanism of modulation of autoimmunity by atorvastatin. J Exp Med 2006;203:401-12.

53. Bae YS, Kang SW, Seo MS, Baines IC, Tekle E, Chock PB, et al. Epidermal growth factor (EGF)-induced generation of hydrogen peroxide. Role in EGF receptor-mediated tyrosine phosphorylation. J Biol Chem 1997; 272:217-21.

54. Bae YS, Sung JY, Kim OS, Kim YJ, Hur KC, Kazlauskas A, et al. Platelet-derived growth factor-induced H(2)O(2) production requires the activation of phosphatidylinositol 3-kinase. J Biol Chem 2000;275:10527-31.

55. Maack C, Kartes T, Kilter H, Schafers HJ, Nickenig G, Bohm M, et al. Oxygen free radical release in human failing myocardium is associated with increased activity of rac1-GTPase and represents a target for statin treatment. Circulation 2003;108:1567-74.

56. Wassmann S, Laufs U, Baumer AT, Muller K, Konkol C, Sauer H, et al. Inhibition of geranylgeranylation reduces angiotensin II-mediated free radical production in vascular

smooth muscle cells: involvement of angiotensin AT1 receptor expression and Rac1 GTPase. Mol Pharmacol 2001;59: 646-54.

57. Yasunari K, Maeda K, Minami M, Yoshikawa J. HMG-CoA reductase inhibitors prevent migration of human coronary smooth muscle cells through suppression of increase in oxidative stress. Arterioscler Thromb Vasc Biol 2001;21:937-42.

58. Shishehbor MH, Brennan ML, Aviles RJ, Fu X, Penn MS, Sprecher DL, et al. Statins promote potent systemic antioxidant effects through specific inflammatory pathways. Circulation 2003;108:426-31.

59. Oktem M, Esinler I, Eroglu D, Haberal N, Bayraktar N, Zeyneloglu HB. High-dose atorvastatin causes regression of endometriotic implants: a rat model. Hum Reprod 2007; 22:1474-80.

Mohamed FM Mitwally, Robert F Casper

Chapter 29

Aromatase Inhibitors for Endometriosis

Introduction

This chapter discusses the theory and available evidence for the use of the group of medications called "aromatase inhibitors" in managing health problems associated with endometriosis. The chapter is meant for clinicians dealing with women suffering from endometriosis. For that reason, emphasis will be placed on clinical aspects rather than theories and hypotheses with focus on practical guidelines for the use of aromatase inhibitors in the management of endometriosis.

The aromatase enzyme catalyzes a terminal steroidogenesis step that leads to estrogen synthesis, by converting androgens into estrogens in a unidirectional pathway. The third-generation aromatase inhibitors include medications that halt estrogen synthesis by specifically inhibiting the aromatase enzyme. Aromatase inhibitors have been approved for women with *"postmenopausal"* breast cancer, an estrogen-dependant cancer that would benefit from suppression of estrogen synthesis. Endometriosis is an estrogen-dependant disease often encountered in *"premenopausal"* women who frequently suffer from pain and associated infertility.

The pioneering work of Bulun[1-3] and other investigators[4] confirmed the expression of aromatase in endometriotic tissues and highlighted the significant role played by local estrogen synthesis in the progress of endometriosis. We had previously reported the effectiveness of one of the third generation aromatase inhibitors in suppressing estrogen levels in *"premenopausal"* women[5-12] suggesting that aromatase inhibitors might also be a successful tool in the management of estrogen-dependant disorders such as endometriosis, outside the traditional postmenopausal indication.

This chapter has two parts: first part discusses the underlying theory behind the potential role for aromatase inhibitors in managing endometriosis, while the second part discusses the available evidence in the literature for the success of such clinical application. From a clinical perspective, pain and infertility, the two predominant health issues associated with endometriosis will be the key points for discussion.

We will try to answer the following questions;
- Is there a sound scientific hypothesis to support the use of aromatase inhibitors in managing endometriosis?
- What is the existing clinical evidence that supports this novel application?
- Is there a difference among various aromatase inhibitors for such application?
- What is the optimal regimen for managing endometriosis with aromatase inhibitors?

Scientific Hypothesis Behind using Aromatase Inhibitors for Endometriosis

Estrogen Synthesis and Production

Estrogens are C-18 steroids (contain 18 carbon atoms), characterized by the presence of an *"aromatic"* ring, with estradiol, the strongest estrogen, containing a *"hydroxyl"* group at C-17 while, estrone, a much weaker estrogen, has a *"ketone"* group at the C-17 position.[13,14] In premenopausal women, the ovaries are the principal source of estrogen production, mainly estradiol, which functions as a circulating hormone to act on distal target tissues. On the other hand, in postmenopausal women when the ovaries cease to produce estrogen, estrogen is produced in a number of extragonadal sites from the circulating C-19 steroids (androgens), a step catalyzed by the aromatase enzyme. Estrogen produced in extragonadal tissues acts locally at these sites as a paracrine or even intracrine factor. These sites include the mesenchymal cells of adipose tissue, breast, osteoblasts and chondrocytes of bone, the vascular endothelium and aortic smooth muscle cells, and numerous sites in the brain. Thus, circulating levels of estrogens in postmenopausal women are not the drivers of estrogen action; they are a spillover from local tissue production. Therefore, circulating levels reflect rather than regulate estrogen action in postmenopausal women.

Interestingly, the control of local estrogen production is modulated through the changes of aromatase. There are distinct tissue-specific promoters of aromatase, each of which is regulated by different hormonal factors and second messenger signaling pathways.[15] Estrogen production is most commonly thought of as an endocrine product of the gonads. However, as mentioned above, there are many tissues that express the aromatase enzyme, and thus have the capacity to synthesize estrogens from circulating androgens. A non-gonadal source of estrogen, in addition to its local action, can sometimes contribute significantly to the circulating pool of estrogens, e.g. adipose tissue estrogen contribution. There is increasing evidence that in both men and women extraglandular production of estrogens from androgens is important in normal physiology, as well as in pathophysiologic states.[16]

Aromatase expression in adipose tissue, and possibly in the skin primarily accounts for the extraglandular (peripheral) formation of estrogen and increases as a function of *body weight* and *advancing age*. Sufficient circulating levels of the biologically active estrogen, estradiol, can be produced as a result of extraglandular aromatization of androstenedione to estrone that is subsequently reduced to estradiol in peripheral tissues. Such biologically active estradiol can activate several estrogen-dependant reproductive disorders including endometriosis, abnormal uterine bleeding, endometrial hyperplasia and cancer.[16, 17]

Aromatase Inhibitors

Blocking estrogen production by inhibiting the enzyme catalyzing the main step of its synthesis from androgens (aromatase enzyme) is an exciting treatment modality for estrogen-dependant disorders. Such treatment has been in clinical application for more than half a century since the development of the first generation of aromatase inhibitors such as aminoglutethimide. However, the clinical applications of the aromatase inhibitors in managing estrogen-dependant disorders had not achieved significant success until recently. This was due to several problems encountered with the clinical use of early generations of the aromatase inhibitors. Those problems were successfully overcome to a great extent by the development of the third generation of aromatase inhibitors. **Table 29-1** summarizes the different generations of the aromatase inhibitors. **Box 29-1** summarizes the main problems associated with the early-generations of the aromatase inhibitors, while **Box 29-2** summarizes the advantages of the third generation aromatase inhibitors.

Development of Aromatase Inhibitors

The location of the estrogen synthesis catalyzed by aromatase at the far end of steroidogenesis cascade makes this terminal step a good target for selective inhibition without significant effect on substrate accumulation. Several aromatase inhibitors have been developed over the last five decades with the third generation aromatase inhibitors licensed in the last decade for suppressing

Table 29-1: Different generations of aromatase inhibitors		
Generation	*Nonsteroidal Aromatase Inhibitors*	*Steroidal Aromatase Inhibitors (Sometimes called suicidal inhibitors of the aromatase enzyme)*
	Work by temporary (reversible) inactivation of the aromatase enzyme	Work by permanent (irreversible) inactivation of the aromatase enzyme.
First Generation	Aminoglutethimide (Cytadren®)	N/A
Second Generation	Rogletimide Fadrozole	Formestane
Third Generation	Letrozole (Femara® 2.5 mg/tablet) Anastrozole (Arimidex® 1mg/tablet) Vorozole	Exemestane (Aromasin® 25 mg/tablet)

estrogen synthesis in postmenopausal women with breast cancer. The third generation aromatase inhibitors were developed after the clinical failure of the earlier generations of aromatase inhibitors as explained in **Boxes 29-1 and 29-2.**

Third Generation Aromatase Inhibitors

The third generation aromatase inhibitors effectively block estrogen synthesis without exerting effects on other steroidogenic pathways and have been heralded as a "triumph of translational oncology". This group includes the non-steroidal letrozole (Femara®) and anastrozole (Arimidex®), and the steroidal exemestane (Aromasin®). These aromatase inhibitors are currently available for clinical use as oral tablets. They have been approved for estrogen suppression in postmenopausal women with breast cancer.[18]

Structure: Third generation non-steroidal aromatase inhibitors are nitrogen-containing triazole derivatives that bind to iron in the heme moiety of the aromatase enzyme resulting in reversible inhibition.[19]

Box 29-1: Problems associated with early generations aromatase inhibitors

Pharmacodynamic:
1. Low potency in inhibiting the aromatase enzyme particularly in premenopausal women (very low potency)
2. Lack of specificity in inhibiting the aromatase enzyme with significant inhibition of other steroidogenesis enzymes leading to medical adrenalectomy.

Pharmacokinetic:
1. Not all members are available orally (some require parentral administration
2. Variable bioavailability after oral administration
3. Variable half-life that changes with the period of administration due to induction of its metabolism.

Clinical:
1. Poorly tolerated on daily administration with more a third of patients discontinued treatment due to adverse effects
2. Significant side effects related to both the aromatase inhibitors, e.g. drowsiness, morbilliform skin rash, nausea and anorexia, and dizziness and side effects secondary to the steroids used for replacement therapy, e.g. glucocorticoids
3. Interaction with alcohol with significant potentiation of its action
4. Significant interactions with other medications, e.g. coumarin and warfarin.
5. Need for replacement therapy due to medical adrenalectomy, e.g. glucocorticoid and mineralocorticoid replacement
6. Long-term possible carcinogenesis (at least in animals)

Box 29-2: Advantages of third generation aromatase inhibitors

Pharmacodynamic Advantages:
1. Extreme potency in inhibiting the aromatase enzyme (up to thousand times potency of the first generation aminoglutethimide)
2. Very specific in inhibiting the aromatase enzyme without significant inhibition of the other steroidogenesis enzymes. This is true even at high doses
3. Absence of estrogen receptor depletion

Pharmacokinetic Advantages:
1. Orally administered (other routes of administration are also possible, e.g. vaginal and rectal)
2. Almost 100% bioavailability after oral administration
3. Rapid clearance from the body due to short half-life, (~ 8 hours for the Aromasin® to ~ 45 hours for the Femara® and Arimidex®)
4. Absence of tissue accumulation of the medications or any of their metabolites
5. No significant active metabolites

Clinical Advantages:
1. Well tolerated on daily administration for up to several years (in post-menopausal women with breast cancer) with few adverse effects
2. Few mild side effects
3. Very safe without significant contraindications
4. Absence of significant interactions with other medications
5. Very wide safety margin (toxic dose is several thousand times higher than recommended efficacious therapeutic dose)
6. Relatively inexpensive

Potency: Aromatase inhibition and estradiol suppression show good correlation and are consistently significantly higher (more than a thousand times) for third-generation aromatase inhibitors when compared with first-generation and second-generation aromatase inhibitors.[20] In cell-free aromatase system experiments (human placental microsomes), letrozole has been found equipotent to anastrozole in inhibiting the aromatase enzyme. However, letrozole was found to be 10–30 times more potent than anastrozole in inhibiting intracellular aromatase in "intact" rodent cells, human adipose fibroblasts, and human cancer cell lines.[21] Compared to other aromatase inhibitors, letrozole has consistently demonstrated greater potency.[22, 23]

Selectivity: Third generation aromatase inhibitors are highly selective for the aromatase enzyme and unlike first- and second-generation aromatase inhibitors do not affect glucocorticoids, mineralocorticoids, or thyroxine secretion. *In vivo* adrenocorticotrophic hormone (ACTH) stimulation tests in rats showed that letrozole had no significant effect on either aldosterone or corticosterone levels, even at a dose 1,000 times greater than that required for inhibition of aromatase.[24] The vast majority of patients treated with letrozole have a normal response to synthetic ACTH.[25]

Pharmacokinetics: Third generation aromatase inhibitors enjoy several pharmacokinetic advantages that make them convenient for clinical practice. This includes almost 100% absorption following oral administration with large apparent volume of distribution due to extensive distribution to various body tissues. The terminal half-life is usually around two days with steady-state concentrations reached usually in less than one week of daily administration. Such steady state is maintained for long periods with no evidence of drug accumulation.[26]

Another major pharmacokinetic advantage that third generation aromatase inhibitors have over the first-generation aromatase inhibitor aminoglutethimide, is the absence of significant drug interactions except when combined with tamoxifen as the case with letrozole. Its plasma concentration is reduced by between 35% and 40% when combined with tamoxifen.[27] However, hepatic impairment can markedly increase the terminal half-life.[26]

Is there a Difference in Response to Individual Aromatase Inhibitors?

This is an important question that is difficult to answer, because the third generation aromatase inhibitors suppress estrogen synthesis strongly enough to bring down estrogen levels below the detection limits of the currently available hormonal assays.[28] However, in a cross-over study between anastrozole and letrozole, the latter was found to be the more potent inhibitor of total body aromatization, and plasma estrogen.[29] In a recent study, the same group recorded a more potent suppression of tissue estrogens with letrozole compared to previous results with anastrozole, without significant inter-individual variability.[30] However, whether such difference in estrogen suppression potency is translated into clinical differences, is still a matter of controversy and awaits future studies.

Non-aromatase Inhibition Actions of Third Generation Aromatase Inhibitors

The presence of other mechanisms of action for the aromatase inhibitors that are not dependant on inhibiting the aromatase enzyme and suppressing estrogen synthesis have been suggested. One such suggestion comes from a three-dimensional fibrin matrix model for *in vitro* study of endometrial explant growth. In this model, letrozole was found to have a growth stimulatory effect on normal human endometrium rather than a suppression of proliferation and angiogenesis as would be expected from aromatase inhibition and estrogen suppression.[31] The authors suggested a possible mechanism though an effect on insulin-like growth factor 1 (IGF-1), known to be synthesized locally in endometrium. All three IGF-1 isoforms are expressed in eutopic endometrium and in endometriomas.[32] Also, the human endometrium is known to have high-affinity receptors for IGF-1,[33] and proliferative activity of uterine cells may be regulated by IGF-1.[34] These speculations of a direct endometrial effect of letrozole or other members of the third generation aromatase inhibitors are still unconfirmed and await further studies.

Differences among Aromatase Inhibitors

Potency of different third generation aromatase inhibitors
There is usually a correlation between the *in vitro* and *in vivo* efficacy of the aromatase inhibitors. However, *in vivo* measurements of the efficacy of an aromatase inhibitor depends on other important factors including drug metabolism e.g. terminal half-life and tissue distribution. This may result in a significant difference between what is seen in *in vitro* experiments and *in vivo* effects.[35] A clear example is the second-generation aromatase inhibitors, which *in vitro* revealed a higher biochemical efficacy when compared with the third-generation inhibitors, but *in vivo* showed a significantly lower suppression of plasma estrogens that translated into an inferior clinical efficacy.[36]

Letrozole was found to have greater potency (both *in vivo* and *in vitro*) than all the other aromatase inhibitors, including anastrozole, exemestane, formestane, and aminoglutethimide. Moreover, letrozole produced near complete inhibition of aromatase in peripheral tissues and was associated with greater suppression of estrogen than other aromatase inhibitors.[37]

Adverse Effects Associated with Third Generation Aromatase Inhibitors

Almost all available data on the side effects and adverse reactions associated with third generation aromatase inhibitors come from clinical trials involving postmenopausal women with advanced breast cancer. In general, third generation aromatase inhibitors have been found very well tolerated with few significant side affects and a low rate of discontinuation due to adverse reactions. If this is the case in such a vulnerable elderly population (post-menopausal women with advanced breast cancer), the use of third generation aromatase inhibitors in premenopausal women during the reproductive age, would be expected to be very well tolerated.

When considering side effects and adverse reactions associated with third generation aromatase inhibitors we should consider two groups of problems:

First: problems related to the medications themselves rather than their estrogen action. There are no known serious side effects reported with third generation aromatase inhibitors other than mild non-specific ones such as headaches and gastrointestinal symptoms. Arthralgia is an interesting problem that has been seen more frequently with third generation aromatase inhibitors treatment and will be discussed later. Second: problems related to estrogen deprivation due to suppression of estrogen synthesis. Those include menopausal symptoms such as hot flashes and vaginal dryness, as well as long-term effects of estrogen deprivation especially on the bones and lipid profile.[38]

The following is a brief discussion of some significant adverse effects associated with aromatase inhibitors use. It is important to reiterate here that most of those adverse effects were associated with long-term use of third generation aromatase inhibitors administered daily for several years in postmenopausal women with breast cancer.

Arthralgia: An important unique side effect that has been found associated with third generation aromatase inhibitors is joint pain (arthralgia) that appears to be quite prevalent and seen more commonly than with tamoxifen use. In some cases, arthralgia was severe enough to be a reason for discontinuation of aromatase inhibitor treatment. The possible mechanisms of aromatase inhibitor-associated arthralgia are still unclear. Treatment options for arthralgia including non-steroidal anti-inflammatory drugs are currently inadequate. High-dose vitamin D and new-targeted therapies to inhibit bone loss are being investigated.[39]

Effect on bone: Third generation aromatase inhibitors were found to increase bone turnover and induce bone loss particularly at sites rich in trabecular bone. In these sites, bone loss averaged 1–3% per year leading to an increase in fracture incidence compared to that seen during tamoxifen use. Such adverse bone effect was found more in younger women with rates of bone loss averaging 7–8% per year of daily use. To reduce the severity of bone loss, osteoporosis, and the risk of fracture, randomized clinical trials in postmenopausal women found bisphosphonates to significantly reduce bone loss caused by aromatase inhibitor therapy. This treatment along with a healthy lifestyle and adequate intake of calcium and vitamin D are currently the treatments of choice to prevent bone loss.[40] However, for younger women in the reproductive age, the use of bisphosphonates should be avoided in those still desiring fertility. Add-back estrogen is a more appealing option to prevent bone loss associated with long-term use of aromatase inhibitors in young women.

Effects on blood lipids: There are concerns about increasing cardiovascular risks from estrogen deprivation caused by aromatase inhibitors, through adverse effect on blood lipids. Concerns about negative lipid changes associated with aromatase inhibitors that could increase cardiovascular adverse events are still unclear. The available data on effects of third generation aromatase inhibitors on serum lipids are limited to short-term studies that found different effects exerted by different aromatase inhibitors. Exemestane was suggested to have little or possibly a slight beneficial effect on serum lipids. This could be due to its steroid nature, while anastrozole appeared to have possibly a little adverse effect; letrozole was suggested to have a detrimental effect. However, the data are limited and long-term studies are still needed.[40]

Aromatase Enzyme in Endometriotic Tissues

Significant levels of aromatase enzyme activity and expression have been detected in the stromal cell component of endometriosis.[1] In addition, the eutopic endometrium of women with endometriosis has been found to contain low but significant levels of aromatase enzyme activity and expression. The authors suggested that upon retrograde menstruation followed by implantation of this inherently abnormal tissue (cells from eutopic endometrium) on the peritoneal surfaces, expression and activity of the aromatase enzyme are amplified.[1, 2]

There are tissue-specific promoters that enhance the expression of the aromatase enzyme. Extraovarian endometriotic tissue and ovarian endometrioma cells almost exclusively use promoter II, which is the proximal promoter responsive to prostaglandin E2 (PGE2) and cyclic adenosine monophosphate (cAMP), for aromatase expression *in vivo*.[2, 3] Other molecular abnormalities have been demonstrated including the presence of significant levels of StAR in addition to aromatase activity both in ectopic and eutopic endometrium of patients with endometriosis. Prostaglandin E2 is a potent inducer of both StAR and aromatase in endometriotic stromal cells. In addition, a transcription factor, steroidogenic factor 1, is also aberrantly expressed and binds to steroidogenic promoters in endometriotic tissues. Steroidogenic factor 1 mediates PGE2–cAMP dependent co-activation of multiple steroidogenic genes, most notably StAR and aromatase.[3]

The enzyme cyclooxygenase-2 (COX-2) that catalyzes the conversion of arachidonic acid to PGE2 is significantly up-regulated in stromal cells of both endometriotic tissue and endometrium of women with endometriosis.[41, 42] Estradiol is a potent stimulator of COX-2 in uterine endothelial cells, which may create a vicious circle of positive feedback involving StAR and aromatase expression. Increased synthesis of E2 stimulates COX-2 leading to PGE2 synthesis that in turn promotes the expression and activity of both StAR and aromatase, thereby leading to the further formation of estrogen.

Aromatase Inhibitors in Premenopausal Women

As indicated earlier, endometriosis is most often encountered in reproductive age women. Use of aromatase inhibitors to suppress estrogen production in reproductive age women has two significant problems due to the presence of functioning ovaries:

First: Aromatase expression and potency in functioning ovaries (mainly the granulosa cells) is known to be much greater compared to postmenopausal women.

Second: In response to estrogen deprivation by aromatase inhibition, endogenous gonadotropins rise and lead to stimulation of *de novo* aromatase synthesis in the ovaries. This will lead to escape from the aromatase inhibitor effect on estrogen synthesis. In addition, follicular cysts may develop.

In contrast to the brain, endometriotic tissue, or adipose tissue, there are overwhelming levels of aromatase expression in the ovaries of premenopausal women (granulosa cells of the growing follicles particularly the Graafian follicle). Thus, it is expected that aromatase inhibitors in premenopausal women would inhibit aromatase activity in peripheral tissues such as the brain, endometriosis, and adipose tissues totally. On the other hand, only partial aromatase activity blockade may be expected in the ovary.[43] Therefore, higher doses of aromatase inhibitors are required in premenopausal women than those successfully applied in postmenopausal women to achieve comparable total body aromatase inhibition.

As mentioned earlier, the compensatory rise in endogenous gonadotropins, particularly FSH leads to *de novo* aromatase synthesis that will overcome the inhibitory effect on estrogen production by aromatase inhibitors in premenopausal women. For that reason, in premenopausal women, using an aromatase inhibitor *"alone"* would not be effective in inhibiting estrogen production, and another agent to prevent the rise in endogenous gonadotropins is required. GnRH analogues (GnRH agonists or antagonists), as well as exogenous sex steroids are expected to be effective agents in blocking the endogenous rise in gonadotropins associated with aromatase inhibitor administration.

When aromatase inhibitors were used alone in premenopausal women with breast cancer, both failure of significant reduction of estrogen levels and elevated levels of gonadotropins were observed.[44-46] This was true even with the use of supratherapeutic levels of formestane.[47] However, third-generation aromatase inhibitors suppressed plasma estradiol concentrations more efficiently, although a near-complete suppression could not be achieved as is the case in postmenopausal women.[48] When the rise in endogenous gonadotropins was prevented (by GnRH agonist), aromatase inhibitors were found to be effective in suppressing circulating estrogen concentrations to levels comparable to those achieved in postmenopausal women.[49]

Evidence for Success of Aromatase Inhibitors for the Treatment of Endometriosis

It is not in the scope of this chapter to discuss medical treatment of endometriosis. Instead, the role of aromatase inhibitors in treating endometriosis-associated pain and infertility will be the focus of discussion.

Aromatase Inhibitors for Postmenopausal Women with Endometriosis

To our knowledge, the first case in the literature that reported the use of an aromatase inhibitor in treating endometriosis was in a postmenopausal woman. The patient had severe recurrent endometriosis and was previously operated three times including bilateral oophorectomy and resection of endometriosis. The patient had a 3-cm polypoid tumor in the vagina and severe pain. She continued to suffer from endometriosis-associated pain even after she underwent definitive treatment in the form of total hysterectomy with bilateral salpingo-oophorectomy. Obviously with the removal of both ovaries, the main source of estrogen production, there would be no role for GnRH agonist use. Treatment with progesterone for 4 months was not successful. The authors thought that peripheral and local estrogen production were the underlying causes for activating her endometriotic lesions. The use of the aromatase inhibitor, anastrozole, proved successful in alleviating the woman's pain and inducing regression of the endometriotic lesions. After 9 months of treatment with anastrozole, the endometriotic lesion was reduced to a scar, and she had no pain.[50] In another report by Fatemi et al, a 55-year-old woman had a laparotomy due to subacute intestinal obstruction caused by endometriosis. After surgery, a mass about 4 to 8 cm was found in the rectovaginal septum. She was treated with the aromatase inhibitor, letrozole. After 1 year of treatment, she had no pain and the mass had shrunk to 1 cm.[51]

It is important to reiterate here that endometriosis is primarily a disease of women in the reproductive age group and postmenopausal women with endometriosis constitute a small fraction of women suffering from endometriosis-associated pain.

A recent review of the available literature on post-menopausal endometriosis found 32 case reports in Medline. The most commonly reported site for postmenopausal endometriosis was the ovaries. The risk of both recurrence and *de novo* occurrence of endometriosis was increased in women on hormone replacement therapy, in particular, estrogen only. The authors recommended that despite the rarity of endometriosis in postmenopausal women, it is important to be aware of this possibility, as well as the risk of ovarian cancer that is believed to be around 1%. For that reason, primary treatment should be surgical while medical treatment including aromatase inhibitors should be considered on an individual basis with very close follow-up.[52]

Aromatase Inhibitors for Premenopausal Women with Endometriosis

Endometriosis-associated Pain

Unfortunately, many women with endometriosis-associated chronic pelvic pain are refractory to currently available medical treatments that aim at creating a pseudopregnant or hypoestrogenic state, e.g. oral contraceptive pills, Depot Provera, oral progestins, and GnRH analogues.[53-55] In addition, significant side effects may cause patients to decline a potentially effective treatment, such as danazol for example, since the drug may have some androgenic activity.[56] On the other hand, conservative surgical excision of endometriosis usually provides significant pain relief. However, the degree and duration of pain relief following surgical treatment varies extensively among patients. Outcome of surgery depends

on many factors including the experience of the surgeon, previous treatment history, and the use of adjuvant medical treatment.[57-60] Recurrence of endometriosis-associated pain unfortunately occurs in a good proportion of women following medical and/or surgical treatments. The last resort in many of these cases is definitive treatment by total hysterectomy and bilateral salpingo-oophorectomy. Even after this definitive treatment, pelvic pain has been reported in 3-17% of women within a year following surgery.[61] For these reasons, the search continues for more effective treatments, particularly for women failing to respond to currently available treatment modalities. As explained earlier, the rationale for using aromatase inhibitors is scientifically plausible since suppressing the continued local estrogen production in endometriotic implants should make these lesions inactive. Local estrogen production in endometriosis would not be suppressed by currently available treatments such as GnRH analogues.[62-64] **Table 29-2** summarizes the clinical studies that have reported the use of aromatase inhibitors for endometriosis-associated pain.

In almost all those studies, one of two aromatase inhibitors belonging to the third generation (anastrozole or letrozole) has been used. High doses of calcium and vitamin D have been invariably administered to patients while receiving the aromatase inhibitors to minimize the risk of bone loss, particularly when long duration of treatment is considered. The concept of add-back of exogenous estrogen seems to be an exciting one that may reduce side effects without reducing the efficacy of pain relief. However, there is not much data in the literature to test this concept. Almost all reported patients who used an aromatase inhibitor were those who failed to respond to other currently available treatment modalities. In most of those studies, the response to aromatase inhibitors has been very encouraging with significant improvement in pain.

An adverse effect that has been reported with aromatase inhibitors use for endometriosis treatment in premeno-pausal women was the formation of ovarian cysts. Interestingly, significant pain relief occurred despite the formation of those cysts.[65] Formation of ovarian cysts seemed to have resulted from inadequate suppression of the rise in endogenous gonadotropins induced by with-drawal of estrogen negative feedback on the hypotha-lamus and/or pituitary. We have proposed another interesting mechanism through estrogen-mediated effects at the level of the anterior pituitary cells involving the local activin-inhibin-follistatin system. This system is responsible for an estrogen-selective modulation of the FSH

Table 29-2: Outline of reports on use of aromatase inhibitors in treating endometriosis-associated pain in premenopausal women

Study (year)	Study design	Aromatase inhibitor used	Dose	Duration of treatment (months)	Adjuvant to suppress rise in endogenous gonadotropins	Number of women	Reference
2004	Non-randomized	Letrozole	2.5 mg/day	6	Norethindrone 2.5 mg/day	10	Ailawadi et al[68]
2004	Case report	Letrozole	2.5 mg/day	3	Patient had bilateral oophorectomy	1	Razzi and Fava[69]
2004	Case report	Anastrozole	1 mg/day	6	Prometrium 200 mg/day	2	Shippen and West[70]
2004	Randomized trial Vs. GnRH agonist alone	Anastrozole	1 mg/day	6	GnRH agonist, goserlin 3.6 mg	97	Soysal et al[71]
2005	Non-randomized	Anastrozole	0.25 mg/day (vaginally)	6	Non reported	10	Hefler et al[72]
2005	Case series	Anastrozole	1 mg/day	6	Oral contraceptive pills (Ethinyl Estradiol 20 microgram and Levonorgestrel 0.1 mg)	15	Amsterdam et al[73]
2007	Case report	Exemestane then Letrozole	Letrozole 2.5 mg/day	Less than 3 months	Patient had already bilateral oophorectomy	1	Mousa et al[74]
2007	Case series	Letrozole	2.5 mg/day	About 3	Desogestrel 0.075 mg	12	Remorgida et al[75]
2009	Case series	-Letrozole for 4 patients -Anastrozole for one patient	-Letrozole 2.5 mg/day -Anastrozole 1mg/day	6	None reported	4	Verma and Konje[76]

(but not LH) production by the anterior pituitary that is independent of GnRH.[66]

Using an aromatase inhibitor to treat other problems associated with endometriosis such as adhesions, has been tried but without success. In a recent case report anastrozole was found to be unsuccessful for treatment of endometriosis causing ureteral obstruction leading to hydronephrosis. A period of fifteen months of anastrozole treatment (1mg/day) did not improve renal function, and surgical intervention was required to alleviate pressure on the kidneys.[67]

Endometriosis-associated Infertility

The treatment of endometriosis-associated infertility is beyond the scope of this chapter and is discussed elsewhere. Here, we discuss the particular role of aromatase inhibitors in helping infertile women achieve pregnancy. There are different theories for endometriosis-associated infertility including ovulatory dysfunction, problems with the interaction between sperm and oocytes, and endometrial dysfunction, as well as interference with tubal motility or patency caused by pelvic adhesions. Aromatase

inhibitors are believed to have the following roles in endometriosis-associated infertility:

1. Suppressing endometriotic lesions
2. Ovarian stimulation agents

1. **Suppressing endometriotic lesions:** As discussed earlier, there is evidence for the success of aromatase inhibitors in suppressing endometriosis and alleviating endometriosis-associated pain. Whether endometriosis suppression before infertility treatment improves the outcome of such treatment or not is still controversial. A recent report found combined down-regulation by an aromatase inhibitor and GnRH agonist to result in favorable IVF-ET outcome in women with *"endometriomas"*. In this study, 20 women received the aromatase inhibitor anastrozole 1 mg daily for about 10 weeks with GnRH agonist depot (three doses of goserelin 3.6 mg every 4 weeks). During the combined down-regulation, the *"endometriomal"* volume and the serum CA125 level decreased by 29% (3-39%) and 61% (21-74%), respectively. Ovarian stimulation started on day 70 following combined down-regulation. In the IVF/ICSI cycle, the number of oocytes retrieved was 7.5

(6.0-10.0) and the fertilization rate was 78% (38-100%). Nine patients (45%) conceived, five (25%) had a clinical pregnancy, and three (15%) delivered healthy children (two singletons and one twin).[77] Despite the favorable outcome regarding the significant regression of endometriomas and reduction in CA125 levels, as well as acceptable IVF-ET outcomes, the study suffered from significant drawbacks, namely the small sample size and lack of a control group.

2. **Ovarian stimulation agents:** To our knowledge, there are no studies in the literature that looked at aromatase inhibitors as an ovarian stimulation agent exclusively in women with endometriosis. After we reported the success of an aromatase inhibitor in ovarian stimulation,[7-12] several other investigators confirmed our observations.[78-80] In those studies, women with endometriosis-associated infertility were included with women with other infertility factors, but were not analyzed separately.

In addition to the obvious value associated with low estrogen levels achieved during ovarian stimulation with aromatase inhibitors that might be of benefit in an estrogen-dependent disease such as endometriosis, we propose another interesting mechanism. The estrogen receptor subtype beta (ERβ) is the predominantly expressed estrogen receptor in endometriotic tissues.[81] Contrary to the estrogen receptor subtype alpha (ERα) that is up-regulated in the presence of *low* estrogen levels, the ERβ is down-regulated in *low* estrogenic milieu.[82] Low estrogen levels and the local hypo-estrogenic milieu expected with aromatase inhibitor use during ovarian stimulation might help suppression of endometriosis through an effect mediated by down-regulated ERβ.

The most commonly used oral ovulation agent, clomiphene citrate has an agonistic effects on the ERbβ. In addition, the high circulating estradiol levels associated with clomiphene citrate treatment should upregulate ERβ. Of historical interest, older literature dating back to the discovery and early use of clomiphene citrate in clinical practice recommended against the use of clomiphene citrate in women with endometriosis. Particularly, the presence of endometriomas was suggested as a contraindication for using clomiphene citrate as an ovarian stimulation agent.[83] An interesting study[84] found endometriosis in significant number of women (about two thirds) who had been treated by clomiphene citrate for several cycles without achievement of pregnancy. More recently, we reported treatment with clomiphene to significantly reduce the chance of pregnancy in women with endometriosis when compared to timed intercourse

without clomiphene citrate treatment. In a cohort of 271 women with surgically-diagnosed endometriosis, after conservative endometriosis surgery, women were given the option of trying on their own with timed intercourse or receiving ovarian stimulation with clomiphene citrate. A total of 193 couples opted for timed intercourse without further intervention, while 78 preferred trying ovarian stimulation with clomiphene and timed intercourse. After controlling for stage of endometriosis, age and duration of infertility, clomiphene citrate treatment was associated with significantly lower clinical pregnancy rates compared to spontaneous pregnancy achieved by timed intercourse without ovarian stimulation.[85] In addition, the beneficial role of clomiphene ovarian stimulation in ovulatory infertility, particularly unexplained infertility, found to be minimal and has been questioned.[86] This could be simply because many women with unexplained infertility may have undiagnosed underlying endometriosis, especially with the recent trend towards less frequent use of diagnostic laparoscopy in evaluating infertility factors.

Aromatase Inhibitors to Prevent Flare Associated with GnRH Agonist

An important potential benefit from aromatase inhibitors during the management of endometriosis is to prevent the estrogen flare associated with the initiation of GnRH agonist treatment. As explained above, GnRH agonist-induced hypoestrogenism is a successful treatment for endometriosis-associated pain and other estrogen-dependant disorders, e.g. leiomyomas. However, a problem associated with GnRH agonist treatment is the initial flare-up of endogenous gonadotropins with subsequent increase in estradiol secretion by the ovaries and elevation in the circulating estradiol levels. This estrogen flare up usually lasts about one week before full suppression of the pituitary is achieved leading to the desired hypoestrogenic state.[87]

The flare of estradiol associated with GnRH agonist results in undesired adverse effects including irregular endometrial bleeding, accentuated pelvic pain or even potential growth of estrogen-dependent tumors. Moreover, incidents of grave complications, such as intestinal obstruction and perforation due to sudden growth of intestinal endometriosis have been reported.[88, 89]

A recent preliminary study found that the use of the aromatase inhibitor, letrozole, when given at a dose of 2.5 mg/day starting on the day of GnRH agonist administration was successful in alleviating the initial estrogen flare up. Letrozole was administered for five days and successfully prevented any rise in estradiol levels in all

14 patients included in the study (GnRH agonist was administered in 9 patients for endometriosis and 5 for leiomyomas).[90]

Aromatase Inhibitors for Adenomyosis

Adenomyosis or endometriosis interna (endometriosis of the uterine wall) is frequently associated with significant debilitating symptoms including pelvic pain and excessive menstrual bleeding. The exact prevalence of this condition is unclear. The diagnosis and management of adenomyosis are still significant challenges to clinicians. Hysterectomy is often the ultimate treatment because conservative treatments to prevent pain or bleeding while retaining fertility are extremely difficult.[91] Recently, there have been reports of significant aromatase activity in uterine adenomyosis.[92] Therefore, the inhibition of estrogen production by an aromatase inhibitor is a logical approach. A recent case report describes a 34-year-old woman with adenomyosis who had severe clinical symptoms and a strong desire to retain fertility. After the failure of adequate response to GnRH agonist and danazol treatment, a concomitant treatment of an aromatase inhibitor (anastrozole 1 mg daily) and a GnRH agonist was found effective. The patient's symptoms were almost eradicated after four months of treatment and remained under contol for six months after anastrozole was discontinued while continuing administration of GnRH agonist.[93]

Conclusion

We hope that the above review succeeded in clarifying the answers to the following questions:

Is there a sound scientific hypothesis to support the success of aromatase inhibitors in managing endometriosis?

It seems that the answer to this question is yes and that there is enough scientific evidence to support aromatase inhibitors as a new tool in the fight against endometriosis-associated health problems. This is based on the significant expression of aromatase and synthesis of local estrogen inside the endometriotic tissues, suppression of which might have a positive effect on alleviating endometriosis-associated symptoms of pain and infertility.

What is the existing clinical evidence that supports such novel application?

Despite the lack of large properly designed randomized trials, the available evidence is strong enough to conclude that aromatase inhibitors are useful for an alternative treatment in managing endometriosis. This is particularly true when considering:

• First: the wide safety profile and high tolerability of the third-generation aromatase inhibitors
• Second: the significant success in reported cases of women with severe endometriosis-associated symptoms who failed to respond to currently available treatment modalities.

Is there a difference among various aromatase inhibitors for such application?

We do not believe there is enough evidence for or against the presence of significant difference among aromatase inhibitors. Even though there is some evidence for possible superiority of one aromatase inhibitor over another when it comes to potency, there is not enough evidence that such difference would translate into a significant difference in clinical efficiency.

What is the optimum regimen for managing endometriosis with aromatase inhibitors?

At the present time, there is no answer to this question. We believe that an important question to consider is what would be the optimum and most cost-effective approach to prevent the rise in endogenous gonadotropins associated with aromatase inhibitors use in premenopausal women. In postmenopausal women, we believe that a combined regimen of an aromatase inhibitor together with hormone replacement (estrogen alone or with progesterone) as add-back therapy seems to be the optimum when it comes to preventing drawbacks associated with long-term hypoestrogenism at the level of the bones, and blood lipids, as well as menopausal symptoms, e.g. vaginal dryness and hot flashes.

References

1. Noble LS, Simpson ER, Johns A, Bulun SE. Aromatase expression in endometriosis. J Clin Endocrinol Metab 1996;81:174-79.
2. Noble LS, Takayama K, Putman JM, Johns DA, Hinshelwood MM, Agarwal VR, Zhao Y, Carr BR, Bulun SE. Prostaglandin E2 stimulates aromatase expression in endometriosis-derived stromal cells. J Clin Endocrinol Metab 1997;82:600-06.
3. Zeitoun K, Takayama K, Michael MD, Bulun SE. Stimulation of aromatase P450 promoter (II) activity in endometriosis and its inhibition in endometrium are regulated by competitive binding of SF-1 and COUP-TF to the same cis-acting element. Mol Endocrinol 1999;13:239-53.
4. Kitawaki J, Noguchi T, Amatsu T, Maeda K, Tsukamoto K, Yamamoto T, Fushiki S, Osawa Y, Honjo H. Expression of aromatase cytochrome P450 protein and messenger

ribonucleic acid in human endometriotic and adenomyotic tissues but not in normal endometrium. Biol Reprod 1997;57(3):514-19.

7. Mitwally MFM, Casper RF. Aromatase Inhibition: a novel method of ovulation induction in women with polycystic ovarian syndrome. Reprod Technol 2000;10:244-47.

8. Mitwally MFM, Casper RF. Use of an aromatase inhibitor for induction of ovulation in patients with an inadequate response to clomiphene citrate. Fertil Steril 2001;75: 305-09.

9. Mitwally MFM, Casper RF. Aromatase inhibition improves ovarian response to follicle-stimulating hormone in poor responders. Fertil Steril 2002;774:776-80.

10. Mitwally MF, Casper RF. Aromatase inhibition reduces gonadotrophin dose required for controlled ovarian stimulation in women with unexplained infertility. Hum Reprod 2003;188:1588-97.

11. Mitwally MF, Casper RF. Aromatase inhibition reduces the dose of gonadotropin required for controlled ovarian hyperstimulation. J Soc Gynecol Investig 2004;11:406-15.

12. Mitwally MFM, Casper RF. Single dose administration of the aromatase inhibitor, letrozole: a simple and convenient effective method of ovulation induction. Fertil Steril 2005;83:229-31.

13. Carr BR. Disorders of the ovaries and female reproductive tract. In: Wilson JD, Foster DW, Kronenberg HM, Larsen PR (Editors): Williams Textbook of Endocrinology (9th edn), WB Saunders, Philadelphia 1998;751-817.

14. Barbieri R, Ryan K. The menstrual cycle. In: Ryan K, Berkowitz R, Barbieri R, Dunaif A (Editors): Kistner's Gynecology and Women's Health (7th edn), Mosby, St Louis 1999;32-34.

15. Simpson ER. Sources of estrogen and their importance. The Journal of Steroid Biochemistry and Molecular Biology 2003;86(3-5):225-30.

16. Nelson LR, Bulun SE. Estrogen production and action. J Am Acad Dermatol 2001;45 (Suppl):S116-S124.

17. Cole PA, Robinson CH. Mechanism and inhibition of cytochrome P-450 aromatase. J Med Chem 1999; 33:2933-44.

18. Buzdar A, Howell A. Advances in aromatase inhibition: clinical efficacy and tolerability in the treatment of breast cancer. Clin Cancer Res 2001; 7:2620-35.

19. Lang M, Batzl C, Furet P, Bowman R, Häusler A, Bhatnagar AS. Structure-activity relationships and binding model of novel aromatase inhibitors. J Steroid Biochem Mol Biol 1993;44:421-28.

20. Sainsbury R. Aromatase inhibition in the treatment of advanced breast cancer: is there a relationship between potency and clinical efficacy? British Journal of Cancer 2004 ;90:1733-39.

21. Bhatnagar AS, Brodie AMH, Long BJ, Evans DB, Miller WR. Intracellular aromatase and its relevance to the pharmacological efficacy of aromatase inhibitors. J Steroid Biochem Mol Biol 2001;76:199-202.

22. Bhatnagar AS, Häusler A, Schieweck K, Lang M, Bowman R. Highly selective inhibition of estrogen biosynthesis by CGS 20267, a new non-steroidal aromatase inhibitor. J Steroid Biochem Mol Biol 1990;37:1021-27.

23. Miller WR. Biology of aromatase inhibitors: pharmacology/endocrinology within the breast. Endocr Relat Cancer 1999;6:187-95.

24. Bhatnagar AS, Häusler A, Schieweck K, Lang M, Bowman R. Highly selective inhibition of estrogen biosynthesis by CGS 20267, a new non-steroidal aromatase inhibitor. J Steroid Biochem Mol Biol 1990;37:1021-27.

25. Demers LM. Effects of fadrozole (CGS 16949A) and letrozole (CGS 20267) on the inhibition of aromatase activity in breast cancer patients. Breast Cancer Res Treat 1994;30:95-102.

26. Lønning P, Pfister C, Martoni A, Zamagni C. Pharmacokinetics of third-generation aromatase inhibitors. Semin Oncol 2003;30(Suppl 14):23-32.

27. Dowsett M, Pfister CU, Johnston SRD, Houston SJ, Miles DW, Verbeek JA, Smith IE. Pharmacokinetic interaction between letrozole and tamoxifen in postmenopausal patients with advanced breast cancer. The Breast 1997;6:245.

28. Geisler J, Detre S, Berntsen H, Ottestad L, Lindtjørn B, Dowsett M, Lønning PE. Influence of neoadjuvant anastrozole (Arimidex) on intratumoral estrogen levels and proliferation markers in patients with locally advanced breast cancer. Clin Cancer Res 2001;7:1230-36.

29. Geisler J, Haynes B, Anker G, Dowsett M, Lønning PE. Influence of letrozole (Femara) and anastrozole (Arimidex) on total body aromatization and plasma estrogen levels in postmenopausal breast cancer patients evaluated in a randomized, cross-over-designed study. J Clin Oncol 2002;20:751-57.

30. Geisler J, Helle S, Ekse D, Duong N, Evans D, Lonning P. Letrozole (Femara) causes potent suppression of breast cancer tissue estrogen levels in the neoadjuvant setting. J Clin Oncol 2006;24 :570s.

31. Khazaei M, Montaseri A, Casper R. Letrozole stimulates the growth of human endometrial explants cultured in three-dimensional fibrin matrix. Fertil Steril 2008;8. Epub ahead of print

32. Bajetta E, Ferrari L, Celio L, Mariani L, Miceli R, Di Leo A, et al. The aromatase inhibitor letrozole in advanced breast cancer: effects on serum insulin-like growth factor (IGF)-I and IGF-binding protein-3 levels. J Steroid Biochem Mol Biol 1997;63:261-67.

33. Talavera F, Reynolds RK, Roberts JA, Menon MJ. Insulin-like growth factor I receptors in normal and neoplastic human endometrium. Cancer Res 1990;50:3019-24.

34. Murphy LJ, Murphy LC, Friesen HG. Estrogen induces insulin-like growth factor-I expression in rat uterus. Mol Endocrinol 1987;1:445-50.

35. Geisler J, Lønning PE. Aromatase inhibition: transaltion into a successful therapeutic approach. Clinical Cancer Research 2005 ;11:2809-21.

36. Tominaga T, Adachi I, Sasaki Y, Tabei T, Ikeda T, Takatsuka Y, Toi M, Suwa T, Ohashi Y. Double-blind randomised trial comparing the non-steroidal aromatase inhibitors letrozole and fadrozole in postmenopausal women with advanced breast cancer. Annals of Oncology 2003;14: 62-70.

37. Ajay S. Bhatnagar. The discovery and mechanism of action of letrozole. Breast Cancer Research and Treatment, 2007;105 (Suppl 1):2-17.

38. Ponzone R, Mininanni P, Cassina E, Pastorino F, Sismondi P. Aromatase inhibitors for breast cancer: different structures, same effects? Endocr Relat Cancer 2008; 15(1): 27-36.

39. Harold J Burstein. Aromatase inhibitor-associated arthralgia syndrome. The Breast 2007;16(3): 223-34.

40. Reid DM, Doughty J, Eastell R, Heys SD, Howell A, McCloskey EV, Powles T, Selby P, Coleman RE. Guidance for the management of breast cancer treatment-induced bone loss: a consensus position statement from a UK Expert Group. Cancer Treat Rev. 2008;34 Suppl 1:S3-18. Epub 2008 Jun 2.

41. Wu M, Wang C, Lin C, Chen L, Chang W, Tsai S. Distinct regulation of cyclooxygenase-2 by interleukin-1(beta) in normal and endometriotic stromal cells. J Clin Endocrinol Metab 2005;90(1):286-95.

42. Ota H, Igarashi S, Sasaki M, Tanaka T. Distribution of cyclooxygenase-2 in eutopic and ectopic endometrium in endometriosis and adenomyosis. Hum Reprod 2001;16: 561-66.

43. Moudgal NR, Shetty G, Selvaraj N, Bhatnagar AS. Use of a specific aromatase inhibitor for determining whether there is a role for oestrogen in follicle/oocyte maturation, ovulation and preimplantation embryo development. J Reprod Fertil Suppl 1996;50:69-81.

44. Santen RJ, Samojlik E, Wells SA. Resistance of the ovary to blockade of aromatization with aminoglutethimide. J Clin Endocrinol Metab 1980;51:473-77.

45. Harris AL, Dowsett M, Jeffcoate SL, McKinna JA, Morgan M, Smith IE. Endocrine and therapeutic effects of aminoglutethimide in premenopausal patients with breast cancer. J Clin Endocrinol Metab 1982;55:718-22.

46. Wander HE, Blossey HC, Nagel GA. Aminoglutethimide in the treatment of premenopausal patients with metastatic breast cancer. Eur J Cancer Clin Oncol 1986;22:1371-74.

47. Stein RC, Dowsett M, Hedley A, Davenport J, Gazet JC, Ford HT, et al. Treatment of advanced breast cancer in postmenopausal women with 4-hydroxyandrostenedione. Cancer Chemother Pharmacol 1990;26:75-78.

48. Wouters W, De Coster R, Krekels M, van Dun J, Beerens D, Haelterman C, et al. R 76713, a new specific non-steroidal aromatase inhibitor. J Steroid Biochem 1989;32: 781-88.

49. Stein RC, Dowsett M, Hedley A, Gazet JC, Ford HT, Coombes RC. The clinical and endocrine effects of 4-hydroxyandrostenedione alone and in combination with goserelin in premenopausal women with advanced breast cancer. Br J Cancer 1990;62:679-83.

50. Takayama K, Zeitoun K, Gunby RT, Sasano H, Carr BR, Bulun SE. Treatment of severe postmenopausal endometriosis with an aromatase inhibitor. Fertil Steril. 1998;69(4):709-13.

51. Fatemi HM, Al-Turki HA, Papanikolaou EG, Kosmas L, DeSutter P, Devroey P. Successful treatment of an aggressive recurrent postmenopausal endometriosis with an aromatase inhibitor. Reprod Biomed Online 2005;11(4): 455-57.

52. Oxholm, Dorthe, Knudsen, Ulla Breth, Kryger-Baggesen, Niels and Ravn, Pernille. Postmenopausal endometriosis. Acta Obstetricia et Gynecologica Scandinavica 2007;86(10): 1158-64.

53. Vercellini P, Trespidi L, Colombo A. A gonadotropin-releasing hormone agonist versus a low-dose oral contra-ceptive for pelvic pain associated with endometriosis. Fertil Steril 1993;60:75-9.

54. Waller KG, Shaw RW. Gonadotropin-releasing hormone analogues for the treatment of endometriosis: long-term follow-up. Fertil Steril 1993; 59:511-15.

55. Vercellini P, Trespidi L, DeGiorgi O, Cortesi I, Parazzini F, Crosignani PG. Endometriosis and pelvic pain. Relation to disease stage and localization. Fertil Steril 1996;65:299-304.

56. Kauppila A. Changing concepts of medical treatment of endometriosis. Acta Obstet Gynecol Scand 1993;72:324-36.

57. Vercellini P, Fedele L, Bianchi S, Candiani GB. Pelvic dener-vation for chronic pain associated with endometriosis: fact or fancy? Am J Obstet Gynecol 1991;165:745-49.

58. Wilson ML, Farquhar CM, Sinclair OJ, Johnson NP. Surgical interruption of pelvic nerve pathways for primary and secondary dysmenorrhoea. Cochrane Database Syst Rev 2000;(2):CD001896.

59. Gambone JC, Mittman BS, Munro MG, Scialli AR, Winkel CA. Consensus statement for the management of chronic pelvic pain and endometriosis:proceedings of an expert-panel consensus process. Fertil Steril 2002;78:961-72.

60. Olive DL, Pritts EA. The treatment of endometriosis: a review of the evidence. Ann NY Acad Sci 2002;955:360 -72.

61. Vercellini P, De Giorgi O, Pisacreta A, Pesole AP, Vicentini S, Crosignani PG. Surgical management of endometriosis. Baillieres Best Pract Res Clin Obstet Gynaecol 2000;14:501-23.

62. Shippen ER, West WJ Jr. Successful treatment of severe endometriosis in two premenopausal women with an aromatase inhibitor. Fertil Steril 2004;81:1395-98.

63. Takayama K, Zeitoun K, Gunby RT, Sasano H, Carr BR, Bulun SE. Treatment of severe postmenopausal endometriosis with an aromatase inhibitor. Fertil Steril 1998;69:709-13.

64. Razzi S, Fava A, Sartini A, De Simone S, Cobellis L, Petraglia F. Treatment of severe recurrent endometriosis with an aromatase inhibitor in a young ovariectomised woman. Br J Obstet Gynaecol 2004;111:182-84.

65. Remorgida V, Abbamonte HL, Ragni N, Fulcheri E, Ferrero S. Letrozole and norethisterone acetate in recto-vaginal endometriosis. Fertil Steril. 2007 Sep;88(3):724-6. Epub 2007 Feb 28.

66. Mitwally MF, Casper RF, Diamond MP. Oestrogen-selective modulation of FSH and LH secretion by pituitary gland. Br J Cancer 2005 ;92(2):416-17.

67. Bohrer J, Chen CC, Falcone T. Persistent bilateral ureteral obstruction secondary to endometriosis despite treatment with an aromatase inhibitor. Fertil Steril 2008;90(5): 2004.e7-9. Epub 2008 Jun 16.

68. Ailawadi R, Jobanputra S, Kataria M, Gurates B, Bulun SE. Treatment of endometriosis and chronic pelvic pain with letrozole and norethindrone acetate: a pilot study. Fertil Steril 2004;81:290-96.

69. Razzi S, Fava A. Treatment of severe recurrent endometriosis with an aromatase inhibitor in a young ovariectomised woman. BJOG 2004;81:290-96.

70. Shippen ER, West WJ Jr. Successful treatment of severe endometriosis in two premenopausal women with an aromatase inhibitor. Fertil Steril 2004;81:1395-98.

71. Soysal S, Soysal M, Ozer S, Gul N, Gezgin T. The effects of post-surgical administration of goserelin plus anastrazole compared to goserelin alone in patients with severe endometriosis: a prospective randomized trial. Hum Reprod 2004;19:160-67.

72. Hefler L, Grimm C, van Trotsenburg M, Nagele F. Role of the vaginally administered aromatase inhibitor anastrozole in women with rectovaginal endometriosis: a pilot study. Fertil Steril 2005;84:1033-36.

73. Amsterdam LL, Gentry W, Jobanputra S, Wolf M, Rubin SD, Bulun SE. Anastrazole and oral contraceptives: a novel treatment for endometriosis. Fertil Steril 2005;84:300-304.

74. Mousa NA, Bedaiwy MA, Casper RF. Aromatase inhibitors in the treatment of severe endometriosis. Obstet Gynecol 2007;109(6):1421-23.

75. Remorgida V, Abbamonte LH, Ragni N, Fulcheri E, Ferrero S. Letrozole and desogestrel-only contraceptive pill for the treatment of stage IV endometriosis. Aust N Z J Obstet Gynaecol 2007;47(3):222-25.

76. Verma A, Konje JC. Successful treatment of refractory endometriosis-related chronic pelvic pain with aromatase inhibitors in premenopausal patients. Eur J Obstet Gynecol Reprod Biol. 2009 Feb 20. [Epub ahead of print.]

77. Lossl K, Loft A, Freiesleben NL, Bangsbøll S, Andersen CY, Pedersen AT, Hartwell D, Andersen AN. Combined down-regulation by aromatase inhibitor and GnRH-agonist in IVF patients with endometriomas-A pilot study. Eur J Obstet Gynecol Reprod Biol. 2009 Mar 2. [Epub ahead of print.]

78. Healey S, Tan SL, Tulandi T, Biljan MM. Effects of letrozole on superovulation with gonadotropins in women undergoing intrauterine insemination. Fertil Steril 2003;806:1325-29.

79. Cortinez A, De Carvalho I, Vantman D, et al. Hormonal profile and endometrial morphology in letrozole-controlled ovarian hyperstimulation in ovulatory infertile patients. Fertil Steril 2005;83(1):110-15.

80. Fatemi HM, Kolibianakis E, Tournaye H, et al. Clomiphene citrate versus letrozole for ovarian stimulation: a pilot study. Reprod Biomed Online 2003;75:543-46.

81. Harris HA. Mol Endocrinol. Estrogen receptor-beta: recent lessons from in vivo studies. 2007;21(1):1-13. Epub 2006 Mar 23.

82. Acconcia F, Kumar R. Signaling regulation of genomic and nongenomic functions of estrogen receptors. Cancer Lett 2006 8;238(1):1-14 Epub 2005 Aug 3.

83. Gabos P. Clomiphene citrate therapy and associated ovarian endometrial cysts. Obstet Gynecol 1979;53(6):763-65.

84. Capelo FO, Kumar A, Steinkampf MP, Azziz R. Laparoscopic evaluation following failure to achieve pregnancy after ovulation induction with clomiphene citrate. Fertil Steril 2003;80(6):1450-53.

85. Mitwally MFM, Albuarki H, Ashraf M, Diamond MP, Abuzeid M. Clomiphene reduces chance of pregnancy in infertile women with endometriosis following laparoscopic surgery. J Soc Gynecol Investig 2006;13(2): Abstract 646: page 277A.

86. Practice Committee of the American Society for Reproductive Medicine. Effectiveness and treatment for unexplained infertility. Fertil Steril 2006;86(5 Suppl): S111-14.

87. Dupont A, Dupont P, Belanger A, Mailoux J, Cusan L, Labrie F. Hormonal and biochemical changes during treatment of endometriosis with the luteinizing hormone-releasing hormone (LH-RH) agonist D-Trp6,des-Gly-NH2(10). LH-RH ethylamide. Fertil Steril 1990;54: 227-32.

88. Saito S, Murakami T, Suzuki K, Terada Y, Fukushima K, Moriya T. Intestinal endometriosis complicated by ileal perforation after initiation of gonadotropin-releasing hormone agonist therapy. Fertil Steril 2007;88:969.e7-9.

89. Hall LLH, Malone JM, Ginsburg KA. Flare-up of endometriosis induced by gonadotropin-releasing hormone agonist leading to bowel obstruction. Fertil Steril 1995;64:1204-06.

90. Bedaiwy MA, Mousa NA, Casper RF. Aromatase inhibitors prevent the estrogen rise associated with the flare effect of gonadotropins in patients treated with GnRH agonists. Fertil Steril. 2009 Apr;91(4 Suppl):1574-77.

91. Fong YF, Singh K. Medical treatment of a grossly enlarged adenomyotic uterus with the levonorgestrel-releasing intrauterine system. Contraception 1999;60:173-75.

92. Kitawaki J, Noguchi T, Amatsu T, Maeda K, Tsukamoto K, Yamamoto T. Expression of aromatase cytochrome P450 protein and messenger ribonucleic acid in human endometriotic and adenomyotic tissue but not in normal endometrium. Biol Reprod 1997;57:514-19.

93. Fuminori Kimura, Kentaro Takahashi, Koichi Takebayashi, Mutsuko Fujiwara, Nobuyuki Kita, Yoichi Noda, Nobuhiro Harada. Concomitant treatment of severe uterine adenomyosis in a premenopausal woman with an aromatase inhibitor and a gonadotropin-releasing hormone agonist. Fert Sterility 2007;87(6):1468-69.

Friedrich Wieser, Robert N Taylor

Chapter
30

Botanical Therapies

Introduction

Endometriosis, a chronic inflammatory disease, affects about 10% of all reproductive-aged women (approximately 70 million worldwide) and the prevalence rises to 20-50% in infertile women.[1] Endometriosis is defined by the presence of endometrial cells outside the uterine cavity (ectopic endometrial cells), which are postulated to arise due to retrograde menstrual dissemination. The implantation hypothesis is the most widely accepted,[2] supported by observations that retrograde menstruation and intraperitoneal spillage of viable endometrial cells occur frequently in cycling women and more commonly in those with genital outflow tract anomalies.

Local inflammation is activated in endometriosis as shown by significantly elevated levels of peritoneal inflammatory and angiogenic cytokines. In endometriotic tissues key anti-inflammatory transcription factors (e.g. progesterone receptor B (PR-B)) are downregulated, whereas pro-inflammatory transcription factors (e.g. NF-kB) are upregulated; as a consequence, expression of pro-inflammatory cytokines and chemokines is increased. Endometriosis seems to be a systemic disease. Women with endometriosis report local and systemic symptoms such as pelvic pain, dysmenorrhea, depression, headache, anxiety, sleeping disorders, and bowel symptoms.

Endometriosis has societal effects in terms of cost, lost work productivity and comorbidity. More than 20% of symptomatic women with endometriosis have associated diseases including migraine, endocrine disorders, autoimmune diseases, and chronic fatigue syndrome.[3] Endometriosis has a profound effect on women's health; with some women reporting symptoms for as many as 20 years until successful treatment of endometriosis.[4]

While traditionally a surgically-treated disorder, endometriosis is a complex, systemic disease that begs for a multi-faceted therapeutic approach. Current treatment strategies involve initial management by NSAIDs and oral contraceptives for several years. Unfortunately, the use of more potent therapeutics like GnRH agonists, medroxyprogesterone acetate (MPA), and danazol, occasions untoward side effects including vasomotor symptoms, headache, insomnia, lipid alterations, and osteoporosis. MPA is partly inefficient because of observed progesterone insensitivity in endometriosis. Moreover, these hormonal agents bear side effects that limit their long-term use. Physicians are particularly reluctant to prescribe drugs that result in osteoporosis in adolescent women with endometriosis for symptoms that are anticipated to continue for many years.

Among the newer strategies are botanical preparations that are being considered as potentially safer and promising therapeutic agents. The increasing popularity of natural products has stimulated scientific and clinical studies assessing the composition and clinical usefulness of botanical treatments of inflammatory diseases such as endometriosis. In this summary the mechanisms and efficacy of several botanicals with exciting potential to treat endometriosis are presented.

Nuclear Factor-KappaB (NF-κB) Pathway – A Target for Treatment of Endometriosis

NF-kB is a family of closely related protein dimers that bind to a common sequence motif in DNA called the κB site.[5] The NF-κB pathway activates many of the target genes that are critical to the initiation and establishment of the early and late stages of endometriosis including the induction of gene expression of several key pro-inflammatory, chemokine, angiogenic, prostanoid, and cell-cycle genes **(Figure 30-1)**. NF-κB is an excellent potential

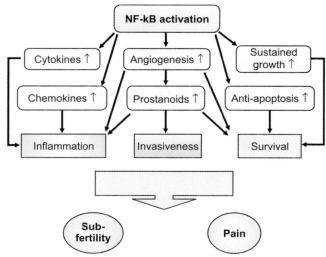

FIGURE 30-1: A postulated model that illustrates NF-κB mediated molecular and cellular aberrations leading to endometriosis-associated symptoms.

drug target to diminish inflammatory and angiogenic responses in endometriosis **(Figure 30-1)**.[6] Physiological suppression of NF-κB activity and the downstream inhibition of associated cytokine expression by functional progesterone receptors (PR) are essential to the physiological regulation of inflammatory processes in the endometrium during the menstrual cycle. In women with endometriosis, the NF-κB pathway is constitutively activated in eutopic endometrium, and ectopic lesions, and peritoneal macrophages.[6-8]

Activation of the NF-κB pathway and disturbance of other anti-inflammatory mechanisms lead to an overall inflammatory/angiogenic response with the upregulation of several cytokines (e.g. tumor necrosis factor (TNF-α), chemokines (regulated on Activation, Normal T Cell Expressed and Secreted (RANTES), and monocyte chemoattractant protein (MCP-1)), and angiogenic factors (vascular endothelial growth factor (VEGF)) that are controlled by NF-κB. Interestingly, TNF-α is itself an inducer of NF-κB, propagating the establishment, growth and persistence of endometriotic implants directly and indirectly. TNF-α is a potent inducer of new vessel growth and propagates endometriosis by generating a cascade of cytokines (interleukin (IL-6, and IL-8), matrix metallo-proteinases (MMPs), prostanoids and other mediators, including TNF-α itself. Increased production of chemokines such as RANTES in endometriosis tissues promotes immune cell recruitment. It is widely accepted that increased angiogenesis plays an essential role in the growth and survival of endometriotic lesions. VEGF plays a major role in inductions of inflammation by promoting

angiogenesis in women with endometriosis. Increased angiogenic activity has been demonstrated in endometriotic lesions of women with endometriosis.

The NF-κB regulated inflammatory/angiogenic responses in endometriosis, which are postulated to lead to endometriosis associated symptoms including pain and infertility, are under direct or indirect influence by ovarian steroid hormones. Standard hormonal endometriosis therapies, including progestagens, danazol, and GnRH-agonists appear to suppress the NF-κB pathway by inhibiting LH and FSH secretion and preventing follicular growth and estrogen production. Unfortunately, the use of these hormonal standard endometriosis treatments occasions untoward side effects that limit long-term adherence. Dietary components and botanicals provide an alternative source of NF-κB inhibitors such as polyphenols (genistein, emodin), terpenes (eugenol, lycopene, glycyrrhizin), alkaloids (piperine), flavonoids (flavopiridol), phenolics (ethyl gallate, gingerol), and others (resveratrol, vitamin C, vitamin E).[5]

Treatment Strategies

Pharmaceutical scientists are currently focusing on the development and application of new drugs exhibiting higher efficacy, fewer side effects and better safety profiles for long-term treatment, especially in young women with severe endometriosis. Hormonal agents, including selective estrogen receptor modulates (SERMs), selective proges-terone receptor modulators (SPRMs), aromatase inhibitors, as well as non-hormonal agents such as thiazolidi-nediones, cyclooxygenase (COX)-2 selective antagonists, anti-angiogenic agents, MMP-inhibitors, recombinant human TNF-α binding proteins, and interferon-α-2b have been investigated. Although, evidence from pre-clinical trials suggests beneficial effects of these compounds, efficient therapeutic options for long-term management of the treatment of endometriosis-associated symptoms are seriously needed.

Experimental endocrine therapies continue to exhibit untoward side effects. Surprisingly, the SERM, raloxifene, when prescribed following ablative endometriosis surgery, actually shortened the time to recurrence of pelvic pain.[9] The SPRM, asoprisnil (J867), showed excellent anti-proliferative effects on the endometrium of subhuman primates and effectively reduced non-menstrual pain and dysemenorrhea in women with endometriosis. However, asoprisnil was observed to induce cystically dilated glands called a 'non-physiologic secretory effect' in the eutopic endometrium of treated women.[10] Thiazolidinediones and

COX-2 inhibitors have been investigated as potential endometriosis treatments because of their anti-inflammatory and anti-proliferative effects. However, some of these trials have been suspended because of unanticipated cardiovascular side effects.

In general, women with endometriosis experience symptoms over an average of 20 years duration. Because of the limitations and side effects of conventional therapy, patients and scientists are exploring alternative options to allopathic medicine for the treatment of endometriosis. Complementary alternative medicine (CAM) pain therapies have gained popularity among women with endometriosis. In some populations of women with endometriosis, CAM used in combination with allopathic medicine or even as the sole treatment has completely replaced standard pharmacological options.[11] Common alternative approaches are dietary modifications, intake of nutritional supplements and use of herbal therapies. CAM treatments including nutraceuticals (e.g. vitamins E, B1 and omega-3 fatty acids) and herbal therapies have been shown to have anti-inflammatory and antinociceptive effects and are being evaluated for the treatment of endometriosis associated symptoms. We will review their efficacy below.

Herbal Therapies

Clinical Trials of Herbal Therapies for Endometriosis

Recently, medicinal herbal treatments have gained popularity in Western cultures for inflammatory diseases such as endometriosis. Historically, many Asian cultures (e.g. India, Japan, China, Korea) have depended on herbal treatment of many illnesses. There are numerous anecdotal reports on the successful use of botanicals for endometriosis associated infertility and pain.[12] Clinical studies have been performed with herbal formulae consisting of 4 to 11 different medicinal herb constituents **(Table 30-1)**.[12] Examples of herbal combinations or recipes that have been used to treat endometriosis-associated symptoms include: Dan'e recipe, Keishi-bukuryo-gan (KBG), Neiyi recipe, Neiyixiao recipe, Shaofu Zhuyu Tang, Shixiao Guijie Tang, and Yiweining.[12] Herbal mixtures have gained popularity because they are effective and lack the untoward hormonal side effects of standard endometriosis agents. In a recent meta-analysis, promising evidence in the literature supported that herbal mixtures are useful in the treatment of primary dysmenorrhea.[13] Yang et al showed that Yiweining (consisting of Chinese angelica, corydalis,

curcuma, persica, red peony, safflower, salvia root, and tortoise shell) was safe and its efficacy was similar to a synthetic progestin, gestrinone, in the prevention of postoperative recurrences of endometriosis.[14] and symptoms including pain and infertility.

Herbs used for the treatment of endometriosis associated symptoms have been generally prescribed for infertility and other menstrual disorders in Chinese medicine. As a result, several of the formulae used for endometriosis and infertility are interchangeable. Medicinal herbs used for infertility include bupleurum, Chinese angelica, cnidium fruit, gentiana, litchi seed, cinnamon, poria and white peony **(Table 30-1)**. However, some of the formulae for endometriosis associated infertility contain exotic materials including deer antler and sea horse (NB, the authors do not recommend use of products derived from endangered species).

Unfortunately, the standards of objective evaluation have been only sporadically applied in published clinical studies of herbal medicine and few studies of herbal treatments of endometriosis meet Western guidelines of evidence-based medicine. Further, a major difficulty in the study of clinical effects of herbal combinations is that traditional health care providers tend to individualize herbal compositions for each woman according to her unique endometriosis symptoms.

Nevertheless, there have been recent efforts at the US National Institute of Health by the National Center of Complementary and Alternative Medicine (NCCAM) to apply methods of evidence-based medicine on the study of botanicals. The NCCAM Institute of the NIH was established in 2000 in an attempt to validate popular and effective traditional herbal treatments.[15] While NCCAM has funded several studies of herbal therapy in the field of cancer, infectious diseases, and inflammatory disorders, to date, only a single NCCAM clinical trial has been carried out to evaluate the use of traditional Chinese medicine for endometriosis. Protocol NCT00034047 at Oregon Health Sciences University and the Oregon College of Oriental Medicine was funded by NCCAM and recently completed, and it is hoped that it will serve as a landmark study in endometriosis therapy.

An intricate challenge to the objective analysis of CAM therapies is the complexity of therapy with herbal mixtures. However, this complexity is grounded in 3000 years of empiric evidence and represents a synergistic approach that was designed to reduce side effects and increase efficacy when compared to single agent therapies. Rigorous interpretation of nutritional studies regarding the effects of dietary patterns on cancer and cardiovascular

Table 30-1: Botanicals used in the treatment of endometriosis				
English name	Pinyin Name	Literal Name	Botanical Name	Pharmaceutical Name
Bupleurum	Chai Hu	Kindling of the barbarians	Bupleurum chinense DC.	Radix Bupleuri
Chinese angelica	Dang Gui	State of return	Angelica sinensis	Radix Angelica Sinensis
Cattail pollen	Pu Huang	Cattail pollen	Typha angustifolia	Pollen Typhae
Cinnamon twigs	Gui zhi	Cinnamon twigs	Cinnamoomum cassia	Ramulus Cinnamomi
Cnidium	Chuang Xiong	-	Ligusticum chuanxiong	Rhizoma Ligustici
Corydalis	Yan Hu Suo	-	Corydalis turtschaninovii	Rhizoma Corydalis
Curcuma	Yu Jin	Constrained metal	Curcuma aromatica	Radix Curcumae
Cyperus	Xiang Fu	Aromatic appendage	Cyperus rotundus	Rhizoma Cyperi
Dahurian angelica	Bai Zhi	White rootlet	Angelica Dahurica	Radix Angelicae Dahuricae
Frankincense	Ru Xiang	Fragrant breast	Boswellia carterii	Gummi Olibanum
Licorice root	Gan Cao	Sweet herb	Glycyrrhiza uralensis	Radix Glycyrrhizae
Myrrh	Mo Yao	-	Commiphora myrha	Myrrha
Persica	Tao Ren	Persia seed	Prunus persica	Semen Persicae
Poria	Fu Ling	-	Poria cocos	Poria
Red peony root	Chi Shao	Bright red peony	Paeonia veitchii Lynch.	Radix Paeoniae Rubrae
Rhubarb	Da Huang	Big yellow	Rheum plamatum L.	Radix et Rhizoma Rhei
Salvia root	Dan Shen	-	Salvia miltiorrhiza	Radix Salvia Miltiorrhizae
Scutellaria	Huang Qin	-	Scutellaria baicalensis	Radix Scutellaria
Sparganium	San Leng	Three edges	Sparganium stoloniferum	Rhizoma Sparganii
Turmeric	Jiang Huang	Ginger yellow	Curcuma longa L.	Rhizoma Curcumae Longae
White peony root	Bai Shao	White peony	Paeonia lactiflora Pall.	Radix Paeonia Alba

disease prevention has led to the definition of the "whole food" concept. This principle, that benefits of the entire diet may exceed more than the sum of its parts, also is likely to hold for synergistic herbal therapies. Nevertheless, researchers need to recognize that better analytical tools are needed to delineate optimal dietary/therapeutic regimens.

In vitro and In vivo Studies of Herbal Therapies for Endometriosis

To establish proof-of-principle, many investigators have used models of endometriosis to evaluate the potential efficacy of these botanical therapies. Herbal mixtures used for endometriosis treatment consist of several potential candidate herbs that have been shown to exert anti-inflammatory and antinociceptive effects. For example, Yiweining is a traditional herbal formula composed of Chinese angelica, corydalis, curcuma, persica, red peony,

safflower, salvia root, and tortoise shell. Yiweining decreased serum cytokine levels (e.g. TNF-α, IL-6, and IL-8) and reduced expression of COX-2 mRNA in rodent endometriosis models.[16] We have studied a commonly used endometriosis herbal mixture (Channel Flow®) consisting of nine different herbs (Chinese angelica, dahurian angelica, cinnamon, corydalis extract, frankincense, licorice, myrrh, salvia, and white peony) in an *in vitro* model of endometriosis.[17] We showed that the herbal mixture has anti-inflammatory effects on human endometriotic cells, resulting in decreased RANTES production.[17] We originally chose this formula because of its traditional use in gynecologic health-related conditions, its commercial over-the-counter availability, and also based on numerous anecdotal reports of its beneficial effects in endometriosis. Moreover, all the botanicals within the formula were reported to exhibit some anti-inflammatory properties **(Table 30-2)**.[12] In addition to its

Table 30-2: Botanicals and their anti-inflammatory effects					
Botanicals	*Major active component*	*Antioxidant*	*COX-2↓*	*Cytokines ↓*	*NF-kB ↓*
Bupleurum	Triterpenoids			+	+
Chinese angelica	Ferulic acid	+		+	
Cattail pollen	Palmitic acid			+	
Cinnamon twigs	Cinnamonaldehyde		+	+	+
Cnidium	Alkaloids				
Corydalis	Tetrahydropalmitine			+	
Curcuma	Curcumin	+	+	+	+
Cyperus	Cyperene	+			
Dahurian angelica	Coumarins		+	+	+
Frankincense	Boswellic acids			+	+
Licorice root	Triterpenoids		+	+	+
Myrrh	Terpenoids	+		+	
Persica	Essential oils			+	
Poria	Pachymose		+	+	
Red Peony	Paeoniflorin	+			
Rhubarb	Emodin			+	+
Salvia root	Tanshinone	+			+
Scutellaria	Baicalin		+	+	+
Sparganium	Essential oils			+	
Turmeric	Curcumin	+	+	+	+
White peony root	Paeoniflorin		+	+	+

anti-inflammatory effects, the herbal mixture has anti-proliferative and pro-apoptotic effects *in vitro*, similar to hormonal drugs including MPA and danazol. Efficacy of less complex endometriosis formulae such as Neiyi or KBG is also promising. The anti-endometriosis herbal recipe Neiyi, consisting of persica, rhubarb, succinum, and tortoise shell, decreased prostaglandin (e.g. PGE_2) levels in clinical settings in women with endometriosis.[18] Another relatively simple formula, KBG (consisting of cinnamon, poria, red peony, persica, and tree peony bark) suppressed spontaneous development of adenomyosis in a murine endometriosis model.[19] The beneficial effects of Neiyi and KBG appear to be attributed to their COX-2 inhibiting effect.

Clinical Application of Plant-derived Pharmaceuticals

Several important drugs in our allopathic pharmacopeia are derived from natural products, including aspirin (from willow bark), penicillin (from fungus), artemisinin (from quinghaosu), mevacor (from fungus), taxol (from the pacific yew tree) and byetta (from Gila monster saliva). In the years between 1981 and 2002 more than 800 small molecule drugs were introduced worldwide, and more than half are of natural origin. It is suggested that plant-derived drugs will treat diseases with less side effects. Most of the natural analogs that have been investigated to date have little or no toxicity. As a result, plant-based products are seen to be more acceptable to patients than exotic synthetic drugs.

Several medicinal herbs with long-standing efficacy in the treatment of endometriosis-associated symptoms are currently in use **(see Table 30-1)**.[12, 20] Each of the herbs used to treat endometriosis is likely composed of multiple active components with anti-inflammatory properties **(Table 30-2)**. Popular botanicals used in various concentrations in Chinese herbal mixtures for the treatment of endometriosis include Chinese angelica, cinnamon, corydalis, curcuma, frankincense, myrrh, persica, prunella vulgaris, and white peony.[12] Many of these herbs have beneficial antioxidant and cytokine-suppressive effects as well as, anti-proliferative, pain-relieving effects in *in vitro* and/or *in vivo* models **(Table 30-2)**. Curiously, many of the medicinal herbs used to treat endometriosis associated pain were shown to suppress the NF-kB pathway, and its downstream cytokines and prostanoids.[12]

The pharmacological activities derived from these medicinal herbs modulate the inflammatory/angiogenic response. Several isolated components have been identified as active moieties, including alkaloids, terpenes, flavonoids, polyphenols, phenolics, and others. We will review their specific activities below.

Curcuma (Curcumin)

Curcuma belongs to the plant family Zingiberaceae, which consists of about 80 different Curcuma species such as Curcuma longa (turmeric) and Curcuma zeodaria. It is commonly used in Chinese and Indian (Ayurvedic) medicine to treat inflammatory diseases including rheumatoid arthritis and endometriosis.[12] Curcuma, one of the best studied medicinal herbs, exerts its prominent beneficial effects via suppression of the NF-kB pathway and NF-kB target genes; it also has a low toxicity profile.[21]

The main active components in Curcuma is curcumin (diferuloylmethane).[21] There are substantial *in vitro* and animal data indicating that curcumin has significant anti-inflammatory activity. That curcumin has potential against endometriosis was first reported in 2005. Cao et al demonstrated anti-inflammatory effects of curcumin in an *in vitro* endometriosis model, where NF-kB induction of the macrophage migration inhibitory factor (MIF) was prevented.[22] Recent studies corroborate that curcumin influences several important molecular targets, including cytokines (e.g. TNF-α, IL-1, IL-6), transcription factors (e.g. NF-kB, AP-1, Egr-1, beta-catenin, and PPAR-gamma), enzymes (e.g. COX-2, iNOS), growth factor receptors (e.g. EGFR and HER2) and cell regulatory proteins (e.g. cyclin D1 and D1 and p21) **(Table 30.2)**. In addition, curcumin has been shown to exert antinociceptive effects.[22] Newly developed synthetic analogs of curcumin (e.g. EF24-tripeptide chloromethyl ketone) have been introduced to treat cancer and chronic inflammatory diseases.[23, 24] These synthetic analogs of curcumin promise to have better bioavailability while retaining cytokine-modulating effects and may provide low-toxicity alternatives to treat endometriosis-associated symptoms.[23]

Dahurian Angelica (Coumarins)

Dahurian angelica is a root that contains various coumarin and furocoumarin derivatives, phenolic compounds with multiple biological activities, including inhibition of lipid peroxidation and neutrophil-dependent anion superoxide generation. Furanocoumarin, one of the active components of dahurian angelica, inhibited cycoloxygenase (COX)-2 and microsomal PGE2 synthase in rat peritoneal macrophages. Dahurian angelica is commonly used as an analgesic and antipyretic in conditions such as athralgia, headache, and sinusitits; dahurian angelica is a component of several Chinese anti-endometriosis herbal formulae and alleviates chronic pain and dysmenorrhea associated with endometriosis. Extracts of dahurian angelica have inhibitory effects on LPS-induced TNF-α, NO and PGE$_2$ production, and phosphorylation of MAPKs, following I-kBα degradation and NF-kB activation. All these described anti-inflammatory effects of dahurian angelica predict benefit in the treatment of endometriosis-associated symptoms.

Chinese Angelica (Ferulic Acid)

Dang Gui or Angelica sinensis, also has been used for thousands of years in traditional Chinese, Japanese, and Korean medicine. One of the active components of Chinese angelica is ferulic acid. Ferulic acid is a phytochemical commonly found in fruits and vegetables such as tomatoes, sweet corn and rice bran. Ferulic acid is observed to exert anti-inflammatory, antioxidant, and analgesic effects. Ferulic acid significantly inhibits the edema induced by carrageenin. Despite the fact that an estrogen-like activity was shown for Dang Gui, it is used in formulae to treat endometriosis symptoms. Its other indication is the treatment of peri- and menopausal symptoms in Chinese Medicine. Estrogenic effects of botanicals such as Dang Gui warrant caution for endometriosis therapy, particularly in risk populations. A water extract of Dang Gui dose-dependently and significantly stimulated the proliferation of MCF-7 cells with a weak estrogen-agonistic activity in the presence of 17β-estradiol.

Corydalis (Tetrahydropalamatine)

Corydalis is a medicinal herb that is commonly used in many formulae for the treatment of endometriosis and other pain syndromes. Tetrahydropalamatine is a major active pharmacologic component of Corydalis rhizome extract and has been shown to block post synaptic dopaminergic receptors. Corydalis was shown to be effective in adjuvant-induced inflammation and hyperalgesia in rats. In addition, Corydalis rhizome extract has also been shown to exhibit sedative, analgesic, hypnotic, and muscle relaxant properties, which are consistent with its dopamine receptor antagonism.

Salvia Root (Tanshinone)

Salvia root is known as red sage in traditional Chinese medicine and it has antioxidant and anti-inflammatory properties. Salvia root increases the activity of superoxide dismutase in platelets, thereby reducing oxygen-free radicals and platelet aggregation. One of the active components of Salvia root is Tanshinone IIA, a diterpene. Tanshinone IIA was shown to inhibit the phosphorylation of Ik-Bα in a dose dependent manner in activated RAW 264.7 macrophages, and to reduce the translocation of NF-kB from cytosol to nucleus.

Frankincense (Boswellic Acids)

Frankincense contains boswellic acids that are known to have anti-inflammatory and analgesic properties and make them useful in the treatment of endometriosis. In animal and *in vitro* studies, boswellic acids have been shown to inhibit lipoxygenase (LOX), an enzyme responsible for leukotriene synthesis. Other *in vitro* and *in vivo* studies have shown that boswellic acid suppresses NF-κB and COX-2. Boswellic acids have been studied in clinical trials for other inflammatory diseases including asthma and ulcerative colitis, where they have been shown to be effective. The potential of boswellic acids in the treatment of endometriosis appears to reflect their anti-inflammatory properties mediated through inhibition of NF-kB, COX-2 and LOX.

Cinnamon (Cinnamonaldehyde)

In traditional Chinese medicine, cinnamon is used to treat a variety of female reproductive disorders such as endometriosis and abdominal pain as well as peptic ulcer disease, diarrhea and flu symptoms. Cinnamonaldehyde was shown to inhibit COX-2 mediated PGE_2 secretion. Since recent data suggest that chronic use of selective COX-2 blockers is associated with increased cardiovascular risk, cinnamonaldehyde-based compounds may represent a potentially safer alternative source for the development of COX-2 selective inhibitors.

Drawbacks and Pitfalls of Herbal Therapies

Plant derived products are promising as new therapeutics because of their efficacy and low toxicity and based on their longstanding acceptance in traditional practice. However, one of the limiting factors of herbal products is their low bioavailability. The reasons for reduced bioavailability of natural products are manifold: low intrinsic activity, poor absorption from the gastrointestinal tract, high rate of metabolism, and rapid elimination and clearance. Poor absorption and rapid metabolism and elimination have led to the development of certain strategies to overcome these obstacles. Herb administration using adjuvants, liposomes, or nanoparticles have been considered, as has the clinical synthesis of analogs. Adjuvants can block metabolic pathways of natural products and have been shown to increase bioavailability up to 2000%. Liposomes, nanoparticles, micelles or phospholipid complexes are alternative ways to increase bioavailability by increasing gastrointestinal absorption, providing longer circulation times and resistance to metabolic processes. Another effective way to increase bioavailability of natural drugs is structural modification. Structural modification has led to the development of synthetic herbal analogs with higher potency and better bioavailability than their natural parent compounds. Structural modification of curcumin has led to one lead compound, EF24. EF24 showed higher intrinsic anti-tumor activity and better bioavailability than curcumin.[23] Novel delivery strategies and structural modifications of natural products promise to enhance efficacy and bioavailability of natural products and offer the means to generate develop new classes of drugs.

Another pitfall is that some herbal products are contaminated. As these compounds are typically not regulated by the FDA, production standards are more lax. Therefore, independent laboratories should be employed to screen for heavy metals, pesticide residues, and microbiological contamination of botanicals. Furthermore, the manufacturing of medicinal herbs should be conducted at state and federally licensed facilities that are regularly inspected, and have a regulated Quality Control department. Auditing at state and federally licensed facilities is usually conducted to make sure that methods and procedures meet or exceed all statutory requirements. Most of the herbs described in this review have been tested extensively in humans and animals. However, safety and effectiveness have generally not been proven according to standards of evidence-based medicine.

Unfortunately, evaluation of herb-drug interactions has been sparse and more studies need to be performed. It is our view that investigations of the efficacy, toxicity, absorption, distribution, metabolism, and excretion of potential botanicals should include testing in *in vitro* (cell culture) and *in vivo* (rodents, subhuman primates) models of endometriosis prior to their introduction in clinical trials. *In vitro* models can include primary endometriosis stromal cells and immortalized cell lines (e.g. EM42 and Ishikawa cell lines, models for epithelial endometrial cells). These are good models because the cells recapitulate the aggravated increased inflammatory response observed in women with endometriosis. Further, comparative analyses can be performed as *in vitro* models have been utilized previously to investigate anti-inflammatory and anti-proliferative effects of standard endometriosis treatments including GnRH-agonists, MPA, danazol, and oral contraceptives. A major limitation of *in vitro* endometriosis models is that absorption and metabolism kinetics of orally administered therapeutics, such as herbal mixtures, is bypassed and hence, may not be fully representative of the anticipated *in vivo* drug action. Surgically transplanted endometrial tissue in rodents provides another model to study the effects of experimental drugs on ectopic endometrial tissue. Rat endometriotic implants show histological transformations similar to those seen in human endometriotic lesions and are large enough for reproducible mRNA and protein preparations. In addition, although it is expensive and labor-intensive to perform, and requires more ethical oversight, surgically transplanted endometrial tissue in the baboon provides a primate model to study the effects of experimental drugs. We propose that knowledge gained from pre-clinical models will provide evidence to optimize the design of clinical trials for botanical therapies.

Conclusions

We have attempted to highlight the limitations of current regimens for endometriosis: untoward side effects, poor efficacy, and high costs. Given the natural history of the disease, in general, endometriosis treatment lasts throughout a woman's reproductive life, and necessitates well-tolerated approaches. Natural therapies, such as herbal mixtures or synthetic analogs, may have higher efficacy and fewer side effects than current hormonal anti-endometriosis treatment regimens. Many of the apparently effective natural therapies can interfere with multiple cell-signaling pathways including the NF-kB pathway, without suppression of estrogen levels, and hence should avoid the severe hypoestrogenic side effects that plague conventional treatments. In addition, herbal combinations with synergistic effects may augment the potential benefits of higher efficacy while minimizing toxicity. Once the

underlying molecular mechanisms for the observed anti-inflammatory and anti-proliferative effects of botanicals are elucidated, we believe that their health benefits can be exploited to develop new and better modalities for treating endometriosis. In the future, we expect that more women with endometriosis will be using phytotherapies to treat endometriosis associated-symptoms.

References

1. Guo SW, Wang Y. The prevalence of endometriosis in women with chronic pelvic pain. Gynecol Obstet Invest 2006;62 :121-30.
2. Sampson JA. Peritoneal endometriosis due to menstrual dissemination of endometrial tissue into the peritoneal cavity. Am J Obstet Gynecol 1927;14:442-69.
3. Sinaii N, Cleary SD, Ballweg ML, Nieman LK, Stratton P. High rates of autoimmune and endocrine disorders, fibromyalgia, chronic fatigue syndrome and atopic diseases among women with endometriosis: a survey analysis. Hum Reprod 2002;17:2715-24.
4. Sinaii N, Cleary SD, Younes N, Ballweg ML, Stratton P. Treatment utilization for endometriosis symptoms: a cross-sectional survey study of lifetime experience. Fertil Steril 2007;87:1277-86.
5. Aggarwal BB, Shishodia S. Molecular targets of dietary agents for prevention and therapy of cancer. Biochem Pharmacol 2006;71:1397-1421.
6. Wieser F, Vigne JL, Ryan I, Hornung D, Djalali S, Taylor RN. Sulindac Suppresses Nuclear Factor-(kappa)B Activation and RANTES Gene and Protein Expression in Endometrial Stromal Cells from Women with Endometriosis. J Clin Endocrinol Metab 2005;90:6441-47.
7. Lousse JC, Van Langendonckt A, Gonzalez-Ramos R, Defrere S, Renkin E, Donnez J. Increased activation of nuclear factor-kappa B (NF-kappaB) in isolated peritoneal macrophages of patients with endometriosis. Fertil Steril 2007;90:217-20.
8. Gonzalez-Ramos R, Donnez J, Defrere S, Leclercq I, Squifflet J, Lousse JC, et al. Nuclear factor-kappa B is constitutively activated in peritoneal endometriosis. Mol Hum Reprod 2007;13 :503-09.
9. Stratton P, Sinaii N, Segars J, Koziol D, Wesley R, Zimmer C, et al. Return of chronic pelvic pain from endometriosis after raloxifene treatment: a randomized controlled trial. Obstet Gynecol. 2008 ;111 :88-96.
10. Mutter GL, Bergeron C, Deligdisch L, Ferenczy A, Glant M, Merino M, et al. The spectrum of endometrial pathology induced by progesterone receptor modulators. Mod Pathol. 2008 ;21 :591-8.
11. Cox H, Henderson L, Wood R, Cagliarini G. Learning to take charge: women's experiences of living with endometriosis. Complement Ther Nurs Midwifery 2003;9:62-68.
12. Wieser F, Cohen M, Gaeddert A, Yu J, Burks-Wicks C, Berga SL, et al. Evolution of medical treatment for endometriosis: back to the roots? Hum Reprod Update 2007;13:487-99.

13. Zhu X, Proctor M, Bensoussan A, Wu E, Smith CA. Chinese herbal medicine for primary dysmenorrhoea. Cochrane Database Syst Rev 2008(2):CD005288.

14. Yang DX, Ma WG, Qu F, Ma BZ. Comparative study on the efficacy of Yiweining and Gestrinone for post-operational treatment of stage III endometriosis. Chin J Integr Med. 2006;12 :218-20.

15. Stokstad E. Alternative medicine. Stephen Straus's impossible job. Science. 2000 ;288 :1568-70.

16. Qu F, Zhou J, Ma B. The effect of Chinese herbs on the cytokines of rats with endometriosis. J Altern Complement Med 2005 ;11 :627-30.

17. Wieser F, Burks-Wicks C, Vigne JL, Cohen M, Gaeddert A, Taylor RN (Editors). An herbal remedy inhibits the expression of the chemokine regulated upon activation, normal T cell expressed, and secreted in endometriotic cells. World Conference of Endometriosis 2005; Maastricht, Netherlands.

18. Wang D, Wang Z, Yu C. Endometriosis treated by the method of resolving blood stasis to eliminate obstruction in the lower-jiao. J Tradit Chin Med 1998;18:7-11.

19. Mori T, Sakamoto S, Singtripop T, Park MK, Kato T, Kawashima S, et al. Suppression of spontaneous development of uterine adenomyosis by a Chinese herbal medicine, keishi-bukuryo-gan, in mice. Planta Med 1993; 59:308-11.

20. Chen J, Chen T. Chinese Medical Herbology and Pharmacology. City of Industry, CA, USA: Art of Medicine Press; 2004.

21. Anand P, Kunnumakkara AB, Newman RA, Aggarwal BB. Bioavailability of curcumin: problems and promises. Mol Pharm 2007;4:807-18.

22. Cao WG, Morin M, Metz C, Maheux R, Akoum A. Stimulation of macrophage migration inhibitory factor expression in endometrial stromal cells by interleukin 1, beta involving the nuclear transcription factor NF-kappaB. Biol Reprod 2005;73:565-70.

23. Adams BK, Ferstl EM, Davis MC, Herold M, Kurtkaya S, Camalier RF, et al. Synthesis and biological evaluation of novel curcumin analogs as anti-cancer and anti-angiogenesis agents. Bioorg Med Chem 2004;12: 3871-83.

24. Sun A, Shoji M, Lu YJ, Liotta DC, Snyder JP. Synthesis of EF24-tripeptide chloromethyl ketone: a novel curcumin-related anticancer drug delivery system. J Med Chem 2006;49:3153-58.

Edurne Novella-Maestre, Antonio Pellicer

Chapter 31

Antiangiogenic Agents in Endometriosis

Introduction

Endometriosis, defined as the presence of functional endometrium, composed of glands and stroma, outside the uterine cavity, is a common benign disease, causing abdominal pain, dysmenorrhea and dyspareunia in about 10–15% of all women in reproductive age and more than 30% of women attended in infertility clinics.[1]

There are a number of theories to explain how endometriosis occurs. Out of them, the implantation theory of Sampson (1927)[2] is the most widely accepted. According to Sampson,, the endometrial tissue is retrogradely shed through the Fallopian tubes into the peritoneal cavity, where it attaches and proliferates at ectopic sites during menstruation. However, endometriosis is a condition showing congenital tendencies and a polygenic/multifactorial etiology has been suggested. The cause for the adherence of the eutopic endometrium in ectopic locations remains unknown in these patients. In addition there are several factors like etiopathogenic, genetic, environmental, hormonal, immunologic, oxidative stress and growth factors which are implicated in the establishment, development and maintenance of endometriosis.

It is absolutely necessary to continue the research in this field to understand the mechanisms involved in endometriosis progression and to discover new treatments to relieve their symptoms. One of the main reasons to adopt this attitude is the absence of any wholly successful medical or surgical therapy and the unacceptable side effects provoked by long-term medical treatments, the epidemiological and social impact of endometriosis, and the disability suffered by each individual patient. Although endometriotic lesions can be removed at surgery improving the pain symptoms,[3] the disease may recur after surgical excision and a second approach should be necessary. As a result, some women may seek medical therapy in order to avoid or delay surgery.

The endometrium has the ability to adhere, attach, and implant ectopically.[4] For the survival in an ectopic location, the acquisition of an adequate blood supply is essential.[5] Thus, the endometrium has angiogenic potential and endometriotic lesions tend to expand in areas with a rich blood supply.[6] Consequently, disproportionate endometrial angiogenesis is proposed as a mechanism in the pathogenesis as well as a new therapeutic target for endometriosis treatment.

In order to study the initiation of endometriotic lesion formation, *ex vivo* and *in vitro* experimental animal models, have been developed.[7] Revascularization of endometriosis lesions has been analyzed in these models demonstrating that an adequate angiogenic response is critical for the successful survival and growth of endometrial tissue in ectopic locations.[8, 9] Various endometriosis models have shown that blocking the angiogenic cascade impairs the development of endometriosis-like lesions in animals[10-16] and in the chicken chorioallantoic membrane.[17] These animal models have provided crucial information on factors triggering angiogenesis and ectopic endometrial tissue revascularization. The continuous angiogenic stimulus and impulses for vascular remodeling to meet the needs of developing endometriotic tissue are guaranteed by the chronic inflammatory environment and the innate properties of the human endometrium.[8, 9] The existence of an imbalance between pro- and antiangiogenic growth factors in peritoneal fluid from endometriosis patients has been reported.[7, 18] In this context, inflammatory cells contribute to this proangiogenic environment.[19, 20] Recent studies have shown that dendritic cells also promote angiogenesis in experimental endometriotic lesions.[21]

Angiogenesis

Angiogenesis involves the formation of new blood vessels released by pre-existing vessels. Depending on their metabolic activity, any group of cells larger than 1 mm^3 may require to be feed by functioning blood vessels, as they cannot receive sufficient oxygen or nutrients by diffusion alone. There are at least 4 different mechanisms that may induce angiogenesis: sprouting, intussusception (internal division of vessels resulting in vessel splitting), elongation/widening, and incorporation of circulating endothelial cells into vessels.[22-25] The maturation of newly formed angiogenic blood vessels implies the recruitment of pericytes and smooth muscle cells, which are essential to stabilize vessels. In sprouting angiogenesis, the vascular endothelial cell activation along with the breakdown of the basement membrane, migration and proliferation of endothelial cells and tube formation are induced by the angiogenic stimulus **(Figure 31-1)**.

Endometriosis and Angiogenic Factors

The endometrium of women with endometriosis has an increased capacity to proliferate, implant, and grow in the peritoneal cavity. In human endometrium, blood vessels grow and regress every menstrual cycle under the overall control of estrogens and progesterone due to the similarity between the angiogenic mechanisms and those found in endometriotic lesions. The emerging evidence that estrogens can both promote and inhibit endometrial vessel growth under different circumstances, demonstrates the complex regulation of endometrial angiogenesis.[26] When the shed menstrual tissue arrives to the abdominal cavity, the induction of an inflammatory process takes place, in which several growth factors and cytokines (mainly secreted by the polymorph nuclear neutrophils (PMNs) population and activated macrophages) are concentrated in the peritoneal fluid (PF) takes place.[27-30] The aim of this inflammatory response is to eliminate the ectopic tissue and cells from the peritoneal cavity. These cells contribute to increase and elevate the oxidative stress and concentrations of inflammatory cytokines, chemoattractants and vasoactive substances. These substances certainly have an effect on the shed endometrial tissue improving its ectopial locations attachment.

During the angiogenic process endothelial cells proliferate, migrate and attach to the External Cellular Matrix (ECM), inducing matrix remodeling, and formation of a new lumen in the endometrium of women with endometriosis.[31, 32]

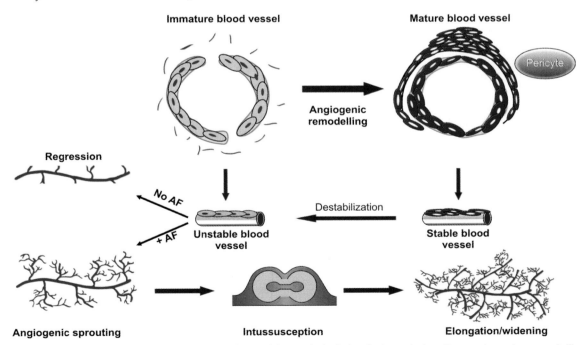

FIGURE 31-1: Angiogenesis. The blood vessels are formed by endothelial cells but, during the angiogenic remodelling process a recruitment of the pericytes and smooth muscle cells rounding the blood vessels exists, that confer stability and insensitivity to angiogenic factors (AF) and vasoactive signals, giving rise to mature blood vessels. However, before the formation of new blood vessels from pre-existing vessels, the mature blood vessels are destabilized. The absence of AF induces blood vessels regression but the presence of AF activates the angiogenic process (sprouting, intussusception, elongation/widening and incorporation of circulating endothelial cells into vessels).

Endometrial angiogenesis is regulated by several factors being particularly important the vascular endothelial growth factor (VEGF) family.[33] The human VEGF gene has been mapped to chromosome 6p12 and is made up of eight exons.[34] Exons 1–5 and 8 are always present in VEGF mRNA, whereas the expression of exons 6 and 7 is regulated by alternative splicing. This phenomenon produces various VEGF isoforms. In humans, five different VEGF mRNAs have been detected encoding the isoforms VEGF121, VEGF145, VEGF165, VEGF189, and VEGF206.[35] The isoforms VEGF121 and VEGF165 appear to be mainly involved in the process of angiogenesis.[36] Five endothelial cell-specific receptor tyrosine kinases, Flt-1 (VEGFR-1), KDR/Flk-1 (VEGFR-2), Flt4 (VEGFR-3), Tie and Tek/Tie-2, have so far been described, which possess the intrinsic tyrosine kinase activity essential for signal transduction.[37,38] The receptor Flk-1/KDR appears to be mainly involved in regulating angiogenesis and vasculogenesis.[39, 40]

VEGF is produced in huge quantities by activated macrophages and T-cells[41, 42] in menstrual effluent and mesothelial cells[43] besides by hypoxic endometrial cells during the menstrual phase.[44] VEGF is able to increase the vascular permeability of blood vessels inducing vascular changes in the peritoneal lining. The vascular permeability increment induces the fibrinogen extravasation into the peritoneum lining, after injection of tumor ascites or tumor cells,[45] leads to the generation of vascularized connective tissue. The fibrin deposits promote the adherence of leukocytes, cellular debris and endometrial cells to the peritoneal lining. Employing the CAM assay, it has been demonstrated that angiogenesis can be induced by the presence of soluble components in PF.[4]

Several reports demonstrate that the PF factors can provoke systemic effects supporting that the presence of factors in the PF, in enough quantity, can enter the circulation and exert their influence on endometriotic lesions in a systemic way. Dunselman et al (1988)[46] reported that proteins with a molecular weight <40 kDa could move between the vasculature and the PF. Intraperitoneal injection with interleukin (IL)-4 inhibits basic fibroblast growth factor (bFGF) induced corneal neovascularization.[47] Ogawa et al (2000)[48] observed a significant decrease in tumor growing when an antibody against macrophage inhibitory factor (MIF) was administered by intraperitoneal injection in mice bearing tumors. Bruner et al (1997)[47] were able to reduce lesion formation by intraperitoneal injection of tissue inhibitor of matrix metalloproteinase (TIMP-1) in an animal model.

Apart from VEGF, a number of factors with pro-angiogenic properties have been shown to be elevated in the peritoneal fluid of endometriosis patients, which are released in a stage-dependent pattern dependent of the disease. These factors include: interleukin 8 (IL-8),[49-52] hepatocyte growth factor (HGF),[53, 54] tumor necrosis factor-alpha (TNF-α),[4, 5] erythropoietin,[55] neutrophil-activating factor,[56] macrophage migration inhibitory factor,[57] interleukin 15 (IL-15),[58] and angiogenin.[59]

It is well known that endometriosis is an estrogen-dependent disease and exist evidences suggesting that estrogen can directly affect angiogenesis or vascular development. The increment of the local estrogen production can be due to the expression of 17β-hydroxysteroid dehydrogenase II, the enzyme that converts the active estradiol into the less active estrone, is suppressed in endometriotic tissue,[60] as well as, aromatase, the rate-limiting enzyme in estrogen biosynthesis, is expressed high levels in endometriotic lesions.[61]

It has been reported that estrogens are able to promote the increment of several proangiogenic factors such as TNF-α, stimulating endothelial cells via an increase in TNF-induced adhesion molecules E-selectin[62] or the induction of endothelial cell proliferation, VEGF expression[26] and nitric oxide synthase.[63]

The increment of several inflammatory factors such as macrophages,[64] T lymphocytes,[65] and mast cells[66, 67] are involved in the progression of the disease, in fact endometriosis is also considered a chronic inflammatory disease. A reduction of granulocytes number,[65] fibromuscular differentiation[68, 69] and active ECM remodeling and synthesis[70, 71] have been also described.

Elevated levels of cyclooxygenase-2 (COX-2) in endometriotic lesions[72, 73] have been reported as the result of the local inflammatory environment and the elevated levels of locally produced estrogen.[61, 74] COX-2 has angiogenic properties by modulation the VEGF production,[75] however it has been shown that COX-2 is able to antagonize VEGF-induced vascular permeability, and to upregulate the integrin αvβ3.[76]

CCN1 (Cyr61, cysteine-rich protein 61) gene, which belongs to a growing family of ECM-associated signalling proteins, has also an angiogenic function promoting the cell adhesion, migration, and neovascularization,[77] so continued expression of CCN1 in endometriosis patients may be important for the acquisition of a vasculature and lesion survival and growth.[78] It has been observed that CCN1 function is through integrin αvβ3,[79, 80] Comparing the endometriotic lesions and endometria gene expression profile of women with versus without endometriosis it was shown that CCN1 is one of the most up-regulated genes in endometria of women with endometriosis and in ectopic endometrium.[78] This expression has been shown to be much higher in the menstrual endometrium than in late proliferative endometrium.[81] The CCN1 is transcriptionally activated by TGF-b1 and bFGF, and in turn it regulates the production and/or activity of other angiogenic molecules as well as molecules that affect the ECM integrity.[77]

The CCN1 protein expression level in the endometrial epithelium is higher during the proliferative and in the epithelial and endothelial cells of the endometriotic lesions.[78] It is suspected a CCN1 estrogen-dependency expression due to its expression is clearly higher during the proliferative phase in endometria of women without endometriosis and it is also induced by estradiol in estradiol-dependent breast cancer cells.[82]

Antiangiogenic Therapy in Endometriosis

Different antiangiogenic treatments such as Anti-VEGF agents and other angiostatic drugs have been tested in experimental models of cancer and endometriosis with successful results inhibiting new vessel formation. These drugs, mainly with cytotoxic properties, target specifically the endothelial cells without penetrate in the tissues.

Angiostatic therapy can affect to various angiogenic response stages, i.e. TNP-470 inhibit endothelial cell proliferation, vitaxin (a humanized anti-avb3-integrin antibody) blocks endothelium-specific integrin survival signalling, batimastat (a MMP inhibitor) blocks extracellular matrix breakdown whereas others such as bevacizumab (a humanized VEGF-neutralizing antibody) neutralize activators of angiogenesis.[83] Recently, the use of bevacizumab, an anti-VEGF agent, has been approved for the treatment of certain defined cancer indications.[84]

The $VEGF_{165}$ is expressed in human ectopic endometrium,[85, 86] but there are another angiogenic factors that are expressed in endometriosis, showing alternative action points to shatter angiogenesis, for example angistatin[10] or angiopoietin 1 and 2.[87]

The initial experimental anti-VEGFR approaches to target angiogenesis, in endometriosis models *in vivo*, were carried out by Hull et al (2003)[11] using the Nude Mouse model. They observed that the administration a soluble truncated receptor that antagonizes VEGF and anti-VEGF-A antibody, induced a vascular destruction decreasing significantly the endometriotic explants. One year later, Nap et al (2004)[12] through the administration of several antiangiogenic agents in an heterologous mice model of endometriosis, demonstrated that avastin (a specific VEGF A inhibitor), and other general efficient angiogenesis

inhibitors, such as TNP-470, endostatin and anginex, significantly decreased the number of endometriosis lesions and blood vessels compared to the controls.

Employing the chicken chorioallantoic membrane (CAM) model, it was confirmed that the implantation of endometrium in ectopic locations induces a strong angiogenic response which seems to be decisive for the establishment, survival and growth of the lesions.[17] Furthermore, the antiangiogenic action of TNP-470, endostatin, anginex and anti-human VEGF antibody was tested in CAM model. The administration of these agents significantly inhibited the angiogenic response induced after the human endometrial tissue transplantation onto the CAM and abundant necrosis areas were observed.[17]

The efficacy of anti-VEGF agents in the treatment of endometriosis was confirmed in the Rhesus monkeys autograft model,[88] actually, the administration of an immunopurified antibody blocking VEGF receptor (anti-Flk1 antibody) determined a significant inhibition of endometriosis explants formation.

The inhibitory effect of Endostatin, an antiangiogenic agent used by Nap et al[12, 17] upon the growth of endometriotic lesions, was subsequently evaluated on a mouse homologous model. Although of the growth of surgically induced endometriosis was inhibited by approximately 50% when the endostatin treatment was initiated immediately after surgical transplantation, this therapy was uneffective when being applied in established lesions.[13] Further studies have demonstrated that two synthetic fragments of the endostatin molecule show an inhibitory activity on the growth of endometriotic lesions.[89]

Novel endometriosis model studies in rodents equipped with dorsal skinfold chambers as means to analyze *in vivo* the angiogenic process in ectopic endometrial tissue established that the administration of rapamycin, an immunosuppressant drug used to prevent rejection in organ transplantation, induced in a significant manner the regression of endometriotic lesions.[14, 90] This effect was associated with the inhibition of VEGF-mediated angiogenesis as indicated by a suppression of endothelial cell sprouting *in vitro* and a reduction of microvessel density in endometriotic lesions *in vivo*.

The angiogenic inhibition effectiveness of TNP-470, previously tested by Nap et al (2004)[12] in an endometriosis mouse model, has been recently tested in a cancer model.[91] The TNP-470 conjugated to monomethoxy-polyethylene glycol-polylactic can be absorbed by the intestine and selectively accumulate in tumors. This acid which forms nanopolymeric micelles was able to inhibit the tumor growth, without causing neurological impairment in tumor-bearing mice. When this oral nontoxic antiangiogenic drug is orally administered, it is particularly effective in preventing the development of liver metastasis in mice proving that it could be chronically administered for cancer therapy or metastasis prevention.[91]

In humans, these agents have been tested to inhibit angiogenesis in oncology patients, specifically when employing avastin, a human anti-VEGF antibody employed for this purpose[92, 83] or rapamycin another antibody currently used for the prevention of allograft rejection following renal and other solid organ transplantation[93-96] and for incorporating into drug-eluting stents to prevent re-stenosis following coronary angioplasty.[97]

However, the systemic administration of these agents inhibits other important physiologic processes, inducing severe side effects that may be accepted by oncological and transplanted patients under critical situations.[98] Nevertheless, although these agents can be helpful to decrease the angiogenesis and recover experimental endometriosis lesions, their clinical use as an endometriosis treatment it is not advisable.

Dopamine Agonist in the Treatment of Endometriosis

The physiopathology associated to infertility in mild-moderate endometriosis remains unknown and there are several hypothesis to explain it. Interestingly, the severity of endometriosis has been directly correlated with spontaneous hiperprolactinemia or after stimulation with

different agents.[99, 100] Prolactin (PRL) is a powerful angiogenic inductor that is present in the decidualization process, inducing the breast growth during pregnancy.[101] Experimentally, PRL induces angiogenesis in other tissues as muscle.[102, 103] Proangiogenic effect of PRL exerts its properties into blood vessels receptors.[104]

The PRL antagonist endostatin is a fusion protein that combines a proapoptotic agent and antiangiogenic agent. This protein has been successfully employed in the breast cancer treatment.[105] It is important to consider that endostatin is one of the successful agents used in Nap's experimental endometriosis nude model.[12]

Apart from antiangiogenic substances, it has been shown that other products are effective in the VEGF system regulation. The dopamine neurotransmitter, used in nontoxic levels, is able to promote the VEGFR-2 endocitosis in endothelial cells, preventing the VEGF- VEGFR-2 union, a critical step in the neoangiogenesis process[106] avoiding receptor phosphorilation and signal cascade (**Figure 31-2**). Similarly, dopamine agonists, as Bromocriptin (Bro), extensively used in gynecology even during pregnancy, exerts the same action.[106] Moreover, if the relationship between neoangiogenesis and PRL is considered together with the relationship between PRL and endometriosis, and the effect of endostatin and the expression of VEGF in ectopic endometrium, dopamine agonists are obvious candidates for the treatment of endometriosis.

In a recent study, the antiangiogenic effect of Cabergoline (Cb2) on experimentally-induced endometriosis was tested.[16] A heterologous animal model of endometriosis

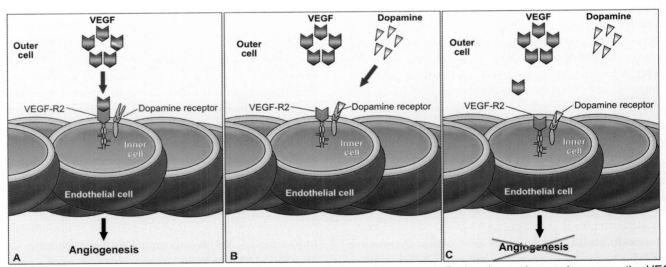

FIGURES 31-2A to C: Anti-angiogenic mechanism action of dopamine agonist. During the angiogenesis process the VEGF binds to the VEGFR-2 located on the epithelial cell surface promoting the receptor phosphorilation and initiating the angiogenic signal cascade (A). The dopamine neurotransmitter, used at non-toxic levels, binds to the Dp-r2 (B) promoting the VEGFR-2 endocitosis in endothelial cells and preventing VEGF-VEGFR-2 to bind, a critical step in the neoangiogenesis. As a consequence, there is no receptor phosphorilation and signal cascade (C).

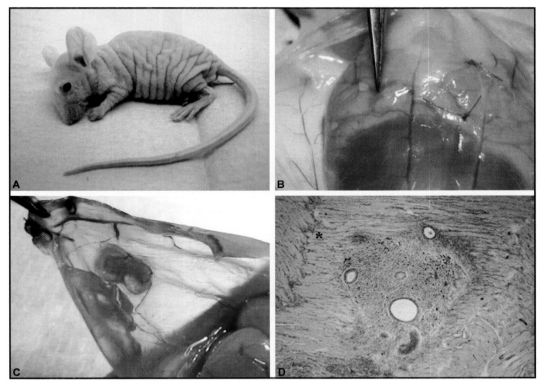

FIGURES 31-3A to D. Experimental model of endometriosis in nude mice. Nude mouse used in the experiments (A). Human endometrial tissue inside mouse peritoneal cavity after 5 weeks (3 weeks of implantation + 2 weeks of cabergoline treatment) (B, C). Microscopic appearance of the lesions (haematoxilyneosin staining). The endometrial stroma, surrounding glandular areas, was easily differentiated to the muscular-conjunctive murine tissue*(D).

was developed introducing human endometrial samples from oocyte donors into the peritoneum of each mouse **(Figures 31-3A and B)**. The human endometrium fragments were stuck into the peritoneum mice wall by n-butyl-ester cyanoacrylate adhesive **(Figure 31-3C)**. Three weeks later, Cb2 was administered at different doses during two weeks. After treatment, the implants were removed and processed for different techniques.

After an exhaustive histological study by optical microscopy, it was observed that the endometriotic lesions of untreated mice presented a high cellular stroma and a histological aspect of complete reorganization and structure, as seen in a typical endometriosis lesions. The human endometrial stroma surrounding the glandular areas was easily differentiated from the muscular-conjunctive murine tissue **(Figure 31-3D)**. However, in

treated lesions a lax stroma with lost cellularity and organization was observed. A significant decrease in the percentage of active lesions in mice treated with low and high doses of Cb2 with respect to the control group was observed **(Table 31-1)**. These results were confirmed by morphometric analysis which revealed a significant difference among the groups in the ratio of glands/stroma showing fewer glands in mice treated with different doses of Cb2 than in controls and demonstrating that Cb2 treatment produced a decrease in the amount of endometrial glands.

The proliferative status of endometriotic cells was investigated using immunohistochemistry and morphopetry techniques. The proliferative index proved to be significantly lower in mice treated with low and high doses of Cb2 than in untreated animals **(Table 31-1)**.

Table 31-1: Antiangiogenic action of dopamine agonist cabergoline on endometriosis in mice determined by percent active lesions, proliferative index, angiogenesis and VEGF activity				
	% Active lesions	*Proliferation index*	*% New blood vessels*	*VEGF activity*
Control	89.6±5.7	0.12±0.02	75.4±1.6	66.9±1.9
Low Dose	58.6±9.7*	0.02±0.01**	13.5±1.1*	12.5±1.0*
High Dose	60.4±8.4*	0.03±0.01**	10.8±3.2*	8.3±1.6*

Data expressed mean±SEM; *P < 0.05 compared to control; **P < 0.001 compared to control

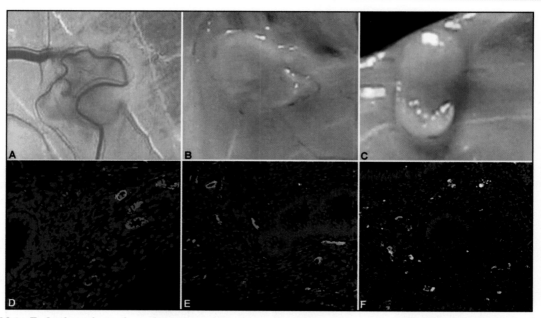

FIGURES 31-4A to F: Anti-angiogenic action of dopamine agonist in experimentally induced endometriosis. Untreated nude mice lesions (A) showed a rich vascular net compared to the lesions of the mice treated with low (B) and high (C) doses of cabergoline, which presented a white aspect and a less developed vascularization. To test the antiangiogenic action of cabergoline, the lesions vascularization was analyzed by confocal microscopy (D, E, F). The presence of double stained blood vessels could be analyzed by using the von Willebrand factor (*vWF*, red) as a maker of endothelial cells and alpha smooth muscle actin (*αSMA*, green) as a maker of mature blood vessels. It can be observed that not all vWF positive blood vessels, was αSMA positive indicating that mature as well as newly formed vessels are present in endometriosis lesions (D). In lesions of the mice treated with low (E) and high (F) doses of cabergoline, most of the blood vessels were both vWF and αSMA positive, indicating inhibition of the angiogenic process.

Macroscopic lesions were observed on the peritoneal wall in all experimental groups with the difference that a rich vascular net was observed in the endometriotic lesions of the control animals **(Figure 31-4A)**, whereas those of Cb2-treated animals were of a whitish color and revealed a less developed vascularization **(Figures 31-4B and C)**.

To test the antiangiogenic action of Cb2, immuno-fluorescence technique and confocal microscopy employing antibodies raised against the von Willebrand factor (vWF) present in endothelial cells and vascular smooth muscle cells (α-SMA) was used to evaluate the number of mature (vWF+/α-SMA+), immature(vWF+/α-SMA-) blood vessels in the different groups **(Figures 31-4D to E)**, showing a significant difference among groups in the ratio newly formed/mature blood vessels **(Table 31-1)** and indicating that Cb2 treatment is associated with a decrease in the amount of newly formed blood vessels. Different factors involved in the angiogenesis process were also studied at the molecular level showing that Cb2 treatment was clearly associated with a decrease in the amount of newly formed blood vessels.

The molecular mechanism by which the Cb2 exerts its antiangiogenic action was also demonstrated by the study of the degree of VEGFR-2 phosphorylation in the experimentally induced lesions. A significant lower VEGFR-2 phosphorylation degree was revealed in Cb2-treated animals, confirming that the dopamine agonist induces VEGFR-2 endocytosis, preventing VEGF binding and receptor phosphorylation blocking the angiogenesis cascade.

In summary, the results of this study demonstrate that the treatment of established experimentally induced endometriotic lesions with different doses of Cb2 produces a significant decrease in the percentage of active lesions. Neoangiogenesis was affected at a morphological and molecular level in treatment groups. The action of Cb2 on the experimental lesions was guided through the angiogenic process inhibiting the new vascular nets developed by blocking the VEGF system.

The use of angiogenesis inhibitors may also have some disadvantages. They require chronic administration and are likely to be particularly favorable in early-stage disease as are prone to prevent recurrence after surgery as well as interfere with new vessel formation conferring a preventive effect. Endometriotic lesions diagnosed at early stages have not yet progressed beyond the superficial lesion, which is usually highly angiogenic.[6, 55]

Several anticancer drugs with antiangiogenic potential have been found to have a detrimental effect on reproductive function in both animal models and patients.[107,108] However, the most important concern remains the risk of teratogenic effects associated with antiangiogenic therapies in case of pregnancy and the side effects of these drugs. VEGFR-2-mediated endothelial cell signals are critical to maintain the functionality of luteal blood vessels during pregnancy.[108] Treatment with TNP-470 was found to completely inhibit embryonic growth.[107]

Moreover, a recent research consistently associates the use of cabergoline and pergolide (another dopamine agonist) for the treatment of chronic conditions, such as Parkinson's disease, hyperprolactinemia and the restless leg syndrome, with an elevated incidence of cardiac valve regurgitation.[109, 110] In the context of endometriosis, it would be important to explore the use of other dopamine agonist, which may not carry the same side effects profile.

References

1. Cramer DW, Missmer SA. The epidemiology of endometriosis. Ann N Y Acad Sci. 2002; 955:11-22. The Practice Committee of the American Society for Reproductive Medicine, 2004.
2. Sampson JA. Peritoneal endometriosis due to menstrual dissemination of endometrial tissue into the pelvic cavity. Am J Obstet Gynecol 1927; 14:422-69.
3. Ford J, English J, Miles WA, Giannopoulos T. Pain, quality of life and complications following the radical resection of rectovaginal endometriosis. BJOG 2004; 111:353-56.
4. Maas JW, Groothuis PG, Dunselman GA, de Goeij AF, Struijker-Boudier HA, Evers JL. Development of endometriosis-like lesions after transplantation of human endometrial fragments onto the chick chorioallantoic membrane. Hum Reprod 2001a;16:627-31.
5. Maas, JW, Groothuis PG, Dunselman GA, de Goeij AF, Struijker-Boudier HA, Evers JL. Endometrial angiogenesis throughout the human menstrual cycle. Hum Reprod 2001b;16:1557-61.
6. Nisolle M, Casanas-Roux F, Anaf V, Mine JM, Donnez J. Morphometric study of the stromal vascularization in peritoneal endometriosis. Fertil Steril 1993; 59:681-84.
7. Laschke MW, Menger MD. In vitro and in vivo approaches to study angiogenesis in the pathophysiology and therapy of endometriosis. Hum Reprod Update 2007;13:331-42.
8. Groothuis PG, Nap AW, Winterhager E, Grümmer R. Vascular development in endometriosis. Angiogenesis 2005; 8147-56.
9. Becker CM, D'Amato RJ. Angiogenesis and antiangiogenic therapy in endometriosis. Microvasc Res. 2007; 74:121-30.
10. Dabrosin C, Gyorffy S, Margetts P, Ross C, Gauldie J. Therapeutic Effect of Angiostatin Gene Transfer in a Murine Model of Endometriosis. Am J Pathol 2002; 909-18.
11. Hull ML, Charnock-Jones DS, Chan CLK, Bruner-Tran KL, Osteen KG, Tom BDM, Fan T-PD, Smith SK.

Antiangiogenic Agents are Effective Inhibitors of Endometriosis. J Clin Endocrin Metab 2003; 86:2889-99.
12. Nap AW, Griffioen AW, Dunselman GAJ, Bouma-Ter Steege JCA, Thijssen VLJL, Evers JLH, Groothuis PG. Antiangiogenesis Therapy for Endometriosis. J Clin Encocrin Metab 2004; 89:1089-95.
13. Becker CM, Sampson DA, Rupnick MD, Rohan RM, Efstathiou JA, Short SA, Taylor GA, Folkman J, D'Amato RJ. Endostatin inhibits the growth of endometriotic lesions but does not affect fertility. Fertil Steril 2005; 84:1144-55.
14. Laschke MW, Elitzsch A, Scheuer C, Holstein JH, Vollmar B, Menger MD. Rapamycin induces regression of endometriotic lesions by inhibiting neovascularization and cell proliferation. Br J Pharmacol 2006;149:137-44.
15. Laschke MW, Elitzsch A, Vollmar B, Vajkoczy P, Menger MD. Combined inhibition of vascular endothelial growth factor (VEGF), fibroblast growth factor and platelet-derived growth factor, but not inhibition of VEGF alone, effectively suppresses angiogenesis and vessel maturation in endometriotic lesions. Hum Reprod 2006; 21:262-68.
16. Novella-Maestre E, Carda C, Noguera I, Ruiz-Saurý A, Garcýa-Velasco JA, Simon C, Pellicer A. Dopamine agonist administration causes a reduction in endometrial implants through modulation of angiogenesis in experimentally induced endometriosis. Human Reprod 2009 (in press).
17. Nap AW, Dunselman GA, Griffioen AW, Mayo KH, Evers JL, Groothuis PG. Angiostatic agents prevent the development of endometriosis-like lesions in the chicken chorioallantoic membrane. Fertil Steril 2005; 83:793-95.
18. Koninckx PR, Kennedy SH, Barlow DH. Endometriotic disease: the role of peritoneal fluid. Hum Reprod Update 1998;4:741-51.
19. Gazvani R, Templeton A. Peritoneal environment, cytokines and angiogenesis in the pathophysiology of endometriosis. Reproduction. 2002; 123:217-26.
20. Lin YJ, Lai MD, Lei HY, Wing LY. Neutrophils and macrophages promote angiogenesis in the early stage of endometriosis in a mouse model. Endocrinology. 2006; 147:1278-86.
21. Fainaru O, Adini A, Benny O, Adini I, Short S, Bazinet L, Nakai K, Pravda E, Hornstein MD, D'Amato RJ, Folkman J. Dendritic cells support angiogenesis and promote lesion growth in a murine model of endometriosis. FASEB J 2008; 22:522-29.
22. Folkman J, D'Amore PA. Blood Vessel Formation: What is Its Molecular Basis? Cell 1996: 87:1153-55.
23. Risau W. Mechanisms of Angiogenesis. Nature 1997; 386:671-74.
24. Asahara T, Masuda H, Takahashi T, Kalka C, Pastore C, Silver M, Kearne M, Magner M, Isner JM. Bone marrow origin of endothelial progenitor cells responsible for postnatal vasculogenesis in physiological and pathological neovascularization. Circ Res 1999; 85:221-28.
25. Burri PH, Djonov V. Intussusceptive angiogenesis – the alternative to capillary sprouting. Mol Aspects Med 2002; 23:S1-27.
26. Girling JE, Rogers PA. Recent advances in endometrial angiogenesis research. Angiogenesis. 2005; 8:89-99.

27. Haney AF, Muscato JJ, Weinberg JB. Peritoneal fluid cell populations in infertility patients. Fertil Steril 1981; 35: 696-98.

28. Haney AF. Endometriosis macrophages, and adhesions. Prog Clin Biol Res 1993; 381:19-44.

29. Hill JA, Faris HM, Schiff I, Anderson DJ. Characterization of leukocyte subpopulations in the peritoneal fluid of women with endometriosis. Fertil Steril 1988; 50:216-22.

30. Ho HN, Wu MY, Yang YS. Peritoneal cellular immunity and endometriosis. Am J Reprod Immunol 1997; 38:400-12.

31. Folkman J, Shing Y. Angiogenesis. J Biol Chem 1992; 267: 10931-34.

32. Donnez J, Smoes P, Gillerot S, Casanas-Roux F, Nisolle M. Vascular endothelial growth factor (VEGF) in endometriosis. Hum Reprod 1998; 13:1686-90.

33. Gargett C, Weston G, Rogers P. Mechanisms and regulation of endometrial angiogenesis. Reprod Med Rev 2002; 10:45-61.

34. Wei MH, Popescu NC, Lerman MI, Merrill MJ, Zimonjic DB. Localization of the human vascular endothelial growth factor gene, VEGF, at chromosome 6p12. Hum Genet 1996; 97:794-99.

35. Neufeld G, Cohen T, Gengrinovitch S, Poltorak Z. Vascular endothelial growth factor (VEGF) and its receptors. FASEB J 1999; 13:9-22.

36. Watkins RH, D'Angio CT, Ryan RM, Patel A, Maniscalco WM. Differential expression of VEGF mRNA splice variants in newborn and adult hyperoxic lung injury. Am J Physiol 1999; 276:858-67.

37. Mustonen T, Alitalo K. Endothelial receptor tyrosine kinases involved in angiogenesis. J Cell Biol 1995; 129: 895-98.

38. Shibuya M. Role of VEGF-flt receptor system in normal and tumor angiogenesis. Adv Cancer Res 1995; 67:281-316.

39. Shalaby F, Rossant J, Yamaguchi TP, Gertsenstein M, Wu XF, Breitman ML, Schuh AC. Failure of blood island formation and vasculogenesis in Flk-1-deficient mice. Nature 1995; 376:62-66.

40. Verheul HM, Hoekman K, Jorna AS, Smit EF, Pinedo HM. Targeting vascular endothelial growth factor blockade: ascites and pleural effusion formation. Oncologist 2000; 5:45-50.

41. Harmey JH, Dimitriadis E, Kay E, Redmond HP, Bouchier-Hayes D. Regulation of macrophage production of vascular endothelial growth factor (VEGF) by hypoxia and transforming growth factor beta-1. Ann Surg Oncol 1998; 5:271-78.

42. Freeman MR, Schneck FX, Gagnon ML; Corless C, Soker S, Niknejad K, Peoples GE, Klagsbrun M. Peripheral blood T lymphocytes and lymphocytes infiltrating human cancers express vascular endothelial growth factor: A potential role for T cells in angiogenesis. Cancer Res 1995; 55:4140-45.

43. Selgas R, del Peso G, Bajo MA, Castro MA, Molina S, Cirugeda A, Sanchez-Tomero JA, Castro MJ, Alvarez V, Corbí A, Vara F. Spontaneous VEGF production by cultured peritoneal mesothelial cells from patients on peritoneal dialysis. Perit Dial Int 2000; 20:798-801.

44. Sharkey AM, Day K, McPherson A, Malik S, Licence D, Smith SK, Charnock-Jones DS. Vascular endothelial growth factor expression in human endometrium is regulated by hypoxia. J Clin Endocrinol Metab 2000; 85:402-09.

45. Nagy JA, Masse EM, Herzberg K, Meyers MS, Yeo KT, Yeo TK, Sioussat TM, Dvorak HF. Pathogenesis of ascites tumor growth: Vascular permeability factor, vascular hyperpermeability, and ascites fluid accumulation. Cancer Res 1995; 55:360-68.

46. Dunselman GA, Bouckaert PX, Evers JL. The acute-phase response in endometriosis of women. J Reprod Fertil 1988; 83:803-08.

47. Bruner KL, Matrisian LM, Rodgers WH, Gorstein F, Osteen KG. Suppression of matrix metalloproteinases inhibits establishment of ectopic lesions by human endometrium in nude mice. J Clin Invest 1997; 99:2851-57.

48. Ogawa H, Nishihira J, Sato Y, Kondo M, Takahashi N, Oshima T, Todo S. An antibody for macrophage migration inhibitory factor suppresses tumour growth and inhibits tumour-associated angiogenesis. Cytokine 2000; 12:309-14.

49. Ryan IP, Tseng JF, Schriock ED, Khorram O, Landers DV, Taylor RN. Interleukin-8 concentrations are elevated in peritoneal fluid of women with endometriosis. Fertil Steril 1995; 63:929-32.

50. Arici A, Tazuke SI, Attar E, Kliman HJ, Olive DL. Interleukin-8 concentration in peritoneal fluid of patients with endometriosis and modulation of interleukin-8 expression in human mesothelial cells. Mol Hum Reprod 1996;2:40-45.

51. Iwabe T, Harada T, Tsudo T, Tanikawa M, Onohara Y, Terakawa N. Pathogenetic significance of increased levels of interleukin-8 in the peritoneal fluid of patients with endometriosis. Fertil Steril 1998; 69:924-30.

52. Barcz E, Rózewska ES, Kaminski P, Demkow U, Bobrowska K, Marianowski L. Angiogenic activity and IL-8 concentrations in peritoneal fluid and sera in endometriosis. Int J Gynaecol Obstet 2002; 79:229-35.

53. Osuga Y, Tsutsumi O, Okagaki R, Takai Y, Fujimoto A, Suenaga A, Maruyama M, Momoeda M, Yano T, Taketani Y. Hepatocyte growth factor concentrations are elevated in peritoneal fluid of women with endometriosis. Hum Reprod 1999; 14:1611-13.

54. Khan KN, Masuzaki H, Fujishita A, Kitajima M, Hiraki K, Miura S, Sekine I, Ishimaru T. Peritoneal fluid and serum levels of hepatocyte growth factor may predict the activity of endometriosis. Acta Obstet Gynecol Scand 2006;85: 458-66.

55. Matsuzaki S, Murakami T, Uehara S, Yokomizo R, Noda T, Kimura Y, Okamura K. Erythropoietin concentrations are elevated in the peritoneal fluid of women with endometriosis. Hum Reprod 2001; 16:945-48.

56. Szamatowicz J, Laudañski P, Tomaszewska I, Szamatowicz M. Chemokine growth-regulated-alpha: a possible role in the pathogenesis of endometriosis. Gynecol Endocrinol 2002; 16:137-41.

57. Kats R, Metz CN, Akoum A. Macrophage migration inhibitory factor is markedly expressed in active and early-stage endometriotic lesions. J Clin Endocrinol Metab 2002; 87:883-89.

58. Arici A, Matalliotakis I, Goumenou A, Koumantakis G, Vassiliadis S, Selam B, Mahutte NG. Increased levels of interleukin-15 in the peritoneal fluid of women with endometriosis: inverse correlation with stage and depth of invasion. Hum Reprod 2003;18:429-32.

59. Suzumori N, Zhao XX, Suzumori K. Elevated angiogenin levels in the peritoneal fluid of women with endometriosis correlate with the extent of the disorder.Fertil Steril 2004; 82:93-96.

60. Attia GR, Zeitoun K, Edwards D, Johns A, Carr BR, Bulun SE. Progesterone receptor isoform A but not B is expressed in endometriosis. J Clin Endocrinol Metab 2000; 85: 2897-2902.

61. Zeitoun KM, Bulun SE. Aromatase: A key molecule in the pathophysiology of endometriosis and a therapeutic target. Fertil Steril 1999; 72:961-69.

62. Cid MC, Kleinman HK, Grant DS, Schnaper HW, Fauci AS, Hoffman GS. Estradiol enhances leukocyte binding to tumor necrosis factor (TNF)-stimulated endothelial cells via an increase in TNF-induced adhesion molecules E-selectin, intercellular adhesion molecule type 1, and vascular cell adhesion molecule type 1. J Clin Invest 1994; 93:17-25.

63. Weiner CP, Lizasoain I, Baylis SA, Knowles RG, Charles IG, Moncada S. Induction of calciumdependent nitric oxide synthases by sex hormones. Proc Natl Acad Sci USA 1994; 91:5212-16.

64. Khan KN, Masuzaki H, Fujishita A, Kitajima M, Sekine I, Ishimaru T. Differential macrophage infiltration in early and advanced endometriosis and adjacent peritoneum. Fertil Steril 2004; 81:652-61.

65. Jones RK, Bulmer JN, Searle RF. Phenotypic and functional studies of leukocytes in human endometrium and endometriosis. Hum Reprod Update 1998; 4:702-09.

66. Matsuzaki S, Canis M, Darcha C; Fukaya T, Yajima A, Bruhat MA. Increased mast cell density in peritoneal endometriosis compared with eutopic endometrium with endometriosis. Am J Reprod Immunol 1998; 40:291-94.

67. Fujiwara H, Konno R, Netsu, Sugamata M, Shibahara H, Ohwada M, Suzuki M. Localization of mast cells in endometrial cysts. Am J Reprod Immunol 2004; 51: 341-4.

68. Anaf V, Simon P, Fayt I, Noel J. Smooth muscles are frequent components of endometriotic lesions. Hum Reprod 2000; 15: 767-71.

69. Itoga T, Matsumoto T, Takeuchi H, Yamasaki S, Sasahara N, Hoshi T, Kinoshita K. Fibrosis and smooth muscle metaplasia in rectovaginal endometriosis. Pathol Int 2003; 53:371-75.

70. Spuijbroek MD, Dunselman GA, Menheere PP, Evers JL. Early endometriosis invades the extracellular matrix. Fertil Steril 1992; 58:929-33.

71. Matsuzaki S, Canis M, Darcha C; Dechelotte P, Pouly JL, Bruhat MA. Fibrogenesis in peritoneal endometriosis. A semi-quantitative analysis of type-I collagen. Gynecol Obstet Invest 1999; 47:197-99.

72. Van Voorhis BJ, Huettner PC, Clark MR, Hill JA. Immunohistochemical localization of prostaglandin H synthase in the female reproductive tract and endometriosis. Am J Obstet Gynecol 1990; 163:57-62.

73. Chishima F, Hayakawa S, Sugita K, Kinukawa N, Aleemuzzaman S, Nemoto N, Yamamoto T, Honda M. Increased expression of cyclooxygenase-2 in local lesions of endometriosis patients. Am J Reprod Immunol 2002; 48:50-56.

74. Zeitoun K, Takayama K, Michael MD, Bulun SE. Stimulation of aromatase P450 promoter (II) activity in endometriosis and its inhibition in endometrium are regulated by competitive binding of steroidogenic factor-1 and chicken ovalbumin upstream promoter transcription factor to the same cis-acting element. Mol Endocrinol 1999; 13:239-53.

75. Williams CS, Tsujii M, Reese J, Dey SK, DuBois RN. Host cyclooxygenase-2 modulates carcinoma growth. J Clin Invest 2000; 105:1589-94.

76. Ruegg C, Dormond O, Mariotti A. Endothelial cell integrins and COX-2: Mediators and therapeutic targets of tumor angiogenesis. Biochim Biophys Acta 2004; 1654:51-67.

77. Brigstock DR. Regulation of angiogenesis and endothelial cell function by connective tissue growth factor (CTGF) and cysteinerich 61 (CYR61). Angiogenesis 2002; 5:153-65.

78. Absenger Y, Hess-Stumpp H, Kreft B, Krätzschmar J, Haendler B, Schütze N, Regidor PA, Winterhager E. Cyr61, a deregulated gene in endometriosis. Mol Hum Reprod 2004; 10: 399-407.

79. Leu SJ, Chen N, Chen CC; Todorovic V, Bai T, Juric V, Liu Y, Yan G, Lam SC, Lau LF. Targeted mutagenesis of the angiogenic protein CCN1 (CYR61): Selective inactivation of integrin alpha 6beta 1-heparan sulfate proteoglycan coreceptormediated cellular functions. J Biol Chem 2004; 279:44177-87.

80. Chen N, Leu SJ, Todorovic, Lam SC, Lau LF. Identification of a novel integrin alpha vbeta 3 binding site in CCN1 (CYR61) critical for pro-angiogenic activities in vascular endothelial cells. J Biol Chem 2004; 279: 44166-76.

81. Punyadeera C, Dassen H, Klomp J, Dunselman G, Kamps R, Dijcks F, Ederveen A, de Goeij A, Groothuis P. Oestrogen-modulated gene expression in the human endometrium. Cell Mol Life Sci 2005; 62:239-50.

82. Rivera-Gonzalez R, Petersen DN, Tkalcevic G, Thompson DD, Brown TA. Estrogen induced genes in the uterus of ovariectomized rats and their regulation by droloxifene and tamoxifen. J Steroid Biochem Mol Biol 1998; 64:13-24.

83. McCarty MF, Liu W, Fan F, Parikh A, Reimuth N, Stoeltzing O, Ellis LM. Promises and pitfalls of anti-angiogenic therapy in clinical trials. Trends Mol Med 2003; 9:53-58.

84. Lien S, Lowman HB. Therapeutic anti-VEGF antibodies. Handb Exp Pharmacol 2008; 181:131-50.

85. Kressin P, Wolber EM, Wodrich H, et al. Vascular endothelial growth factor mRNA in eutopic and ectopic endometrium. Fertil Steril 2001; 76:1220-24.

86. Tan XJ, Lang JH, Liu DY, et al. Expression of vascular endothelial growth factor and thrombospondin-1 mRNA in patients with endometriosis. Fertil Steril 2002;78: 148-53.

87. Drenkhahn M, Gescher DM, Wolber EM, et al.Expression of angiopoietin 1 and 2 in ectopic endometrium on the chicken chorioallantoic membrane. Fertil Steril 2004; 81:869-75.

88. Park A, Chang P, Ferin M, Xiao E, Zeitoun K. Inhibition of endometriosis development in Rhesus monkeys by blocking VEGF receptor: a novel treatment for endometriosis. Fertil Steril 2004; 82: S71.

89. Becker CM, Sampson DA, Short SA, Javaherian K, Folkman J, D'Amato RJ. Short synthetic endostatin peptides inhibit endothelial migration in vitro and endometriosis in a mouse model. Fertil Steril 2006; 85: 71-77.

90. Laschke MW, Elitzsch A, Vollmar B, Menger MD. In vivo analysis of angiogenesis in endometriosis-like lesions by intravital fluorescence microscopy. Fertil Steril 2005; 84: 1199-209.

91. Benny O, Fainaru O, Adini A, Cassiola F, Bazinet L, Adini I, Pravda E, Nahmias Y, Koirala S, Corfas G, D'Amato RJ, Folkman J. An orally delivered small-mollecule formulation with antiangiogenic and anticancer activity. Nat Biotechnol. 2008; 26:799-807.

92. Ferrara N. Role of vascular endothelial growth factor in physiologic and pathologic angiogenesis: therapeutic implications. Semin Oncol 2002; 29:10-14.

93. McAlister VC, Peltekian KM, Malatjalian DA, Colohan S, MacDonald S, Bitter-Suermann H, MacDonald AS. Orthotopic liver transplantation using low-dose tacrolimus and sirolimus. Liver Transpl 2001; 7:701-08.

94. Chueh SC, Kahan BD. Clinical application of sirolimus in renal transplantation: an update. Transpl Int 2005; 18: 261–77.

95. Lee VW, Chapman JR. Sirolimus: its role in nephrology. Nephrology (*Carlton*) 2005; 10:606-14.

96. Mota A. Sirolimus: a new option in transplantation. Expert Opin Pharmacother 2005; 6:479-87.

97. Kastrati A, Dibra A, Eberle S, Mehilli J, Suarez de Lezo J, Goy JJ, Ulm K, Schömig A. Sirolimus-eluting stents vs paclitaxel-eluting stents in patients with coronary artery disease: meta-analysis of randomized trials. JAMA 2005; 294:819-25.

98. Via LE, Gore-Langton RE, Pluda JM. Current clinical trials administering the antiangiogenesis agent SU5416. Oncology 2000; 14:1312-23.

99. Gregoriou G, Bakas P, Vitoratos N, Papadias K, Goumas K, Chryssicopoulos A, Creatsas G. Evaluation of serum prolactin levels in patients with endometriosis and infertility. Gynecol Obstet Invest 1999; 48:48-51.

100. Cunha-Filho JS, Gross JL, Lemos NA, Brandelli A, Castillos M, Passos EP. Hyperprolactinemia and luteal insufficiency in infertile patients with mild and minimal endometriosis. Horm Metab Res. 2001; 33:216-20.

101. Reese J, Binart N, Brown N, Ma WG, Paria BC, Das SK, Kelly PA, Dey SK. Implantation and decidualization defects in prolactin receptor (PRLR)-deficient mice are mediated by ovarian but not uterine PRLR. Endocrinology 2000; 141:1872-81.

102. Ko JY, Ahn YL, Cho BN. Angiogenesis and white blood cell proliferation induced in mice by injection of a prolactin-expressing plasmid into muscle. Mol Cell 2003; 15:262-70.

103. Malaguarnera L, Pilastro MR, Quan S, Ghattas MH, Yang L, Mezentsev AV, Kushida T, Abraham NG, Kappas A. Significance of heme oxygenase in prolactin-mediated cell proliferation and angiogenesis in human endothelial cells. Int J Mol Med 2002; 10:433-40.

104. Merkle CJ, Schuler LA, Schaeffer RC Jr, Gribbon JM, Montgomery DW. Structural and functional effects of high prolactin levels on injured endothelial cells: evidence for an endothelial prolactin receptor. Endocrine 2000;13: 37-46.

105. Beck MT, Chen NY, Franek KJ, Chen WY. Prolactin antagonist-endostatin fusion protein as a targeted dual-functional therapeutic agent for breast cancer. Cancer Res 2003; 63:3598-604.

106. Basu S, Nagy JA, Vasile E, et al. The neurotransmitter dopamine inhibits angiogenesis induced by vascular permeability factor/vascular endothelial growth factor. Nat Med 2001; 7:569-74.

107. Klauber N, Parangi S, Flynn E, Hamel E, D'Amato RJ. Inhibition of angiogenesis and breast cancer in mice by the microtubule inhibitors 2-methoxyestradiol and taxol. Cancer Res 1997; 57:81-86.

108. Pauli SA, Tang H, Wang J, Bohlen P, Posser R, Hartman T, Sauer MV, Kitajewski J, Zimmermann RC. The vascular endothelial growth factor (VEGF)/VEGF receptor 2 pathway is critical for blood vessel survival in corpora lutea of pregnancy in the rodent. Endocrinology 2005; 146:1301-11.

109. Schade R, Andersohn F, Suissa S, Haverkamp W, Garbe E. Dopamine agonists and the risk of cardiac-valve regurgitation. N Engl J Med 2007; 356:29-38.

110. Zanettini R, Antonini A, Gatto G, Gentile R, Tesei S, Pezzoli G. Valvular heart disease and the use of dopamine agonists for Parkinson's disease. N Engl J Med 2007; 356:39-46.

Felice Petraglia, Stefano Luisi

Chapter 32
New Delivery for Classical Drugs: Intrauterine or Intravaginal

Introduction: New Routes of Administration for Hormones

In the recent years, new treatments for endometriosis have been investigated. Following the recent evidences that hormonal treatment by vaginal or intrauterine route are becoming of current use for hormonal postmenopausal replacement treatment, contraception or menorrhagia, the administration of progestins, such as levonorgestrel and danazol, answers to some problems related to the long-term management of endometriosis.

Intrauterine Device Releasing Levonorgestrel

Levonorgestrel, derived from 19-nortestosterone, is a potent progestin with androgenic and anti-estrogenic activity on the endometrium[1] used for various gynecological disturbances. An intrauterine device releasing 20 mg/day of levonorgestrel (Lng-IUD), has been developed and used for contraception and for abnormal uterine bleeding. The local administration of levonorgestrel has a profound effect on the endometrium, which becomes atrophic and inactive, although ovulation is generally not suppressed. Since to be safe and an effective treatment constitutes an essential element in the current clinical research on symptomatic endometriosis, it has been studied for treating these patients.

Intrauterine administration of levonorgestrel with a direct distribution to pelvic tissues implies a local concentration greater than its plasma levels. This could translate into a superior effectiveness with limited adverse effects, due to the absence of the hepatic first-pass effect and to the low dosage of the drug administered. However, side effects typical of progestins are reported and related to a relative uterine absorption of levonorgestrel. In fact, Lockhat et al[2] observed levonorgestrel concentrations in the order of 300–400 pg/mL months after Lng-IUD insertion, suggesting that the progestin released by the IUD is partially absorbed by the subendometrial vascular network. The Lng-IUD has been used in patients with peritoneal, superficial ovarian, rectovaginal and recurrent endometriotic lesions, and also as a postoperative measure.

Lockhat et al studied a group of women of reproductive age with clinically suspected and laparoscopically confirmed symptomatic minimal to moderate endometriosis. They received the Lng-IUD inserted for 6 months. Significant improvements in severity and frequency of pain and menstrual symptoms as well as staging were achieved, with 68% of cases electing to continue with the device after 6 months of therapy.[2]

The 3-year follow-up data on the subjects enrolled in the 6-month trial requesting continuation of therapy with the Lng-IUD showed an improvement in symptoms.[3] The greatest changes in pain (assessed by either the VAS or VRS) or blood loss were recorded between the pretreatment and 12 months evaluation. A multicenter randomized controlled trial compared the efficacy of the Lng-IUD vs the leuprolide depot, (3.75 mg/28 days), in the control of endometriosis related pain over a period of 6 months, and showed a pelvic pain decrease substantially from the first month of treatment throughout the study period without significant between-group differences **(Figure 32-1)**.[4]

Lng-IUD has been proposed as a treatment of choice for symptomatic endometriosis, since it does not provoke hypoestrogenism and it only requires one medical intervention for its introduction (every 5 years). Vercellini et al studied a group of women who did not wish to conceive, who were operated conservatively for endometriosis in the previous 12 months and did not want to

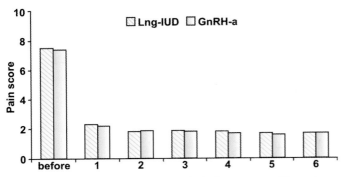

FIGURE 32-1: Control of pelvic pain in women with endometriosis undergoing to Lng-IUD or GnRH-a.[4,20]

undergo further surgery: they showed a reduced dysmenorrhea severity as well as a good patients' satisfaction assessed after 1 year of therapy.[5] A pilot study revealed that the frequency and severity of dysmenorrhea recurrence is reduced at 1-year follow-up in women in whom an Lng-IUD is inserted immediately after laparoscopic surgery for endometriosis (90%) compared with women treated with laparoscopic surgery alone (55%).[6] Also dyspareunia and non-menstrual pain scores were reduced to a greater extent with the postoperative use of Lng-IUD. Side effects were reported by eight of the 20 patients allocated to Lng-IUD insertion (bloating in six patients, weight gain in six patients, headache in three patients, seborrhea and acne in two patients, breast tenderness in one patient, decreased libido in one patient and pelvic pain in one patient) but were deemed to be tolerable. At 12 months, 75% of subjects in the surgery plus Lng-IUD group were satisfied or very satisfied compared with 50% in the surgery-alone group.

The use of an Lng-IUD in women with endometriosis confers several advantages over other conventional systemic therapies (avoidance of the need for repeated administration, effective contraception, fewer side effects) and shows high patients' compliance during long-term treatments. Although it may be expensive at the outset, the cumulative final costs is less than other medications. Women should be informed that during the first 3–4 months of use, major menstrual disorders are expected, including spotting, prolonged or continuous bleeding, and even menorrhagia. After the first year of use, few women report intermenstrual bleeding and about 20–30% are amenorrheic. This is relevant as dysmenorrhea is the most frequent symptom in patients with endometriosis. The expulsion rate of the device is over 5% and the risk of pelvic infection is about 1.5%.[7] Accordingly, the recommended patient profile is parous women with no history of pelvic inflammatory disease. Nulliparity is not

a contraindication, but the use of IUDs in smaller uteri may be associated with increased uterine cramping. This could be particularly worrisome in patients with severe dysmenorrhea associated with endometriosis. Finally, limited information is available on the risk of endometrioma formation during long periods of therapy. In fact, it has been demonstrated that development of endometriotic ovarian cysts is associated with ovulation and since the Lng-IUD does not generally inhibit ovulation this may constitute a specific drawback of the Lng-IUD in comparison with other forms of progestin treatment.[8]

In current practice, it is erroneously taken for granted that medical treatments are not efficacious for rectovaginal endometriosis. This uncritical belief, based on a reportedly different receptor pattern from eutopic endometrium, leads to the obvious conclusion that surgery is the only reasonable therapeutic choice, and thus exposes women to potentially severe morbidity, especially if procedures are performed by gynecologists who are not specifically trained in this difficult and technically demanding field.[9] This clinical approach should be challenged as, in these patients, good results are obtainable with safe, tolerable and inexpensive drugs that can be used for prolonged periods of time.

The Lng-IUD resulted an effective therapy for rectovaginal endometriosis in a group of symptomatic women who had previously undergone conservative surgery without excision of deep lesions.[10] At 1-year follow-up, dysmenorrhea, which had been moderate or severe in all cases, and non-menstrual pelvic pain were absent, with a reduction of deep dyspareunia to absent or mild in all subjects throughout treatment. Transrectal ultrasonography showed a slight but significant reduction in rectovaginal lesions after 6 months of therapy.

The mechanism of action of the Lng-IUD is a receptor mediated effect of levonorgestrel that may reach endometriotic foci through blood circulation or direct diffusion from the uterus.[11] Other mechanism of action could be secondary oligoamenorrhea and the consequent reduction in cyclic bleeding at ectopic endometrial sites. Relief of organic symptoms such as deep dyspareunia and rectal tenesmus is probably due to a decrease in size of the fibronodular rectovaginal plaques, and a decrease in the intra- and perilesional inflammatory condition.

Intrauterine Device Releasing Danazol

Danazol is an oral androgenic agent that interferes on progesterone receptors on endometrial or endometriosic cells, associated with increased serum androgen levels and modulation on estrogen receptors.[12] The rationale of this approach is to interfere with ovarian cyclic activity, thus disrupting the pathogenetic mechanisms leading to the development of endometriosis-associated pain symptoms. The effect may be also related to an immune, antiangiogenic, and anti-inflammatory function.[12]

Danazol represented the gold standard of treatment in the 1980s. Multiple studies demonstrated its efficacy in reducing endometriosis-associated pain symptoms.[12-14] Danazol acts directly on endometriotic tissue *in vitro* to inhibit DNA synthesis and induce apoptosis.

However, similar to other suppressive treatments, symptoms typically resume after discontinuation; moreover, although danazol is less expensive than GnRH analogues, its use is associated with remarkable androgenic/anabolic effects. The most common side effects include weight gain, fluid retention, breast atrophy, acne, oily skin, hot flushes and hirsutism.[12] Therefore, danazol administered orally has been commonly used in the medical treatment of pain associated with endometriosis but its use is heavily limited by the severity of side effects, particularly in long-term therapies, with a consequent low patient compliance.

Since it is known that danazol acts directly on endometriotic tissue *in vitro* to inhibit DNA synthesis and to induce apoptosis, and also that it may be adsorbed, a local administration, intrauterine or vaginal, was investigated. The first report showed that danazol administered in the uterine cavity is transported directly to the adenomyotic tissue and then in the surrounding tissues and serum concentrations are lower than after oral administration.[15]

The insertion of danazol-loaded intrauterine device in women with adenomyosis showed a good efficacy not only in the remission of dysmenorrhea and hypermenorrhea but also in infertile patients allowing conception after its removal.[15]

Later a prospective study showed the effectiveness of continuous (6 months) intrauterine release of danazol on dysmenorrhea, chronic pelvic pain and dyspareunia associated with moderate or severe endometriosis diagnosed at a laparoscopy previously performed for the presence of ovarian cysts or unexplained infertility.[16]

The danazol-loaded intrauterine system containing 400 mg of danazol (Fuji Latex, Tokyo, Japan) was inserted into the uterine cavity within 7 days of the menstrual cycle, using local anesthesia and the device was then maintained for 6 months without any additional medical treatments.[15-16] Dysmenorrhea, dyspareunia, and pelvic pain showed a statistically significant decrease after the first month of therapy (p<0.01), with a persistent effect during 6 months

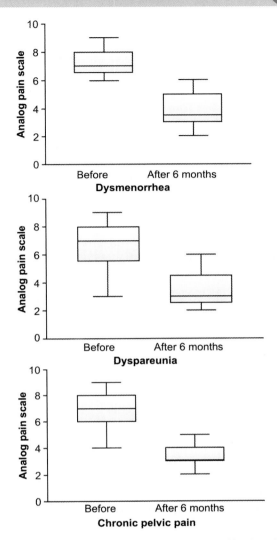

FIGURE 32-2: Analog pain score in women with chronic pain before and at 6 month-follow-up after therapy with danazol-loaded IUD.[16]

(Figure 32-2). The only local side effect was spotting during the first month of application in two cases. In one case the IUD was removed and replaced 2 months later because it had become dislodged. These results showed that this danazol intrauterine system represents an effective and conservative treatment for the relieve of all painful symptoms associated to endometriosis and for the control of menorrhagia related to adenomyosis. However, some chemical- pharmaceutical difficulties does not allow to continue these investigations.

Vaginal Administration of Danazol

The vaginal administration of danazol has been tested with encouraging results in women with endometriosis.

Vaginal danazol for the treatment of endometriosis has been administered by ring, gel or capsule.

Danazol administered via the vagina by using a vaginal ring drug delivery system contained 1500 mg. This therapy was effective for treatment of deeply infiltrating endometriosis, resulting in a cure of dysmenorrhea and tenderness in the cul-de-sac within 3 months, and of induration or nodularity in the cul-de-sac within 7 months.[17] No endometrial atrophy was observed during vaginal danazol ring therapy and conception occurred during insertion of vaginal danazol ring in 17 out of 31 infertile women with deeply infiltrating endometriosis, and in two out of eight infertile women with ovarian endometriotic cysts. Serum danazol concentrations, resulted almost undetectable during vaginal danazol ring therapy, thus explaining why ovulation and conception could occur and general side effects were very rare. Danazol is absorbed through the vaginal mucosa and reaches the deeply infiltrating endometriosis via diffusion.[17]

In a case-control study, the vaginal administration of a gel containing danazol (100 mg/day in 0.2 ml) for four months effectively reduced dysmenorrhea and chronic pelvic pain related to endometriosis in 24 women.[18]

The effectiveness of danazol pill by vaginal route (200 mg/day) self-administered for 12 months has been also evaluated.[19] Following a previous laparoscopic surgery, these patients referred recurrent severe dyspareunia, dysmenorrhea and pelvic pain due to deep infiltrating endometriosis. Before and every three months during the treatment a visual analog pain scale was used. Transvaginal and transrectal ultrasound were performed before and after 6 and 12 months of treatment.

Dysmenorrhea, dyspareunia and pelvic pain significantly decreased within 3 months and disappeared after 6 months of treatment, with a persistent effect during the 12 months of treatment **(Figure 32-3)**. Ultrasound showed a reduction of the nodularity in the rectovaginal septum within 6 months **(Figure 32-4)**. The medical treatment did not affect metabolic or trombophilic parameters; few local vaginal adverse effects were referred.

Vaginal danazol resulted an effective medical treatment for the various painful symptoms in women with recurrent deeply infiltrating endometriosis, and since the lack of significant adverse effects it may be proposed in alternative to repeat surgery.

The advantages of vaginal danazol therapy compared with the oral danazol and GnRH analogue therapy are as follows: (i) dysmenorrhea and severe pelvic pain, induced by deeply infiltrating endometriosis, are cured more rapidly by vaginal therapy; (ii) it has no general

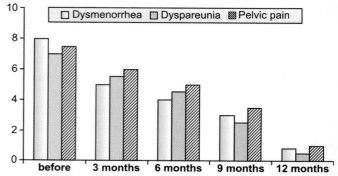

FIGURE 32-3: Pain symptoms as assessed by a visual analog scale during the 12 month-follow-up therapy with vaginal danazol.[19]

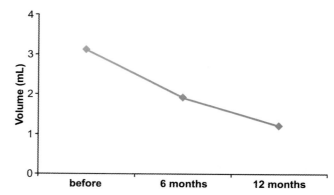

FIGURE 32-4: Mean ± SD volume of rectovaginal plaques evaluated by ultrasound before and during the treatment with vaginal danazol (p<0.05).[19]

associated side-effects; (iii) conception may occur even during therapy.

Vaginal danazol therapy on uterine adenomyosis and ovarian endometriotic cysts remain to be investigated.

Conclusion

In conclusion, local danazol administration, both intrauterine and vaginal, has been shown to be an effective and conservative treatment for dysmenorrhea, chronic pelvic pain and dyspareunia associated with adenomyosis and deep endometriosis. Nevertheless, the intrauterine administration of levonorgestrel showed good effectiveness, limited adverse effects and an increased patient compliance during endometriosis long-term treatment. Moreover, as additional advantages, Lng-IUD does not provoke hypo-estrogenism, so becoming the treatment of choice in cases of chronic pelvic pain associated endometriosis in women who do not want to conceive.

References

1. Salmi A, Pakarinen P, Peltola AM, et al. The effect of intrauterine levonorgestrel use on the expression of C-Jun, oestrogen receptors, progesterone receptors and Ki-67 in human endometrium. Mol Hum Reprod 1998; 4: 1110-15.

2. Lockhat FB, Emembolu JO, Konje JC. The evaluation of the effectiveness of an intrauterine-administered progestogen (levonorgestrel) in the symptomatic treatment of endometriosis and in the staging of the disease. Hum Reprod 2004; 19: 179-84.

3. Lockhat FB, Emembolu JO, Konje JC. The efficacy, side-effects and continuation rates in women with symptomatic endometriosis undergoing treatment with an intra-uterine administered progestogen (levonorgestrel): a 3 year follow-up. Hum Reprod 2005; 20: 789-93.

4. Petta CA, Ferriani RA, Abrao MS, et al. Randomized clinical trial of a levonorgestrel-releasing intrauterine system and a depot GnRH analogue for the treatment of chronic pelvic pain in women with endometriosis. Hum Reprod 2005; 20: 1993-98.

5. Vercellini P, Aimi G, Panazza S, et al. A levonorgestrel-releasing intrauterine system for the treatment of dysmenorrhoea associated with endometriosis: a pilot study. Fertil Steril 1999; 72: 505-08.

6. Vercellini P, Frontino G, De Giorgi O, et al. Comparison of a levonorgestrel-releasing intrauterine device versus expectant management after conservative surgery for symptomatic endometriosis: a pilot study. Fertil Steril 2003; 80: 305-09.

7. Shulman LP, Nelson AL, Darney PD. Recent developments in hormone delivery system. Am J Obstet Gynecol 2004; 190: 39-48.

8. Vercellini P, Vigano' P, Somigliana E. The role of the levonorgestrel-releasing intrauterine device in the management of symptomatic endometriosis. Curr Opin Obstet Gynecol 2005; 17: 359-65.

9. Ford J, English J, Miles WA, et al. Pain, quality of life and complications following the radical resection of rectovaginal endometriosis. BJOG 2004; 111: 353-56.

10. Fedele L, Bianchi S, Zanconato G, et al. Use of levonorgestrel-releasing intrauterine device in the treatment of rectovaginal endometriosis. Fertil Steril 2001; 75: 485-88.

11. Maruo T, Laoag-Fernandez JB, Pakarinen P, Murakoshi H, Spitz IM, Johansson E. Effects of the levonorgestrel-releasing intrauterine system on proliferation and apoptosis in the endometrium. Hum Reprod 2001; 16: 2103-08.

12. Crosignani P, Olive D, Bergqvist A, et al. Advances in the management of endometriosis: an update for clinicians. Hum Reprod Update 2006; 12: 179-89.

13. Royal College of Obstetricians and Gynaecologists (RCOG) Guidelines n. XX, 2005. The investigation and management of endometriosis.

14. Selak V, Farquhar C, Prentice A, et al. Danazol for pelvic pain associated with endometriosis. Cochrane Database Syst Rev 2001; 4. CD000068.

15. Igarashi M, Abe Y, Fukuda M, et al. Novel conservative medical therapy for uterine adenomyosis with a danazol-loaded intrauterine device. Fertil Steril 2000; 74: 412-13.

16. Cobellis L, Razzi S, Fava A, et al. A danazol-loaded intrauterine device decreases dysmenorrhea, pelvic pain, and dyspareunia associated with endometriosis. Fertil Steril 2004; 82: 239-40.

17. Igarashi M, Iizuka M, Abe Y, et al. Novel vaginal danazol ring therapy for pelvic endometriosis, in particular deeply infiltrating endometriosis. Hum Reprod 1998; 13: 1952-56.

18. Janicki TI, Dmowsky WP. Intravaginal danazol significantly reduces chronic pelvic pain in women with endometriosis. Supplement to the Journal of the Society for Gynecologic Investigation (SGI) 2004 Annual Meeting, abs n. 266.

19. Razzi S, Luisi S, Calonaci F, et al. Efficacy of vaginal danazol treatment in women with recurrent deeply infiltrating endometriosis. Fertil Steril 2007; 88: 789-94.

20. The ESHRE Capri Workshop Group. Intrauterine devices and intrauterine systems. Hum Reprod Update 2008; 14: 197-208.

Future Trends

David Smart, Marc Princivalle

Chapter 33

New Drugs in the Pipeline

Introduction

Earlier chapters in this book have demonstrated endometriosis to be an extremely common disorder with a broad spectrum of symptoms from asymptomatic (often only identified during investigation of infertility) through to intense pain. Endometriosis is characterized by the presence of an estrogen responsive ectopic growth of endometrial tissue within the peritoneal cavity. Common sites for the endometrial explants include the peritoneum and ovaries, although any organ within the peritoneal cavity is a potential target. In some incidences endometrial tissue has been demonstrated to move further a field with localization in the lungs and very rarely the arms or brain. By its nature this condition is typically associated with its outward signs and symptoms and as such is usually characterized by a spectrum of pain, dependant on the severity and/or location of lesions, with endometriosis also acting as a common cause of infertility. Until recently a lack of good biomarkers had left laparoscopy as the only true diagnostic tool for this condition, further promoting the 'black box' approach to treatment of endometriosis and the lack of progress in new therapeutics.

As we have also seen in the previous chapters, there are already a large number of therapies available in this indication however, broadly speaking, these fall into three categories; surgical, pain relief or hormonal therapies. Surgical intervention in this indication may be both therapeutic and diagnostic in the form of laparoscopy. Therapeutic surgery still has a significant role to play in current treatment, with endometriosis being a frequent source of infertility. Surgery provides a therapeutic option for women wishing to become pregnant as it is independent of hormone modulators which themselves disrupt fertility. Therapeutic surgery in endometriosis is quite often a quick fix, with repeat surgery being required

in 36% of patients who undergo procedures; as a result this is often used in combination with endocrine therapy. Ultimately endometriosis accounts for a significant number of performed hysterectomies. This mode of treatment represents a highly invasive and drastic course of action that we should be striving to move away from with any new therapies.

Medicinal therapies for this condition have, broadly speaking, changed little over the last two decades. Endometriosis has been largely overlooked in drug discovery as a primary indication, with many of the current therapies being based on a symptomatic approach, such as pain relief. Although pain relief is obviously a major concern, prevention of irreversible damage should also be a priority even if fertility is not currently of importance to the patient. Moreover, most therapies target this diseases progression by blockade of estrogen mediated endometrial growth, to which this tissue is highly responsive. All the current medicinal therapies targeting progression utilize the endocrine pathways for mode of action and as such many of those available have come directly from oncology indications. These agents offer a broad spectrum hormonal modulation to total ablation which, while effective, leads to alternative unpleasant side effects. The majority of such therapies are incompatible with fertility and some result in premature, all be it reversible, menopause.

One reason for the current approach to medicinal endometriosis therapy is the long established dogma attributing the condition to retrograde menstruation (RM). RM was proposed as a cause for endometriosis by Samson in 1927, suggesting that the incidence of this condition was due to the passage of endometrial tissue up the fallopian tubes into the peritoneal cavity during menstruation.[1] While this concept is in part true, for decades this gave endometriosis an anatomical rather than a mechanistic cause. The result is a general acceptance that it may be impossible to treat patients 'prone' to endometriosis without disruption of their normal monthly cycle, as there is no difference in their tissue. More recently however endometrial tissue from RM has been observed to occur in 90% of women.[2] This high incidence of RM suggests that it is not the passage of endometrial tissue into the peritoneal cavity of sufferers that distinguishes them from 'normal' women. While there is no doubt that endometriosis is reliant on RM passage as a source of endometrial material, its aggressive growth, survival and the development of symptomatic endometriosis are due to additional factors. Thus, the discrepancy in the incidence of RM and endometriosis is highly suggestive of either an increase in a survival factor/s or the lack of an apoptotic signal in the sufferers of this condition. Evidence appears to suggest that there is a substantial inflammatory/ immune constituent to endometriosis, with large numbers of infiltrating leukocytes, in particular macrophages. These observations are also combined with both localized and circulating increases in chemokines. Differences are seen in the way the immune system responds to RM; in patients with no endometriosis the immune system completely removes endometrial material from the peritoneal cavity, whereas in endometriosis the tissue is associated with a profound immune response but there is a failure to remove these cells. Moreover, some observers have also identified that endometriosis is often associated with other pathological conditions, which are anatomically unrelated but known to have significant immune system related factors.[3] Currently there is no definitive answer to the question of survival and growth of the tissue explants, although there are possible molecular targets which could prevent the deterioration from RM into endometriosis, without the use of drastic hormonal therapies. There is a clear unmet medical need in this indication, with new therapies targeted to prevent the survival of endometrial cells outside the uterus.

Current Pipeline Therapy

Drug Development

The major focus of this chapter is new targets in endometriosis, however, a number of the most developed pipeline treatments have already been discussed in depth in previous chapters; in particular those associated with GnRH analogues, anti-angiogenesis (VEGF) and aromatase inhibitors. As a result of the overlap in these chapters these areas will not be discussed, concentrating instead on earlier

targets and the pipeline. An exception to this is the area of GnRH analogues which will be touched on as an example.

Drug development is unsurprisingly governed by cost and risk; as such many pipeline treatments represent refinements of previously utilized pathways and targets. The GnRH analogue situation discussed below presents a good example of this situation. New targets and ultimately successful therapeutic projects are dependant not only on whether the drug will work but also on whether its sales will cover the costs of development and production. The average cost of drug production has been estimated at $1 billion, a figure which includes the large number of projects (>20% of projects) which fail in the clinical setting.[4,5] It is not surprising that the industry is very conservative in the targets which it pushes. Most drugs fail because they either don't work or are toxic. With the vast majority of the investment made in the later clinical stages of development this represents a large risk, which explains the refinement of drugs and reuse of established therapeutic pathways.

GnRH Analogues

The clear regulation of endometrial growth by estrogen continues to make steroid modulation a primary target for the treatment of endometriosis. The side effects of any ablation are obviously unsatisfactory, but the process provides a profound alleviation of symptoms, at the cost of menopause and or infertility. It is, however, possible to find a half-way house in ablation; improve drug product profile and remove some of the other contraindications of these treatments.

Endocrine therapy is extremely effective at blocking endometrial growth while at the same time reducing the lesions size. Its affects are, however, not necessarily limited to the endometriosis tissue. Although already discussed elsewhere in this book it is important to mention the use of gonadotrophin-release hormone (GnRH) analogues which continue to have a role in drug discovery. The analogues of GnRH act directly on the pituitary to block the circadian release of gonadotrophins. As a result GnRH analogues lead to complete ablation akin to premature menopause, resulting in hot flushes, bloating, fat redistribution and infertility. The current licensed GnRH peptide analogues Goserelin and Leuprolide used in endometriosis are examples of agonists of the GnRH receptor (GnRHR). The agonists appear to work by initially desensitizing the pituitary receptors then by down-regulating them with continued exposure due to lack of feedback. The downside of the use of a receptor agonist in this way is that there is an initial 'flare' resulting in increased gonadotrophin production, leading to an initial phase of increased growth. The use of agonist therapy takes a number of days to down-regulate the GnRHR and block downstream steroidal production. In addition upon removal of the therapy it also takes some time before the pathway is restored.

More recently advances have been made in the development of a number of GnRHR antagonists and examples include Cetrorelix and Degarelix.[6] The advantage of the antagonist over the agonist therapy is that there is an almost immediate down-regulation in gonadotrophin release, resulting in a rapid reduction in endometrial tissue size and corresponding pain, without the 'flare' of the agonist analogues. Also this therapy is far more rapidly reversible than agonist drugs, as the receptor remains. Unlike the agonist, antagonists of the GnRHR also provide more possibilities in dosing and treatment regimens. The agonists, while cheaper, are inflexible, requiring a high therapeutic dose to desensitize the receptors for any beneficial effect. Earlier attempts with antagonists led to histamine release issues associated with their non-host sequence but these have been overcome with the latest analogues. A disadvantage of both the agonists and antagonists therapies is that they are peptides restricting administration routes.

Survival and Growth Factor Targets

Tumor Necrosis Factor-Alpha (TNF-α)

Tumor necrosis factor-alpha (TNF-α) is a key regulator in inflammatory response, occurring as both a circulating and surface factor **(Figure 33-1)**. There are two TNF-α receptors; TNF-α type I (TNFRI) and TNF-α type II (TNFRII), the former has an intracellular death domain, while the latter's function is harder to define. The two receptors are differentially expressed leading to a context dependant cell growth, death, migration and differentiation.[7] TNF-α represents a significant alternative target in endometriosis, appearing as a result of the current interest in the immune systems role in the clinical manifestation of the condition. Primarily produced by the macrophages, TNF-α demonstrates increased local expression in endometriosis and is known to be both involved in the inflammatory process and in increasing expression of the cytokines IL-1, IL-6 and gamma Interferon. TNF-α is also suggested to be involved in the process of endometrial invasion through the up-regulation of MMP-1 and MMP-3 expression. The higher average levels of TNF-α present in endometriosis may also have direct effects on fertility as this cytokine has been shown to have detrimental effects on sperm survival. A number of studies have examined the use of (TNF) blockers, however the results of these studies have been mixed.[8,9] Studies using various different blockers have identified sepsis and exacerbation of lung infection as the most serious adverse reactions. Examples of current therapies under development for the targeting of TNF-α include Onecept soluble recombinant TNFRI receptor, Etancept TNF-α blocker, recombinant TNFRII receptor combined with Fc portions of human immune globulin IgG1 and Infliximab a chimeric humanized murine anti-TNF antibody with human IgG1 Fc portions.[10]

While TNF blocker therapy appears to be beneficial in early disease, showing improvements in severity with reductions in size and numbers of lesions, it appears not

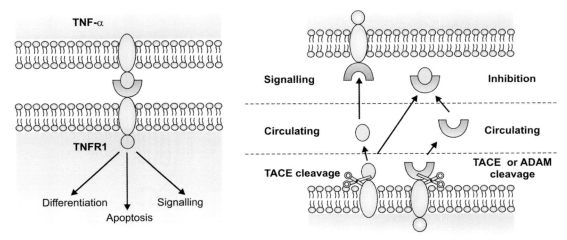

FIGURE 33-1: TNF-α Signalling (A) Cell contact-mediated signalling via surface bound TNF-α and TNFR. (B) Cleavage of the TNF-α extracellular domain by TACE leads to circulating TNF-α and peripheral activity. Cleavage of TNFR receptor by either TACE or another ADAMs leads to soluble endogenous inhibitor of circulating TNF-α

to help in more severe cases. As with the GnRH peptide analogues, monoclonal antibody therapy suffers from issues associated with stability and the route of administration, which could make it unpopular. Studies have also demonstrated potential risk factors in this therapy. Tests in baboons and monkeys have demonstrated that this treatment could be compounded by the immunosuppressive effects with increased incidence of pneumonia. There is also a strong suggestion from animal studies that the use of TNF blockers can lead to severe cardiac and liver effects. Altogether these treatments may require a high level of medical intervention.

Tumor Necrosis Factor Alpha Converting Enzyme (TACE)

An alternative method of targeting the TNF-α pathway in endometriosis may be to inhibit tumor necrosis factor alpha converting enzyme (TACE) also known as sheddase and a disintergrin and metalloproteinase 17 (ADAM-17). TACE acts to selectively cleave TNF-α from the cell surface leading to a circulatory form. TACE may also cleave the surface receptors of TNF-α, TNFRI and TNFRII; these cleaved receptors act as endogenous inhibitors of circulating TNF-α **(Figure 33-2)**. Unlike the cleavage of TNF-α, the cleavage of the receptors is not exclusive to TACE.[7] An elevated level of TACE expression has been demonstrated in endometriosis, consistent with it having an active function.[11] Unfortunately no mechanistic evidence is available to support its pathological role in endometriosis; this target does, however, appear in a number of patients for TACE inhibitors. There appears to be no developmental research focusing on TACE as a target in endometriosis. The context dependant nature of the TNF pathway may allow this therapeutic route to show improvements in the contraindications over the TNF-α blockers and maintain apoptotic while removing the growth factor pathways. A further function of TACE that may be of significance in its use as a target is its function in the cleavage of MUC1. This surface bound mucin is abundant in reproductive tissue, in particular the uterus, where it is responsible for lubrication, tissue hydration and, more importantly, microbial and enzyme resistance. One certain advantage of any potential TACE inhibitor therapy over those currently under investigation for the TNF-α pathway is that current small molecule drugs are available so an oral therapy is entirely possible in the future.

Telomerase

Telomerase has been recently proposed as a target for endometriosis as expression of this protein has been identified by immuno-histochemistry in the ectopic endometrial tissue. It is suggested that it is this expression which may lead to increased survival and proliferation of RM tissue in sufferers.[12] It seems unlikely that direct inhibition of telomerase may prove useful in endometriosis due to toxic effects, however, selectively down-regulating telomerase expression via tissue directed pathways may prove possible.

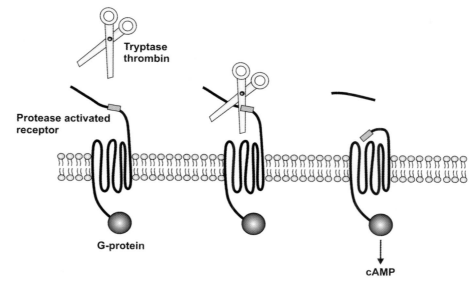

FIGURE 33-2: PARs are activated by thrombin or mast cell tryptase. Cleavage of the N-terminus domain leads to availability of self-activation domain and subsequent signalling.

Cyclooxygenase-2 (COX-2)

The primary feature of endometriosis is pain and as such nonsteroidal anti-inflammatory drugs (NSAIDs) provide the first line of treatment. With the incidence of endometriosis believed to be as high as 10%, much of this NSAID therapy may well be self-proscribed. Generic mixed cyclooxygenase (COX) 1 and 2 inhibitors such as acetylsalicylic acid, indomethacin and ibuprofen have been previously mentioned as current therapy due to their pain relief and NSAID functions. However, selective COX-2 antagonists also constitute one area of development in the endometriosis pipeline.[10] The two currently identified COX enzymes differ in their distribution; COX-1 is believed to be constitutive and account for baseline levels of prostaglandins, whereas COX-2 is inducible, mediating many of the effects of prostaglandin. Prostaglandin's local effects include inflammation, platelet aggregation, vascular dilation or constriction and cell proliferation. Current research demonstrates a detectable increase in cyclooxygenase-2 (COX-2) expression in lesions and also in the peritoneal macrophages of endometriosis patients. COX-2 is responsible for the generation of the prostaglandins, in particular prostaglandin E2 (PGE2), which acts as a survival factor for endometrial tissue. The expression of COX-2 is regulated by the action of estrogens, which leads to the production of a positive feedback in endometriosis, with PGE2 also acting to increase aromatase expression thus leading to increased estrogen production. It is for this reason that a number of drugs are currently being investigated to tease apart this pathway, notably the COX-2 inhibitors Nimesulide, Valdecoxib RO-346 and the aromatase inhibitor Anastrazole. So far mixed results have been seen in animal models for COX-2 inhibitors in endometriosis.[13,14] Unfortunately, recent results have shown chronic use of COX-2 inhibitors may be linked to an increased prevalence of stroke and heart attack. While these adverse reactions should be a consideration when approaching this therapy, they are likely to pose less of a risk when considering the likely treatment group in this indication.

Relaxin

The peptide relaxin was originally described by function in 1926 by Frederick Hisaw. Consisting of a number of family members, slow progress in the field was due to problems associated with the identification of the receptors binding these peptides, the LGR7 and LGR8 receptors only being de-orphanized in 2002. One of the reasons for the delay in identifying the receptors was the similarity of the peptide to insulin. Ultimately the receptor turned out to be a 7 trans-membrane GPCR rather than a single span insulin like receptor.

The secretory phase in the menstrual cycle is associated with an increased expression of the H2 relaxin receptor LGR7. The relaxin peptide H2 is responsible in pregnancy for a localized reduction in immune response and increased stability, leading to increased endometrial expression of VEGF receptors thus making the uterus more receptive to placental implantation.[15] A number of companies have attempted to produce a small molecule LGR7 agonist, currently without success probably due to the receptors similarity to the follicle stimulating hormone (FSH) receptor. However, antagonists are easier to identify, which makes this a possible future target.[16]

Serotonergic Modulators

Melatonin is produced by the pineal gland and results in the arrest of lipid peroxidation and leads to a reduction in MMP-9 activity and expression in a time dependant manner. Exposure to melatonin results in protection against and regression of peritoneal endometriosis in a mouse model, duplicating the result seen previously in rats.[17] It is highly likely that this effect is due to the disruption of the circadian release of FSH and resultant reduction in estradiol release.

Peroxisome Proliferators-activated Receptors (PPARs)

Peritoneal macrophages have been demonstrated to express peroxisome proliferator-activated receptors (PPARs) in particular PPAR-α and PPAR-γ. Endometrial cell cultures demonstrated a response to PPAR-γ ligand, increasing the expression of IL-6, IL-8 and colony stimulating factor-1 (CSF-1).[18] PPAR ligand Rosiglitazone has been shown to reduce angiogenesis, probably through its down-regulation of VEGF. Rosilitazone has also been shown to suppress the formation of endometriosis lesions and reduce those already formed.[19] Significantly Rosilitazone has also been shown to reduce endometriosis burden in baboons without effect on menstrual cycle and leads to no reduction in fertility in mice. The apparent lack of effect on fertility represents a significant therapeutic advantage over other hormonal based therapies.

Hepatocyte Growth Factor (HGF)

Hepatocyte growth factor (HGF), also known as scatter factor (SF) due to its function in metastasis, binds the receptor c-Met of the tyrosine kinase (TK) receptor family

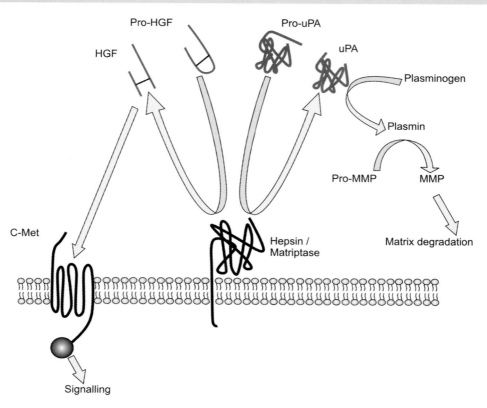

FIGURE 33-3: Hepsin or matriptase can lead to the local activation of HGF signalling. Hepsin also can act on the uPA and plasmin pathway to activate MMPs, resulting in local matrix degradation.

(Figure 33-3). HGF is produced in an inactive long form by mesenchymal cells; its cleavage results in an alpha and beta chain, linked by a single disulphide bond. As well as its physiological function of organ regeneration, HGF acts directly on most cells of epithelial linage. HGF is known to affect many cellular phenotypic changes, including cell growth, survival, angiogenesis, invasion and metastasis, which has made it a popular oncology target. A high level of HGF immune reactivity has been demonstrated in the stroma adjacent to endometriosis lesions.[20] HGF release has also been demonstrated in endometriosis in response to IL-6 and TNF-α and the macrophages from endometriosis patients produce significantly more HGF than controls when exposed to estradiol. There are currently a number of second generation selective c-Met antagonists in clinical testing for oncology indications. HGF may be a possible target for the future in endometriosis; the main potential problem is that the large size of the TK family of receptors makes selectivity an issue.

Protease Targets

Matrix Metalloproteinases (MMPs)

Endometriosis is a highly invasive condition and as such is associated with the increased localized expression of MMPs, in particular MMP-2 (gelatinase A), MMP-3 (stromlysin) and MMP-9 (gelatinase B).[21] Recent evidence has identified a promoter polymorphism for MMP-2 in deep infiltrating disease in north Chinese patients with endometriosis. An association has also been identified with superficial endometriosis and polymorphisms in MMP-12 (macrophage elastase) and MMP-13 (interstitial collagenase-3) (P=0.004). It is interesting to note, however, that no incidence was identified for MMP-12 and 13 in deep infiltration, suggesting that these polymorphisms are associated with limiting the disease rather than being causative factors in endometriosis.[22] The issue with the use of MMP inhibitors in this indication is the same as all other indications in which they have been tested. MMPs are not only at the end of the mechanistic pathological pathway but also they are not as substrate specific as is often suggested. Work in other indications has demonstrated both in models and the clinic, that inhibition often leads to compensation in expression or activity of other family members and/or down-regulation of endogenous inhibitors to restore the balance. Broad spectrum inhibitors may prove too toxic in this indication to consider and would not address either the inflammatory process, serine proteases or growth factor mediated changes in tissue morphology.

Tryptase

The serine protease tryptase is highly abundant in mast cells and as such is often used as a cell marker. Tryptase has been implicated in the cleavage of the protein activated receptor -2 (PAR-2). The PAR receptors are a family of g protein couple receptors (GPCRs), which self activate via a tethered ligand following the selective cleavage of a pre-peptide region **(Figure 33-3)**. Tryptase following the cleavage of PAR-2 has demonstrated the release of IL-6 and IL-8 by the endometrial stoma.[23] Sites of endometriosis are associated with elevated levels of mast cells and the numbers of activated and degranulating mast cells correlate highly in the deep infiltrating lesions.[24] Both PAR-1 and PAR-2 have been implicated as possible future targets in endometriosis with functions in pain and inflammation, PAR-1 may be cleaved by thrombin.[25] As GPCRs, the PAR receptors could well prove good therapeutic targets.

Hepsin and Matriptase

Unlike the pathways pursued with the MMP targets, the serine proteases may be used to actively target more obvious upstream events in the progression of this condition. An important example of such a pathway is those proteases involved in the local activation of hepatocyte growth factor (HGF), which has been mentioned above. HGF circulates in an inactive long form and is selectively cleaved by either matriptase or the more recently identified hepsin to form a disulphide linked dimer **(Figure 33-3)**. While the literature does not link either enzyme directly with endometriosis, the role of HGF in endometriosis indicates that at least one is likely to be involved. The literature and unpublished data also demonstrate localization of hepsin to the endometrium in histological samples and matriptase more broadly to the uterus. While c-Met may prove a difficult target due to toxicity in endometriosis, hepsin/matriptase may prove to be a more easy way into the same pathway. In addition to its role in HGF activation, urokinase plasminogen activator (uPA) has also been identified as a further substrate of hepsin making it a possible upstream target for the inhibition of multiple MMPs. There are at present a number of companies developing matriptase inhibitors and the similarity of hepsin makes it highly likely that the same companies also have hepsin and dual inhibitors in early stage development in search of an indication.

Conclusion

It can be clearly seen from the literature that there are plenty of potential new avenues to pursue when it comes to the development of therapies for the treatment of endometriosis. However, it would still appear that endometriosis is dependant on drug 'hand me downs' from other diseases. As a result many of the available therapies are drastic, leading to many unsatisfactory side effects. Unfortunately, although endometriosis represents a potentially huge market, many of the current therapies, while far from perfect, do work and are in the main generic. There is a clear unmet medical need in this indication due to the implications of present therapy. Current drugs in the pipeline pose new possibilities for improvement to the treatment of sufferers; with the third generation of endocrine drugs having considerable improvements over those from the past. It appears that the invasive nature of endometriosis still leads to an overlap with cancer therapies and chronic inflammatory conditions. There is an opportunity in endometriosis, although to get a truly bespoke therapy for which there is both a sizable market and unmet medical need it may be necessary for a small company to raise interest. As a result of this, there has probably never been an indication more suited to transitional pharma. The main reason for failure of drugs is either that they do not work or are too toxic. In order to be successful in the passage of a compound to release, every new drug must address a clear unmet medical need or represent a significant refinement of current therapies, especially where cheap off license generics provide some disease coverage. The minimal drug product profile is a further consideration both in terms of marketability and function; given the severity of the condition, what course duration, dosing regimen or route of administration are acceptable? There is a real opportunity/need for transitional pharma to take the lead in endometriosis, combining new academic ideas from research with *in situ* knowledge from the clinic, to create new directions in this poorly supported indication. The transitional option could provide the necessary high quality product validation and as such any subsequent package would undoubtedly prove highly attractive to the larger pharmaceutical industry.

References

1. Sampson JA. Peritoneal endometriosis due to the menstrual dissemination of endometrial tissue into the peritoneal cavity. Am J Obstet Gynecol 1927;14: 422–69.

2. Halme J, Hammond MG, Hulka JF, et al. Retrograde menstruation in healthy women and in patients with endometriosis. Obstet Gynecol 1984; 64: 151-54.

3. Matorras R, Ocerin I, Unamuno M, et al. Prevalence of endometriosis in women with systemic lupus erythematosus and Sjogren's syndrome. Lupus 2007; 16: 736-40.

4. Smith C. Drug target validation: Hitting the target. Nature 2003; 422; 341-47.

5. Mark Moran. Cost of Bringing New Drugs To Market Rising Rapidly. Psychiatric News 2003; 38: 25.

6. Broqua P, Riviere PJ, Conn PM, et al. Pharmacological profile of a new, potent, and long-acting gonadotropin-releasing hormone antagonist: Degarelix. J Pharmacol Exp Ther 2002; 301:95-102.

7. Bradley JR. TNF-mediated inflammatory disease. J Pathol 2008;214:149-60.

8. Koninckx PR, Craessaerts M, Timmerman D, et al. Anti-TNF-alpha treatment for deep endometriosis-associated pain: a randomized placebo-controlled trial. Hum Reprod 2008; 23:2017-23.

9. Kyama CM, Overbergh L, Mihalyi A, et al. Effect of recombinant human TNF-binding protein-1 and GnRH antagonist on mRNA expression of inflammatory cytokines and adhesion and growth factors in endometrium and endometriosis tissues in baboons. Fertil Steril 2008; 89: 1306-13.

10. Kyama CM, Mihalyi A, Simsa P, et al. Non-Steroidal Targets in the Diagnosis and Treatment of Endometriosis. Curr Med Chem 2008; 15: 1006-17.

11. Gottschalk C, Malberg K, Arndt M, et al. Matrix metalloproteinases and TACE play a role in the pathogenesis of endometriosis. Adv Exp Med Biol 2000;477:483-86.

12. Kim CM, Oh YJ, Cho SH, et al. Increased telomerase activity and human telomerasse reverse transcriptase mRNA expression in the endometrium of patients with endometriosis. Hum Reprod 2007; 22: 843-49.

13. Laschke MW, Elitzsch A, Scheuer C, et al. Selective cyclooxygenase-2 inhibition induces regression of autologous endometrial grafts by down-regulation of vascular endothelial growth factor-mediated angiogenesis and stimulation of caspase-3-dependent apoptosis. Fertil Steril 2007;87:163-71.

14. Hull ML, Prentice A, Wang DY, et al. Nimesulide, a COX-2 inhibitor, does not reduce lesion size or number in a nude mouse model of endometriosis. Hum Reprod 2005; 20: 350-58.

15. Kaczmarek MM, Blitek A, Kaminska K, et al. Assessment of VEGF-receptor system expression in the porcine endometrial stromal cells in response to insulin-like growth factor-I, relaxin, oxytocin and prostaglandin E2. Mol Cell Endocrinol 2008; 291: 33-41.

16. Gui Y, Zhang J, Yuan L, et al. Regulation of HOXA-10 and its expression in normal and abnormal endometrium. Mol Hum Reprod 1999; 5: 866-73.

17. Paul S, Sharma AV, Mahapatra PD, et al. Role of melatonin in regulating matrix metalloproteinase-9 via tissue inhibitors of metalloproteinase-1 during protection against endometriosis. J Pineal Res 2008; 44: 439-49.

18. Wanichkul T, Han S, Huang RP, et al. Cytokine regulation by peroxisome proliferator-activated receptor gamma in human endometrial cells. Fertil Steril 2003; 79: 763-69.

19. Hornung D, Waite LL, Ricke EA, et al. Nuclear peroxisome proliferator-activated receptors alpha and gamma have opposing effects on monocyte chemotaxis in endometriosis. J Clin Endocrinol Metab 2001; 86: 3108-14.

20. Ishimaru T, Khan KN, Fujishita A, et al. Hepatocyte growth factor may be involved in cellular changes to the peritoneal mesothelium adjacent to pelvic endometriosis. Fertil Steril 2004; 81: 810-18.

21. Salata IM, Stojanovic N, Cajdler-Łuba A, et al. Gelatinase A (MM-2), gelatinase B (MMP-9) and their inhibitors (TIMP 1, TIMP-2) in serum of women with endometriosis: Significant correlation between MMP-2, MMP-9 and their inhibitors without difference in levels of matrix metalloproteinases and tissue inhibitors of metalloproteinases in relation to the severity of endometriosis. Gynecol Endocrinol 2008; 24: 326-30.

22. Borghese B, Chiche JD, Vernerey D, et al. Genetic polymorphisms of matrix metalloproteinase 12 and 13 genes are implicated in endometriosis progression. Hum Reprod 2008; 23: 1207-13.

23. Hirota Y, Osuga Y, Hirata T, et al. Possible involvement of thrombin/protease-activated receptor 1 system in the pathogenesis of endometriosis. J Clin Endocrinol Metab 2005; 90: 3673-79.

24. Anaf V, Chapron C, El Nakadi I, Pain, mast cells, and nerves in peritoneal, ovarian, and deep infiltrating endometriosis. Fertil Steril 2006; 86: 1336-43.

25. Hirota Y, Osuga Y, Hirata T, et al. Activation of protease-activated receptor 2 stimulates proliferation and interleukin (IL)-6 and IL-8 secretion of endometriotic stromal cells. Hum Reprod 2005; 20: 3547-53.

Jacques Donnez, Pascale Jadoul, Marie-Madeleine Dolmans,
Jean Squifflet, Jean-Christophe Lousse

Chapter 34

Fertility Preservation in Women with Endometriosis

Introduction

Endometriosis is one of the most frequently encountered benign diseases in gynecology. It is the cause of pelvic pain (dysmenorrhea, dyspareunia) and infertility in more than 35% of women of reproductive age.[1] Complete resolution of endometriosis is not yet possible, but therapy has essentially three main objectives: (1) to preserve and improve fertility; (2) to reduce pain; and (3) to delay recurrence for as long as possible. The aim of this chapter is to focus on fertility preservation in women with severe endometriosis.

Treatment of endometriosis-associated infertility has been investigated with medical and surgical therapeutic modalities, individually and in combination.[2] In moderate and severe endometriosis, a medico-surgical approach remains the gold standard.[2,3]

The most important surgery in endometriosis-associated infertility is ovarian surgery (hemorrhagic cysts or endometriomas), but there are some concerns. Indeed, excessive surgery may lead to normal ovarian tissue destruction, while incomplete surgery is associated with a much higher risk of recurrence. As reported below, more and more papers are describing a low ovarian reserve after laparoscopic cystectomy for endometriomas.[4-9] Indeed, very frequently, normal ovarian tissue is excised together with the endometrioma wall.[10] Ovarian surgery in endometriosis patients should therefore be performed by experienced surgeons in order to both preserve and improve fertility. We very recently reported a laparoscopic procedure that combines the advantages, while avoiding the corresponding risks, of current techniques used in endometrioma surgery (cystectomy and ablative surgery).[11] This new technique, called the 'combined' technique, will be described in this chapter.

Moreover, in severe pelvic endometriosis and/or recurrent endometriomas, normal residual ovarian tissue and/or ovarian vascularization may be compromised. Preservation of ovarian tissue should therefore be considered in these patients with seriously impaired fertility, particularly before any treatment viewed as high risk for ovarian endometriosis recurrence techniques of autotransplantation of human ovarian tissue (fresh or cryopreserved) technique will be presented in this chapter. Research into isolation of primordial follicles from cryopreserved tissue will also be discussed.

Laparoscopic Management of Endometriomas Using a Combined Technique of Excisional and Ablative Surgery

There are two main risks associated with the surgical treatment of endometriomas: (1) the risk of excessive surgery (removal or destruction of normal ovarian cortex together with the endometrioma); and (2) the risk of incomplete surgery (with subsequent early recurrence of endometriomas). Depending on the risk, two techniques are currently used, with both advantages and disadvantages: either cyctectomy involving removal of the endometrioma wall, or ablative surgery that entails opening the endometrioma and destroying the internal cyst wall by laser vaporization or bipolar coagulation.

Ablative surgery may prove difficult because of the thickness and hypervascularization of the cyst wall. Recently, a Cochrane Review reported a higher rate of recurrence after ablative surgery than cystectomy.[12] On the other hand, recent data in the literature appear to indicate that excisional surgery of endometriomas may be deleterious for ovarian function, causing ovarian trauma and removal of follicles. According to Muzii et al,[10] recognizable ovarian tissue was inadvertently excised together with the endometriotic cyst wall in most cases during stripping for endometrioma excision. Close to the ovarian hilus, ovarian tissue removed along the endometrioma wall contained primordial, primary and secondary follicles in 69% of cases. Away from the hilus, the presence of follicles was infrequent.[10]

In view of these data, we set out to develop a new approach that combines the techniques of cystectomy and ablative surgery, in order to take the best elements from both, while avoiding the corresponding risks (excessive surgery or incomplete surgery respectively). As illustrated in **Figure 34-1**, a large part of the endometrioma is first excised according to the cystectomy technique. The endometrial cyst is opened and washed out with irrigation fluid. After identifying the correct plane of cleavage between the cyst wall and ovarian tissue by applying opposite bimanual traction and countertraction with two grasping forceps, providing strong but non-traumatic force, the inner lining of the cyst is stripped from the normal ovarian tissue. When approaching the hilus, where the ovarian tissue is more functional, partial cystectomy is performed by resecting the excised tissue with scissors

(Figures 34-1A and B). The stripping technique allows removal of 80-90% of the cyst. If the excision provokes bleeding or the plane of cleavage is not clearly visible, the cystectomy is stopped because of the risk of removing normal ovarian tissue containing primordial, primary and secondary follicles along with the endometrioma. After this first step (partial cystectomy), CO_2 laser (Storz, Lumenis, USA) is used to vaporize the remaining 10-20% of the endometrioma close to the hilus. Care must be taken to vaporize all the residual cyst wall in order to avoid recurrence **(Figures 34-1C and D)**.

This combined technique was applied in 52 patients with ovarian endometriosis.[11] They all received GnRH agonist therapy for three months postoperatively. Six months after surgery, vaginal ultrasound was carried out in order to evaluate the ovarian volume and antral follicle count (AFC) on day 2-5. In 20 women who had unilateral endometriomas, a comparison was made with the contralateral healthy ovary. Data were also compared with those from women of similar age with normal ovaries and regular ovulatory cycles presenting for IVF because of male factor infertility.

The combined technique was possible in all cases. The volume of the ovary after the combined technique was similar to that of the contralateral normal ovary, as well as

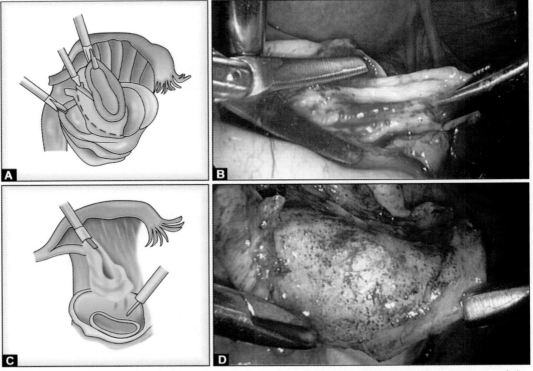

FIGURE 34-1: Combined technique: schematic and laparoscopic views. Partial cystectomy of the endometrioma is first carried out (A, B). To avoid excessive surgical damage close to the hilus, vaporization of the residual cyst is then performed (C, D).

Table 34-1: Ovarian volume and antral follicle count (AFC) six months after surgery in women treated for endometriomas by the combined technique and women of similar age with normal ovaries and regular ovulatory cycles presenting for IVF because of male factor infertility.

	Ovarian volume (cm³)	Antral follicle count (AFs)
Combined technique (n=31)	7.64 ± 2.95	6.1 ± 3.2
Women without endometriosis (n=20)	7.99 ± 5.33	6.2 ± 4.8

Table 34-2: Ovarian volume and antral follicle count (AFC) six months after surgery in women with unilateral endometriomas and contralateral normal ovaries serving as controls.

	Ovarian volume (cm³)	Antral follicle count (AFs)
Combined technique (n=20)	7.45 ± 2.93	5.5 ± 2.4
Contralateral normal ovaries (n=20)	7.82 ± 3.91	5.7 ± 1.6

that observed in infertile women without endometriosis presenting for male factor infertility. The AFC on day 2-5 showed the same number of antral follicles in all subgroups (**Tables 34-1 and 34-2**). Histopathology of the excised part of the endometrioma revealed the presence of follicles in only one case (2%).

According to our present data, this new technique appears to combine the best results of the stripping technique in terms of recurrence outcomes, since most of the cyst wall is excised, and the ablation technique, since the hilus area of the ovary is spared from surgical damage.

Autotransplantation of Human Ovarian Tissue in Endometriosis Patients

Normal residual ovarian tissue and/or ovarian vascularization may be compromised in patients with severe endometriosis and/or recurrent endometriomas. In case of radical treatment (oophorectomy), but also if there is a risk of recurrence after conservative treatment, preservation of ovarian tissue with future autotransplantation should be seriously considered. We report our experience with autotransplantation of human ovarian tissue (fresh or cryopreserved). Current research into isolation of primordial follicles from cryopreserved tissue is also discussed, as transplantation of isolated follicles may prove to be an alternative option in the future.

Orthotopic Transplantation of Fresh Ovarian Cortex in Endometriosis Patients

Silber et al[13] reported successful reimplantation of fresh ovarian tissue using ovarian cortex donated by a monozygotous twin. In 2005, we reported the first two cases of orthotopic transplantation of fresh ovarian tissue in humans with ovarian endometriosis.[14] Two 25- and 27-year-old women were diagnosed with recurrent large unilateral left-sided endometriomas. At laparoscopy, the left part of the pelvis was found to be frozen in both cases and, after careful dissection, left ovarian vascularization appeared to be compromised. Left oophorectomy was performed. However, before removal of the ovary, two to four strips of ovarian cortex (measuring 3-4 × 12 mm) were taken from residual healthy ovarian tissue. A window was created beneath the healthy right ovarian hilus close to the ovarian blood vessels. One strip of fresh ovarian cortex was placed in the window and fixed (**Figures 34-2A to F**). The remaining healthy tissue of both patients was cryopreserved.

At second-look laparoscopy, macroscopically viable-looking ovarian tissue of ± 1 cm in size was visible in the grafted area of the two patients and biopsies were taken (**Figures 34-3A and B**). In one patient, a small cystic structure (follicle) not covered with peritoneum was seen on the grafted ovarian tissue.

Biopsies of reimplanted tissue were studied by histology and vital fluorescent staining (calcein-AM and ethidium homodimer-1), according to the technique used by Donnez et al.[15]

In both patients, primordial follicles and active angiogenesis (demonstrated by the presence of numerous small vessels in the grafted tissue) were observed. Viability of the primordial follicles was proved by vital fluorescent staining. Biopsy of the small cystic structure seen in one patient at laparoscopy revealed granulosa cells, but the oocyte was not recovered. Finally, in part of the biopsy from one patient, six viable follicles were detected after collagenase isolation and vital fluorescent staining (**Figures 34-3C and D**).

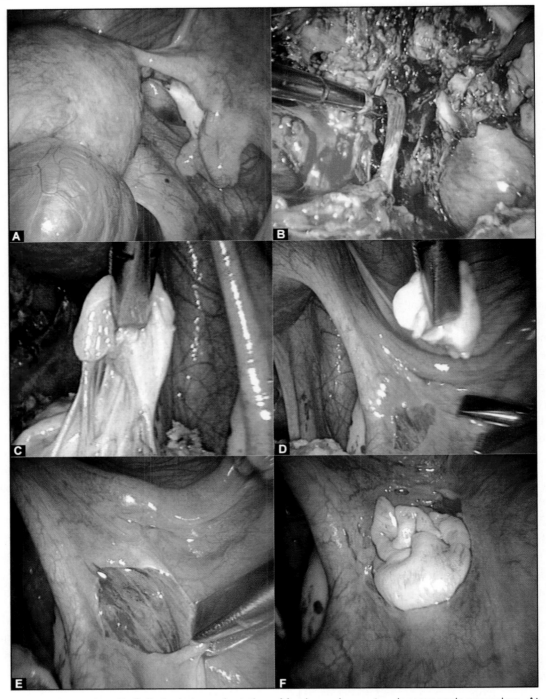

FIGURES 34-2A to F: Orthotopic transplantation of fresh ovarian cortex: laparoscopic procedure. At laparoscopy, the left part of the pelvis was found to be frozen, while the right part was free of adhesions (A). After careful dissection, left ovarian vascularization appeared to be compromised (B). Before removal of the ovary, strips of ovarian cortex were taken from residual healthy ovarian tissue (C and D). A window was created beneath the healthy right ovarian hilus close to the ovarian blood vessels (E). One strip of fresh ovarian cortex was placed in the window and fixed (F).

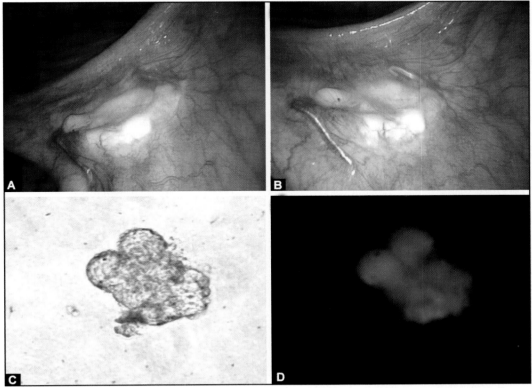

FIGURES 34-3A to D: At second-look laparoscopy, macroscopically viable-looking ovarian tissue of ± 1 cm in size was visible in the grafted area of the two patients and a biopsy was taken (A and B). In part of the biopsy from one patient, six viable follicles were detected after collagenase isolation and vital fluorescent staining (C and D).

This study provides histological data after orthotopic autotransplantation of fresh ovarian cortex, proving the survival of primordial follicles and the presence of a neovascular network. This technique could therefore be used to preserve ovarian tissue in case of severe and/or recurrent ovarian endometriosis, when normal residual ovarian tissue is compromised.

Orthotopic Transplantation of Cryopreserved Ovarian Tissue

As already stated, fertility preservation is a priority in the treatment of endometriosis in patients at risk of impaired future fertility. During surgery, cryopreservation of healthy ovarian tissue may be an option in case of severe endometriosis. Orthotopic autotransplantation of cryopreserved ovarian cortex has already proved to be efficient in cancer patients, leading to restoration of ovarian function, pregnancy and live birth.[15-20]

The different cryopreservation options available for fertility preservation in cancer patients or patients at risk of premature ovarian failure (family history, recurrent ovarian surgery,...) are embryo cryopreservation, oocyte cryopreservation and ovarian tissue cryopreservation, the choice depending on various parameters such as the type and timing of chemotherapy, the type of cancer, the patient's age and the partner status.[16] The only established method of fertility preservation is embryo cryopreservation according to the Ethics Committee of the American Society for Reproductive Medicine,[21] but this option requires the patient to be of pubertal age, have a partner or use donor sperm, and be able to undergo a cycle of ovarian stimulation.

In our department, cryopreservation of ovarian tissue has also been proposed for benign diseases, including severe endometriosis. The indications for cryopreservation of ovarian tissue in case of malignant and non-malignant diseases are summarized in **Table 34-3**. The age of the patient should be taken into consideration, since the follicular reserve of the ovary is age-dependent. Because a decline in fertility is now well documented after the age of 38 years, the procedure should probably be restricted to patients below this limit.

Table 34-3: Indications for ovarian tissue cryopreservation in case of malignant and non-malignant diseases *(from Donnez et al, Hum Reprod Update 2006, with permission).*

Malignant	*Non-malignant*

Extrapelvic diseases
  Bone cancer (osteosarcoma – Ewing's sarcoma)
  Breast cancer
  Melanoma
  Neuroblastoma
  Bowel malignancy
Pelvic diseases
  Non-gynecological malignancy
    Pelvic sarcoma
    Rhabdomyosarcoma
    Sacral tumors
    Rectosigmoid tumors
  Gynecological malignancy
    Early cervical carcinoma
    Early vaginal carcinoma
    Early vulvar carcinoma
    Selected cases of ovarian carcinoma (stage IA)
    Borderline ovarian tumors
  Systemic diseases
    Hodgkin's disease
    Non-Hodgkin's lymphoma
    Leukemia
    Medulloblastoma
	Uni/bilateral oophorectomy
	  Benign ovarian tumors
	  Severe and recurrent endometriosis
	  BRCA-1 or BRCA-2 mutation carriers
	Risk of premature menopause
	  Turner's syndrome
	  Family history
	  Recurrent ovarian surgery
	  Benign diseases requiring chemotherapy: autoimmune diseases (systemic lupus erythematosus, rheumatoid arthritis, Behçet's disease and Wegener's disease)
	
	Bone marrow transplantation
	  Benign hematological diseases: sickle cell anemia, thalassemia major and aplastic anemia
	  Autoimmune diseases unresponsive to immunosuppressive therapy

The aim of this strategy is to reimplant cortical ovarian tissue into the pelvic cavity (orthotopic site), or a heterotopic site like the forearm or abdominal wall in case of premature ovarian failure, in patients with severe and recurrent endometriosis. So far, only orthotopic transplantation of cryopreserved ovarian cortical fragments has resulted in pregnancies and live births in cancer patients. However, other strategies, such as transplantation of isolated cryopreserved primordial follicles, may prove to be alternative options in the future, as discussed below.[16,22]

Ovarian Biopsy Samples

Follicles are located inside the ovarian cortex, and thus tissue samples collected for cryopreservation have to come from the surface of the organ. A biopsy can be taken during any gynecological procedure, by laparoscopy or laparotomy, and may be composed of one or several cortical fragments. Palmer forceps are inserted through one of the 5-mm trocars placed in the iliac fossa, and are used to grasp the ovary and cut a fragment from its surface. Cortical biopsy can also be easily carried out with laparoscopic scissors. The number of samples taken varies according to the size of the patient's ovaries and the estimated risk of premature ovarian failure. Biopsy samples are immediately transferred to the laboratory in Leibovitz

L-15 medium supplemented with Glutamax™ (Invitrogen, Paisley, UK) on ice. To minimize any tissue damage due to ischemia, the samples are transferred within minutes to the laboratory for processing.

Freezing and Thawing Procedures

Freezing of ovarian tissue is undertaken according to the protocol described by Gosden et al.[24] In the laboratory, the remaining stromal tissue is gently removed. The cortical samples are cut into small cubes (2 x 2 mm) or strips (10 x 3 mm). These fragments of ovarian tissue are suspended in cryoprotective medium and then placed into precooled 2 ml cryogenic vials (Simport, Quebec, Canada) filled with L-15 medium supplemented with 4 mg/ml of human serum albumin (Red Cross, Brussels, Belgium) and 1.5 mol/l of dimethylsulphoxide (Sigma, St Louis, MO, USA). The cryotubes are cooled in a programmable freezer (Kryo 10, Series III; Planer, Sunbury-on-Thames, UK) with the following program: cooled from 0°C to -8°C at -2°C/min; seeded manually by touching the cryotubes with forceps pre-chilled in liquid nitrogen; cooled to -40°C at -0.3° C/min; cooled to -150°C at -30°C/min; and transferred to liquid nitrogen (-196°C) immediately for storage.

The thawing procedure is as follows: the cryogenic vials are thawed at room temperature (between 21°C and 23°C)

for 2 min and immersed in a water bath at 37°C for another 2 min. Ovarian tissue is immediately transferred from the vials to tissue culture dishes (Becton Dickinson, NY, USA) in L-15 medium and subsequently washed three times at room temperature with fresh medium to remove cryoprotectant before further processing. Thawed ovarian cortical tissue is then placed in sterile medium and immediately transferred to the operating theater.

Orthotopic Transplantation Techniques

Nine cases of orthotopic transplantation have so far been carried out in our department, using two techniques of ovarian cortex reimplantation.

The first technique involved creating a peritoneal window before reimplantation in order to induce angiogenesis and neovascularization in that area. This procedure was clearly described in our publication reporting the first pregnancy and live birth after orthotopic transplantation of cryopreserved ovarian tissue.[15] We performed the first laparoscopy 7 days before reimplan-

tation to create a peritoneal window by means of a large incision just beneath the ovarian hilus, followed by coagulation of the edges of the window **(Figure 34-4A)**. Seven days later, during a second laparoscopy, small cubes of frozen-thawed ovarian tissue were pushed into the furrow created by the peritoneal window very close to the ovarian vessels and fimbria. An extensive neovascular network was clearly visible in this space **(Figure 34-4B)**.

We used another technique to reimplant ovarian cortex in the other eight cases. By laparotomy or laparoscopy, ovarian tissue was reimplanted onto the remaining ovary after removal of the native cortex **(Figure 34-4C)**. In some cases, large strips of ovarian tissue were attached to the decorticated medulla with stitches **(Figure 34-4D)**. In other cases, small ovarian fragments were placed on the decorticated medulla and an absorbable adhesion barrier was used to cover and fix the thawed fragments to the ovary.

In our experience, the peritoneal window created close to the ovarian hilus, as well as the ovarian medulla, were both found to be equally efficient sites of reimplantation.

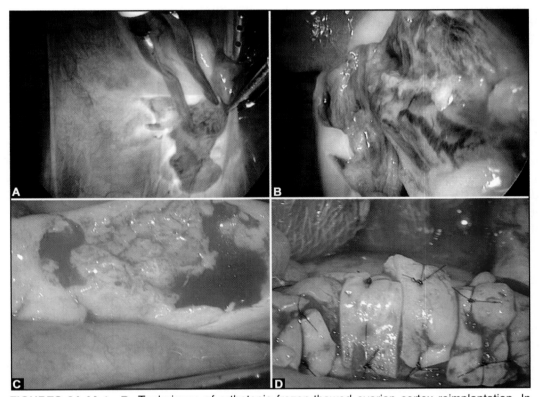

FIGURES 34-4A to D: Techniques of orthotopic frozen-thawed ovarian cortex reimplantation. In one case, a peritoneal window was created 7 days before reimplantation in order to induce angiogenesis in this area (A). On the day of reimplantation, an extensive neovascular network was clearly visible in this space (B).

In the other eight cases, ovarian tissue was reimplanted onto the remaining ovary after removal of the native cortex (C). In most cases, large strips of ovarian tissue were attached to the decorticated medulla with stitches (D).

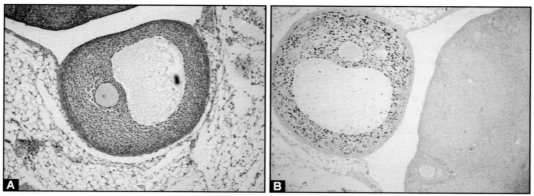

FIGURES 34-5A and B: Histological sections of isolated human follicles xenografted for 5 months to severe combined immunodeficient (SCID) mice.[22] Hematoxylin-eosin-stained histological section of a 600-μm antral follicle (A). H = human ovarian graft, M = mouse ovary. The oocyte with a visible nucleolus is surrounded by an intact zona pellucida. The antral cavity is encapsulated by multiple layers of apparently normal granulosa cells and a few theca cells. Anti-human Ki-67 immunostaining of an antral follicle (B). Intensive brown staining of the granulosa cells indicates proliferation.

Large strips (8-10 mm x 5 mm) or small cubes (2 mm) were reimplanted. Both sizes effectively restored ovarian endocrine function. From a microsurgical point of view, however, it is easier to attach large strips to the medulla rather than small cubes, which cannot be sutured. Since reimplantation of large strips is easier and just as effective as small cube reimplantation, we suggest that large strips be taken from the ovarian cortex for cryopreservation purposes.

Isolation of Primordial Follicles from Cryopreserved Ovarian Tissue

In case of microscopic endometriotic foci in apparently normal ovarian tissue, reimplantation of fresh or cryopreserved ovarian tissue may lead to recurrence of the disease, although the risk is probably very low. The same risk is present in cancer patients (particularly in case of breast cancer and leukemia), in whom the possibility of reintroducing malignant cells cannot be excluded.

To decrease the risk of transferring endometriotic cells, *in vitro* follicle maturation could be performed after follicle isolation. Culturing isolated follicles from the primordial stage is an attractive proposition because they represent >90% of the total follicular reserve and show high cryotolerance.[22,25] However, isolated primordial follicles do not grow properly in culture.[26] Another approach could be to transplant a suspension of isolated follicles.[22] As the follicular basal lamina encapsulating the membrana granulosa excludes capillaries, white blood cells and nerve processes from the granulosa compartment,[22,26] grafting fully isolated follicles could be considered safer. Moreover, this would allow the introduction of a high and known

number of follicles, obtaining faster angiogenesis and minimizing ischemic and reperfusion damage.[27]

In a murine model, Dolmans et al recently demonstrated the development of antral follicles after xenografting of isolated small human preantral follicles.[22] Human ovarian biopsies were enzymatically using collagenase to obtain purified isolated follicles that were xenografted to severe combined immunodeficient (SCID) mice for 5 months. After sacrifice euthanasia, follicular morphology was assessed by histology, and follicular proliferation by Ki-67 immunohistochemistry. Four grafts containing a total of 84 follicles were recovered. This follicular population was composed of 11 primordial follicles, 38 primary follicles, 31 secondary follicles and four antral follicles **(Figure 34-5A)**. Finally, Ki-67 was found to intensively stain granulosa cells in antral follicles **(Figure 34-5B)**.

Conclusion

The most important surgery in endometriosis-associated infertility is ovarian surgery. Because surgery has to be effective (decrease the risk of recurrence) and protective (avoid normal ovarian tissue destruction), we propose a new surgical procedure that combines the best results of the stripping technique in terms of recurrence outcomes, since most of the cyst wall is excised, and the ablation technique, since the hilus area of the ovary is spared from surgical damage.

In case of severe endometriosis and/or recurrent endometriomas, normal residual ovarian tissue and/or ovarian vascularization may be compromised. In case of radical treatment (oophorectomy) in particular, but also conservative treatment as there is a risk of recurrence, preservation of ovarian tissue should be considered with a view to future autotransplantation. Orthotopic autotransplantation of fresh ovarian cortex is one option, as our results provide proof of the survival of primordial follicles and the presence of a neovascular network. Cryopreservation and autotransplantation of frozen-thawed ovarian tissue is another valuable technique, as demonstrated by the live births obtained in cancer patients.

References

1. Nisolle M, Donnez J. Peritoneal endometriosis, ovarian endometriosis, and adenomyotic nodules of the rectovaginal septum are three different entities. Fertil Steril 1997; 68:585-96.
2. Donnez J, Chantraine F, Nisolle M. The efficacy of medical and surgical treatment of endometriosis-associated infertility: arguments in favour of a medico-surgical approach. Hum Reprod Update 2002; 8:89-94.
3. Donnez J, Nisolle M, Gillet N, Smets M, Bassil S, Casanas-Roux F. Large ovarian endometriomas. Hum Reprod 1996; 11 ;641-46.
4. Nargund G, Cheng W, Parsons J. The impact of ovarian cystectomy on ovarian response to stimulation during in-vitro fertilization cycles. Hum Reprod 1996; 11:81-83.
5. Loh F, Tan A, Kumar J, Ng S. Ovarian response after laparoscopic ovarian cystectomy for endometriocitic cysts in 132 monitored cycles. Fertil Steril 1999; 72:316-21.
6. Ho H, Lee R, Hwu Y, Lin M, Su J, Tsai Y. Poor response of ovaries with endometrioma previously treated with cystectomy to controlled ovarian hyperstimulation. J Assist Reprod Genet 2002; 19:507-11.
7. Geber S, Ferreira D, Spyer Prates L, Sales L, Samaio M. Effects of previous ovarian surgery for endometriosis on the outcome of assisted reproduction treatment. Reprod Biomed Online 2002; 5:162-66.
8. Somigliana E, Ragni G, Benedetti F, Borroni R, Vegetti W, Crosignani P. Does laparoscopic excision of endometriotic ovarian cysts significantly affect ovarian reserve? Insights from IVF cycles. Hum Reprod 2003;18:2450-53.
9. Exacoustos C, Zupi E, Amadio A, Szabocs B, De Vivo B, Marconi D et al. Laparoscopic removal of endometriomas: sonographic evaluation of residual functioning ovarian tissue. Am J Obstet Gynecol 2004; 191:68-72.
10. Muzii L, Bellati F, Bianchi A, Palaia I, Manci N, Zullo M, et al. Laparoscopic stripping of endometriomas: a randomized trial on different surgical techniques. Part II: pathological results. Hum Reprod 2005; 20:1987-92.
11. Donnez J, Lousse JC, Jadoul P, Donnez O, Squifflet J. Laparoscopic management of endometriomas using a combined technique of excisional (cystectomy) and ablative surgery. Fertil Steril.
12. Hart R, Hickey M, Maouris P, Buckett W. Excisional surgery versus ablative surgery for ovarian endometriomata. Cochrane Database Syst Rev 2008; 16:CD004992.
13. Silber S, Lenahan K, Levine D, Pineda J, Gorman K, Friez M, Crawford E, Gosden R. Ovarian transplantation between monozygotic twins discordant for premature ovarian failure. N Engl J Med 2005; 353:58-63.
14. Donnez J, Squifflet J, Dolmans MM, Martinez-Madrid B, Jadoul P, Van Langendonckt A. Orthotopic transplantation of fresh ovarian cortex: a report of two cases. Fertil Steril 2005; 84:1018.
15. Donnez J, Dolmans M, Demylle D, Jadoul P, Pirard C, Squifflet J, Martinez-Madrid B, Van Langendonckt A. Livebirth after orthotopic transplantation of cryopreserved ovarian tissue. Lancet 2004; 364:1405-10.
16. Donnez J, Martinez-Madrid B, Jadoul P, Van Langendonckt A, Demylle D, Dolmans MM. Ovarian tissue cryopreservation and transplantation: a review. Hum Reprod Update 2006; 12:519-35.
17. Donnez J, Squifflet J, Van Eyck A, Demylle D, Jadoul P, Van Langendonckt A. Restoration of ovarian function in orthotopically transplanted cryopreserved ovarian tissue: a pilot experience. Reprod Biomed Online 2008; 16:694-704.
18. Meirow D, Levron J, Eldar-Geva T, Hardan I, Fridman E, Zalel Y, Schiff E, Dor J. Pregnancy after transplantation of cryopreserved ovarian tissue in a patient with ovarian failure after chemotherapy. N Engl J Med 2005; 353:318-21.
19. Demeestere I, Simon P, Emiliani S, Delbaere A, Englert Y. Fertility preservation: Successful transplantation of cryopreserved ovarian tissue in a young patient previously treated for Hodgkin's disease. Oncologist 2007;12: 1437-42.
20. Andersen C, Rosendahl M, Byskov A, Loft A, Ottosen C, Dueholm M, Schmidt K, Andersen A, Ernst E. Two successful pregnancies following autotransplantation of frozen/thawed ovarian tissue. Hum Reprod 2008:23: 2266-72.
21. Ethics Committee of the American Society for Reproductive Medicine. Fertility preservation and reproduction in cancer patients. Fertil Steril 2005; 83:1622-28.
22. Dolmans M, Yuan W, Camboni A, Torre A, Van Langendonckt A, Martinez-Madrid B, Donnez J. Development of antral follicles after xenografting of isolated small human preantral follicles. Reprod Biomed Online 2008; 16:705-11.
23. Gosden R, Baird D, Wade J, Webb R. Restoration of fertility to oophorectomized sheep by ovarian autografts stored at -196 degrees C. Hum Reprod 1994; 9:597-603.
24. Smitz J, Cortvrindt R. The earliest stages of folliculogenesis in vitro. Reproduction 2002; 123:185-202.
25. Hovatta O, Wright C, Krausz T, Hardy K, Winston R. Human primordial, primary and secondary ovarian follicles in long-term culture: effect of partial isolation. Hum Reprod 1999; 14:2519-24.
26. Rodgers R, Irving-Rodgers H, Russell D. Extracellular matrix of the developing ovarian follicle. Reproduction 2003; 126:415-24.
27. Laschke M, Menger M, Vollmar B. Ovariectomy improves neovascularization and microcirculation of freely transplanted ovarian follicles. J Endocrinol 2002; 172:535-44.

Jose Schneider

Chapter 35

The Link Between Endometriosis and Cancer

Introduction

Endometriosis shares some features with cancer, among which the most striking are its ability to grow at distant sites from its origin in the endometrial cavity, to proliferate, and to invade adjacent tissues. There even exists reports in the literature of "metastatic" spread of endometriosis to regional lymph nodes.[1] Molecular events which underlie the genesis of cancer, such as the activation of oncogenes or loss of heterozygosity (LOH) at specific chromosomal regions are also known features of endometriosis.[2-4] Nevertheless, endometriosis, however, puzzling in its behavior and incapacitating due to its clinical manifestations, is definitely not a malignant disease. Quite another aspect is its possible association with cancer, most notably endometrioid and clear cell ovarian cancer,[5] although an elevated incidence of other types of cancer, e.g. breast cancer has also been postulated in carriers of the disease.[6,7] There exists a growing number of reports linking epidemiologically endometriosis and ovarian cancer, and it is now accepted that the relative risk of developing the latter is slightly higher in endometriosis patients than in the general population, and varies between 1.3 and 1.9.[8,9] A cascade of molecular events marking the transition from endometriosis to borderline ovarian neoplasm and finally to cancer has been postulated based on immuno-histochemical studies of surgical specimens containing all three lesions in close proximity.[10,11] The notion that endometriosis might thus be a precursor lesion of ovarian cancer has been, however, heavily challenged in later times.[12-14] The strongest argument against it is that endometriosis is an extraordinarily widespread disease among women, whereas ovarian cancer is fortunately not, and ovarian cancer associated with endometriosis even less so. In fact, it has been convincingly argued that ectopic endometrium may indeed undergo malignant transfor-

mation, albeit with the same frequency that its normal, eutopic counterpart does.[14] The higher incidence of cancer in endometriosis patients might thus be simply explained by the higher availability of tissue liable to undergo malignant transformation under the appropriate hormonal influence, among other causes. Alternatively, and following the now widely accepted "seed and soil" theory of cancer, it might well be that environmental (or genetic) conditions favoring endometriosis might also favor the development of cancer, without a direct causal relationship between both. On the other hand, it is also true that a transgenic, mutant K-ras carrying mouse model has been developed in which spontaneously arising endometriosis-like lesions undergo malignant transformation after an additional genetic manipulation (PTEN-inactivation).[15] However, this transition model is not automatically transposable to human endometriosis, not even in those few cases where human ovarian carcinoma does indeed seem to have arisen from endometriosis. In fact, K-ras mutations have never been detected in either normal or atypical endometriosis surrounding endometrioid or clear cell ovarian cancer, as we will comment further on.

In the following chapter, we will analyze the available evidence (epidemiological, histological and molecular/genetic) linking endometriosis with the subsequent development of cancer, in order to discuss whether endometriosis may be considered a premalignant condition or not.

Epidemiological Evidence

At least two large Swedish population-based cohort studies using the same data from the Swedish National Registries have addressed the question of the increased risk for developing malignancies in endometriosis patients.[8,16,17] They are the largest epidemiological studies carried out up to date. In the first study, data from 20.686 women hospitalized for endometriosis were checked for the incidence of cancer during their long-term follow-up (mean: 11.4 years) after hospital discharge. A total of 738 malignancies were detected, with significantly increased risks for breast cancer (1.3; 95% CI, 1.1-1.4), ovarian cancer (1.9; 95% CI, 1.3-2.8) and non-Hodgkin´s lymphoma (1.8; 95% CI, 1.2-2.6), this latter one limited to patients older than 40. The second study was an extension of the just cited one, involving data from 64.492 women. It confirmed the increased risk for ovarian cancer (1.4; 95% CI, 1.2-1.7) and a borderline significant risk for non-Hodgkin´s lymphoma, since the confidence interval contains the unity (1.2; 95% CI, 1.0-1.5). Intriguingly, a significantly reduced risk for cervical cancer also emerged from this second study (0.6; 95% CI, 0.5-0.8). A subsequent study including a subset of 15.844 women from this same register identified a higher than three-fold risk of breast cancer in women whose sole indication for surgery had been endometriosis.

A strong epidemiological link between ovarian cancer and endometriosis has emerged from several studies carried out on infertile women.[9,18] Direct causality is extremely difficult to elicit from these studies, however, given the high incidence of endometriosis as a cause of infertility. In the study by Ness et al,[18] for instance, both endometriosis as a known cause of infertility, and infertility from an unknown cause were independently associated with a higher incidence of ovarian cancer. Further confounders in all these studies are the use or not of oral contraceptives, tubal ligation or previous parity, all known to be protective against the development of ovarian cancer, and, on the other hand, age and family history of breast and/or ovarian cancer, known to favor it. Some studies have tried to stratify by all these factors, in order to assess the independent impact of endometriosis on ovarian cancer risk, and indeed Modugno et al[19] still found a higher incidence of ovarian cancer in women whose sole purported risk factor was endometriosis (1.3; 95% CI, 1.1-1.6).

All in all, however, the increase in risk derived from all these studies is less than two-fold if compared to that of the general population, which, in epidemiological terms, indicates a weak association, which may as well be explained by bias. If we add this to the fact that evidence from retrospective cohort or case-control studies suffers from an inherent weakness when trying to establish a causal link, the case for a direct relationship between endo-metriosis and ovarian cancer based on epidemiological data alone is at best weak. The same can be said of the

relationship with other cancers. The association between endometriosis and breast cancer found in the two large Swedish studies has not been convincingly duplicated in other similar ones. One plausible explanation for this association, furthermore, might be that the same hormonal environment favoring the development of endometriosis, which is acknowledgedly a hormone-dependent disease, also favors the development of breast cancer, which is the paradigm of hormone-related cancer. Wyshak et al reported for the first time an association between endometriosis and melanoma,[20] and this same research group has repeatedly confirmed its findings in several workups of its original data.[21,22] However, the results are based on data from a limited number of cases and those from other groups addressing the same question are inconclusive.[8,23] The only association that has been independently confirmed in large studies conducted by different groups has been the one between endometriosis and non-Hodgkin´s lymphoma.[8,24] Among the explanations ventured are a common immunological predisposition to both conditions (the most plausible one), medication prescribed for treating endometriosis as a trigger of lymphoma or a common etiological agent.[25] **Table 35-1** summarizes the most relevant epidemiological studies conducted on the relationship between endometriosis and the development of ovarian and other cancers, disclosing a statistically significant association. For every study depicted on the table, there exists at least one carried out with the same methodology which does not obtain the same results (in most cases, the confidence interval includes the unit). This notwithstanding, the associations described must not be dismissed as simple chance findings, since future studies may confirm them.

Table 35-1: Studies reporting statistically significant differences in incidence of cancer between endometriosis-carriers and normal population

Study	Reference	Type of cancer	Risk	95% CI
Brinton et al	8	Ovarian	1.9	1.3 – 2.8
Ness et al	18	Ovarian	1.7	1.1 – 2.7
Modugno et al	19	Ovarian	1.3	1.1 – 1.6
Schairer et al	15	Breast	3.2	1.2 – 8.0
Wyshak et al	20	Melanoma	3.9	1.2 – 12.4
Brinton et al	8	Lymphoma	1.8	1.2 – 2.6
Borgfeldt and Andolf	17	Cervical	0.6	0.4 – 0.9

Histological Evidence

A small number of ovarian cancers seems to arise from ectopic endometrium which has undergone malignant transformation. According to Scott,[26] to be able to diagnose such an eventuality, it is not enough to see the tumor in close proximity to endometriosis, i.e. to tissue showing the presence of endometrial glands and endometrial stroma (what is known as "Sampson´s criteria"), but it is also necessary to observe in the same specimen variable degrees of endometrial hyperplasia, metaplasia and atypia leading from normal endometrium to cancer. Applying retrospectively such stringent criteria to large series, the largest including 1.000 patients,[27] the incidence of ovarian cancer in patients operated upon primarily for endometriosis has been reported to lie between 0.8% and 8.9%. The most consistent among these findings is atypia. In the largest series contemplating this aspect, Prefumo et al[28] found significantly more severe atypia in endometriotic lesions from patients with ovarian cancers apparently arising from endometriosis if compared to lesions from patients with plain endometriosis (14/14 cases, 100%, vs. 5/325 cases, 2%).

There is unanimity in that the most frequent histological varieties of ovarian carcinoma associated with endometriosis are the clear cell and endometrioid ones. In this respect, one of the most important studies is the first report by Sainz de la Cuesta et al,[29] who limited their investigation to stage-I cancers, the tumors most likely to reflect the biological features of the original oncogenic clone giving rise to them. Their series is the one in which the association of endometriosis almost exclusively with clear cell and endometrioid carcinoma is more clear-cut. This shift towards two relatively infrequent histological varieties, especially the clear cell one, together with the fact that the concomitant finding of endometriosis in ovarian carcinoma (4-29%) does not differ significantly from the expected one in the general population, does indeed suggest some kind of etiological link between both entities. Another histopathological feature further reinforces this notion: unilateral endometriotic ovarian cysts, at variance with all other ovarian cysts, which are evenly distributed between the right and left hemipelvis, are more frequently left- than right-sided, and this difference is statistically significant.[30] It has been postulated that this is due to preferential entrapment in the left hemipelvis of tubal reflux containing viable endometrial cell clusters. The same significant imbalance towards the left hemipelvis has been reported by Vercellini et al for endometrioid ovarian carcinoma,[31] who also found

a similar trend for clear cell carcinoma, which in this case did not reach statistical significance.

Molecular/Genetic Evidence

Biological features at the molecular and genetic level shared by endometriosis and cancer can throw light on the malignant potential of endometriotic lesions. The present state of knowledge about this question has been reviewed in depth by Viganò et al.[12] According to these authors, cancer is defined biologically by monoclonal growth, specific genetic changes, mutations in tumor suppressor genes and replicative advantage. It is now in fact widely accepted that the origin of cancer is monoclonal. Following this theory, a single cell at a certain point acquires through mutation a growth advantage that is transmitted to daughter cells. Subsequent genetic changes in the offspring (four to six is thought to be the necessary minimum) ultimately give rise to a malignant tumor. Thus, if monoclonality is convincingly demonstrated in a proliferative lesion, its potential for malignant transformation is much higher than, say, that of scar tissue, or for that matter, normal endometrium, which also proliferates, but in an absolutely controlled way. The classical genetic tool for assessing clonality in females is the phenomenon of X-chromosome inactivation. Women, from the molecular genetic point of view, are a mosaic of cells in which either X-chromosome is randomly inactivated, since both cannot be activated at a time (if they were, women would have a double set of active X-chromosome genes if compared to men). Inactivation is triggered in the embryonic phase of development and maintained in daughter cells throughout life. There exists tools which are beyond the scope of his chapter to know if, in a given cell, the inactivated X-chromosome is the paternal or the maternal one. In a monoclonal tissue, the inactivated chromosome is, obviously, always the same in every cell. Although several reports seem to indicate that endometriotic lesions are indeed of monoclonal origin, the present evidence is still not conclusive. The investigation is hampered by the fact that the monoclonal portion of endometriotic foci is the epithelial component, whereas the surrounding stroma is always polyclonal. Laser capture microdissection techniques will help to solve this dilemma in the immediate future.

As has been mentioned above, the "multiple-hit" theory of cancer[31] implies that several genetic changes (at least four to six) are necessary for cancer to develop from normal tissues. Basically, they result in the abnormal activation by a number of mechanisms of otherwise normal genes called protooncogenes, which in that way are transformed into oncogenes, and the mutation or loss of tumor suppressor genes. Such models of oncogenic activation are rather well known for a number of cancers, such as colon carcinoma, where the molecular steps marking the transition from a benign polyp to invasive cancer are clearly defined. This is, however, not the case for the transition from endometriosis to ovarian cancer, and it is even not clear if such a transition ever takes place at all. The most gross genetic alterations that can be studied during oncogenic activation are cytogenetic ones. Chromosomal gains or losses, leading to rearrangement of genetic material or loss thereof, and by which, e.g. a promoter region can be relocated near a protooncogene, or a region containing a tumor suppressor gene may be completely lost, can be studied by relatively simple means, such as classical cytogenetic techniques, or slightly more sophisticated ones, such as fluorescent *in situ* hybridization (FISH) with probes specific for especially vulnerable chromosomal regions, or PCR-based loss of heterozygosity (LOH) studies. No alterations have been found up-to-date in endometriosis by means of standard cytogenetics.[32] By means of FISH, specific alterations in the region of chromosome 17 containing the p53 locus, one of the main players in ovarian carcinogenesis, have been found in advanced endometriosis.[33] Although the number of cases and chromosomes studied was low, this is the first hint at a molecular level that an alteration commonly found in ovarian cancer is also involved in endometriosis progression. These findings have not been confirmed in subsequent specific studies of p53 mutations or LOH in the p53-containing region of chromosome 17. Only Sáinz de la Cuesta et al[10] found a transition in mutant p53 protein accumulation from normal endometriotic lesions (12%) through atypical endometriosis (100%) to ovarian carcinoma (100%) in ovarian carcinoma specimens. The general consensus at present is that normal endometriosis, even if adjacent to cancer, only very rarely presents mutations in the p53 gene.

Other LOH studies of endometriosis have spanned a larger set of chromosomal regions, and a gradient of alterations from normal endometriosis through endometriosis adjacent to ovarian cancer to ovarian cancer itself have been identified in several of them.[3,34-36] The results of these studies are summarized in **Table 35-2**.

Comparative genomic hybridization studies, which allow for the detection of genomic imbalances across the whole genome have detected alterations in 83% of samples from patients with advanced endometriosis.[37] The highest

Chromosomal region	Endometriosis %	Endometriosis adjacent to endometrioid ovarian carcinoma%	Endometrioid ovarian carcinoma%
2q	0	0	40
4q	0	8	29
5p	0	0	14
5q	6	20-25	46
6q	0	27-60	29-70
7p	0	0	28
9p21	0-17	31	54
10q23.3	56	40-60	42-43
11q	18	20-25	37-50
17p13.1	0-5	0	42
17q21	0	0	46
22q	15	20-31	45-47
Xq11.2-q12	0	0	38

Table 35-2: PCR based loss of heterozygosity studies demonstrating a gradient of alterations from normal endometriosis through endometriosis adjacent to ovarian cancer

rate of genomic loss (50% of cases) was detected in chromosomes 1p and 22q, and lower rates were also detected in chromosomes 5p, 6q, 7p, 9q, 16 and 17q.

Alterations in specific oncogenes and tumor suppressor genes, besides p53, mentioned above, which might facilitate the passage from normal endometriosis to cancer, have also been studied in endometriosis. If such a transition does indeed take place, PTEN is one of the principal candidates to play a major role in it. As has been mentioned in the introductory paragraph, a mouse model involving K-ras activation and PTEN inactivation has been developed,[15] in which normal endometriosis undergoes malignant transformation. K-ras mutations have been described in clear cell ovarian carcinoma, but not in adjacent atypical or distant endometriosis.[11] PTEN mutations have been described in most endometrial carcinomas,[38] and a high frequency of LOH at 10q23.3 (the locus of PTEN, from which the gene takes its name) has also been found in endometrioid ovarian carcinoma.[36]

Conclusion

In conclusion, there exists (weak) epidemiological and histological evidence linking endometriosis with the development of endometrioid and clear cell ovarian carcinoma in a small number of cases. There also exists an animal model in which a transition from spontaneously arising endometriosis to cancer can be elicited by means of genetic manipulation involving a small number of oncogenes and tumor suppressor genes. However, this model of transition from benign tissue to cancer has still not been fully confirmed in humans. All in all, the available evidence is still very controversial in many aspects, and is not enough for considering endometriosis a premalignant condition at the present time.

References

1. Noel JC, Chapron C, Fayt I, Anaf V. Lymph node involvement and lymphovascular invasion in deep infiltrating rectosigmoid endometriosis. Fertil Steril 2008; 89:1069-72

2. Schneider J, Jiménez E, Rodríguez F, del Tánago J. c-myc, c-erb-B2, nm23 and p53 expression in human endometriosis. Oncol Rep 1998; 5:49-52.

3. Sato N, Tsunoda H, Nishida M, Morishita Y, Yakimoto Y, Kubo T, Noguchi M. Loss of heterozygosity on 10q23.3 and mutation of the tumor suppressor gene PTEN in benign endometrial cyst of the ovary: possible sequence progression from benign endometrial cyst to endometrial carcinoma and clear cell carcinoma of the ovary. Cancer Res 2000; 60:7052-56.

4. Thomas EJ, Campbell IG. Molecular genetic defects in endometriosis. Gynecol Obstet Invest 2000; 50 (Suppl) 1:44-50.

5. Ogawa S, Kaku T, Amada S, Kobayashi H, Hirakawa T, Ariyoshi K, Kamura T, Nakano H. Ovarian endometriosis associated with ovarian cancer: a clinicopathological and immunohistochemical study. Gynecol Oncol 2000; 77: 298-304.

6. Modesitt SC, Tortolero-Luna G, Robinson JB, Gershenson DM, Wolf JK. Ovarian and extraovarian endometriosis-associated cancer. Obstet Gynecol 2002; 100:788-95.

7. Bertelsen L, Mellemkjær L, Frederiksen K, Kjær SK, Brinton LA, Sakoda LC, van Valkengoed I, Olsen JH. Risk for breast cancer among women with endometriosis. Int J Cancer 2006; 120:1372-75.

8. Brinton LA, Gridley G, Persson I, Baron J, Bergkvist A. Cancer risk after a hospital discharge diagnosis of endometriosis. Am J Obstet Gynecol 1997; 176:572-79.

9. Brinton LA, Lamb EJ, Moghissi KS, Scoccia B, Althuis MD, Mabie JE, Westhoff CL. Ovarian cancer risk associated with varying causes of infertility. Fertil Steril 2004; 82:405-14.

10. Sáinz de la Cuesta R, Izquierdo M, Cañamero M, Granizo JJ, Manzarbeitia F. Increased prevalence of p53 expression from typical endometriosis to atypical endometriosis and ovarian cancer associated with endometriosis. Eur J Obstet Gynecol Reprod Biol 2004; 113:87-93.

11. Otsuka J, Okuda T, Sekizawa A, Amemiya S, Saito H, Okai T, Kushima M, Tachikawa T. K-ras mutation may promote

carcinogenesis of endometriosis leading to ovarian clear cell carcinoma. Mod Electron Microsc 2004; 37:188-92.

12. Viganò P, Somigliana E, Chiodo I, Abbiati A, Vercellini P. Molecular mechanisms and biological plausibility underlying the malignant transformation of endometriosis: a critical analysis. Hum Reprod Upd 2005; 12:77-89.

13. Somigliana E, Viganò P, Parazzini F, Stoppelli S, Giambattista E, Vercellini P. Association between endometriosis and cancer: a comprehensive review and a critical analysis of clinical and epidemiological evidence. Gynecol Oncol 2006; 101:331-41.

14. Viganò P, Somigliana E, Parazzini F, Vercellini P. Bias versus causality: interpreting recent evidence of association between endometriosis and ovarian cancer. Fertil Steril 2007; 88:588-93.

15. Dinulescu DM, Ince TA, Quade BJ, Shafer SA, Crowley D, Jacks T. Role of K-ras and Pten in the development of mouse models of endometriosis and endometrioid ovarian cancer. Nat Med 2005; 11:63-70.

16. Schairer C, Persson I, Falkenborn M, Næssen T, Troisi R, Brinton LA. Breast cancer risk associated with gynecologic surgery and indications for such surgery. Int J Cancer 1997; 70:150-54.

17. Borgfeldt C, Andolf E. Cancer risk after hospital discharge diagnosis of benign ovarian cysts and endometriosis. Acta Obstet Gynecol Scand 2004; 83:395-400.

18. Ness RB, Cramer DW, Goodman MT, Kjaer SK, Mallin K, Mosgaard BJ, Purdie DM, Risch HA, Vergona R, Wu AH. Infertility, fertility drugs, and ovarian cancer: a pooled analysis of case-control studies. Am J Epidemiol 2002; 155:217-24.

19. Modugno F, Ness RB, Allen GO, Schildkraut JM, Davis FG, Goodman MT. Oral contraceptive use, reproductive history, and risk of epithelial ovarian cancer in women with and without endometriosis. Am J Obstet Gynecol 2004; 191:733-40.

20. Wyshak G, Frisch RE, Albright NL, Albright TE, Schiff I. Reproductive factors and melanoma of the skin among women. Int J Dermatol 1989; 28:527-30.

21. Hornstein MD, Thomas PP, Sober AJ, Wyshak G, Albright NL, Frisch RE. Association between endometriosis, dysplastic nevi and history of melanoma in women of reproductive age. Hum Reprod 1997; 12:143-44.

22. Wyshak G, Frisch RE. Red hair color, melanoma and endometriosis: suggestive associations. Int J Dermatol 2000; 39:795-800.

23. Holly EA, Cress RD, Ahn DK. Cutaneous melanoma in women: III. Reproductive factors and contraceptive use. Am J Epidemiol 1995; 141:943-50.

24. Vercellini P, Parazzini F, Bolis G, Carinelli S, Dindelli M, Vendola N, Luchini L, Crosignani PG. Endometriosis and ovarian cancer. Am J Obstet Gynecol 1993; 169:181-2.

25. Olson JE, Cerhan JR, Janney CA, Anderson KE, Vachon CM, Sellers T. Postmenopausal cancer risk after self-reported endometriosis diagnosis in the Iowa women´s health study. Cancer 2002; 94:1612-18.

26. Scott RB. Malignant changes in endometriosis. Obstet Gynecol 1953; 2:283-89.

27. Stern RC, Dash R, Benley RC, Snyder MJ, Haney AF, Robboy SJ. Malignancy in endometriosis: frequency and comparison of ovarian and extraovarian types. Int J Gynecol Pathol 2001; 20:133-39.

28. Prefumo F, Todeschini F, Fulcheri E, Venturini PL. Epithelial abnormalities in cystic ovarian endometriosis. Gynecol Oncol 2002; 84:280-84.

29. Sáinz de la Cuesta R, Eichhorn JH, Rice LW, Fuller AF, Nikrui N, Goff BA. Histologic transformation of benign endometriosis to early epithelial ovarian cancer. Gynecol Oncol 1996; 60:238-44.

30. Al-Fozan H, Tulandi T. Left lateral predisposition of endometriosis and endometrioma. Obstet Gynecol 2003; 101:164-66.

31. Han WC, Weinberg RA. Modelling of the molecular circuitry of cancer. Nat Rev 2002; 2:321-41.

32. Tamura M, Fukaya T, Murakami T, Uehara S, Yajima A. Analysis of clonality in uman endometriotic cysts based on evaluation of X chromosome inactivation in archival formalin-fixed, paraffin-embedded tissue. Lab Invest 1998; 78:213-18.

33. Simpson JL, Farideh ZB, Kamat A, Buster JE, Carson SA. Genetics of endometriosis. Obstet Gynecol Clin North Am 2003; 30:21-40.

34. Jiang X, Morland SJ, Hitchcock A, Thomas EJ, Campbell IG. Allelotyping of endometriosis with adjacent ovarian carcinoma reveals evidence of a common lineage. Cancer Res 1998; 58:1707-12.

35. Diebold J. Molecular genetics of ovarian carcinomas. Histol Histopathol 1999; 14:269-77.

36. Obata K, Hoshiai H. Common genetic changes between endometriosis and ovarian cancer. Gynecol Obstet Invest 2000; 50:39-43.

37. Gogusev J, Bouquet de Joliniere J, Telvi L, Doussau M, du Manoir S, Stojkoski A, Levardon M. Detection of DNA copy number changes in human endometriosis by comparative genomic hybridization. Hum Genet 1999; 105:444-51.

38. Mutter GL, Lin MC, Fizgerald JT, Kum JB, Baak JP, Lees JA, Weng LP, Eng C. Altered PTEN expression as a diagnostic marker for the earliest endometrial precancers. J Natl Cancer Inst 2000; 92:924-30.

Caroline E Gargett, Sun-Wei Guo

Chapter 36

Stem Cells and Clonality in Endometriosis

Introduction

Adult stem cells are undifferentiated cells present in most adult tissues. They are difficult to identify in many tissues due to their rarity, lack of distinguishing morphological features and the current lack of known specific markers. Adult stem cells are defined by their functions: high proliferative potential, self-renewal, and differentiation into one or more lineages.[1] Adult stem cells also initiate clones of cells in culture when seeded at very low densities. The retention of a DNA synthesis label (BrdU) for prolonged periods of time is another property of adult stem cells, since paradoxically they proliferate less frequently than their non-stem daughter cells.[2] Adult stem cells maintain tissue homeostasis by providing replacement cells in regenerating tissues, in routine cellular turnover, and for repair after acute injury.[3] The balance between adult stem cell self-renewal and differentiation is strictly regulated by the stem cell niche, comprising the adult stem cell, surrounding niche cell(s) and extracellular matrix, ensuring an appropriate balance between stem cell replacement and provision of differentiated mature cells to maintain tissue homeostasis for organ function.[3] Thus the stem cell niche serves to provide a protective environment for the resident stem cell to maintain genetic fidelity over the lifespan, and at the same time maintaining capacity to rapidly respond to tissue needs for cellular replacement.

The successful identification of endometrial stem cells and their cell surface markers will significantly impact on research in endometrial physiology, implantation, pregnancy, reproductive aging, endometrial diseases such as myoma, fibrosis, dysmenorrhea, endometrial cancer, and adenomyosis, and on other gynecological diseases such as endometriosis. This is precisely the impetus for the growing interest in this area.

Endometrial Stem/Progenitor Cells

The concept that basalis endometrium harbours stem/progenitor cells responsible for the remarkable regenerative capacity of endometrium was proposed many years ago (reviewed in Gargett 2007).[2] Attempts to isolate, characterize and locate endometrial stem/progenitor cells have recently been undertaken as experimental approaches to identify adult stem cells in other tissues have been developed,[2] resulting in the identification of rare populations of epithelial stem/progenitor cells and mesenchymal stem-like cells in human endometrium.

Endometrial Epithelial Stem/Progenitor Cells

Cell Cloning Studies

The first published evidence for the existence of endometrial epithelial stem/progenitor cells in human endometrium came from cell cloning studies, where single cell suspensions were seeded at cloning density in culture.[4] Rare clonogenic epithelial cells were identified in normal cycling and inactive perimenopausal endometrium, and in endometrium of women on oral contraceptives, suggesting that clonogenic epithelial cells may be responsible for regenerating glands in cycling and atrophic endometrium.[4,5] These studies found that 0.22% of human endometrial epithelial cells had colony forming unit (CFU) activity. Two types of CFU formed: large (0.09%) and small (0.14%), leading to the hypothesis that large CFU were initiated by a stem/progenitor cell **(Figure 36-1)** possibly located at the base of the glands in the basalis **(Figure 36-2)**. Small CFU are possibly initiated by more differentiated transit amplifying cells, likely located in the functionalis layer and responsible for the extensive proliferation observed in the first half of the menstrual cycle.[2,5] Differential expression of epithelial markers was noted

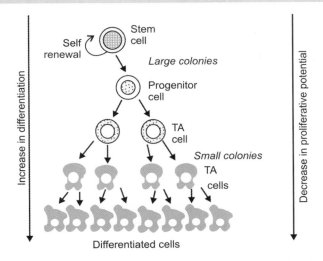

FIGURE 36-1: The relationship of endometrial colony forming cells to the hierarchical model for stem cell differentiation.

Stem cells have the capacity to self-renew and replace themselves as well as differentiate into committed progenitors through asymmetric cell divisions. Progenitors proliferate and give rise to more differentiated rapidly proliferating transit amplifying cells, which finally differentiate to produce a large number of terminally differentiated functional cells with no capacity for proliferation. We postulate that the large colonies are initiated by putative stem/progenitor cells and the small colonies by putative transit amplifying cells. Reproduced with permission from Chan *et al.* 2004.[4]

between large and small CFU. Small CFU expressed epithelial differentiation markers, cytokeratin, epithelial cell adhesion molecule (EpCAM) and α6-integrin, but only the latter was expressed in cells of large CFU, which comprised small cells with a high nuclear:cytoplasmic ratio, suggesting an undifferentiated phenotype.[4] The percentage of endometrial epithelial CFU did not vary with menstrual cycle stage, indicating their persistence in human endometrium.[5] The growth factor requirements of human endometrial epithelial CFU have been characterized in serum free culture conditions.[5]

Clonality of Human Endometrium

A clone is a group of genetically, functionally, and morphologically identical cells that are descended from a common ancestor cell. Clonality, in cell biology, stipulates the state of a cell being derived from one source or the other. Endometrial cells derived from two different stem/ progenitor cells are thus two clones, even though they may seem identical morphologically and functionally.

Convincing evidence for the monoclonal composition of human endometrial epithelial glands was obtained by using a PCR-assay for X-linked androgen receptor gene which undergoes random X-linked inactivation.[6] Adjacent

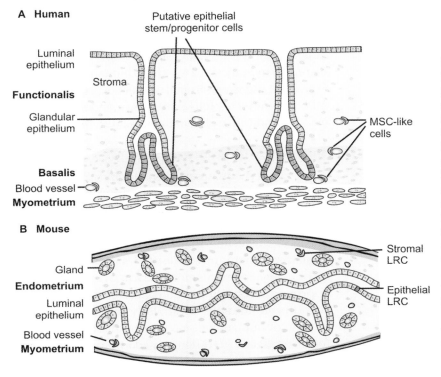

FIGURE 36-2: Schematic showing the possible location of candidate endometrial stem/ progenitor cells in human and mouse endometrium. (A) In human endometrium, it is hypothesized that epithelial stem/progenitors will be located in the base of the glands in the basalis. Recent data indicates that MSC-like cells are located near blood vessels possibly in both the basalis and/or the functionalis. (B) In mouse endometrium, candidate epithelial and stromal stem/progenitor cells (label-retaining cells, LRC) which rapidly proliferate during estrogen-stimulated endometrial growth are located in the luminal epithelium and mainly near blood vessels at the endometrial–myometrial junction, respectively. Reprinted from Molecular and Cellular Endocrinology Vol 288, Gargett CE, Chan RWS, Schwab KE. Hormone and growth factor signalling in endometrial renewal: role of stem/progenitor cells, pages 22-29, 2008, with permission from Elsevier.

glands within a 1 mm^2 area shared the same clonality. Further study using female mice harboring the green fluorescent protein gene on either the maternal or paternal X chromosome indicated that individual endometrial glands consist completely of either fluorescent or non-fluorescent cells and that the surface epithelium exhibited a clear boundary between these cell types.[6] These findings suggest the existence of individual epithelial stem/progenitor cells at the base of individual endometrial glands and that the human endometrium comprises monoclonal glandular units each derived from a single epithelial stem/progenitor cell.

Label Retaining Cells

Label retaining cells (LRC) have been identified as candidate adult stem cells *in vivo* in mouse endometrium.[7-9] The LRC approach identifies adult stem cells by their quiescent, slowly cycling nature. It is based on pulse-labelling the majority of tissue cells with a DNA synthesis label (bromodeoxyuridine (BrdU)) during a time when adult stem cells are proliferating and a subsequent chase of the label over long periods of time. Slow cycling stem cells retain the label, while rapidly dividing transit amplifying cells dilute the label to undetectable levels. Immunohistochemistry localizes bromodeoxyuridine (BrdU$^+$) LRC, revealing their location and the stem cell niche. Epithelial LRC, comprising 3% of mouse endometrial epithelial cells, were observed as well separated ERα^- cells in the luminal but not glandular epithelium, suggesting that luminal epithelial stem/progenitor cells are responsible for the growth of glands during development and in the cycling adult mouse **(Figure 36-2B)**.[7]. In prepubertal mice, the first cells to proliferate in estrogen-stimulated endometrial growth are the epithelial LRC, indicating that the epithelial LRC are functioning as stem/progenitor cells.[7] This suggests that they have an important role in regenerating luminal epithelium which undergoes substantial proliferation and apoptosis during the estrus cycle rather than shedding as in human endometrium. While the location of human endometrial epithelial stem/progenitor cells is currently not known, it is expected that they will be located in the bases of glands in the basalis region **(Figure 36-2A)**.

Endometrial Gland Methylation Patterns

Endometrial epithelial stem/progenitor cell kinetics has been investigated by examining epigenetic errors encoded in the methylation patterns of individual glands from human endometrium.[10] This study demonstrates the power of using molecular "fossil records" to document cell turnover history in endometrium (see section on Reconstituting cellular genealogy in endometrial cells). Through investigation of epithelial stem/progenitor cell kinetics by examining methylation patterns of the CSX and CSX6 genes in 30 women, aged 17-87 years old, with varying parity and body mass index, age-related methylation with stable levels after menopause was observed, as well as significantly less methylation in lean or older multiparous women.[10] These results suggest that a woman's reproductive history (i.e. age at menarche, gravidity, and parity), and, perhaps to a less extent, her life history (body weight, history of oral contraceptive use), are recorded serendipitously in the genome and/or epigenome of her endometrium. Furthermore, mathematical modeling of the data suggested that an individual gland contains a stem cell niche with an unknown number of long-lived stem cells rather than a single stem cell, which would argue against the monoclonality of individual endometrial glands.

Endometrial Stromal/Mesenchymal Stem-like Cells

Cell Cloning Studies

A small population (1.25%) of freshly isolated human endometrial stromal cells possess colony-forming ability.[4] These CFU are not only retained in culture but their proportion increases to 15% of stromal cells after prior expansion in culture at normal seeding densities.[11] Similar to epithelial CFU, two types of stromal CFU formed from freshly isolated cells, with only 0.02% of stromal cells initiating large CFU, thus supporting a stromal cellular hierarchy hypothesized to exist in human endometrium.[2] Both large and small stromal colonies expressed fibroblast markers, with some cells expressing a smooth muscle actin (αSMA), indicative of myofibroblast differentiation.

Multilineage Differentiation

A key property of mesenchymal stem cells (MSC) is the ability to undergo multilineage differentiation. Various human endometrial stromal cell populations can be induced to differentiate into one or more mesenchymal lineages, suggesting that MSC-like cells may reside in human endometrium. Endometrial stromal cells comprise a heterogeneous population and when cultured under the appropriate conditions some differentiated into fat or chondrocyte lineages.[11,12] Similarly, the CD146$^+$PDGF-Rβ$^-$ fraction of human endometrial stromal cells, enriched 8 fold for stromal CFU differentiated into four mesenchymal lineages; adipogenic, chondrogenic, osteoblastic and myogenic.[13] Since mixed populations of stromal cells were examined in all these studies, it was not possible to determine whether individual endometrial stromal cells are multipotent.

Label Retaining Cells

Candidate stromal stem/progenitor cells have been identified in mouse endometrium as stromal LRC.[7-9] Between 6-9% of the stromal cells were identified as LRC. A large proportion of these were located near blood vessels close to the endometrial-myometrial junction,[7,8] correlating with their postulated basalis location in human endometrium (Figure 36-2B). Stromal LRC were further characterized for expression of various markers. They were not leukocytes or of bone marrow origin as they did not express CD45.[7] Some (16%) expressed ERβ [7] and some (0.6%) expressed Oct-4, a pluripotency marker.[8]

Human Endometrial Side Population Cells

Another approach to identify adult stem cells when there are no known markers is to use the Hoechst dye exclusion method, which identifies a small population of cells called the Side Population (SP). Recently, SP cells (0-5%) were identified in freshly isolated human endometrial cell suspensions.[14,15] Similar to CFU activity in human endometrium, the percentage of SP cells was highly variable between subjects, although higher in the menstrual and proliferative stages of the menstrual cycle. They comprise a mixed population of cells, predominantly endothelial cells, although some were of epithelial and stromal origin.[15] The SP population were mainly in G_0 phase of the cell cycle indicating their relative quiescence[15] and did not express endometrial epithelial (CD9) or stromal (CD13) cell differentiation markers.[14] Following fluorescence activated cell sorting (FACS) and long term 3D culture in Matrigel, the SP cells differentiated into CD9+E-cadherin+ gland-like organoids and CD13+ stromal clusters.[14] Both SP and non-SP cells differentiated into prolactin-secreting decidual cells.[15] Clonogenic endometrial cells were also enriched in the SP compared to the non-SP fraction,[15] although toxic levels of Hoechst dye may affect CFU activity in the non-SP cells.

Endometrial Stem/Progenitor Cell Reconstitution of Endometrial Tissue *in vivo*

Demonstrating the regenerative capacity of putative endometrial adult stem cell populations by examining their ability to reconstitute endometrial tissue *in vivo* is an important goal and provides functional proof of adult stem cell activity. Functional endometrium has been regenerated from singly dispersed unfractionated human endometrial cell suspensions xenotransplanted beneath the kidney capsule of ovariectomized and estrogen supplemented NOG mice.[16] Well organized endometrial tissue comprising cytokeratin+ CD9+ glandular structures, CD10+CD13+ stroma and αSMA+ myometrial layers was reconstructed.[16] The endometrial xenografts responded to cyclical sex steroids hormones, forming tortuous glands and decidualized stroma when estrogen and progesterone were administered, as well as large blood-filled cysts similar to red spot lesions of active endometriosis after hormonal withdrawal.[16] This animal model suggests that human endometrial cells have capacity to grow endometriosis-like tissue when transplanted into an ectopic site.

Markers of Endometrial Stem / Progenitor Cells

Investigation of the role of endometrial stem/progenitor cells in endometriosis would be greatly facilitated if there were specific markers that identify their location in shedding endometrium and endometriotic lesions. Currently there are no markers for endometrial epithelial stem/progenitor cells and they cannot be distinguished from their mature progeny, the pseudostratified epithelium comprising the glands and luminal epithelium.

However, MSC-like cells were recently isolated from human endometrium using co-expression of two perivascular cell markers, CD146 and PDGF-receptor-β (PDGF-Rβ).[13] The FACS-sorted CD146+PDGF-Rβ+ subpopulation of endometrial stromal cells was enriched 8 fold for CFU compared to unsorted stromal cells. The CD146+PDGF-Rβ+ cells expressed typical MSC surface markers, CD29, CD44, CD73, CD90 and CD105 and were negative for hemopoietic and endothelial markers (CD31, CD34 and CD45.[13] However, STRO-1, a marker used to prospectively isolate bone marrow MSC was not expressed by CD146+PDGF-Rβ+ cells, nor by clonogenic stromal CFU.[17] The CD146+PDGF-Rβ+ cells underwent multilineage differentiation into adipogenic, myogenic, chondrogenic and osteoblastic lineages when cultured in appropriate induction media.[13] Confocal microscopy demonstrated that CD146+PDGF-Rβ+ cells were located perivascularly in both the functionalis and basalis of human endometrium.[13] The CD146+PDGF-Rβ+ subpopulation of endometrial stromal cells appear to be similar to bone marrow and fat MSC in differentiation potential and perivascular location. This finding also indicates that it is possible that endometrial MSC-like cells are shed during menstruation.

A number of studies have examined stem cell marker expression in human and mouse endometrium by immunotechniques. Oct-4 (POU5F1), a marker of pluripotent human embryonic stem cells and some adult stem cells, was demonstrated in some human endometrial samples but the cell types and location was not determined.[18] Musashi-1, an RNA binding protein in neural stem cells and an epithelial progenitor cell marker that regulates stem cell self-renewal signalling pathways was recently localized to single epithelial and small clusters of stromal cells in human endometrium.[19] Musashi-1[+] cells were mainly found in the basalis in the proliferative stage of the menstrual cycle, suggesting their possible stem/progenitor cell function. Stromal Musashi-1[+] cells were not found in a perivascular location, although some were in a periglandular region, similar to some stromal LRC in mouse endometrium.[7] A large proportion of endometriotic glands expressed Musashi-1. Whether Musashi-1[+] endometriotic cells represent basalis-derived epithelium or stem/progenitor cells with CFU activity remain to be determined. It is also important to determine whether Musashi-1 is expressed in CD146[+]PDGF-Rβ[+] stromal cells and SP cells.

Cells with a hematopoietic stem cell phenotype (CD34[+]CD45[+]) co-expressing CD7 and CD56 have been identified in human endometrial cell suspensions and may be lymphoid progenitors.[20] Whether these cells function as hemopoietic stem cells and generate endometrial leukocytes in the endometrium or contribute to the SP population is unknown. Neither is it known whether the cells expressing these markers function as endometrial stem/progenitor cells.[2]

Source of Endometrial Stem/Progenitor Cells

It is thought that endometrial epithelial and stromal stem/progenitor cells may be derived from residual fetal stem cells,[2] however, there is increasing evidence that bone marrow derived cells may also be a potential source of cells for endometrial regeneration.[21] Significant chimerism ranging from 0.2-52% was detected in the endometrial glands and stroma of 4 women who received single antigen HLA mismatched bone marrow transplants, suggesting that bone marrow stem cells contributed to endometrial regeneration in a setting of cellular turnover and inflammatory stimuli.[21] Most glands consisted entirely of host or entirely donor-derived cells indicating their monoclonality. However, some individual glands contained a fraction of cells of each origin or only a few cells of donor origin,[21] suggesting that a single gland may be comprised of multiple clones. The gland methylation study investigating epithelial stem/progenitor cell kinetics confirms this finding.[10]

It is not known if the source of the donor bone marrow cells contributing to chimeric endometrial tissue is hemopoietic or mesenchymal stem cells or even myeloid cells. Further evidence for bone marrow stem cell contribution to endometrial repair comes from gender mismatch bone marrow transplant studies in mice, where <0.01% of cytokeratin positive endometrial epithelial cells and <0.1% of stromal cells contained a Y chromosome.[22] Bone marrow cell contribution to endometrial repair is very modest and engraftment of the endometrium seems more likely during repair after injury. In a novel double reporter *CD45/Cre-Z/EG* transgenic mouse model used to track the fate of CD45[+]- green fluorescent protein, circulating CD45[+] bone marrow cells were shown to contribute small numbers of GFP[+] endometrial luminal epithelial cells, ranging from 0% in 6-week old to 6% in 20-week old mice.[23] Although there were insufficient animals for statistical analysis, these data suggest increasing contribution of bone marrow-derived cells to the endometrial epithelium over time. A lack of CD45 expression in epithelial and stromal LRC may be due to transdifferentiation into endometrial cells.[7] It is too early to draw conclusions on whether endometrial cells are derived from bone marrow cells or resident stem cells. Furthermore, it is currently unclear if there is an ultimate endometrial stem cell that has capacity to replace all endometrial cells, including epithelial, stromal, vascular cells, or whether there are separate epithelial and MSC. To date, the data suggest that there are two distinct endometrial stem/progenitor cells, an epithelial progenitor cell and a MSC-like cell.

Endometrial Stem/Progenitor Cells and Endometriosis

The pathogenesis of endometriosis is currently poorly understood. The most commonly held theory is that retrograde menstruation deposits viable endometrial fragments into the pelvic cavity which attach to and invade the peritoneal mesothelium to establish ectopic growth of endometrial tissue.[24] It is not known why only 6-10% of

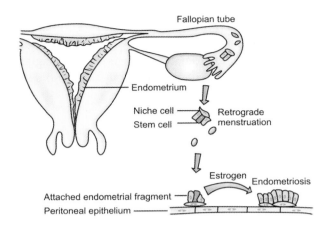

FIGURE 36-3: Possible role of endometrial stem/progenitor cells in the pathogenesis of endometriosis. It is postulated that endometrial stem/progenitor cells together with their niche cells are shed into the peritoneal cavity via retrograde menstruation in women who develop endometriosis.

women develop endometriosis when retrograde menstruation occurs in most women. One seemingly attractive hypothesis is that endometrial stem/progenitor cells are abnormally shed during menses, gaining access to the peritoneal cavity where they establish ectopic implants in those women who develop endometriosis **(Figure 36-3)**.[2,25-27] Although long-term endometriotic lesions may develop from endometrial stem/progenitor cells, those that resolve may have been established by more mature transit amplifying cells. Alternatively, endometrial stem/progenitor cells with intrinsic aberrations, yet to be identified, may have increased propensity to implant and establish an ectopic colony, or, normal stem/progenitor cells implant more readily in an abnormal peritoneal mesothelium. No direct evidence for the role of endometrial stem/progenitor cells in the pathogenesis of endometriosis has been reported to date, however there are numerous experiments reporting that unfractionated human endometrial cells can establish ectopic endometrial growth in the many models used for the study of endometriosis.[26] In baboons which also menstruate, shed menstrual debris induces endometriosis spontaneously or under experimental conditions,[28] suggesting the presence of stem/progenitor cells in the debris.

Clonality of Ectopic Endometrium

There is a strong interest in establishing clonality of endometriotic lesions to provide clues on the pathogenesis of endometriosis, particularly the natural history of lesion development. When a clinical diagnosis of endometriosis is made, the lesion(s) have already been in existence for some time. There are no clues on how long the lesion(s) have existed, the relationship, if any amongst different lesions in the same patient, and how the existence of these lesions correlate with either the onset or the severity of symptoms such as dysmenorrhea or other type of pelvic pain.

If monoclonality of endometriotic lesions can be firmly established, it may be possible to reconstruct lesion histories through molecular genetic means.[29] In addition, if multifocal lesions are polyclonal yet each focus is monoclonal, that would suggest different origins of these lesions, either due to the polyclonality of endometrial cells or sequential viable seeding of endometrial cells. Alternatively, this could mean that the ectopic implants could have been established by fragments of endometrial tissues with multiple endometrial stem/progenitor cells, as shown in a study on a long-term cell culture derived from endometrial cells.[30] Either way, the reconstruction and comparison of lesion histories of multifocal lesions reveals important information on the natural history of lesions, especially if the reconstructed history is linked to symptom history of the patient.

Initial studies reported that epithelial cells from a single endometriotic lesion are mostly monoclonal in origin.[31-35] In 18-40% of cases, however, polyclonality could not be unequivocally ruled out. This apparent polyclonality has been attributed to possible contamination with polyclonal stromal cells, since the tissue samples examined were manually microdissected.[35] It is possible that polyclonality only occurs at some periods during lesion development.[35] It is also difficult to avoid contamination with non-epithelial cells such as macrophages and fibroblasts during manual dissection of endometriotic tissues. However, with laser capture microdissection (LCM), cells from each individual focus of endometriotic lesion can be captured and individually analyzed. With this technique, multifocal lesions often found to be polyclonal turned out to be monoclonal in each focus upon more refined microdissections and further analyses.[36] A later study also using LCM independently confirmed this finding.[37] Thus, it can be concluded that each individual focus of an endometriotic lesion is of monoclonal in origin, yet different lesions are polyclonal in origin. If Sampson's theory of retrograde menstruation is correct, then endometriotic lesions may thus be initiated by transplantation of viable endometrial *fragments* through menstrual regurgitation into the pelvic cavity. Subsequently, the progression of endometriosis may occur through successions of selection and clonal expansion, as in neoplasia.[38]

Reconstruction of Cellular Genealogy in Endometrial Cells

The monoclonality of each individual endometriotic lesion implies that, because all current cells in a single lesion are descendants of a single progenitor cell, its cell genealogy or history could be potentially reconstructed. This history, once reconstructed, would permit a comparison of lesion histories among multiple lesions in a patient, and, once correlated with information on lesion sites and on other clinical variables such as staging, age of onset, and recurrence, would shed new light on how lesions initiate, progress, and cause symptoms.[36] Finally, if it can be proven that these cells are descendants of endometrial stem/progenitor cells, then Sampson's theory can be unequivocally proven.

Given the monoclonality of each individual lesion focus, there is a compelling reason to believe that the progression of a single lesion may be a multistep process involving multiple genetic and possibly epigenetic alterations that stimulate the progressive growth into a lesion, a process similar to tumorigenesis. This multistep process, viewed as a lesion history, is currently inferred from its morphology.[39] However, the progression may be variable between similar appearing lesions, and some events critical to the pathogenesis may be difficult to visualize or conceptualize.

In cancer research, it has become increasingly apparent that the tumor history may be reconstructed from replication errors, in either genome or epigenome, that surreptitiously record cell divisions and ancestry.[40] Hence, the clonal expansion, or evolution preceding a last common progenitor, is represented by a single cell lineage that can be reconstructed in a fashion similar to reconstruction of phylogeny through molecular genetic data. Methylation patterns common to all cells in a silenced gene of a given lesion are more likely to have occurred before the last clonal expansion, whereas methylation patterns present in only some lesion cells probably occur after the final progenitor. Therefore, it may be possible to decipher the past based on these molecular epigenetic "fossil records".

A proof-of-concept study reported recently showed that cellular lineage can be successfully reconstructed from a patch of menstrual debris through the use of the molecular epigenetic clock.[41] This suggests that the history of endometriotic lesions may be feasibly reconstructed by

current molecular genetic tools. The results also showed that the number of stem/progenitor cells in the endometrium is remarkably small, likely to be hundreds. The rarity of endometrial stem/progenitor cells highlights the challenge involved in identifying endometrial stem/progenitor cells **(Figure 36-4)**.

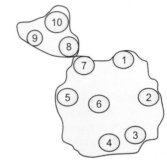

A. The geographical location of each patch

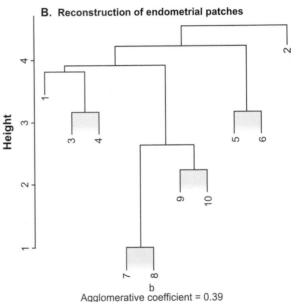

FIGURE 36-4: Reconstructing cellular lineages in endometrial cells. (A) Diagram showing the geographic locations of 10 patches (for demonstration only, not to scale). (B) Dendrogram of 10 patches based on tag data. Reprinted with permission from Wu and Guo.[41]

Menstrual Blood Stem/Progenitor Cells

There is increasing evidence that endometrial stem/progenitor cells may be shed in menstrual blood.[42,43] These cells have broad differentiation capacity with ability to differentiate into skeletal and cardiac muscle cells. Menstrual blood not only contains fragments of shed endometrial functionalis but also peripheral blood which may contain small numbers of hemopoietic stem cells, MSC or endothelial progenitor cells. The shedding of endometrial stem/progenitor cells into menstrual blood requires more investigation to confirm these interesting findings, and determine whether there are differences in their numbers in women with and without endometriosis, or whether women susceptible to endometriosis may have a higher propensity to shed endometrial stem/progenitor cells. Neither is it known whether endometrial stem/progenitor cells are shed in a retrograde manner in women with endometriosis. It is likely that if endometrial stem/progenitor cells are shed in retrograde menstrual debris, they will only establish ectopic lesions when transported with their niche cells.

There is circumstantial evidence to suggest that endometriosis may be caused by dislocation and implantation of basal endometrial fragments into the peritoneal cavity during menstruation.[25] The basalis layer, as judged by ER immunoreactivity in the secretory phase, was significantly thicker in women with endometriosis compared to control women. Endometriotic lesions had similar ER and PR receptor expression patterns as the basalis, and there was a higher prevalence of ER+ epithelium and stroma in shed endometrial fragments collected from vaginal menstrual blood in endometriosis women.[25] Thus endometrial stem/progenitor cells in the basalis of endometriosis women may gain access to the peritoneum to establish endometriotic lesions due to both increased detachment and retrograde transport of basalis tissue fragments.[25]

Transdifferentiation, Metaplasia and Endometrial Stem/Progenitor Cells

An area of controversy in the stem cell field is the concept of adult stem cell plasticity. A substantial body of literature suggests that adult stem cells transdifferentiate into cells of other tissues and across embryonic germ layer boundaries.[1,44] Transdifferentiation involves nuclear reprogramming and represents a form of metaplasia or alteration of key developmental genes. It results from changes in the extracellular environment, and appears to occur in the setting of tissue damage.[44] Metaplasia of the peritoneal lining has been suggested as one possible cause of endometriosis. However, another source of the metaplastic cells with transdifferentiation capacity are bone marrow stem cells transported via the circulation into the pelvic cavity. In a mouse transplant model where genetically marked bone marrow-derived cells can be

tracked, it was demonstrated that a small number incorporated into established endometriosis lesions and transdifferentiated into epithelial (<0.04%) and stromal cells (0.1%).[22] However bone marrow derived cells did not appear to initiate lesions. Bone marrow stem cells may therefore contribute to the progression of endometriosis lesion development rather than initiation.

Changing cell phenotype may involve epithelial mesenchymal transition (EMT) or mesenchymal epithelial transition (MET), processes known to occur during embryogenesis and recapitulated again in carcinogenesis. Changing cell phenotypes within endometriotic lesions may be responsible for the invasiveness of endometriotic cells. For example endometriotic lesions contain a well differentiated CK+E-cadherin+ population, a CK-E-Cadherin–stromal population and a more invasive CK+E-Caderin–N-Cadherin+ epithelial population, the latter with properties similar to early carcinoma micrometastasis.[27] In keeping with the similarity to early carcinoma, endometriotic lesions regress during estrogen depletion therapy but recur on cessation of therapy, suggesting that putative stem/progenitor cells in the lesion remain quiescent or dormant and then reactivate on subsequent estrogen replacement. Endometrial stem/progenitor cells within the lesions may also reseed subsequent lesions. Interestingly, clonogenic endometrial epithelial cells are weakly or negative for cytokeratin[4] and some SP cells do not express the epithelial maturation marker CD9,[14] also suggesting an epithelial-mesenchymal transition in these putative epithelial stem/progenitor cells.

Summary

There is now sufficient evidence to conclude that rare populations of epithelial stem/progenitor cells and MSC-like cells are present in human and mouse endometrium. While there is some evidence for the monoclonality of individual endometrial glands, it is still not clear whether epithelial stem/progenitor cells exist as single or multiple cells in the bases of individual glands. There is much interest in the hypothesis that foci of endometriosis which are monoclonal in origin are initiated by retrogradely shed endometrial stem/progenitor cells and their niche cells in women who develop endometriosis. Genealogy studies on menstruated fragments, the recent evidence for the presence of MSC-like cells in menstrual blood, and the identification of markers that enables the prospective isolation and identification of endometrial MSC-like cells provides impetus for investigating the role of endometrial stem/progenitor cells in the pathogenesis of endometriosis. The eventual goal would be to target self-renewal processes in shed endometrial stem/progenitor cells as novel therapeutic options for the treatment of endometriosis.

Acknowledgments

The authors' work described in this review was supported by grants from the Cancer Council Victoria ID491079 (CEG). C Gargett is supported by an NHMRC RD Wright Career Development Award (465121) and SW Guo is supported by grant 074119517 from the Shanghai Science and Technology Commission, China.

References

1. Eckfeldt CE, Mendenhall EM, Verfaillie CM. The molecular repertoire of the 'almighty' stem cell. Nature Rev Molec Cell Biol 2005; 6: 726-37.

2. Gargett CE. Uterine stem cells: what is the evidence? Hum Reprod Update 2007; 13: 87-101.

3. Li L, Xie T. Stem Cell Niche: Structure and Function. Annu Rev Cell Dev Biol 2005; 21: 605-31.

4. Chan RWS, Schwab KE, Gargett CE. Clonogenicity of human endometrial epithelial and stromal cells. Biol Reprod 2004; 70: 1738-50.

5. Schwab KE, Chan RW, Gargett CE. Putative stem cell activity of human endometrial epithelial and stromal cells during the menstrual cycle. Fertil Steril 2005; 84 (Suppl 2): 1124-30.

6. Tanaka M, Kyo S, Kanaya T, et al. Evidence of the monoclonal composition of human endometrial epithelial glands and mosaic pattern of clonal distribution in luminal epithelium. Am J Pathol 2003; 163: 295-301.

7. Chan RW, Gargett CE. Identification of label-retaining cells in mouse endometrium. Stem Cells 2006; 24: 1529-38.

8. Cervello I, Martinez-Conejero JA, Horcajadas JA, et al. Identification, characterization and co-localization of label-retaining cell population in mouse endometrium with typical undifferentiated markers. Hum Reprod 2007; 22: 45-51.

9. Szotek PP, Chang HL, Zhang L, et al. Adult mouse myometrial label-retaining cells divide in response to gonadotropin stimulation. Stem Cells 2007; 25: 1317-25.

10. Kim JY, Tavare S, Shibata D. Counting human somatic cell replications: Methylation mirrors endometrial stem cell divisions. Proc Natl Acad Sci USA 2005; 17739-44.

11. Dimitrov R, Timeva T, Kyurkchiev D, et al. Characterisation of clonogenic stromal cells isolated from human endometrium. Reprod 2008; 135: 551-8.

12. Wolff EF, Wolff AB, Du H, et al. Demonstration of multipotent stem cells in the adult human endometrium by in vitro chondrogenesis. Reprod Sci 2007; 14: 524-33.

13. Schwab KE, Gargett CE. Co-expression of two perivascular cell markers isolates mesenchymal stem-like cells from human endometrium. Hum Reprod 2007; 22: 2903-11.

14. Kato K, Yoshimoto M, Kato K, et al. Characterization of side-population cells in human normal endometrium. Hum Reprod 2007; 22: 1214-23.

15. Tsuji T, Yoshimoto M, Takahashi K, et al. Side population cells contributed to the genesis of human endometrium. Fert Steril 2008; 90 (suppl 4):1528-37.

16. Masuda H, Maruyama T, Hiratsu E, et al. Noninvasive and real-time assessment of reconstructed functional human endometrium in NOD/SCID/g_c^{null} immunodeficient mice. Proc Natl Acad Sci U S A 2007; 104: 1925-30.

17. Schwab KE, Hutchinson P, Gargett CE. Identification of surface markers for prospective isolation of human endometrial stromal colony-forming cells. Hum Reprod 2008; 23: 934-43.

18. Matthai C, Horvat R, Noe M, et al. Oct-4 expression in human endometrium. Mol Hum Reprod 2006; 12: 7-10.

19. Götte M, Wolf M, Staebler A, et al. Increased experssion of the adult stem cell marker Musashi-1 in endometriosis and endometrial carcinoma. J Pathol 2008; 215: 317-29.

20. Lynch L, Golden-Mason L, Eogan M, et al. Cells with haematopoietic stem cell phenotype in adult human endometrium: relevance to infertility? Hum Reprod 2007; 22: 919-26.

21. Taylor HS. Endometrial cells derived from donor stem cells in bone marrow transplant recipients. JAMA 2004; 292: 81-85.

22. Du H, Taylor HS. Contribution of bone marrow-derived stem cells to endometrium and endometriosis. Stem Cells 2007; 25: 2082-86.

23. Bratincsak A, Brownstein MJ, Cassiani-Ingoni R, et al. CD45-positive blood cells give rise to uterine epithelial cells in mice. Stem Cells 2007; 25: 2820-26.

24. Giudice LC, Kao LC. Endometriosis. Lancet 2004; 364: 1789-99.

25. Leyendecker G, Herbertz M, Kunz G, et al. Endometriosis results from the dislocation of basal endometrium. Human Reprod 2002; 17: 2725-36.

26. Sasson IE, Taylor HS. Stem Cells and the Pathogenesis of Endometriosis. Ann NY Acad Sci 2008; 1127: 106-15.

27. Starzinski-Powitz A, Zeitvogel A, Schreiner A, et al. In search of pathogenic mechanims in endometriosis: the challenge for molecular cell biology. Curr Molec Med 2001; 1: 655-64.

28. Fazleabas AT, Brudney A, Gurates B, et al. A modified baboon model for endometriosis. Ann N Y Acad Sci 2002; 955: 308-17.

29. Salipante SJ, Horwitz MS. Phylogenetic fate mapping. Proc Natl Acad Sci U S A 2006; 103: 5448-53.

30. Tanaka T, Nakajima S, Umesaki N. Cellular heterogeneity in long-term surviving cells isolated from eutopic endometrial, ovarian endometrioma and adenomyosis tissues. Oncol Reports 2003; 10: 1155-60.

31. Nilbert M, Pejovic T, Mandahl N, et al. Monoclonal origin of endometriotic cysts. Int J Gynecol Cancer 1995; 5: 61-63.

32. Jiang X, Hitchcock A, ryan EJ, et al. Microsatellite Analysis of Endometriosis Reveals Loss of Heterozygosity at Candidate Ovarian Tumor Suppressor Gene Loci. Cancer Res 1996; 56: 3534-39.

33. Jimbo H, Hitomi Y, Yoshikawa H, et al. Evidence for monoclonal expansion of epithelial cells in ovarian endometrial cysts. Am J Pathol 1997; 150: 1173-8.

34. Tamura M, Fukaya T, Murakami I, et al. Analysis of clonality in human endometriotic cysts based on evaluation of x chromosome inactivation in archival formalin-fixed, paraffin-embedded tissue. Laboratory Investigation 1998; 78: 213-8.

35. Yano T, Jimbo H, Yoshikawa H, et al. Molecular analysis of clonality in ovarian endometrial cysts. Gynecol Obstet Invest 1999; 47 (Suppl 1): 41-6.

36. Wu Y, Basir Z, Kajdacsy-Balla A, et al. Resolution of clonal origins for endometriotic lesions using laser capture microdissection and the human androgen receptor (HUMARA) assay. Fertil Steril 2003; 79: 710-7.

37. Nabeshima H, Murakami T, Yoshinaga K, et al. Analysis of the clonality of ectopic glands in peritoneal endometriosis using laser microdissection. Fertility and Sterility 2003; 80: 1144-50.

38. Nowell PC. The clonal evolution of tumor cell populations. Science 1976; 194: 23-8.

39. Redwine DB. Age-related evolution in color appearance of endometriosis. Fertil Steril 1987; 48: 1062-3.

40. Nomura S, Suganuma T, Suzuki T, et al. Endometrioid adenocarcinoma arising from endometriosis during 2 years of estrogen replacement therapy after total hysterectomy and bilateral salpingo-oophorectomy. Acta Obstet Gynecol Scand 2006; 85: 1019-21.

41. Wu Y, Guo SW. Reconstructing cellular lineages in endometrial cells. Fertil Steril 2008; 89: 481-4.

42. Cui CH, Uyama T, Miyado K, et al. Menstrual Blood-derived Cells Confer Human Dystrophin Expression in the Murine Model of Duchenne Muscular Dystrophy via Cell Fusion and Myogenic Transdifferentiation. Mol Biol Cell 2007; 18: 1586-94.

43. Hida N, Nishiyama N, Miyoshi S, et al. Novel Cardiac Precursor-Like Cells from Human Menstrual Blood-Derived Mesenchymal Cells. Stem Cells 2008; 26: 1695-704.

44. Tosh D, Slack JMW. How cells change their phenotype. Nature Rev Molec Cell Biol 2002; 3: 187-94.

Emile Daraï, Charles Coutant, Marc Bazot
Gil Dubernard, Roman Rouzier, Marcos Ballester

Chapter 37

Quality of Life Questionnaires

Summary

High recurrence rates have been reported in women treated for endometriosis despite advances in medical and surgical treatments improving both fertility and symptoms. It should therefore be considered a chronic disorder. In this particular setting, the main objectives for practitioners are to limit disease progression, recurrence and to improve quality of life (QOL). Previous studies have demonstrated a relation between an increase in pain intensity and a decrease in QOL. However, visual analogue scales to measure general well-being are insufficient to quantify the impact of endometriosis on QOL. Several generic questionnaires, mainly the SF-36, are available in various languages but are not specifically for women with endometriosis. Some specific questionnaires are available but have been validated in English populations for the most part rending comparison between countries difficult. Despite these limits, QOL should be systematically monitored over time by a validated questionnaire for this chronic disorder.

Keywords: endometriosis, quality of life, validated questionnaire, SF-36 questionnaire, EHP-30 questionnaire.

Introduction

Endometriosis is a well-known gynecological disorder defined by the presence of endometrial gland and stroma outside the uterus. It affects 10% to 15% of women in the reproductive period[1] and has an incidence of up to 50% in infertile women. Endometriosis is classically divided into three types: peritoneal, ovarian and deep infiltrating endometriosis depending on the type of infiltration of anatomical structures and organs. However, these various forms are in fact often associated and demand a global approach in management taking into account the availability of the medicine and patient's profile.

Generalized hypersensitivity has been demonstrated in women with visceral pain such as primary dysmenorrhea[2] and endometriosis.[3] Surgical induction of endometriosis in animal models also demonstrates hyperalgesia, indicating that a state of sensitization is associated with endometriosis.[4, 5] Generalized hyperalgesia in chronic pain conditions may be induced by a decrease in the efficacy of the descending antinociceptive system, central sensitization due to long-lasting activation of receptive fields or heterotopic facilitation caused by active nociceptive fibers outside the receptive fields.[6] It is evident from many studies that chronic pain patients suffer and have substantially reduced quality of life (QOL).[7]

As medical therapies only suppress symptoms and are ineffective on anatomical lesions, surgical management is justified.[8-13] Despite proved efficacy of surgery on both fertility and symptoms, high recurrence rates of endometriosis have been reported depending on the patient's age, the location of endometriosis as well as the completeness of surgery.[14] Hence, endometriosis should be considered a chronic disorder.[11-13] In this particular setting, the main objectives for practitioners are to limit disease progression, post-surgical complications, recurrence and to improve QOL.

Quality of Life Questionnaires

QOL is a multi-dimensional, dynamic variable with high variations over time encompassing physical, psychological and social aspects.[15] Endometriosis negatively impacts psycho-social parameters[16] and leads to a significant reduction in health-related QOL.[17-20] This decreased QOL is a result of the symptoms, their association and intensity as well as associated infertility. In addition, the side effects of medical and surgical treatments, persistence of a certain degree of symptoms, recurrences and the need to continue medical treatment for many years, also impacts QOL.

Age of onset may also contribute to the impact of endometriosis on QOL. Indeed, endometriosis is often diagnosed in young women of reproductive age impairing social, sentimental and professional functioning.[20] Moreover, chronic pain and the potential side effects of treatments can also contribute to decreased QOL by disrupting job performance, social relationships or sexual functioning.[20, 21] Although Laursen et al demonstrated a relation between increased pain intensity of the ongoing pain and a decrease in QOL, visual analog scales to measure the areas of general well-being, work performance, sexual and leisure-time activities are insufficient to quantify the impact of endometriosis on QOL.[19] There is, therefore, a need for appropriate tools to evaluate QOL in endometriosis. In this setting, several questionnaires are available though not all of them are specific to patients with endometriosis.

Generic Questionnaires of Quality of Life

The Short Form 36 (SF-36) is a general health-related QOL survey comprising 36 multiple choice questions sorted in eight categories or subscales which address health constructs considered to be important in most health care situations: physical functioning, role limitations (physical problems), bodily pain, general health, vitality, social functioning, role limitations (emotional problems), and mental health.[22] Item scores are coded, summed, and transformed into a scale from 0 (worst health) to 100 (best health) for each dimension. This instrument was developed to measure health perception in a general population, and its clinical validity and internal consistency have been demonstrated in large samples in many countries. The SF-36 has emerged as being one of the most widely used generic instruments for measuring perceived health status in various diseases and conditions.[23] Moreover, the measurement properties, including the reliability, validity and responsiveness of the measures for women with endometriosis, have been validated.[24]

The Short Form 12 (SF-12) is an even shorter, validated, multipurpose generic measure of health status derived from the SF-36 **(Figure 37-1)**.[25] The 12 items include one or two questions from each of the eight health concepts of the SF-36. The questions are scored and analyzed using a statistical algorithm to obtain two scores; the Physical Component Summary (PCS) and the Mental Component

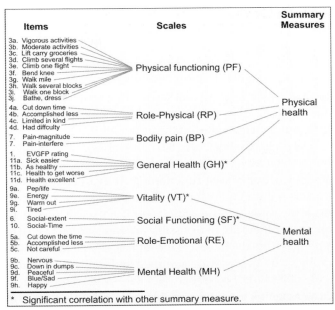

FIGURE 37-1: SF-36 Measurement model

Summary (MCS). These scores can be compared over time. Reliability tests have been carried out in the USA and the UK.

The EuroQOL EQ-5D questionnaire defines health status in terms of five dimensions: mobility, self-care, usual activity, pain/discomfort and anxiety/depression. Each dimension is divided in three levels: no problem, some problem or extreme problem. The health status can be calculated into numerical values with a score 100 for the "best imaginable health" and 0 for the "worst imaginable state of health". The questionnaire has been validated to reflect variations in health status by population subgroups.[26]

Other questionnaires such as the Psychological General Well-Being Index Questionnaire (PGWBI)[27] and the psychological general well-being (PGWB) index have also been used to evaluate QOL in women with endometriosis but have rarely been used in clinical studies.

Quality of Life Questionnaires Evaluating Specific Dimensions

As well as these generic questionnaires, several questionnaires evaluating specific dimensions such as sexuality and anxiety/depression have been used in populations of women with endometriosis.

The Sexual Satisfaction Subscale of the Derogatis Sexual Functioning Inventory (DSFI)[28] is a multidimensional measure of various aspects of psychological and sexual function, and consists of nine items reflecting the individual level of sexual fulfilment. It is one of the most thoroughly studied instruments in sexual research and has been found to have high internal and test–retest reliability as well as discriminative validity.[28] The Global Sexual Satisfaction Index (GSSI) asks subjects to self-rate their overall level of sexual satisfaction on a 9-point scale anchored at the lower extreme by [0] "could not be worse," to[8] "could not be better" at the upper limit.

The revised Sabbatsberg Sexual Rating Scale is a simple but satisfactory 12-item questionnaire suitable for self-assessment of sexual functioning. It evaluates various aspects separately including libido, arousal or pleasure, orgasm capacity, and satisfaction. For each of the 12 questions, there are five possible answers scored from 0 to 4 points (from the lowest to the highest sexual satisfaction rating). The 12 scores are summed and transposed onto a scale of 0 to 100. Scores between these values represent a percentage of the total possible score. The validity and reliability of this instrument have been demonstrated.[29]

The Hospital Anxiety and Depression (HAD) Scale is a self assessment mood scale specifically designed for use in nonpsychiatric hospital outpatients to determine states of anxiety and depression. It comprises 14 items: 7 for the anxiety subscale and 7 for the depression subscale. Five mutually exclusive answers, rated from 0 to 4 according to increasing psychiatric severity, are provided for each of the 14 questions. The points are then summed to give anxiety and depression subtotal scores and a total score. The HAD Scale has been shown to be a reliable screening instrument for clinically significant anxiety and depression and a valid measure of the severity of these mood disorders.[30]

Quality of Life Questionnaires Specific for Women with Endometriosis

The first specific questionnaire to evaluate QOL in women with endometriosis was developed by Colwell et al.[15] Jones et al[18, 31] subsequently developed another specific QOL questionnaire for women with endometriosis: the Endometriosis Health Profile-30 (EHP-30).[15,18,31] This questionnaire is comprised of two parts: a core questionnaire containing 5 scales applicable to all women with endometriosis (30 items) and a modular part containing 6 scales which do not necessarily apply to all women with endometriosis (23 items). Specified EHP-30 scales are composed of different items on pain, emotional well-being, self-image and intercourse as well as two scales on social support, control and powerlessness. Each scale of the EHP-30 is transformed into numerical data from 0 (indicating the best health status) to 100 (indicating the worst health

status) and calculated as follows: scale score is equal to the total of the raw scores of each item in the scale divided by the maximum possible raw score of all the items in the scale, multiplied by 100.

Limits of Quality of Life Questionnaires

To evaluate the quality of the data obtained by health-status instruments studies typically focus on psychometric tests: internal consistency, reliability, secondary factor analysis and item correlations. However, about one quarter of the tools used to evaluate QOL in women with endometriosis are based on nonestablished psychometric properties. Moreover, other variables, such as data completeness, have been identified to influence the scoring and structure of the dimensions of a questionnaire: a high percentage of missing data on a dimension indicates that items may be confusing, aggressive or inappropriate[32] making it difficult to draw conclusions about improvement or deterioration in health status.[33]

One potential limitation for the use of generic questionnaires such as the SF-36 is that they might not be sensitive enough to assess changes in a specific illness because they are designed to evaluate QOL in a wide variety of diseases or conditions. Indeed, the SF-36 only has a limited number of questions on pain. On the other hand, these questionnaires have been validated in several languages and thus allow comparison between one country and another. In contrast, while specific questionnaires for women with endometriosis should be more sensitive to changes in health status because they include more targeted items, they are often only available for English-speaking populations or have only been validated in the USA or the UK.

Impact of Medical and Surgical Therapies on Quality of Life as Evaluated by Questionnaires

Although numerous studies have focused on the efficacy of the medical and surgical treatments of pain and symptoms associated with endometriosis, evaluation of QOL using validated questionnaires has been less extensively studied.

Quality of Life after Medical Treatment of Endometriosis

Several studies evaluating the impact of medical therapies on QOL have been published[34-37] but we will only focus on recent reports of randomized trials in this chapter.

In a 12-month study including 46 women treated with GnRH analog plus add-back therapy, 44 women treated with GnRH analog alone and 43 women treated with estroprogestin, Zupi et al[38] demonstrated that add-back therapy gives better patient QOL as assessed by the SF-36 questionnaire, with reduced bone mineral density loss.

In another trial, Petta et al[27] compared the efficacy of a levonorgestrel-releasing intrauterine system (LNG-IUS) to a depot-GnRH-analog over a period of 6 months. The PGWBI scores of LNG-IUS users increased by 8.3 points and by 6.8 points for GnRH analog users (not significant).

A trial by Crosignani et al[17] comparing depot medroxyprogesterone acetate (DMPA) to leuprolide using the endometriosis-specific EHP-30 scale and the SF-36 questionnaire found a significant improvement in QOL in both groups. Mean scores for both the questionnaires improved significantly in both groups at month 6 compared with pre-treatment, and these improvements were maintained at 12 months of post-treatment follow-up. No attempt was made to correlate the EHP-30 and SF-36 questionnaire.

Quality of Life after Surgery for Endometriosis

Garry et al[39] used the SF-12 and EuroQOL (EQ-5D) questionnaires to determine the effect of radical laparoscopic excision on QOL in a prospective 4-month study. Although significant improvement in QOL was obtained, the short follow-up could not exclude the placebo effect of laparoscopy.

In a randomized blinded trial using the EQ-5D and SF-12 questionnaires, Abbott et al[40] demonstrated that laparoscopic excision of endometriosis was more effective than placebo at improving QOL. Surgery was associated with a 30% placebo response rate that was not dependent on severity of the disease. Approximately 20% of women did not report an improvement after surgery for endometriosis.

In a series of 254 women with endometriosis undergoing laparoscopic excision and with a follow-up up to 5 years, Abbott et al[40] found that QOL was improved using the EQ-5D questionnaire and that the risk of requiring further surgery was 36%. Endometriosis was found histologically in 68% of the women who underwent further surgery.

Again using the EQ-5D questionnaire, Ford et al[41] observed that patients having undergone a hysterectomy or a disc or segmental resection of the rectum reported a normal postoperative QOL. However, QOL scores in the study group remained lower than those of the background population.

In an open randomized clinical trial in women with stage I to IV endometriosis, Vercellini et al[42] compared laparoscopic conservative surgery with or without uterosacral ligament resection. Using the SF-36 questionnaire, the HAD Scale and the revised Sabbatsberg Sexual Rating Scale, uterosacral ligament resection was not found to have additional positive impact on QOL, psychiatric profile, and sexual satisfaction while exposing women to a high risk of bleeding, ureteral lesions, and pelvic support disorders.

Sesti et al[43] used the SF-36 questionnaire in a 6-month trial to compare the effectiveness of placebo versus GnRH-a (tryptorelin or leuprorelin, 3.75 mg every 28 days) or continuous estroprogestin (ethynilestradiol, 0.03 mg plus gestoden, 0.75 mg) versus dietary therapy on painful symptoms in women having undergone surgery for endometriosis. They found that both postoperative hormonal suppression treatment and dietary therapy were more effective than placebo to obtain improvement in QOL.

Using the SF-36 questionnaire in a series of 58 women undergoing laparoscopic colorectal resection for endometriosis, Dubernard et al[44] found that QOL was significantly improved. Surprisingly, these authors also reported a significant improvement of QOL in women experiencing severe complications such as rectovaginal fistulae requiring repeat surgery or those requiring a conversion to laparotomy.

Use of Quality of Life Questionnaires as a Predictor of Outcome after Surgery

Redwine and Wright[45] reported that not all symptoms of endometriotic obliteration of Douglas' cul-de-sac were similarly improved after surgery, and that some symptoms were unchanged or worsened. Qualitative and/or semi-quantitative visual analog symptom scales[9,10] have confirmed that fatigue, diarrhea, constipation, dyspareunia and dysmenorrhea can remain unchanged. In a series of women without rectum involvement undergoing complete laparoscopic excision of deep endometriosis with partial resection of the posterior vaginal fornix, Angioni et al[46] observed that 65% of patients were free of analgesic postoperatively, 38% had total remission of chronic pain and 22% were improved; 38% had total remission of dysmenorrhea and 22% were improved; 45% had total remission of dyspareunia and 25% were improved. Improvement of symptoms was maintained for 5 years without recurrence of the disease or repeated surgery. Nevertheless, a large proportion of women were not, or only slightly, improved by surgery. In the same way, Daraï et al[9] demonstrated that colorectal resection for DIE with bowel involvement improved symptoms and QOL using a visual analogical scale. However, all these authors failed to clearly identify good candidates for surgery so as to rule out patients for whom surgery carries no benefit or whose condition might even worsen.

Redwine and Wright[45] suggested that palpation of a nodule causing tenderness spontaneously felt by the patient was a positive predictive factor of outcome after surgery. However, this finding seems to vary according to the location of endometriosis, the lesion accessibility to clinical examination, the lesion size as well as the surgeon's experience. Therefore, it is clear that objective criteria are required to select patients with a high probability of being improved by surgery which exposes women to potential major postoperative complications such as rectovaginal fistula or *de novo* dysuria.[9, 47] In women with colorectal endometriosis, Dubernard et al[47] used a recursive partitioning to determine SF-36 cut-offs of PCS and MCS scores predicting an improvement in QOL. Women with a preoperative PCS score below 37.5 had an 80.7% probability of having an improved PCS score after surgery. Women with a preoperative PCS score between 46.5 and 37.5 had a 33.3% probability of a score improvement after surgery, whereas no postoperative improvement in PCS could be expected by women with a preoperative score over 46.5. Women with a preoperative MCS score below 44.5 had an 84.2% probability of a score improvement after surgery. Women with a preoperative MCS score between 44.5 and 47.5 had a 30% probability of improving their score after surgery, whereas women with a preoperative MCS score above 47.5 had only a 10.7% probability. These results underline that QOL questionnaires can be used not only to evaluate the efficacy of treatment but also to predict outcome of surgery allowing the selection of good candidates. Further studies are required to validate the use of the SF-36 questionnaire as a predictor of outcome in women with various locations of endometriosis. Moreover, a Markov analysis is needed to evaluate QOL progression over time.

Conclusion

All new studies on endometriosis should systematically include QOL evaluation. In this setting, the SF-36 questionnaire appears particularly relevant and is available in many languages. Moreover, the SF-36 seems to be a useful tool to predict outcome after surgery though further studies are required to definitively validate this point. Although specific questionnaires such as the EHP-30 exist, they would need to be validated in several languages before becoming the gold standard.

References

1. Koninckx PR, Meuleman C, Demeyere S et al. Suggestive evidence that pelvic endometriosis is a progressive disease, whereas deeply infiltrating endometriosis is associated with pelvic pain. Fertil Steril 1991; 55: 759-65.
2. Bajaj P, Madsen H, Arendt-Nielsen L. A comparison of modality-specific somatosensory changes during menstruation in dysmenorrheic and nondysmenorrheic women. Clin J Pain 2002; 18: 180-90.
3. Bajaj P, Madsen H, Arendt-Nielsen L. Endometriosis is associated with central sensitization: a psychophysical controlled study. J Pain 2003; 4: 372-80.
4. Berkley KJ, Cason A, Jacobs H et al. Vaginal hyperalgesia in a rat model of endometriosis. Neurosci Lett 2001; 306: 185-88.
5. Giamberardino MA, Berkley KJ, Affaitati G et al. Influence of endometriosis on pain behaviors and muscle hyperalgesia induced by a ureteral calculosis in female rats. Pain 2002; 95: 247-57.
6. Mense S. Nociception from skeletal muscle in relation to clinical muscle pain. Pain 1993; 54: 241-89.
7. Laursen BS, Bajaj P, Olesen AS, et al. Health related quality of life and quantitative pain measurement in females with chronic non-malignant pain. Eur J Pain 2005; 9: 267-75.
8. Anaf V, Simon P, Fayt I, Noel J. Smooth muscles are frequent components of endometriotic lesions. Hum Reprod 2000; 15: 767-71.
9. Darai E, Thomassin I, Barranger E, et al. Feasibility and clinical outcome of laparoscopic colorectal resection for endometriosis. Am J Obstet Gynecol 2005; 192: 394-400.
10. Thomassin I, Bazot M, Detchev R, et al. Symptoms before and after surgical removal of colorectal endometriosis that are assessed by magnetic resonance imaging and rectal endoscopic sonography. Am J Obstet Gynecol 2004; 190: 1264-71.
11. Child TJ, Tan SL. Endometriosis: aetiology, pathogenesis and treatment. Drugs 2001;61:1735-50.
12. Schweppe KW. Current place of progestins in the treatment of endometriosis-related complaints. Gynecol Endocrinol 2001; 15(Suppl 6): 22-28.
13. Valle RF, Sciarra JJ. Endometriosis: treatment strategies. Ann N Y Acad Sci 2003; 997:229-39.
14. Fedele L, Bianchi S, Zanconato G, et al. Use of a levonorgestrel-releasing intrauterine device in the treatment of rectovaginal endometriosis. Fertil Steril 2001; 75: 485-88.
15. Colwell HH, Mathias SD, Pasta DJ, et al. A health-related quality-of-life instrument for symptomatic patients with endometriosis: a validation study. Am J Obstet Gynecol 1998; 179: 47-55.
16. Low WY, Edelmann RJ, Sutton C. A psychological profile of endometriosis patients in comparison to patients with pelvic pain of other origins. J Psychosom Res 1993; 37: 111-16.
17. Crosignani P, Olive D, Bergqvist A, Luciano A. Advances in the management of endometriosis: an update for clinicians. Hum Reprod Update 2006; 12: 179-89.
18. Jones G, Jenkinson C, Taylor N, et al. Measuring quality of life in women with endometriosis: tests of data quality,

score reliability, response rate and scaling assumptions of the Endometriosis Health Profile Questionnaire. Hum Reprod 2006; 21: 2686-93.

19. Jones GL, Kennedy SH, Jenkinson C. Health-related quality of life measurement in women with common benign gynecologic conditions: a systematic review. Am J Obstet Gynecol 2002; 187: 501-11.

20. Marques A, Bahamondes L, Aldrighi JM, Petta CA. Quality of life in Brazilian women with endometriosis assessed through a medical outcome questionnaire. J Reprod Med 2004; 49: 115-20.

21. Ovarian and endometrial function during hormonal contraception. Hum Reprod 2001;16:1527-35.

22. Ware JE, Jr. Using generic measures of functional health and well-being to increase understanding of disease burden. Spine 2000; 25: 1467.

23. Beaton DE, Hogg-Johnson S, Bombardier C. Evaluating changes in health status: reliability and responsiveness of five generic health status measures in workers with musculoskeletal disorders. J Clin Epidemiol 1997; 50: 79-93.

24. Bodner CH, Garratt AM, Ratcliffe J et al. Measuring health-related quality of life outcomes in women with endometriosis—results of the Gynaecology Audit Project in Scotland. Health Bull (Edinb) 1997; 55: 109-117.

25. Ware JE, Jr., Kosinski M, Bayliss MS et al. Comparison of methods for the scoring and statistical analysis of SF-36 health profile and summary measures: summary of results from the Medical Outcomes Study. Med Care 1995; 33: AS264-79.

26. Brooks R, Kerridge R, Hillman K et al. Quality of life outcomes after intensive care. Comparison with a community group. Intensive Care Med 1997;23:581-86.

27. Petta CA, Ferriani RA, Abrao MS, et al. Randomized clinical trial of a levonorgestrel-releasing intrauterine system and a depot GnRH analogue for the treatment of chronic pelvic pain in women with endometriosis. Hum Reprod 2005; 20: 1993-98.

28. Derogatis LR, Melisaratos N. The DSFI: a multidimensional measure of sexual functioning. J Sex Marital Ther 1979; 5: 244-81.

29. Garratt AM, Torgerson DJ, Wyness J et al. Measuring sexual functioning in premenopausal women. Br J Obstet Gynaecol 1995; 102: 311-16.

30. Zigmond AS, Snaith RP. The hospital anxiety and depression scale. Acta Psychiatr Scand 1983; 67: 361-70.

31. Jones G, Jenkinson C, Kennedy S. Evaluating the responsiveness of the Endometriosis Health Profile Questionnaire: the EHP-30. Qual Life Res 2004; 13: 705-13.

32. Gandek B, Ware JE, Jr., Aaronson NK et al. Tests of data quality, scaling assumptions, and reliability of the SF-36 in eleven countries: results from the IQOLA Project. International Quality of Life Assessment. J Clin Epidemiol 1998; 51:1149-58.

33. Bindman AB, Keane D, Lurie N. Measuring health changes among severely ill patients. The floor phenomenon. Med Care 1990; 28:1142-52.

34. Burry KA. Nafarelin in the management of endometriosis: quality of life assessment. Am J Obstet Gynecol 1992; 166: 735-39.

35. Miller JD. Quantification of endometriosis-associated pain and quality of life during the stimulatory phase of gonadotropin-releasing hormone agonist therapy: a double-blind, randomized, placebo-controlled trial. Am J Obstet Gynecol 2000; 182: 1483-88.

36. Regidor PA, Regidor M, Kato K et al. Long-term follow-up on the treatment of endometriosis with the GnRH-agonist buserelin acetate. Long-term follow-up data (up to 98 months) of 42 patients with endometriosis who were treated with GnRH-agonist buserelin acetate (Suprecur), were evaluated in respect of recurrence of pain symptoms and pregnancy outcome. Eur J Obstet Gynecol Reprod Biol 1997; 73: 153-60.

37. Zhao SZ, Kellerman LA, Francisco CA, Wong JM. Impact of nafarelin and leuprolide for endometriosis on quality of life and subjective clinical measures. J Reprod Med 1999; 44: 1000-06.

38. Zupi E, Marconi D, Sbracia M et al. Add-back therapy in the treatment of endometriosis-associated pain. Fertil Steril 2004; 82: 1303-08.

39. Garry R, Clayton R, Hawe J. The effect of endometriosis and its radical laparoscopic excision on quality of life indicators. BJOG 2000; 107: 44-54.

40. Abbott J, Hawe J, Hunter D et al. Laparoscopic excision of endometriosis: a randomized, placebo-controlled trial. Fertil Steril 2004; 82: 878-84.

41. Ford J, English J, Miles WA, Giannopoulos T. Pain, quality of life and complications following the radical resection of rectovaginal endometriosis. BJOG 2004; 111: 353-56.

42. Vercellini P, Aimi G, Busacca M et al. Laparoscopic uterosacral ligament resection for dysmenorrhea associated with endometriosis: results of a randomized, controlled trial. Fertil Steril 2003; 80: 310-19.

43. Sesti F, Pietropolli A, Capozzolo T et al. Hormonal suppression treatment or dietary therapy versus placebo in the control of painful symptoms after conservative surgery for endometriosis stage III-IV. A randomized comparative trial. Fertil Steril 2007; 88: 1541-47.

44. Dubernard G, Rouzier R, David-Montefiore E et al. Use of the SF-36 questionnaire to predict quality-of-life improvement after laparoscopic colorectal resection for endometriosis. Hum Reprod 2008; 23: 846-51.

45. Redwine DB, Wright JT. Laparoscopic treatment of complete obliteration of the cul-de-sac associated with endometriosis: long-term follow-up of en bloc resection. Fertil Steril 2001; 76: 358-65.

46. Angioni S, Peiretti M, Zirone M et al. Laparoscopic excision of posterior vaginal fornix in the treatment of patients with deep endometriosis without rectum involvement: surgical treatment and long-term follow-up. Hum Reprod 2006; 21: 1629-34.

47. Dubernard G, Rouzier R, David-Montefiore E et al. Urinary complications after surgery for posterior deep infiltrating endometriosis are related to the extent of dissection and to uterosacral ligaments resection. J Minim Invasive Gynecol 2008; 15: 235-40.

Epilogue

The Future: Our Field Could Be World Leaders – Will We Meet the Challenge?

In the epilogue, "The Future," of their text, *Modern Approaches to Endometriosis*, Eric Thomas and John Rock stated that the aim of their book was to provide current thinking in all the major areas of endometriosis. They also wrote that it was their great pleasure to leave the discipline of writing chapters controlled by references and data and to envision where advances in our understanding take us.

Likewise, the distinguished editors of this book, Botros Rizk and Juan Garcia-Velasco, have compiled a text with comprehensive thoughtfulness. It is my pleasure and honor to respond to their invitation to provide this epilogue to an important text and to envision what the future of our field could be. In the tradition of our field, I will take this opportunity, drawing on 30 years of work (having founded the first organization singly devoted to endometriosis – an organization of affected families, doctors, and scientists, solidly based in science) to provide the big picture, the vision, to look at our field and suggest directions for the future.

Developing Nations' Perspective on Endometriosis Will Help the Whole World

I am especially pleased to be invited to this task given that this text is one of the first on endometriosis directed to low-resource countries as well as medically-advanced countries. This recognition of the importance of endometriosis in developing countries is welcome – the suffering of families affected by endometriosis in the global South has for too long gone unacknowledged. Assisting developing nations with the modern epidemic of endometriosis and all its related health problems (cancers, autoimmune diseases, and atopic diseases) will have benefits for all of us. The fact that expensive medications and surgeries are not feasible in these countries opens the door to new perspectives, indigenous – even ingenious – approaches to the disease. Since, as many authors in this text point out, we are currently somewhat stumped in managing this enigmatic disease, the thinking outside the box which developing nations and other medical disciplines can bring is very much needed. We need their help. As I wrote in an often-quoted statement in a medical text in 1992, "endometriosis can be, from the patient's point of view, a nightmare of misinformation, myths, taboos, lack of diagnosis, and problematic hit-and-miss treatments overlaid on a painful, chronic, stubborn disease."

Noninvasive Diagnostic Test Will Open Surprising New Doors

This trend toward worldwide recognition of endometriosis is likely to escalate with the development of noninvasive diagnostic tests for endometriosis. Such tests will not only help so many who currently have no name for their pain but will also revolutionize the very definition of endometriosis as we are able to better define who is affected (impossible now because of the selective and severe under-diagnosis), where prevalence is greatest, and, for the first time, we will have true controls in our clinical and scientific studies, which virtually all suffer from the inclusion of cases, due to diagnostic difficulties. We may also discover that endometriosis, as implied in a number of chapters in this text, is more than a gynecological disease and cannot be defined by lesions, a concept we first wrote about back in 1986. Indeed, we are on the cusp of a whole new era in endometriosis.

With noninvasive diagnostic tests, diagnosis may be so easy that non-specialists can provide it, leading to many more medical specialties becoming interested in treating endometriosis. If our specialty does not rise to the challenge – and admittedly, we have not been able to convince most even in gynecology to care for endometriosis patients in any substantial way – then other specialties will move to fill the void as huge numbers of girls and women are finally diagnosed. If we welcome these new, much-needed specialists into our field, we can reach the greatness that I believe our field offers. If we resist, and continue to insist on the primacy of purely gynecologic approaches to a disease that appears to be systemic, immunological, toxicological, and epigenetic, we are the ones who will be left behind.

As Dmowski and Braun note in Chapter 9, certain immunopathologic changes documented in endometriosis apparently are not affected by either surgical or medical treatment – yet, these well-replicated observations have not led our field to bring in other approaches that could increase our clinical success. The best way to solve this problem, from my perspective, is to open the door to other specialists. Our field would benefit, for example, by teaming up with specialists working with inflammatory diseases to help us understand ways to possibly reduce the proven chronic inflammation in endometriosis. As pointed out in Chapter 4, endo has been linked to "some kind of atypical autoantibody (lupus anticoagulant, antinucleotide, antiphospholipids, antihistones, antithyroids, etc.) in almost 85% of women suffering from endometriosis." What are we waiting for? Despite so much evidence indicating endometriosis is much more than a simple pelvic disease, despite our leaders often being the academicians training new physicians in medical schools worldwide, we seem to insist on continuing to use the same tired tools that have been far less than effective!

Similarly, bringing toxicologists into our field (see Chapters 7 and 9) could open new approaches to understanding and treating endometriosis. As one of the leading scientists in the area of toxins and endo stated, the people in our field don't understand toxicology and don't think they need to understand it. Any serious reading of the voluminous and rapidly-expanding literature on endocrine-disrupting toxicants clearly shows that these toxicants are deeply detrimental to health in numerous ways, including endo, immune disorders, and cancers. Why then are we not advising patients on avoidance (and pushing our governments to act to protect public health as Dominique de Zeigler points out in chapter 7)?

Diagnosing many more of the existing cases will also help better establish the relationships between endo and various cancers. Even with the extreme under-diagnosis of endo, the evidence on the relationships between ovarian endometriosis and three types of deadly ovarian cancer warrants vigilance on behalf of our patients. Knowing that lives are at stake, why are we waiting to counter the move to "watch and wait" for long periods of time when endometriomas are present? And why are we waiting to adopt guidelines that are life-protective of young women with endo, who have a propensity to develop this cancer at a younger age than the general population, making it even more likely it will not be diagnosed early? I was actually told by one medical society in our field that it would not adopt guidelines on this matter because of concern about legal liability. What clearer statement could there be that the lives of women are secondary to the financial concerns of the profession (at least in that country)?

Are Taboos Keeping Us from Taking Endometriosis Seriously?

Perhaps even those in our profession, specializing in endometriosis, are reluctant to accept the seriousness of endometriosis? The Endometriosis Association has written extensively over the last 30 years about the taboos involved in endometriosis. I have come to believe that taboos about the basic biology of women lie at the heart of much of the discrimination against women. Indeed, psychosocial and historical studies (see *The Curse: A Cultural History of Menstruation* and *Blood Magic: The Anthropology of Menstruation*) show an almost primal fear related to menstruation and female sexuality. How can it be a curse to be endowed with the capability of bringing another human being into the world? Our profession is in the best position to help the world realize and respect the normalcy and the beauty of female physiological functions and, by logical extension, abnormal functioning. If even we, in women's health, weren't touched by these same societal taboos and stigmas, we would have many decades ago studied pain as the cardinal symptom of endometriosis – indeed, it was not until 2006 that our field hosted conferences focused on endometriosis and pain! – and the role of dysmenorrhea (important in its own right). Our field could have, some would say, should have, led the way in countering the widespread idea that pain in women is normal – something that 75% of women with endometriosis in North America are told, as if women were designed defectively!

The modern epidemic of pain in women and girls undermines the struggle to attain their full rights worldwide. If our specialty, which professes that the health of females is its primary raison d'être, doesn't take a clear stand and act to create understanding and respect for female biology, how can we be surprised at the horrific practices of female infanticide (11 dead baby girls daily at just one charity in one city in one developing country alone), female genital mutilation (is it really so different than unnecessary "cosmetic" gynec surgery on healthy tissue?), sexual assault and molestation (one in three females before the age of 18 in the U.S.), female and child kidnapping and sexual slavery, child brides and resultant obstetrical damage and ostracization, "honor" killings, dowry burnings, the objectification and dehumanization so rampant in advertising and pornography? Imagine, if instead of images of women, these horrific images were of people of color, bound, gagged, in positions of servitude? Wouldn't our societies be up in arms? With the World Health Organization estimating that over 100 million females are "missing" in the world because of gender-based persecution, isn't it time for our specialty to live up to its calling, its sacred trust on behalf of the women and girls of the world?

What are we waiting for? Endometriosis could be the route through which we counter the fears and taboos related to female biology and help heal the rampant violations of the human rights of women. In the process, we could help reclaim dignity for women and girls and for our profession.

Mary Lou Ballweg
President/Executive Director
Endometriosis Association (International)

Index